LEISHMANIASIS - TRENDS IN EPIDEMIOLOGY, DIAGNOSIS AND TREATMENT

Edited by **David M. Claborn**

Leishmaniasis - Trends in Epidemiology, Diagnosis and Treatment
http://dx.doi.org/10.5772/57067
Edited by David M. Claborn

Contributors

Patricia Sampaio Tavares Veras, Deborah Fraga, Carlos Eduardo Sampaio Guedes, Manuela Da Silva Solcà, A K M Mamunur Rashid, Ikram Guizani, Souheila Guerbouj, Levi Makala, Babak Baban, Faustino Mollinedo, Ana B. Caballero, Juan M. Salas, Manuel Sánchez-Moreno, Alane Beatriz Vermelho, Claudiu Supuran, Veronica Da Silva Cardoso, Daniela Sales Alviano, Ana Claudia Fernandes Amaral, Dayanne Menezes, Celuta Sales Alviano, Igor Almeida Rodrigues, Labrini Athanasiou, Constantina N. Tsokana, George Valiakos, Vassiliki Spyrou, Katerina Manolakou, Charalambos Billinis, Jailson De Andrade, Jairo Magalhaes Junior, Paulo Mesquita, Fabio Oliveira, Frederico Rodrigues, Stella Maria Barrouin-Melo, Elizabeth Ferreira Rangel, Simone da Costa, Bruno Moreira Carvalho, Moncef BenSaid, David Claborn, Norma Galindo-Sevilla, Javier Mancilla, Enrique Segura, Miroslava Avila-Garcia, Mauricio S. Baptista, José Angelo Lindoso, Antero De Andrade, Tales Alexandre Aversi-Ferreira, Roqueline Aversi-Ferreira, Jucimaria Galvao, Ediana Vasconcelos Silva, Sylla Figueredo Silva, Naina Bhatia-Dey, Giovanna Felipe Cavalcante, Luiz Alberto Alves Mota, Roberta Miranda, Anabela Cordeiro-Da-Silva, Javier Moreno, João Carreira, Alba Silva, Mônica de Avelar Figueiredo Mafra Magalhães, Aldo Job, Alexandre Fioravante de Siqueira, Caroline Silva Danna, Felipe Bellucci, Flavio Camargo Cabrera, Leandra Ernst Kerche Silva, Pedro Henrique Benites Aoki, Carlos Jose Leopoldo Constantino

Published by InTech

Janeza Trdine 9, 51000 Rijeka, Croatia

Publishing Process Manager Iva Lipovic

Technical Editor InTech DTP team

Cover InTech Design team

First published March, 2014

Printed in Croatia

Additional hard copies can be obtained from orders@intechopen.com

Leishmaniasis - Trends in Epidemiology, Diagnosis and Treatment, Edited by David M. Claborn

p. cm.

ISBN 978-953-51-1232-7

Meet the editor

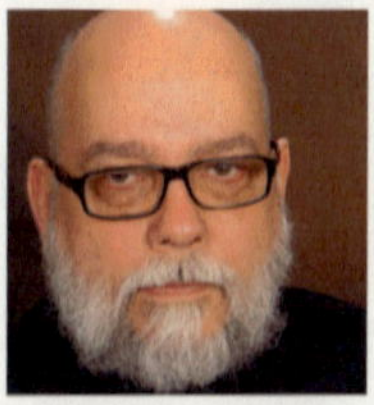

David M. Claborn is the Interim Director of the Master of Public Health Program at Missouri State University in Springfield, Missouri. He completed his Doctor of Public Health degree in 2001 at the Uniformed Services University of the Health Sciences in Bethesda, MD, where his dissertation dealt with the epidemiology and control of malaria near the demilitarized zone in South Korea. He also has degrees in entomology and zoology from Texas Tech University. Dr. Claborn's interests for teaching and research are focused on human health issues associated with disrupted environments, especially as they are related to natural or technological disasters and war. Prior to his academic career, Dr. Claborn was a career military officer, retiring from the U.S. Navy's Medical Services Corps at the rank of Commander.

Contents

Preface

Leishmaniasis is a particularly diverse disease with a wide range of physical manifestations. As a vector-borne disease, it exhibits a complex life cycle as well. The diversity of this disease, especially as it relates to the multiple parasite species which serve as causative agents, has allowed the disease to adapt to a variety of habitats throughout the world. In Central and South America, the disease is often associated with jungle or other heavily vegetated environments, but in the Middle East it is adapted to the desert and its reservoir of rodent hosts. As a result, the disease is quite widespread, affecting humans in Europe, Asia, Africa and the Americas. There is zoonotic infection in Australia though, at present, no evidence of human disease.

Not surprisingly, the clinical manifestations of leishmaniasis are quite varied. They range from relatively minor, self-limiting cutaneous lesions to deadly visceral infections. Other types may cause a mucocutaneous form that, though often not fatal, can result in extreme disfiguration. These clinical manifestations are linked to the specific parasite species causing the infections, but in recent years, researchers have noted that species thought to be limited to cutaneous manifestations may also elicit visceral disease.

The diversity of this disease requires that researchers, physicians, and public health workers address this disease in a way that is appropriate to the region-specific epidemiology and medical needs of the local population. Diagnosis, treatment and prevention may vary depending on the particular parasite species involved, not to mention the biology of the local sand fly vector. Recent developments in the diagnosis and treatment of leishmaniasis, both human and veterinary, have been extensive. This book presents many of these developments along with discussions of possible future utilization of new technologies in the diagnosis and control of leishmaniasis.

A perusal of the chapters in this book will reveal an emphasis on diagnosis and clinical treatment of the disease. Much research remains to be done in these fields, but perhaps even more is left to do in the prevention of the disease. Despite a great deal of research on the subject, there is still a noticeable lack of an effective and available vaccine. Recent experiences by western military forces in Iraq also demonstrate that much remains unknown about effective vector control and personal protection as they apply to prevention of leishmaniasis. This situation will mandate future updates on research and application of technologies for diagnosis, prevention and treatment of this disease.

David M. Claborn
Master of Public Health Program, College of Health and Human Services,
Missouri State University,
Springfield, MO, USA

Section 1

Epidemiology and Ecology of Leishmaniasis

Chapter 1

Environmental Changes and the Geographic Spreading of American Cutaneous Leishmaniasis in Brazil

Elizabeth F. Rangel, Simone M. da Costa and Bruno M. Carvalho

Additional information is available at the end of the chapter

http://dx.doi.org/10.5772/57207

1. Introduction

Global human population is facing the impacts of centuries of constant changes in natural environments. Impacts in the dynamics of infectious diseases are not only expected, but can already be noticed. Vector-borne diseases are particularly susceptible to environmental changes, since their occurrence depends on the ecological balance between different species in complex transmission cycles [1-3]. Leishmaniases are among the vector-borne diseases most affected by this *ecological chaos* driven by human actions [4], and one of the expected impacts is the expansion of its geographical distribution [5-7].

Leishmaniases are among the world's six most neglected diseases, affecting indistinctively men, women and children. Usually they occur among the poorest of the poor, mainly in developing countries, contributing to establishment and maintenance of social inequities [7]. They can be divided in two main clinical forms: visceral leishmaniasis (VL) and cutaneous leishmaniasis (CL). Despite this simple classification, a wide clinical spectrum is observed, mostly because of the high diversity of parasites (Trypanosomatidae of *Leishmania* genus), vectors (Phlebotominae sand flies) and reservoir hosts (mammals of several orders) involved in its transmission cycles [7, 8].

The geographical distribution of leishmaniases includes 98 countries in American, European, Asiatic, African and Australian continents. The World Health Organization estimates the yearly occurrence of about 200,000 to 400,000 VL human cases and 700,000 to 1.2 million CL human cases. More than 90% of global VL cases are recorded in six countries: India, Bangladesh, Sudan, South Sudan, Ethiopia and Brazil. Cutaneous leishmaniasis is more widely distributed, with about one-third of cases occurring in tropical regions of the Americas, the

Mediterranean basin, western and central Asia. In the American continent, Brazil is the country with the highest estimated incidences of both visceral and cutaneous leishmaniases [9].

The distribution of leishmaniases in the world can be partially explained by its widely distributed vectors. The sand flies are small insects (adults of about 3-5 mm) from order Diptera, family Psychodidae, subfamily Phlebotominae. Although occurring mainly in the tropical, hottest areas of the world (Latin America, South Europe, Africa, South Asia and Australia), their distribution stretches north and south to latitudes of over 40°, such as in Germany [10] and Argentinean Patagonia [11]. Sand flies have primarily crepuscular and nocturnal habits, but adults were captured during the day in dense forests [12], caves [13] and dark, humid animal shelters [14]. Only females are haematophagous and thus are related with *Leishmania* transmission. Their broad feeding habits contribute to the transmission of pathogens between hosts in sylvatic and peridomestic areas [15, 16]. Of approximately 900 described sand fly species, no more than 70 have been implicated in leishmaniases transmission [17]. All New World vector species belong to *Lutzomyia* genus, while the Old World vectors are grouped in *Phlebotomus* genus [15, 18].

In Brazil, the concept of leishmaniases as a sylvatic zoonosis is restricted to the Amazon Forest, Atlantic Forest fragments and parts of Cerrado. A new transmission profile has emerged, driven mostly by human-made environmental changes. In past decades, human migration of different origins and purposes resulted in major deforestation and unplanned settlements. These changes favor the dispersion of sylvatic animals (some *Leishmania* reservoir hosts) and sand flies (especially those species with eclectic feeding habits) to peridomestic areas, where new transmission cycles may establish close to human dwellings [19-21].

This new transmission profile is especially evident for American Cutaneous Leishmaniasis (ACL), which is caused by a variety of *Leishmania* parasites. Although some clinical manifestations are more frequently associated with a particular *Leishmania* species or subgenus (*Viannia* or *Leishmania*), none is unique to a species. In addition, a substantial but variable proportion of infections are asymptomatic. Human cases have been occurring with different clinical forms, including localized, disseminated, diffuse and atypical cutaneous and mucosal lesions. Different species of sand flies and reservoirs interact in complex transmission cycles, with particular ecoepidemiological features on each disease focus [22, 23].

According to Brazilian Ministry of Health [23], ACL can be categorized in three epidemiological patterns:

1. Sylvatic: In this case, transmission occurs in primary vegetation areas, where the disease is characterized as a strictly sylvatic zoonosis. Humans get infected occasionally when entering these areas, where the enzootic cycle is maintained;

2. Sylvatic/occupational and impacted areas: This pattern is associated with exploitation of natural environments and deforestation, originated mostly from constructions of roads, hydroelectric power plants, human settlements, wood extraction, agricultural activities, military training and ecotourism. In this case, humans are more intensively exposed to vector contact;

3. Rural/periurban (colonization areas): ACL occurrence is related to human migration, occupation of slopes and aggregation in periurban areas associated with secondary and residual vegetation. Synanthropic and domestic animals such as dogs, horses and rodents are suggested reservoir hosts.

Brazil is currently facing an increasing geographical expansion of ACL, with a shift from the classical predominant epidemiological pattern 1 to frequent observations of pattern 2. All of its states have records of the disease, with a growing number of municipalities affected each year (Figure 1).

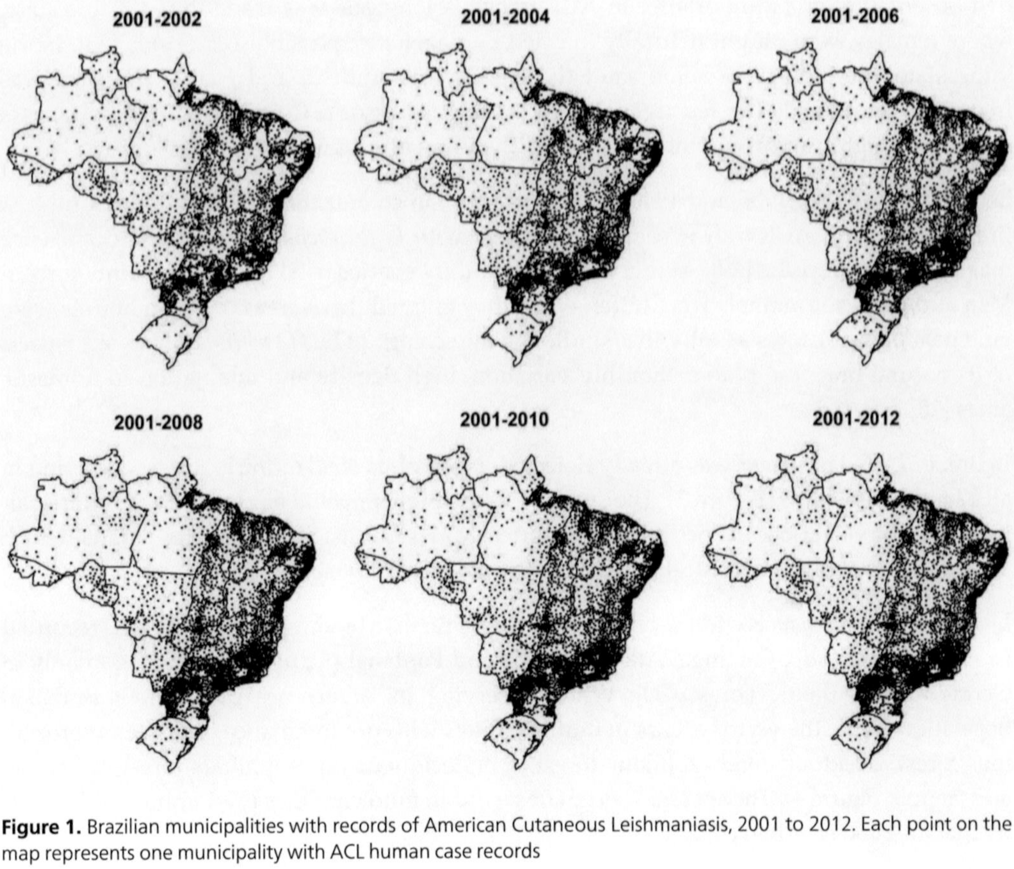

Figure 1. Brazilian municipalities with records of American Cutaneous Leishmaniasis, 2001 to 2012. Each point on the map represents one municipality with ACL human case records

This expansion can probably be explained by the growing environmental changes, which in turn affect vector behavior. Some ACL vector species have been showing evidences of adaptation to man-modified environments, establishing in peridomestic areas, even in outskirts of large cities [22, 23]. In this case, two sand fly species are particularly good examples, in different ecoepidemiological situations: *Lutzomyia (Nyssomyia) whitmani* and *Lutzomyia (Nyssomyia) flaviscutellata*. On the following sections the geographical distribution in Brazil and relation with ACL transmission of these species are presented.

2. *Lutzomyia (Nyssomyia) whitmani* (Antunes & Coutinho 1939)

Lutzomyia (N.) whitmani was described by Antunes & Coutinho in 1939 [24] as *Flebotomus whitmani* in honor of Dr. Whitman, from Rockefeller Foundation, an institute that collaborated with the Brazilian government at the time in the Yellow Fever Service. The new species was described based on male and female specimens captured in Ilhéus municipality, Bahia state. This species can be observed in all five regions of Brazil and, in the American continent it is also present in Argentina, French Guiana, Paraguay and Peru [7, 18].

The role of *L. (N.) whitmani* as ACL vector is evident throughout the Brazilian territory. The first observation of its importance in ACL transmission cycle was made in São Paulo state, where females were caught naturally infected by flagellates, possibly *Leishmania* [25]. In the same state, the biology of some sand fly species was studied, and *L. (N.) whitmani* was frequently found in deforested areas [26]. According to Pessoa & Coutinho [25], this species is considered highly anthropophilic, constantly invading houses for biting humans.

Between decades of 1930 and 1940, during the human colonization of South and Southeast Brazilian regions, ACL transmission was related with *L. (N.) whitmani*, with its occurrence mainly in sylvatic areas [27]. At this time, this sand fly species used to inhabit mainly forests. Man and domestic animals were bitten when they entered these areas or when houses were built near or inside forests [26]. Other studies on the ecology of *L. (N.) whitmani* showed aspects of its natural breeding places, monthly variation, high density and adaptation to domestic areas [28].

In Brazil, *L. (N.) whitmani* was already detected in 634 of its 5566 municipalities, occurring in all 27 federative units (Figure 2). The states with the higher spatial aggregation of municipalities with the vector occurrence are Pernambuco, Minas Gerais, São Paulo and Paraná, which are also areas of high concentration of ACL human cases [29] (see Figure 1).

Lutzomya (N.) whitmani is widely distributed across Brazilian biomes. Its presence was recorded in Amazon, Cerrado, Caatinga, Atlantic Forest and Pantanal (Figure 3), occurring mainly in Cerrado and Atlantic Forest [30]. When observing its occurrence in different Brazilian vegetation types, the vector occurs in municipalities with predominance of dense ombrophilous forest, deciduous ombrophilous forest, semideciduous ombrophilous forest, savannah and steppe (Figure 4). The species was not observed in municipalities predominantly covered by marshes and sandbanks [29].

In São Paulo state, *L. (N.) intermedia* and *L. (N.) whitmani* were the predominant species during deforestation of primary forests [28]. However, as deforestation continued to expand, *L. (N.) whitmani* showed lower abundances, suggesting that this species would be more dependent of primary forest than *L. (N.) intermedia*. On the other hand, *L. (N.) whitmani* was found frequently inside houses built near the forest. In Southeast Region, this species can be found during all months of the year [22, 26]. In São Roque municipality, São Paulo state, *L. (N.) whitmani* was the predominant sand fly species among *Leishmania (V.) braziliensis* transmission areas [31], showing higher abundances in the hotter months of the year [32].

http://dx.doi.org/10.5772/57207

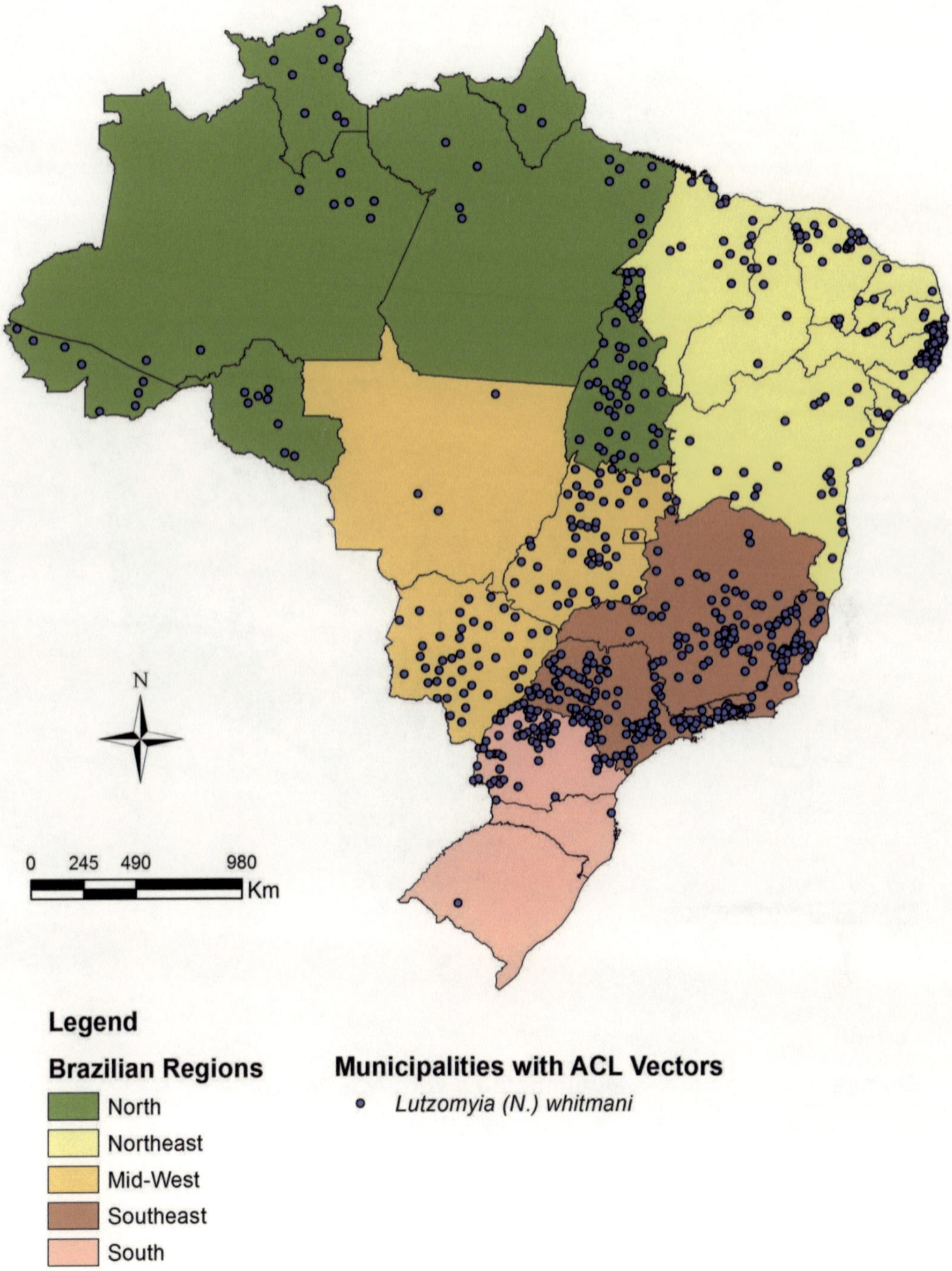

Figure 2. Brazilian municipalities with *Lutzomyia (Nyssomyia) whitmani* occurrence

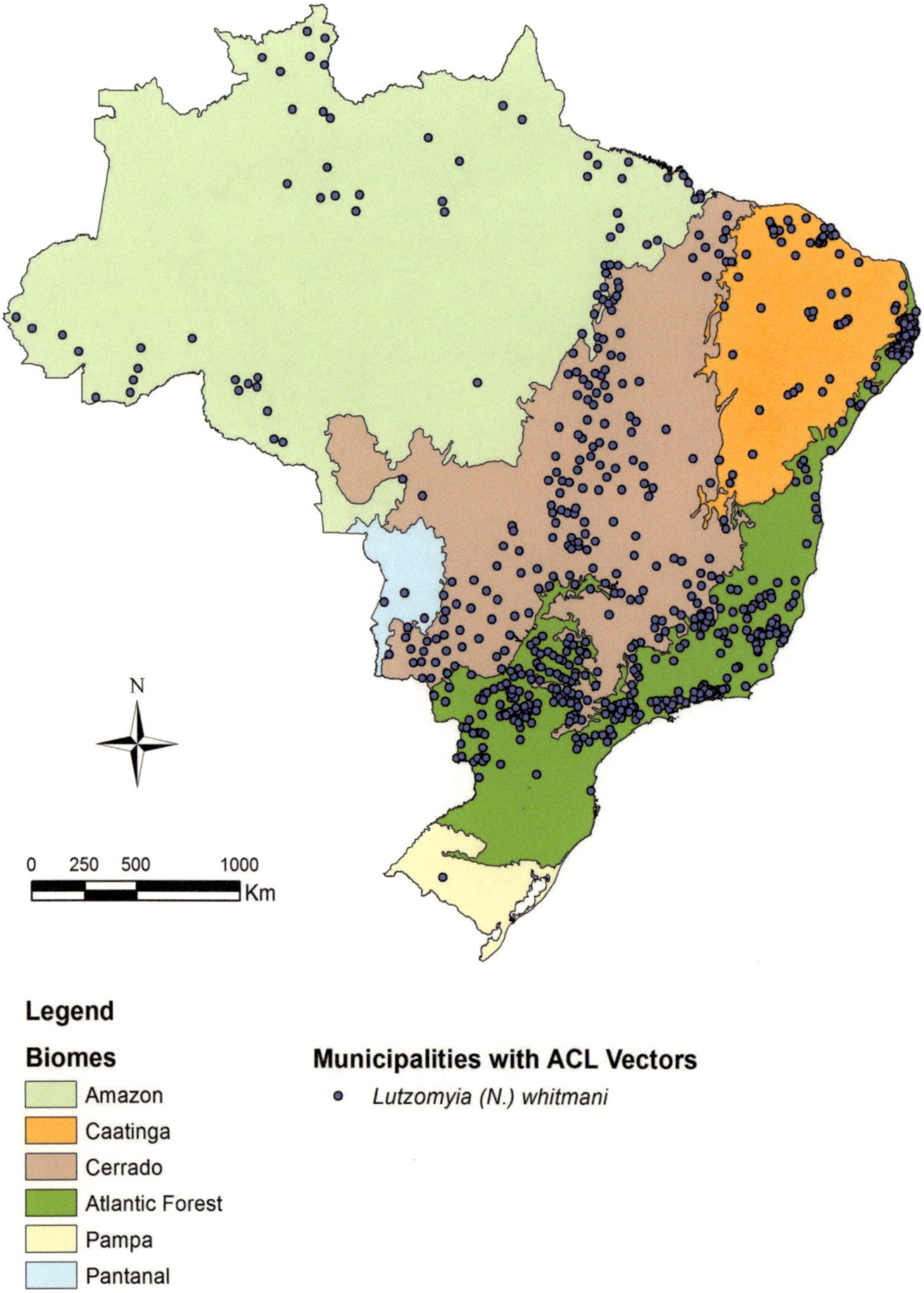

Figure 3. Brazilian municipalities with *Lutzomyia (Nyssomyia) whitmani* occurrence and biomes

http://dx.doi.org/10.5772/57207

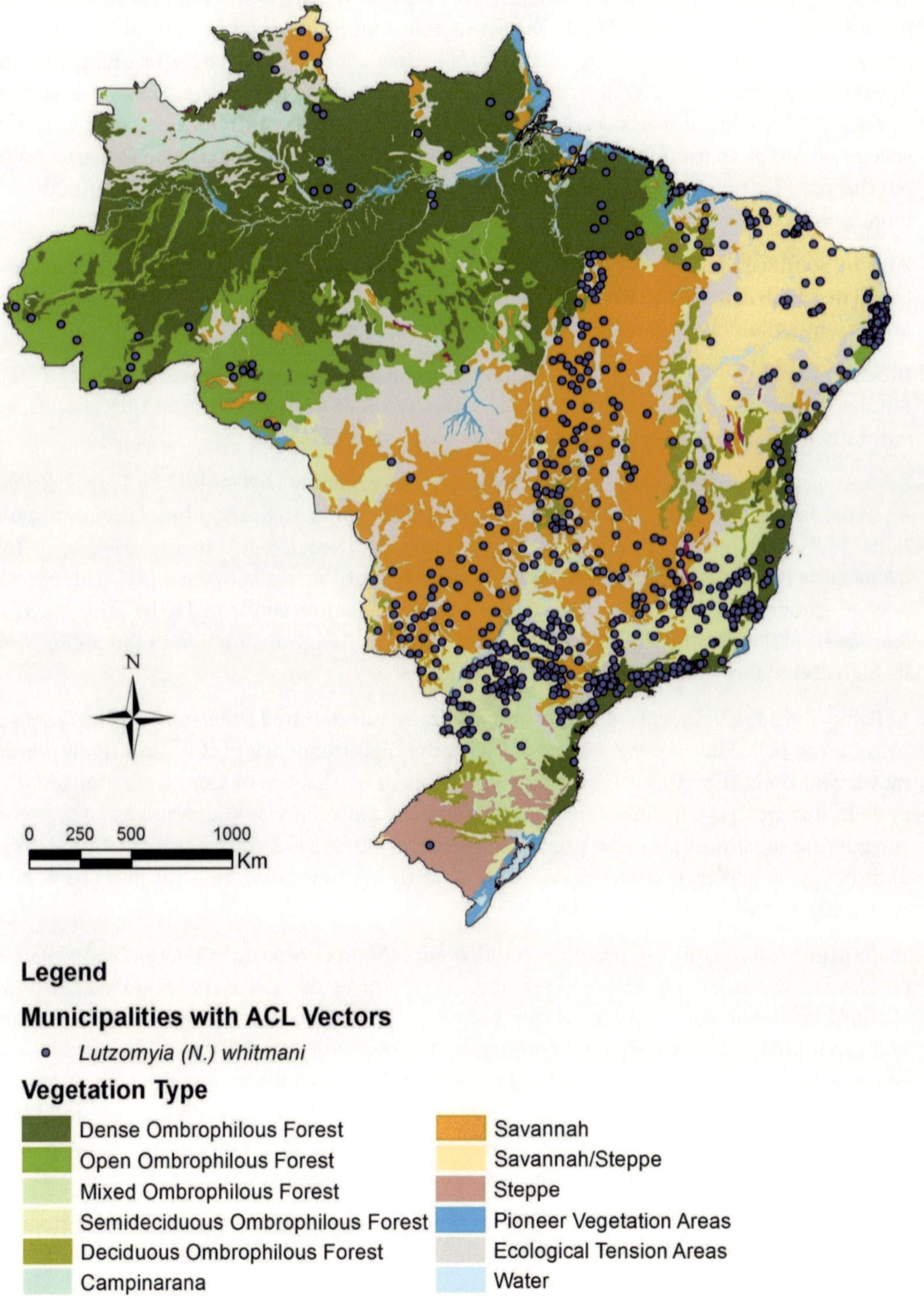

Figure 4. Brazilian municipalities with *Lutzomyia (Nyssomyia) whitmani* occurrence and vegetation types

This species was also observed in Atlantic Forest protected areas and inside houses near the forest in Rio de Janeiro state [33]. In the same state, studies performed in rural areas of ACL transmission showed the co-occurrence of *L. (N.) intermedia* and *L. (N.) whitmani* biting humans. In peridomestic areas, *L. (N). intermedia* was predominant, while *L. (N.) whitmani* was more frequent in the nearest forest. With this spatial separation, the authors suggested that both species would be sharing *Leishmania (V.) braziliensis* transmission on the same focus, throughout the year. *Lutzomyia (N.) whitmani* was captured during all year, but was more frequent in months with lower temperatures [34].

Also in Southeast region, besides São Paulo and Rio de Janeiro states, *L. (N.) whitmani* was associated with *Leishmania (Viannia) braziliensis* transmission in Caratinga (Minas Gerais state) and in a mountainous region of Afonso Cláudio (Espírito Santo state) [35, 36].

In South Brazil, *L. (N.) whitmani* is probably associated to ACL transmission in Paraná state. Studies performed in the north of this state detected it as predominant sand fly species and naturally infected by *Leishmania (V.) braziliensis* parasites [37].

Leishmania (V.) braziliensis in Northeast region is also probably transmitted by *L. (N.) whitmani*. In Bahia and Ceará states this vector shows similar habits to the Southeast region populations: high anthropophily and presence in domestic areas [38-40]. In Ceará state, *L. (N.) whitmani* was found naturally infected by *Leishmania* of *Viannia* subgenus [41]. Afterwards, new infections were detected and the parasite characterization confirmed to be *Leishmania (V.) braziliensis* [42]. Other evidences of this vector's role in ACL transmission in the region were its high abundance and anthropophily [40, 42].

In Bahia state, *L. (N.) whitmani* was found naturally infected by *Leishmania (V.) braziliensis* in Três Braços [43]. This finding, associated with the high frequency of this sand fly in peridomestic and domestic areas allowed the hypothesis of occurrence of a domestic transmission cycle in this area [44]. In Ilhéus municipality, *L. (N.) whitmani* was suggested as ACL vector, considering its almost absolute predominance over other sand fly species (99.7%), its high anthropophily and its occurrence on every sand fly capture point, most of them coincident with areas of ACL human cases [40].

In the Mid-West Region, in Corguinho municipality (Mato Grosso do Sul state), *Leishmania (V.) braziliensis* was isolated from every tested ACL patient by monoclonal antibodies. *Lutzomyia (N.) whitmani* was suggested as vector because it was observed in high abundances and anthropophilic [45]. Furthermore, its predominance over other sand flies was observed in eight of ten ecotopes studied in the locality. *Lutzomyia (N.) whitmani* was present both in ground level and in the forest canopy, suggesting its eclectic feeding habits on mammals and birds. Although in this locality the species is not very common in peridomestic areas, its high abundance and anthropophily are strong evidences of its role in ACL transmission [46].

The behavior of *L. (N.) whitmani* in North region seems to be different from other regions. In these areas, the species was considered mainly sylvatic, being captured on tree trunks and canopies, besides showing low attractiveness for humans [47]. Afterwards, novel studies confirmed such observations and suggested that, if the species were to be anthropophilic, it would be only in some situations [48, 49]. In 1989, in Pará state, a parasite was isolated from

http://dx.doi.org/10.5772/57207

L. (N.) whitmani, and after its characterization as *Leishmania (V.) shawi*, the sand fly species was suggested as its vector [50].

3. *Lutzomyia (Nyssomyia) flaviscutellata* (Mangabeira 1942)

Lutzomyia (N.) flaviscutellata was described by Mangabeira [51] as *Flebotomus flaviscutellatus*, based on two male specimens captured in Belém (Pará state). Later, Sherlock & Carneiro [52] described a female collected in Salvador (Bahia state), although its identification has been questioned by several authors [18, 27, 53]. At the same time, the species *Phlebotomus apicalis* was described by Floch & Abonnenc [54] in French Guiana. Three years later, after a review of the specimens, *P. apicalis* was considered synonym of *L. (N.) flaviscutellata* [55].

In the following years, descriptions of *L. (N.) olmeca* [56], *L. (N.) olmeca bicolor* [53] and *L. (N.) olmeca nociva* [57], all of them morphologically similar to *L. (N.) flaviscutellata*, led some authors to consider these four species as the "*L. flaviscutellata* complex" [58]. However, they are all currently considered valid species, with more recent taxonomic reviews supporting their status [18, 59].

Lutzomyia (N.) flaviscutellata is currently widely distributed across Latin America, occurring in Bolivia, Brazil, Colombia, Ecuador, French Guiana, Peru, Suriname, Trinidad and Venezuela [7, 18].

This sand fly species is associated with *Leishmania (Leishmania) amazonensis* transmission in Brazil. This parasite, when infecting humans, can cause localized cutaneous lesions and eventually develop a more severe clinical form, diffuse cutaneous leishmaniasis (DCL). This clinical form is rare, with chronic development, where the immunodepressed patient shows frequent relapses and insufficient responses to available therapies [60].

The first observation of this sand fly's role in ACL transmission cycle was from a study in the Utinga forest, an Amazon area in Belém municipality (Pará state) [61]. In this area, wild rodents of *Proechimys* and *Oryzomys* genus were captured with cutaneous lesions on tails and feet, from where *Leishmania* parasites were isolated. These rodents were then used as baits and 98% of captured sand flies were *L. (N.) flaviscutellata*. Captured sand flies were dissected and flagellates were isolated from eight females.

Studies of the feeding habits of *L. (N.) flaviscutellata* showed higher preference for small sylvatic rodents (*Proechimys* sp., *Oryzomys* sp.), agoutis (*Dasyprocta* sp.) and porcupines (*Coendou* sp.), having the species also fed on opossums (*Philander* sp.), monkeys (*Saimiri* sp.) and chickens (*Gallus gallus*). Few females fed on humans, so the authors considered the species as having low anthropophily [62]. This preference for biting small rodents indicates that captures of this species tend to be more efficient when using animal baited traps, such as the Disney trap [63].

Despite its strong zoophilic habits and low anthropophily, *Lutzomyia (N.) flaviscutellata* has recently been captured in peridomestic areas, suggesting its dispersion to human dwellings [64-67]. This hypothesis is plausible, since the species also occurs in secondary forests in the

Amazon. In a study performed in the late 1980s in Pará state, *L. (N.) flaviscutellata* was the predominant sand fly species in an area where the primary forest was replaced with exotic trees (*Pinus* and *Gmelina*), with occasional captures in peridomestic areas of houses near the forest [68]. In a review of the Amazonian ACL transmission cycles, *L. (N.) flaviscutellata* was considered one of the few vector species that could adapt to deforestation and become peridomestic [69].

In Brazil, *L. (N.) flaviscutellata* was detected in 131 municipalities, mostly in North and Mid-West regions, with occurrences also in Southwest and Northeast regions (Figure 5).

Lutzomya (N.) flaviscutellata is considered mainly an Amazonian species, although it can also be found in Cerrado and some few occurrences were recorded in Atlantic Forest, Caatinga and Pantanal (Figure 6).

In the Amazon, *L. (N.) flaviscutellata* is more commonly found in seasonally flooded areas of "igapó forests", when compared with non-flooded areas of "terra-firme forests" [70]. Its vertical distribution was also studied in the Amazon. The species has a very low flight, with 26 times more specimens captured 0.2 meters above ground than at 1.2 meters. This observation reinforces its association with small rodents and the fact that human cutaneous lesions caused by *Leishmania (L.) amazonensis* are mainly located in the lowest parts of the body [71].

The species was also captured in peridomestic areas of Manaus (Amazonas state) [72], Ilha de Marajó (Pará state) [73] and Santarém (Pará state) [74]. Other examples of surveyed Amazon forest areas of the North region with records of *L. (N.) flaviscutellata* include the states: Acre [75, 76], Amazonas [13, 76-79], Amapá [80], Pará [61, 62, 68, 70, 81], Rondônia [82, 83] and Roraima [84, 85].

Also in the North region, Tocantins state has most of its area covered by Cerrado. It was in this biome that *L. (N.) flaviscutellata* was captured during a four-year sand fly fauna monitoring in the ACL endemic areas of Porto Nacional and Guaraí municipalities. This vector species was found in peridomestic captures in rural settlements and periurban areas [66, 67] and was suggested as *Leishmania (L.) amazonensis* vector in Porto Nacional [66]. In municipalities of the south of the same state, *L. (N.) flaviscutellata* was captured near houses in areas directly and indirectly impacted by a hydroelectric power plant construction in Tocantins River [86].

In Bela Vista municipality (Mato Grosso do Sul State, Mid-West region), an ACL outbreak associated with *Leishmania (L.) amazonensis* in a military training unit led to a sand fly fauna monitoring during years 2004 to 2006. Using light traps, few specimens of *L. (N.) flaviscutellata* were caught [87]. When a modified Disney trap baited with hamsters (*Mesocricetus auratus*) was used, *L. (N.) flaviscutellata* was the species with the highest female abundance [88]. Despite its capture with these methodologies, some females were also captured in white and black Shannon traps [89], suggesting that the species can also feed on humans, and therefore be a possible *Leishmania (L.) amazonensis* vector in this locality [87].

The sand fly fauna of an ecotourism area in Bonito (Mato Grosso do Sul state) was studied. In Cerrado areas, *L. (N.) flaviscutellata* was caught with light traps mainly inside the forest, but it was also found in yards and kennels of houses [64].

http://dx.doi.org/10.5772/57207

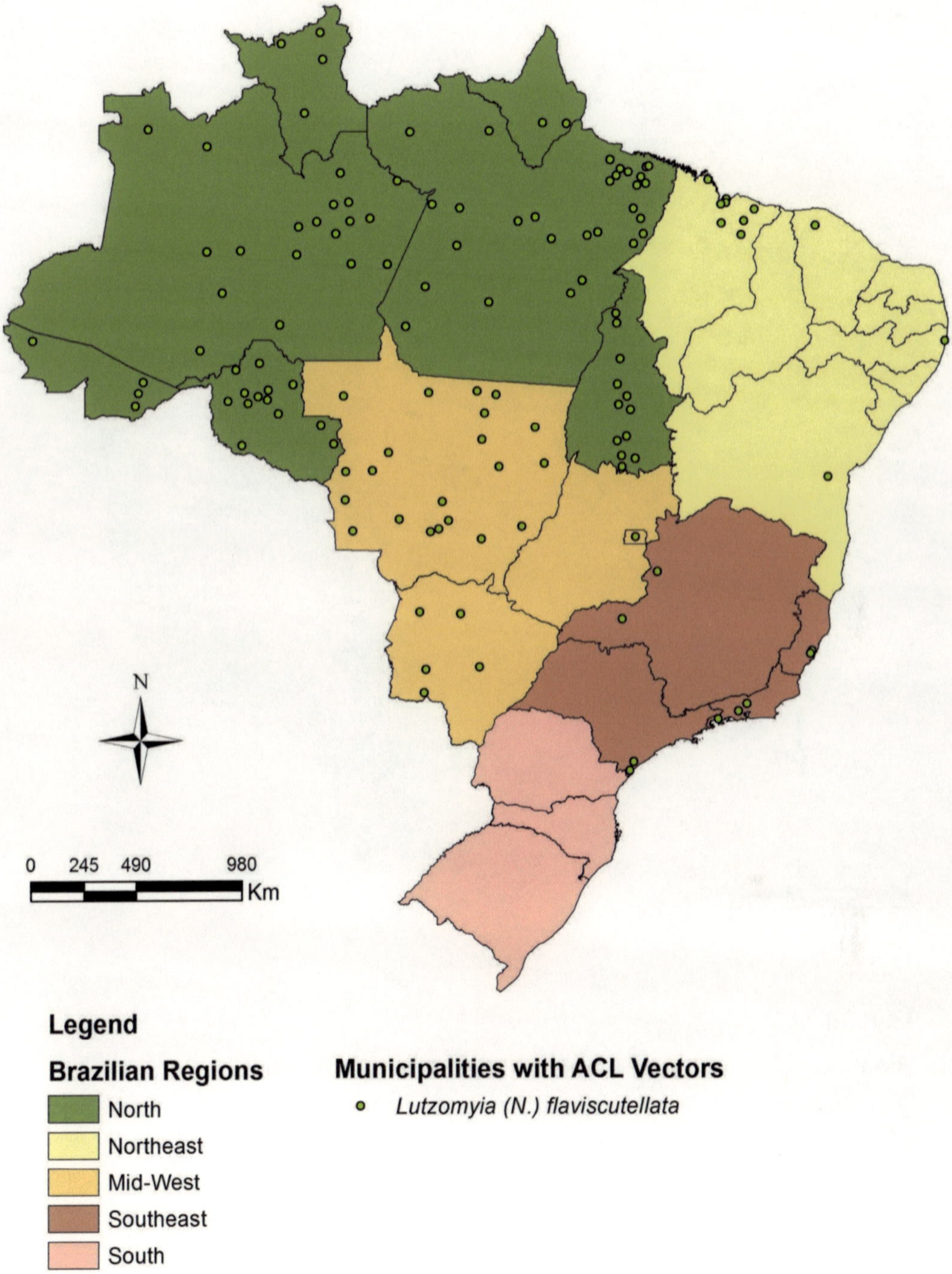

Figure 5. Brazilian municipalities with *Lutzomyia (Nyssomyia) flaviscutellata* occurrence

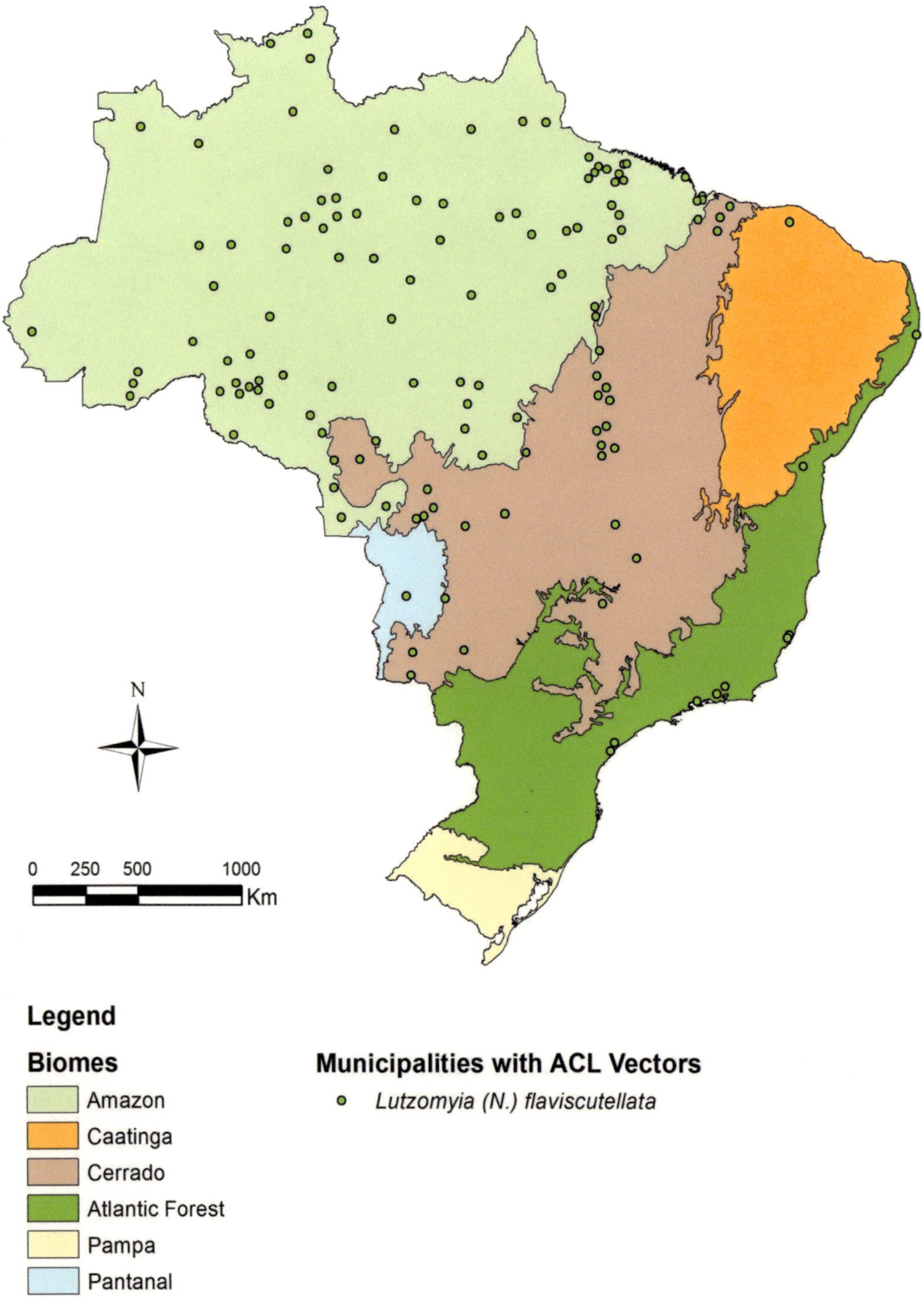

Figure 6. Brazilian municipalities with *Lutzomyia (Nyssomyia) flaviscutellata* occurrence and biomes

In Southeast region, another ecotourism area was surveyed, in Rio de Janeiro state, Atlantic Forest biome. In Angra dos Reis municipality, the state's biggest continental island - Ilha Grande - has records of sporadic ACL cases since the first outbreak in the decade of 1970. At the time of the ACL outbreak, the sand fly fauna was monitored and *L. (N.) flaviscutellata* was captured inside the forest with Disney traps, baited with *Proechimys* rodents [90]. Over three decades later, the same localities were surveyed, and *L. (N.) flaviscutellata* was captured inside the forest and in peridomestic areas of several fisherman villages in Ilha Grande [65]. Even though there are no recorded human cases of *Leishmania (L.) amazonensis* infection in Ilha Grande, one DCL case was recorded in 2007 in Paraty, a municipality neighbor to Angra dos Reis [91].

4. Conclusion: Two American cutaneous leishmaniasis vectors as drivers of its geographical expansion in Brazil

Both *Lutzomyia (N.) whitmani* and *L. (N.) flaviscutellata* are widely spread in Brazilian territory. Each one with its particular epidemiological importance, their geographical distributions overlap areas of ACL occurrence in Brazil (Figure 7).

Since it has a wide geographical distribution and it is associated with two ACL parasites (*Leishmania (V.) braziliensis* and *Leishmania (V.) shawi*), currently, *Lutzomyia (N.) whitmani* is considered the most important ACL vector in Brazil. Its importance is due mainly to its role in transmission cycles related with ACL epidemiological pattern 2 (sylvatic/occupational and impacted areas). This sand fly species was found in several localities associated with areas of environmental changes of different origins, such as deforestation, road constructions, human settements and agricultural activities. This epidemiological pattern is frequently observed in Brazil, and constitutes the main evidence of the disease's geographical spreading.

Lutzomyia (N.) flaviscutellata, with evidences of dispersion to peridomestic areas especially in the Cerrado biome, confirms the ruralization process of the previously considered strictly sylvatic cycle of *Leishmania (L.) amazonensis*. The possibility of this enzootic cycle to be maintained in secondary forests and even become peridomestic was previously discussed [69]. This could be happening, in part, because of the adaptation process of the vector to man-modified environments. At first, it would be logical to think that a strictly sylvatic cycle would disappear with deforestation of primary forests [92], but the *Leishmania (L.) amazonensis* cycle shows evidences of occurrence in secondary forests and peridomestic areas, where the vector could be dispersing to domestic animal shelters [22].

Considering the great challenge that is controlling ACL, a disease with complex epidemiology directly associated with environmental changes, studies that aim to characterize and monitor its spatial and temporal trends can support the Epidemiological and Entomological Surveillance actions of Health Departments. These studies can help to identify receptive areas for new ACL outbreaks and population groups at higher risk of infection, so that control actions can be better planned and more effective.

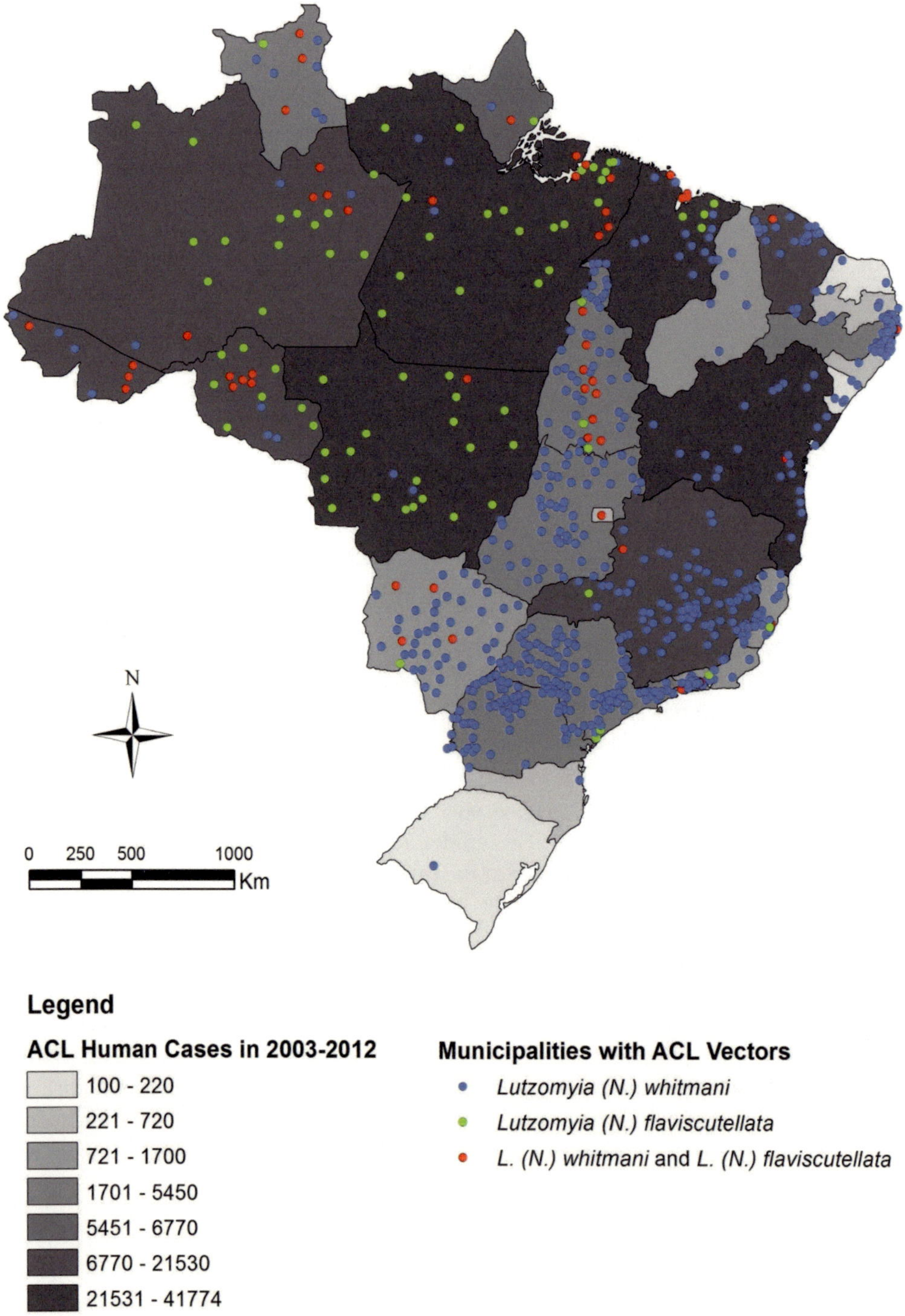

Figure 7. Brazilian municipalities with *Lutzomyia (Nyssomyia) whitmani* and *Lutzomyia (Nyssomyia) flaviscutellata* occurrence and American Cutaneous Leishaniasis human cases recorded by state in the past ten years (2003-2012)

Acknowledgements

To Mônica Magalhães, from Instituto de Comunicação e Informação Científica e Tecnológica em Saúde (FIOCRUZ) and Thiago Vasconcelos, from Instituto Evandro Chagas. To Fundação Carlos Chagas Filho de Amparo à Pesquisa do Estado do Rio de Janeiro (FAPERJ) and Instituto Oswaldo Cruz (FIOCRUZ) for financial support.

Author details

Elizabeth F. Rangel, Simone M. da Costa and Bruno M. Carvalho*

*Address all correspondence to: brunomc@ioc.fiocruz.br

Oswaldo Cruz Institute, FIOCRUZ, Rio de Janeiro, Brazil

References

[1] Walsh JF, Molyneux DH, Birley MH. Deforestation: effects on vector-borne disease. Parasitology 1993;106(Suppl) 55-75.

[2] Patz JA, Thaddeus KG, Geller N, Vittor AY. Effects of environmental change on emerging parasitic diseases. International Journal for Parasitology 2000;30 1395-1405.

[3] McMichael AJ. Environmental and social influences on emerging infectious diseases: past, present and future. Philosophical Transactions of the Royal Society London B 2004;359 1049-1058.

[4] Shaw J. How climatic and environmental variations affect the eco-epidemiology of the leishmaniases and their control. In: III Workshop de Genética e Biologia Molecular de Insetos Vetores de Doenças Tropicais; Recife (PE), Brasil 2008; p13.

[5] Ashford RW. The leishmaniasis as emerging and reemerging zoonoses. International Journal for Parasitol 2000;30 1269-1281.

[6] Dujardin JC. Risk factors in the spread of leishmaniases: towards integrated monitoring? Trends in Parasitology 2006;22(1) 4-6.

[7] WHO – World Health Organization. Control of the leishmaniases: report of a meeting of the WHO Expert Committee on the Control of Leishmaniases, Geneva, 22-26 March 2010 (WHO Technical Report Series, nº 949). Geneva: WHO Press; 2010.

[8] Peters W, Killick-Kendrick R. The Leishmaniasis in Biology and Medicine, London: Academic Press; 1987.

[9] Alvar J, Vélez ID, Bern C, Herrero M, Desjeux P, Cano J, Jannin J, den Boer M. Leishmaniasis worldwide and global estimates of its incidence. PlosOne 2012;7(5) e35671.

[10] Naucke TJ, Pesson B. Presence of *Phlebotomus (Transphlebotomus) mascittii* Grassi, 1908 (Diptera : Psychodidae) in Germany. Parasitolgy Research 2000;86(4) 335-336.

[11] Muzón J, Spinelli GR, Salomón OD, Rossi GC. A first record of Phlebotominae from Argentinean Patagonia (Diptera: Psychodidae: Phlebotominae). Memórias do Instituto Oswaldo Cruz 2002;97(6) 797-798.

[12] Ready PD, Lainson R, Shaw JJ. Habitat and seasonality of *Psychodopygus wellcomei* help incriminate it as a vector of *Leishmania braziliensis* in Amazonia and northeast Brazil. Transactions of the Royal Society of Tropical Medicine and Hygiene 1984;78 543-544.

[13] Alves VR, Freitas RA, Santos FL, Barrett TV. Diversity of sandflies (Psychodidae: Phlebotominae) captured in sandstone caves from Central Amazonia, Brazil. Memórias do Instituto Oswaldo Cruz 2011;106(3) 353-359.

[14] Campbell-Lendrum DH, Brandão-Filho SP, Pinto MC, Vexenat A, Ready PD, Davies CR. Domesticity of *Lutzomyia whitmani* (Diptera: Psychodidae) populations: Field experiments indicate behavioural differences. Bulletin of Entomological Research 2000;90 41-48.

[15] Killick-Kendrick R. The Biology and Control of Phlebotomine Sand Flies. Clinics Dermatology 1999;17(3) 279-289.

[16] Afonso MMS, Chaves SAM, Rangel EF. Evaluation of feeding habits of haematophagous insects, with emphasis on Phlebotominae (Diptera: Psychodidae), vectors of Leishmaniasis - Review. Trends in Entomology 2012;8 125-136.

[17] Ready PD. Biology of Sand Flies as Vectors of Disease Agents. Annual Review of Entomology 2013;58 227-250.

[18] Young DG, Duncan MA. Guide to the identification and geographic distribution of *Lutzomyia* sandflies in Mexico, the West Indies, Central and South America (Diptera:Psychodidae). Memoirs of the American Entomological Institute 1994;54 1-881.

[19] Rangel EF. Tropical Diseases, Society and the Environment. SAREC Documentation/ TDR, 1995; 103-110.

[20] Rangel EF, Lainson R. Ecologia das Leishmanioses: Transmissores de Leishmaniose Tegumentar Americana. In: Rangel EF, Lainson R (eds.) Flebotomíneos do Brasil, Rio de Janeiro: Fiocruz; 2003. p291-310.

[21] Costa, SM, Cechinel M, Bandeira V, Zannuncio JC, Lainson R, Rangel EF. *Lutzomyia (Nyssomyia) whitmani* s.l. (Antunes & Coutinho, 1939) (Diptera: Psychodidae: Phlebotominae) and the Epidemiology of American Cutaneous Leishmaniasis in Brazil. Memórias do Instituto Oswaldo Cruz 2007;102(2) 149-153.

[22] Rangel EF, Lainson R. Proven and putative vectors of American cutaneous leishmaniasis in Brazil: aspects of their biology and vectorial competence. Memórias do Instituto Oswaldo Cruz 2009;104(7) 937-954.

[23] Brasil. Ministério da Saúde. Secretaria de Vigilância em Saúde. Departamento de Vigilância Epidemiológica. Manual de Vigilância da Leishmaniose Tegumentar Americana 2a. ed. Brasília: Editora do Ministério da Saúde; 2007.

[24] Antunes PCA, Coutinho JO. Notas sobre flebótomos sul-americanos. II. Descrição de *Flebotomus whitmani* n. sp. e da armadura bucal de algumas espécies. Boletim de Biologia de São Paulo 1939;4 448-453.

[25] Pessoa SB, Coutinho JO. Infecção natural e experimental dos flebótomos pela *Leishmania braziliensis* no Estado de São Paulo. O Hospital 1941;20 25-35.

[26] Barretto MP. Observações sobre a biologia em condições naturais dos flebótomos do estado de São Paulo (Diptera, Psychodidae). PhD thesis. University of Public Health São Paulo; 1943.

[27] Forattini OP. Entomologia Médica, 4º Volume: Psychodidae. Phlebotominae. Leishmanioses. Bartonelose. São Paulo: Edgard Blücher and Universidae de São Paulo; 1973.

[28] Forattini OP. Novas observações sobre a biologia de flebótomos em condições naturais (Diptera, Psychodidae). Arquivos da Faculdade de Higiene e Saúde Pública 1960;25 209-215.

[29] Costa SM, Cechinel M, Magalhães MAFM, Barcellos C, Rangel EF. Use of geoprocessing techniques in the analysis of the distribution of *Lutzomyia (Nyssomyia) whitmani* (Diptera:Psychodidae:Phlebotominae) in association with vegetation and the epidemiological circuits of American Cutaneous Leishmaniasis (ACL) in Brazil. In: International Symposium on Phlebotomine Sandflies, 25-30 Apr 2011, Kuşadası, Turkey. 2011.

[30] Costa SM, Cordeiro JP, Rangel EF. Distribuição espacial de *Lutzomyia (Nyssomyia) whitmani* (Diptera;Phychodidae;Phlebotominae), vetor de Leishmaniose Tegumentar Americana, em associação com os diferentes biomas brasileiros. In: 1ª Conferência Brasileira em Saúde Silvestre e Humana, 24-26 Oct 2012, Rio de Janeiro, Brazil. 2012.

[31] Taniguchi HH, Tolezano JE, Corrêa FMA, Morales RAP, Veiga RMO, Marassa AM. Epidemiologia da leishmaniose tegumentar americana no Estado de São Paulo, Brasil. I. Composição da fauna flebotomínica no Município de São Roque, Região de Sorocaba. Revista do Instituto Adolfo Lutz 1991;51 23-30.

[32] Taniguchi HH, Tolezano JE. American cutaneous Leishmaniasis in São Paulo State. II Seasonal fluctuation of Phlebotominae sandflies species in São Roque Country. Memórias do Instituto Oswaldo Cruz 1988;83(Supp.1) 201.

[33] Souza NA, Vilela ML, Andrade-Coelho CA, Rangel EF. The Phlebotominae sand fly (Diptera: Psychodidae) fauna of two Atlantic Rain Forest Reserves in the State of Rio de Janeiro,Brazil. Memórias do Instituto Oswaldo Cruz 2001;96(3): 319-324.

[34] Souza NA, Andrade-Coelho CA, Vilela ML, Peixoto AA, Rangel EF. Seasonality of *Lutzomyia intermedia* and *Lutzomyia whitmani* (Diptera: Psychodidae: Phlebotominae), occurring sympatrically in area of Cutaneous Leishmaniasis in the State of Rio de Janeiro, Brazil. Memórias do Instituto Oswaldo Cruz 2002;97(6) 759-765.

[35] Mayrink W, Willians P, Coelho MV, Dias M, Martins AV, Magalhães PA, Costa CA, Falcão AR, Melo MN, Falcão AL. Epidemiology of dermal leishmaniasis in the Rio Doce Valley, State of Minas Gerais, Brazil. Annals of Tropical Medicine and Parasitology 1979;73 123-137.

[36] Falqueto A. Especificidade alimentar de flebotomíneos em duas áreas endêmicas de leishmaniose tegumentar no Estado do Espírito Santo. PhD thesis. Fundação Oswaldo Cruz. Rio de Janeiro; 1995.

[37] Luz E, Membrive N, Castro EA, Dereure J, Pratlong F, Dedet JA, Pandey A, Thomaz-Soccol V. *Lutzomyia whitmani* (Diptera: Psychodidae) as vector of *Leishmania (V.) braziliensis* in Paraná state, southern Brazil. Annals of Tropical Medicine & Parasitology 2000;94(6) 623-631.

[38] Barretto AC, Vexenat JA, Cuba-Cuba CA, Marsden PD. Fauna flebotomínica de uma região endêmica de leishmaniose cutâneo-mucosa, no Estado da Bahia. In: IX Reunião Anual sobre Pesquisa Básica em Doenças de Chagas; 1982. p147.

[39] Vexenat JA, Barretto AC, Rosa AC. Infecção experimental de *Lutzomyia whitmani* em cães infectados com *Leishmania braziliensis braziliensis*. Memórias do Instituto Oswaldo Cruz 1986;81 125-126.

[40] Azevedo ACR, Rangel EF. Study of sandfly species (Diptera: Psychodidae: Phlebotominae) in focus of cutaneous leishmaniasis in the Municipality of Baturité, Ceará, Brasil. Memórias do Instituto Oswaldo Cruz 1991;86(4) 405-410.

[41] Azevedo ACR, Rangel EF, Costa EM, David J, Vasconcelos AW, Lepes VG. Natural infection of *Lutzomyia (Nyssomyia) whitmani* (Antunes & Coutinho, 1939) by *Leishmania* of the braziliensis complex in Baturite, Ceará State, northeast Brazil. Memórias do Instituto Oswaldo Cruz 1990;85: 251.

[42] Queiroz RG, Vasconcelos IA, Vasconcelos AW, Pessoa FA, Souza RN, David JR. Cutaneous leishmaniasis in Ceará State in northeasten Brazil: incrimination of *Lutzomyia whitmani* (Diptera: Psychodidae) as a vector of *Leishmania braziliensis* in Baturité municipality. The American Journal of Tropical Medicine and Hygiene 1994;50 693-698.

[43] Hoch A, Ryan L, Vexenet JA, Rosa AC, Barretto AC. Isolation of *Leishmania braziliensis braziliensis* and other trypanosomatids from Phlebotomines in mucocutaneous

leishmaniases endemic area Bahia, Brazil. Memórias do Instituto Oswaldo Cruz 1986;81(Suppl) BI 44.

[44] Ryan L, Vexenet A, Marsdem PD, Lainson R. The importance of rapid diagnoses of new cases of cutaneous leishmaniasis in pinpointing the sand fly vector. Transactions of the Royal Society of Tropical Medicine and Hygiene 1990;84: 786.

[45] Nunes VLB, Dorval MEC, RC, Oshiro ET, Noguchi Arão LB, Filho GH, Espínola MA, Cristaldo G, Rocha HC, Serafini LN, Santos D. Estudo epidemiológico sobre Leishmaniose Tegumentar (LT) no Município de Corguinho, Mato Grosso do Sul – estudos na população humana. Revista da Sociedade Brasileira de Medicina Tropical1995;28(3) 185-193.

[46] Galati EAB, Nunes VLB, Dorval MEC, Oshiro ET, Cristaldo G, Espínola MA, Rocha HCR, Garcia WB. Estudo dos flebotomíneos (Diptera, Psychodidae), em área de leishmaniose tegumentar, no Estado de Mato Grosso do Sul, Brasil. Revista de Saúde Pública 1996;30 115-128.

[47] Lainson R, Shaw JJ, Ward RD, Ready PD, Naiff RD. Lesmmaniases in Brazil: XIII. Isolation of *Leishmania* from armadillos (*Dasypus novemcinctus*), and observation on the epidemiology of cutaneous leismaniasis in north Pará State. Transactions of the Royal Society of Tropical Medicine and Hygiene 1979;73 239-242.

[48] Ready PD, Lainson R, Shaw JJ, Ward D. The ecology of *Lutzomyia umbratilis* (Ward & Fraiha, 1977) (Diptera: Psychodiade), the major vector to man *Leishmania braziliensis guyanensis* in north-eastern Amazonian Brazil. Bulletin of Entomological Research 1986;76 21-40.

[49] Shaw JJ, Ishikawa EAY, Lainson R, Braga RR, Silveira FT. Cutaneous leishmaniasis of man due to *Leishmania (Viannia) shawi* Lainson, De Souza, Póvoa, Ishikawa & Silveira in Pará State, Brazil. Annales de Parasitologie Humaine et Comparée 1991;66 243-246.

[50] Lainson R, Braga RR, De Souza AA, Pôvoa MM, Ishikawa EA, Silveira FT. *Leishmania (Viannia) shawi* sp. n., a parasite of monkeys, sloths and procyonids in Amazonian Brazil. Annales de Parasitologie Humaine et Comparée 1989;64(3) 200-207.

[51] Mangabeira O. 7a. Contribuição ao estudo dos *Flebotomus* (Diptera: Psychodidae). Descrição dos machos de 24 novas espécies. Memórias do Instituto Oswaldo Cruz 1942;37(2) 111-218.

[52] Sherlock IA, Carneiro M. Algumas fêmeas de *Phlebotomus* do Brasil (Diptera, Psychodidae). Memórias do Instituto Oswaldo Cruz 1962;60(3) 421-435.

[53] Fairchild GB, Theodor O. On *Lutzomyia flaviscutellata* (Mangabeira) and *L. olmeca* (Vargas and Diaz-Najera) (Diptera: Psychodidae). Journal of Medical Entomology 1971;8(2) 153-159.

[54] Floch H, Abonnenc E. Phlébotomes de Guyane Française. V. Institute Pasteur de la Guyane, Publ. No. 61. Cayenne: Institute Pasteur; 1943.

[55] Barreto MP. Sôbre a sinonímia de flebótomos americanos (Diptera, Psychodidae). Primeira nota. Revista Brasileira de Biologia 1946;6: 527-536.

[56] Vargas L, Días-Nájera A. *Phlebotomus farilli* n. sp., *Ph. humboldi* n. sp. y *Ph. olmecus* n. sp. de Mexico (Diptera: Psychodidae). Revista del Instituto de Salubridad y Enfermedades Tropicales1959;19 141-149.

[57] Young DG, Arias JR. A new phlebotomine sand fly in the *Lutzomyia flaviscutellata* complex (Diptera: Psychodidae) from northern Brazil. Journal of Medical Entomology 1982;19(2) 134-138.

[58] Lewis DJ. The *Lutzomyia flaviscutellata* complex (Diptera: Psychodidae). Journal of Medical Entomology 1975;12(3) 363-368.

[59] Galati EAB. Classificação de Phlebotominae. In: Rangel EF, Lainson R (eds.) Flebotomíneos do Brasil. Rio de Janeiro: Editora Fiocruz; 2003. p23-52.

[60] Costa JML, Cunha AK, Gama MEA, Saldanha ACR. Leishmaniose cutânea difusa (LCD) no Brasil: revisão. Anais Brasileiros de Dermatologia 1998;73(6) 565-576.

[61] Lainson R, Shaw JJ. Leishmaniasis in Brazil I. Observations on enzootic rodent leishmaniasis - Incrimination of *Lutzomyia flaviscutellata* (Mangabeira) as the vector in the lower Amazonian Basin. Transactions of the Royal Society of Tropical Medicine and Hygiene 1968;62 385-395.

[62] Shaw JJ, Lainson R. Leishmaniasis in Brazil: II. Observations on enzootic rodent leishmaniasis in the lower Amazon region – the feeding habits of the vector, *Lutzomyia flaviscutellata*, in reference to man, rodents and other animals. Transactions of the Royal Society of Tropical Medicine and Hygiene 1968;62(3) 396-405.

[63] Disney RHL. A trap for phlebotomine sandflies attracted to rats. Bulletin of Entomological Research 1966;56 445-451.

[64] Andrade ARO, Nunes VLB, Galati EAB, Arruda CCP, Santos MFC, Rocca MEG, Aquino RB. Epidemiological study on leishmaniasis in an area of environmental tourism and ecotourism, State of Mato Grosso do Sul, 2006-2007. Revista da Sociedade Brasileira de Medicina Tropical 2009;42(5) 488-493.

[65] Carvalho BM. Aspectos da ecologia de potenciais vetores de leishmanioses (Diptera: Psychodidae: Phlebotominae) na Ilha Grande, Angra dos Reis, Rio de Janeiro. MS dissertation. Instituto Oswaldo Cruz. Rio de Janeiro; 2011.

[66] Vilela ML, Azevedo CG, Carvalho BM, Rangel EF. Phlebotomine fauna (Diptera: Psychodidae) and putative vectors of leishmaniases in impacted area by hydroelectric plant, state of Tocantins, Brazil. PLoS One 2011;6(12) e27721.

[67] Vilela ML, Pita-Pereira D, Azevedo CG, Godoy RE, Britto C, Rangel EF. The phlebotomine fauna (Diptera: Psychodidae) of Guaraí, state of Tocantins, with an emphasis

on the putative vectors of American cutaneous leishmaniasis in rural settlement and periurban areas. Memórias do Instituto Oswaldo Cruz 2013;108(5) 578-585.

[68] Ready PD, Lainson R, Shaw JJ. Leishmaniasis in Brazil. XX: Prevalence of "enzootic rodent leishmaniasis" (*Leishmania mexicana amazonensis*) and apparent absence of pian-bois (*Le. braziliensis guyanensis*), in plantations of introduced tree species and in other non-climax forests in eastern Amazonia. Transactions of the Royal Society of Tropical Medicine and Hygiene 1983;77 775-785.

[69] Lainson R, Shaw JJ, Silveira FT, de Souza AA, Braga RR, Ishikawa EA. The dermal leishmaniases of Brazil, with special reference to the eco-epidemiology of the disease in Amazonia. Memórias do Instituto Oswaldo Cruz 1994;89(3) 435-443.

[70] Shaw JJ, Lainson R. Leishmaniasis in Brazil: VI. Observations on the seasonal variations of *Lutzomyia flaviscutellata* in different types of forest and its relationship to enzootic rodent leishmaniasis (*Leishmania mexicana amazonensis*). Transactions of the Royal Society of Tropical Medicine and Hygiene 1972;66(5) 709-717.

[71] Shaw JJ, Lainson R, Ward RD. Leishmaniasis in Brazil. VII. Further observations on the feeding habitats of *Lutzomyia flaviscutellata* (Mangabeira) with particular reference to its biting habits at different heights. Transactions of the Royal Society of Tropical Medicine and Hygiene 1972;66(5) 718-723.

[72] Feitosa MAC, Castellon EG. Fauna de flebotomíneos (Diptera: Psychodidae) em fragmentos florestais ao redor de conjuntos habitacionais na cidade de Manaus, Amazonas, Brasil. II. Estratificação horizontal. Acta Amazônica 2004;34(1) 121-127.

[73] Lainson R, Shaw JJ, Silveira FT, Fraiha H. Leishmaniasis in Brazil. XIX. Visceral leishmaniasis in the Amazon region, and the presence of *Lutzomyia longipalpis* on the Island of Marajó, Pará State. Transactions of the Royal Society of Tropical Medicine and Hygiene 1983;77(3) 323-330.

[74] Arias JR, Freitas RA. The known geographical distribution of sand flies in the State of Acre, Brasil (Diptera: Psychodidae). Acta Amazonica 1982;12 401-408.

[75] Azevedo ACR, Costa SM, Pinto MCG, Souza JL, Cruz HC, Vidal J, Rangel EF. Studies on the sandfly fauna (Diptera: Psychodidae: Phlebotominae) from transmission areas of American Cutaneous Leishmaniasis in state of Acre, Brazil. Memórias do Instituto Oswaldo Cruz 2008;103(8) 760-767.

[76] Castellón EG, Arias JR, Freitas RA, Naiff RD. Os flebotomíneos da região amazonica, estrada Manaus-Humaitá, Estado do Amazonas, Brasil (Diptera: Psychodidae; Phlebotominae). Acta Amazônica 1994;24(1-2) 91-102.

[77] Castellón EG, Fé NF, Buhrnheim PF, Fé FA. Flebotomíneos (Diptera, Psychodidae) na Amazônia. II. Listagem das espécies coletadas na bacia petrolífera no Rio Urucu, Amazonas, Brasil, utilizando diferentes armadilhas e iscas. Revista Brasileira de Zoologia 2000;17(2) 455-462.

[78] Silva DF, Freitas RA, Franco AMR. Diversidade e abundância de flebotomíneos do gênero *Lutzomyia* (Diptera: Psychodidae) em áreas de mata do nordeste de Manacapuru, AM. Neotropical Entomology 2007;36(1) 138-144.

[79] Alves VR, Freitas RA, Santos FL, Oliveira AFJ, Barrett TV, Shimabukuro PHF. Sand Flies (Diptera, Psychodidae, Phlebotominae) from Central Amazonia and four new records for the Amazonas state, Brazil. Revista Brasileira de Entomologia 2012;56(2) 220-227.

[80] Freitas RA, Naiff RD, Barrett TV. Species diversity and flegellate infections in the sand fly fauna near Porto Grande, state of Amapá, Brazil (Diptera: Psychodidae. Kinetoplastida: Trypanosomatidae). Memórias do Instituto Oswaldo Cruz 2002;97(1) 53-59.

[81] Ryan L. Flebótomos do Estado do Pará, Brasil (Diptera: Psychodidae: Phlebotominae). Tech Doc No. 1, Instituto Evandro Chagas, Belém, Pará, Brazil; 1986.

[82] Gil LHS, Basano AS, Souza AA, Silva MGS, Barata I, Ishikawa EA, Camargo LMA, Shaw JJ. Recent observations on the sand fly (Diptera: Psychodidae) fauna of the state of Rondônia, Western Amazonia, Brazil: the importance of *Psychodopygus davisi* as a vector of zoonotic cutaneous leishmaniasis. Memórias do Instituto Oswaldo Cruz 2003;98(6) 751-755.

[83] Gil LHS, Araújo MS, Villalobos JM, Camargo LMA, Ozaki LS, Fontes CJF, Ribolla PEM, Katsuragawa TH, Cruz RM, Silva AA, Silva LHP. Species structure of sand fly (Diptera: Psychodidae) fauna in the brazilian western Amazon. Memórias do Instituto Oswaldo Cruz 2009;104(7) 955-959.

[84] Castellón EG, Araújo Filho NA, Fé NF, Alves JMC. Flebotomíneos (Diptera: Psychodidae) no Estado de Roraima, Brazil. II. Espécies coletadas na região Norte. Acta Amazônica 1991;21 45-50.

[85] Castellón EG, Araújo Filho NA, Fé NF, Alves JMC. Flebotomíneos (Diptera: Psychodidae) no Estado de Roraima. III. Listagem das espécies no Estado. Acta Amazônica 1991;21 51-54.

[86] Vilela ML, Azevedo ACR, Costa SM, Costa WA, Motta-Silva D, Grajauskas AM, Carvalho BM, Brahim LRN, Kozlowsky D, Rangel EF. Sand fly survey in the influence area of Peixe Angical hydroeletric plant, state of Tocantins, Brazil. In: 6th International Symposium on Phlebotomine Sandflies, 27-31 Oct 2008, Lima, Peru; 2008.

[87] Dorval MEC, Cristaldo G, Rocha HC, Alves TP, Alves MA, Oshiro ET, Oliveira AG, Brazil RP, Galati EAB, Cunha RV. Phlebotomine fauna (Diptera: Psychodidae) of an American cutaneous leishmaniasis endemic area in the state of Mato Grosso do Sul, Brazil. Memórias do Instituto Oswaldo Cruz 2009;104 695-702.

[88] Dorval MEC, Alves TP, Cristaldo G, Rocha HC, Alves MA, Oshiro ET, Oliveira AG, Brazil RP, Galati EAB, Cunha RV. Sand Fly Captures with Disney traps in area of occurrence of *Leishmania (Leishmania) amazonensis* in the State of Mato Grosso do Sul,

mid-western Brazil. Revista da Sociedade Brasileira de Medicina Tropical 2010;43(5) 491-495.

[89] Galati EAB, Nunes VLB, Dorval MEC, Cristaldo G, Rocha HC, Gonçalves-Andrade RM, Naufel G. Attraction of black Shannon trap for phlebotomines. Memórias do Instituto Oswaldo Cruz 2001;96 641-647.

[90] Araújo Filho NA, Sherlock IA, Coura JR: Leishmaniose Tegumentar Americana na Ilha Grande, Rio de Janeiro. V. Observações sobre a biologia dos transmissores em condições naturais. Revista da Sociedade Brasileira de Medicina Tropical 1981;14(4-6) 171-183.

[91] Azeredo-Coutinho RB, Conceição-Silva F, Schubach A, Cupolillo E, Quintela LP, Madeira MF, Pacheco RS, Valete-Rosalino CM, Mendonça SC. First report of diffuse cutaneous leishmaniasis and *Leishmania amazonensis* infection in Rio de Janeiro State, Brazil. Transactions of the Royal Society Tropical Medicine and Hygiene 2007;101 735-737.

[92] Campbell-Lendrum D, Dujardin JP, Martinez E, Feliciangeli MD, Perez JE, Silans LNMP, Desjeux P. Domestic and peridomestic transmission of American cutaneous leishmaniasis: Changing epidemiological patterns present new control opportunities. Memórias do Instituto Oswaldo Cruz 2001;96(2) 159-162.

Chapter 2

Transmission to Humans

Miroslava Avila-García, Javier Mancilla,
Enrique Segura-Cervantes and
Norma Galindo-Sevilla

Additional information is available at the end of the chapter

http://dx.doi.org/10.5772/57271

1. Introduction

Tissue parasites such as *Leishmania* are transmitted from host to host through a vector species, and transmission can be from human to vector to animal or vice versa (zoonotic transmission), which occurs in rural and periurban environments or from human to vector to human (anthroponotic transmission), which occurs in urban environments. *Lutzomyia* and *Phlebotomus* species have long been known as the primary transmitters of leishmaniasis. However, in recent decades, evidence has been building for the existence of alternative transmission pathways. These pathways involve direct contact with infected tissues, such as may be encountered during surgical/therapeutic procedures, biological/reproductive activities, certain work-related practices and by unsafe drug use, all of which are reviewed below.

2. Transmission forms

2.1. The life cycle of *Leishmania* spp.: the vector transmission

Leishmania spp. is a parasite with a dimorphic life cycle that is controlled by the passage from vector to host [1]. As such, the parasite has developed novel adaptations to survive within the vector [2]. The vector phase of the life cycle begins when the vector ingests blood containing the parasites. Following ingestion, the parasites eventually reach the midgut, where they are held for approximately 4 hours in the peritrophic matrix. There, the amastigote cells differentiate into small, motile cells with short flagella, a form known as the procyclic promastigote. Next, *Leishmania* initiates the first stage of the vector life cycle, which occurs over the following 24-48 hours. The body of the parasite elongates in the next 72 hours to form the nectomonad promastigote, and the microorganism then breaks down the peritrophic matrix to reach the midgut lumen and migrate into the thoracic region of the vector. Once there, the promastigotes differentiate into leptomonad promastigotes by decreasing in size and changing the location of their flagella, which is followed by a second replication cycle during days 5-7. This process produces a massive infection in the anterior portion of the midgut, where the parasites differentiate into metacyclic promastigotes within the stomodeal valve, ensuring a large number of parasites for the purpose of infection. To protect the metacyclic promastigotes, the leptomonads also differentiate into gel-producing promastigotes, which surround the leptomonad and metacyclic promastigotes. The latter cell type is considered to be the infective form of the parasite because it possesses an elongated flagellum, which allows for motility and resistance to complement-mediated lysis. When metacyclic promastigotes differentiate into haptomonad promastigotes, they form parasitic rings that plug the stomodeal valve, eventually leading to its degeneration. Finally, this process allows the parasites to pass into the proboscis [2], where they can inoculate the host during feeding of the vector.

Upon entering the host, the parasite first encounters a host immune reaction following activation of the complement system. With respect to this process, four distinct activation pathways have been identified: the classical pathway, the alternative pathway, the lectin pathway and the extrinsic pathway [3]. In humans, the parasite can evade the immune response by inhibiting complement-mediated lysis, which occurs within the phagolysosomes of macrophages. This protective effect is conferred by the membrane protease gp63, or leishmanolysin, which inhibits attacks against the parasite cell membrane by adhering to complement components [4]. Promastigote-stage parasites differentiate into small, round cells 3-5 μm in size that lack flagella, known as amastigotes. This form can be readily observed within host cells by microscopy, where they are referred to as Leishman-Donovan [5] bodies. Finally, when multiplication of the parasites exceeds the holding capacity of the phagocytic cell, cell lysis occurs, releasing the parasites to infect new cells.

By some conservative estimates, a vector might release between 1-1000 metacyclic promastigotes into the host during feeding [6-7]. However, other estimates based on molecular biology techniques indicate that a vector might release as many as 600 to 100,000 metacyclic promastigotes during a feeding period and that this number varies as function of feeding time. In addition, it is known that large numbers of parasites actually increase vector feeding time, as the parasites physically obstruct proper functioning of the proboscis [8]. Therefore, based on these findings, between 100 and 100,000 metacyclic parasites are commonly used to inoculate the footpads or pinnae of animals in *in vivo* models of infection [8-10].

2.2. Organ transplants, blood transfusions and hemodialysis

Therapeutic advances in a wide variety of medical fields have dramatically improved overall quality of life and life expectancy in modern societies. This has partly been achieved through the development of techniques such as organ transplantation, hemodialysis, and blood transfusion, which are particularly useful for the treatment of chronic disease. However, the transmission of infectious diseases during such procedures must account for and avoided. Furthermore, human migration can easily transport diseases transmitted by vectors from endemic locations to non-endemic locations, as often happens with protozoan parasites of the blood, such as *Leishmania* [11-12], *Trypanosoma* and *Plasmodium* [3].

During organ transplantations, there are several possible ways in which microorganisms such as *Leishmania* can be transmitted, including reactivation of dormant parasites in the recipient following treatment with immunosuppressants, infection by parasites derived from the donor, transmission of parasites through blood transfusions during the surgical procedure and *de novo* transmission [11-12]. *Leishmania* infections have been observed in individuals who have undergone kidney [13-16] and liver [17-18] transplants, as well as in patients that have undergone heart [17, 19-23], lung [24], pancreas [25], stem cell [26-27] and bone-marrow transplants, although these are less common. Overall, the number of leishmaniasis cases resulting from organ transplants is estimated to be fewer than 100 in total [11, 13-16], which were mainly associated with kidney transplants. A primary risk factor for transmission is whether the donor had lived in an area where leishmaniasis was endemic. However, this subject is not commonly addressed during screening processes, and relevant laboratory tests are not usually carried out on organ donors [28]. Therefore, it is important to generate and review epidemiological data concerning leishmaniasis, as the number of infected individuals who are asymptomatic could be even greater than the number of those showing clinical symptoms [17]. There have also been reports of organ donors who were asymptomatic before surgery but who died of leishmaniasis several months after the transplantation procedure. Furthermore, there has been at least one case in which an organ recipient developed leishmaniasis symptoms two years after the transplantation procedure [29]. In cases where individuals show symptoms approximately one month after transplantation, transmission is generally considered to be due to the reactivation of dormant parasites within the recipient [30]. On the other hand, in cases where leishmaniasis symptoms are observed approximately 18 months after receiving a new organ, transmission is generally considered to be due to the *de novo* acquisition of parasites [11-12, 16]. In either case, the suggested course of treatments to favour transplant survival includes corticosteroids [24], immunosuppressants [13-14], or monoclonal antibodies [11], which favor the development of leishmaniasis.

Infrequent or atypical symptoms can cause delayed diagnosis of leishmaniasis. The primary clinical signs and symptoms related to *Leishmania* infections due to organ transplantation are fever, splenomegaly, hepatomegaly, leukopenia and hypoalbuminemia [14, 31-32]. Unfortunately, the therapeutic responses to such cases are often insufficient to save the patient's life, which can be ascribed to late diagnoses, particularly severe infections and other health complications [13] due to prolonged immunosuppressive regimens [16, 24].

Blood volume loss or deficiencies in specific blood components are indicators that a transfusion of blood or blood-derivatives from a donor to a recipient may be necessary. Blood transfusions are frequently performed during or after surgical interventions, and in the case of leishmaniasis patients with a history of organ transplantation and blood transfusion, the disease is generally considered to be a complication of the transplantation process [15, 32-33]. In patients without such a background, infections are generally considered to have occurred through the transfusion of blood or blood-derived products. The first case of *Leishmania* transmission via a blood transfer was documented in China in 1948, when two girls were given 20 mL of blood intramuscularly to stimulate passive immunity against measles and rubella. The blood came from their mother, who was hospitalized days later with symptoms suggestive of visceral leishmaniasis; this diagnosis was made one month after her being hospitalized. Therefore, due to the medical history of the mother, the girls were monitored over the subsequent months. Both girls developed leishmaniasis 9-10 months after the blood transfer [34]. Although this case was not due to blood transfusion *per se*, it is the first documented case in which the use of blood components for therapeutic purposes resulted in the contraction of leishmaniasis.

In general, the causative agents of visceral leishmaniasis belong to the *donovani* complex of species, although there have also been reports of visceralization in species more typically related to the mucocutaneous and cutaneous clinical presentations of the disease. These types of clinical presentations have primarily been observed in individuals with compromised immune systems, such as HIV-positive patients. However, there has been a single reported case of a patient with these characteristics who also had a history of kidney transplantation and blood transfusions. Furthermore, there was no history of vector exposure as the patient was not living in an endemic region. The infection hypothesis was ruled out by searching for signs of *Leishmania* in the blood by PCR and by searching for *Leishmania*-specific antibodies in the donor and in the recipient of the second kidney. The patient's death was caused by complications due to the presence of *T. cruzi*, *S. aureus* and *L. mexicana*. Although the patient's transfusion donors could not be evaluated, based on analysis of other possible transmission pathways, it was concluded that the most likely pathway of infection was through blood transfusion [35].

Among other notable cases of secondary leishmaniasis due to blood products and transfusions, there was the case of a patient with an autoimmune disease, idiopathic thrombocytopenic purpura. The patient was transfused with concentrated platelets on multiple occasions over the 2-3 year period prior to the development of leishmaniasis, a diagnosis that was confirmed by bone marrow aspiration [36].

Another case involved an infant who received a blood transfusion within 7 days of birth due to integument pallor with a subsequent diagnosis of myelofibrosis. The blood donor was a relative who died three months after the donation, after developing hepatosplenomegaly, pyrexia and a fever of unknown origin; the diagnosis was made *postmortem* after the detection of Leishman-Donovan bodies. The infant began to show abdominal distension, fever and integument pallor one month after the transfusion. At 5 months of age, visceral leishmaniasis was diagnosed from a spleen aspirate that scored positive for Leishman-Donovan bodies. Leishmaniasis treatment was initiated without improvement, and two months later, the infant was rehospitalized with anemia, respiratory distress, hepatomegaly and splenomegaly. A liver biopsy revealed changes consistent with steatohepatitis with necrotic foci and lipid granulomas. Furthermore, the biopsy was positive for anti-*Leishmania* antibodies (rK-39), whereas the infant's family members were negative for these antibodies. Due to a severe anemic syndrome, the infant was given a blood transfusion. Despite treatment with antimonials, the infant showed no improvement and indeed worsened with the development of septicemia caused by *Staphylococcus*, *Klebsiella* and *Pseudomonas*. A change of drugs to Amphotericin B only deteriorated the infant's health further, and it died one month after admission [37].

http://dx.doi.org/10.5772/57271

In a case involving an elderly patient, a 77-year-old woman with a history of chronic atrial fibrillation, hypertension and chronic kidney disease with hemodialysis treatment underwent surgery due to cholecystitis, during which time she received two units of blood. A month and a half later, she presented with fever, diaphoresis and chills during a hemodialysis session and over the next 24 hours; she also showed occasional diarrhea and weight loss. These symptoms did not improve despite treatment with antibiotics. In the intensive care unit following hemodialysis, the patient showed thrombocytopenia and hypotension with good ventricular systolic function, requiring volume recovery and vasopressor therapy; hydrocortisone was also included in the treatment. A bone marrow aspirate confirmed the presence of intracellular amastigotes and numerous extracellular promastigotes, although these were not observed in the peripheral blood. Treatment with Amphotericin B increased her platelet numbers, although hemodynamic deterioration continued until the patient's death. Cultures begun previous to death showed the presence of *Acinetobacter baumannii*, a bacterium that is resistant to multiple types of antibiotics. During a *postmortem* examination, the presence of *Leishmania* parasites in the bile was tested for due to prior gastrointestinal symptoms. The transmission of *Leishmania* through the blood was confirmed when one of her donors (to the source of the units transfused during the cholecystectomy) tested positive for *Leishmania*-specific antibodies [38].

Seven U.S. military groups assigned to Operation Desert Storm in the 1990s developed atypical clinical presentations of *L. donovani* infection that were suggestive of Kala-azar. The symptoms included stiffness, nonproductive cough, diffuse abdominal tenderness, diarrhea, nausea, headache, myalgia, and arthralgia without organomegaly. One of the patients was asymptomatic, whereas two had diseases that compromised their immune systems: renal carcinoma and HIV. The diagnoses were performed using an immunofluorescent antibody test (IFAT). In all cases, the onset of symptoms occurred 1-14 months after their time in Saudi Arabia, and none showed lesions that may have aided in the diagnosis of leishmaniasis [39]. These clinical cases led U.S. authorities to recommend that all candidates who had visited the Persian Gulf be rejected as blood donors. This situation was further complicated by the fact that the conditions under which the *Leishmania* parasite might survive in blood products in bank bloods were unknown. As a result, *in vitro* assays were performed on parasites isolated from the soldiers. The *Leishmania* parasites that were isolated from the individuals participating in Operation Desert Storm included *L. tropica*, *L. major* and *L. donovani*. These parasites were maintained in log-phase culture and used to inoculate donated blood samples, which were then stored at 4ºC for 35 days or at 24ºC for 5 days. It was observed that in whole-blood units stored under these common blood-bank conditions, *L. tropica* intracellular parasites within monocytes could survive up to 30 days at 4ºC and up to 5 days at 24ºC, in contrast to promastigotes in stationary phase or free amastigotes that does not. With respect to fresh frozen plasma, it was observed that intracellular parasites could survive inside monocytes for 25 days at 4ºC and for at least 5 days in the platelet fraction at 24ºC. For erythrocyte fractions frozen with glycerol, survival time of the parasite was 35 days at 4ºC [40]. It is clear that *Leishmania* shows low-temperature resistance, highlighting the very real possibility of parasite transmission from infected individuals, either in the preclinical or asymptomatic phase, to immunocompromised individuals via blood products.

Transmission of *Leishmania* via blood transfusions has been demonstrated in domestic animals [41] and model organisms, and these typically present symptoms following treatment with either infected human blood or blood from experimentally infected animals [40, 42-43]. For example, blood transfusions can be carried out in rodents by transferring 0.1-1.0 mL blood via tail-vein [40] or intracardiac injection [43]. In a study involving hamsters, all groups that received infected blood showed symptoms between 90-120 days following transfusion [43]. It was found that 22.1% of the transfused hamsters scored positive for *Leishmania* by PCR analysis, and 14.75% remained positive when the test was performed again after 12 months. All of the monocyte cultures were negative. Furthermore, it was demonstrated that 29.5% of the transfused hamsters tested positive by at least one of the techniques, with PCR being the most sensitive assay [44].

There have also been various clinical studies carried out on individuals attending blood banks in which the presence of the parasite was assessed for using techniques such as ELISA (enzyme-linked immunosorbent assay) [45], IFAT [46], Western blotting, culturing and PCR [44-45]. ELISA experiments showed that 2.4% of the individuals had *Leishmania*-specific antibodies, whereas 3.5% scored positive by Western blotting analysis; both tests showed a seroprevalence of 7.6%.

Furthermore, questioning may be insufficient to exclude donors that have visited endemic areas within the last 12 months or that have had clinical diagnoses of leishmaniasis, as recommended by the WHO publication *Blood donor selection: guidelines on assessing donor suitability for blood donation*. Therefore, there is a clear need to develop laboratory techniques to identify this microorganism in blood or derivatives, and indeed, several studies have been carried out to detect the presence of *Leishmania*-specific antibodies in healthy individuals who have donated blood.

In cutaneous species, such as those belonging to the *L. mexicana* complex, it is unknown whether the parasite can be transmitted through blood in humans under the same conditions as the visceral species. However, as was previously mentioned, it should be noted that there are cases of HIV patients that have developed visceral leishmaniasis when infected with cutaneous species [35].

In individuals with chronic kidney disease, hemodialysis is a therapy that can greatly improve patient prognosis and prolong and improve their quality of life. However, like many other therapeutic procedures, hemodialysis can have adverse effects, including bacteremia and sepsis due to poor aseptic techniques during treatment [47]. Indeed, it has been documented that if proper care is not taken to sterilize hemodialysis equipment, including the cleaning and replacement of disposable parts, there is high risk of acquiring infectious/contagious diseases [47], including parasitic infections. Unlike with the situation with *Toxoplasma,* [48] *Leishmania* has not been directly linked to hemodialysis patients, although large assays for *Leishmania*-specific antibodies have been performed [49-50] that found the parasite in 9-25% of patients in endemic areas [50]. Despite the fact that no studies directly link *Leishmania* infection to hemodialysis treatment, perhaps because most patients with kidney disease who are treated with hemodialysis also have a clinical history of immunosuppressive blood treatment, organ transplantation and multiple blood transfusions [38, 50-51]. All of these conditions increase

http://dx.doi.org/10.5772/57271

the possibility of acquiring leishmaniasis and negatively affect patient health, making the analysis of causal factors difficult.

2.3. Sexual transmission

2.3.1. *Leishmaniasis in sexual organs in humans*

Cases of leishmaniasis of the sexual organs have been reported, manifesting as lesions on the genitals, and such cases have been reported in both humans [52-56] and in animals [57-58]. Three possible mechanisms for the development of leishmaniasis of the sexual organs and genitals have been suggested: (1) local infection derived from a wider systemic infection; (2) infection due to exposure of the genitals to a vector in an endemic area; and (3) infection due to direct contact of the genitals with an ulcerated lesion during intercourse [59].

By questioning patients, such cases of genital leishmaniasis in humans could not always be directly linked to either intercourse [52-53] or to sleeping naked in endemic areas [55]. However, in cases where the lesions were observed on the vulvar regions [53], direct vector-mediated infection can be ruled out, leaving open the possibility for localized infection of systemic origin or from intercourse with a previously infected individual.

It should be noted that genital ulcers can have numerous causes, and thorough diagnoses should be conducted in all cases to avoid confusion with other diseases, such as squamous cell carcinoma or primary syphilis [55]. Likewise, the presence of other types of infectious microorganisms should also be ruled out [59].

2.3.2. *Leishmaniasis in sexual organs in animals*

Among animals, domestic dogs are considered to be the main reservoir of *Leishmania*, and this parasite has been detected in canine sexual organs as well [57-58]. In females, the absence of exposed genitals and internal sex organs suggests that infections are either systemic in origin or sexually transmitted, which is especially true in non-endemic areas [60-61].

It has been observed that when *L. chagasi* infects sexual organs (e.g., the testis, epididymis and prostate) and genitals (e.g., the glans and foreskin), it can induce an inflammatory response. In addition, macrophages infested with parasites accompanied by neutrophils in the foreskin have also been observed in dogs. In one study involving dog semen, the presence of the parasite was detected by PCR in 8 out of 22 samples analyzed [57], a finding which suggests the possibility of sexual infection between animals. Indeed, when 12 serologically negative females were mated to males that tested serologically positive for *L. chagasi*, 165 days after mating, 3 out of the 12 females were serologically positive and 6 out of the 12 females scored positive by PCR [62]. Although the external genitals and the vulva are the most commonly affected areas in symptomatic and asymptomatic females, females that scored positive for *Leishmania* by PCR also showed effects in at least one other region of the reproductive system. Histological changes included perifollicular lymphocytic infiltration with intracellular parasites as well as inflammatory infiltration in the vulvar dermis [58]. Other trials have been carried out in which male and female dogs infected with *Leishmania* were mated to observe vertical transmission.

However, it remains unclear whether sexual transmission plays an important role in vertical transmission [63].

2.4. Congenital transmission

2.4.1. Congenital leishmaniasis in humans

Vertical transmission is defined as the congenital transmission of a pathogenic microorganism, condition, or characteristic from one generation to the next via the placenta, hematogenous, the birth canal, or nursing at the maternal breast [64]. Vertical transmission has been demonstrated for visceral leishmaniasis caused by *L. donovani* and *L. infantum*. The first case of vertical transmission in leishmaniasis was reported in 1926 in a pregnant woman who began to show symptoms suggestive of leishmaniasis during her first trimester. The treatment for visceral leishmaniasis was administered upon the exclusion of malaria and typhoid fever as differential diagnoses by laboratory results. Upon treatment, the symptoms disappeared, and the pregnancy continued to term. The birth took place without complications via the vaginal canal, and the neonate was of normal weight. However, both mother and neonate exhibited a general state of deterioration immediately postpartum. Visceral leishmaniasis was not suspected, and the symptoms were fever, diarrhea, and abdominal pain. Due to the state of the mother, nursing did not occur. The child was tracked during its first year and presented with anemia and splenomegaly. A biopsy of the spleen revealed the presence of Leishman-Donovan bodies [65], indicating that vertical transmission of leishmaniasis had occurred.

The epidemiological antecedents of leishmaniasis are crucial when pediatric patients or those of childbearing age develop symptoms suggestive of leishmaniasis. A mother who was diagnosed with *L. infantum* by ELISA had been on a farm when she was between 28 and 30 weeks pregnant. The child was born by elective caesarean at 38 weeks in a non-endemic zone in the Ukraine. At the age of eight months, the nursing child suddenly exhibited a fever, decreased appetite, weakness, pallor of the integuments, bruising, hepatosplenomegaly, tachypnea, and lymphadenopathy. An aspirate of the bone marrow revealed ovoid cells of 3-5 μm that were identified as Leishman-Donovan bodies [66].

In Germany, there have been two reported cases of leishmaniasis involving mothers who visited endemic zones prior to their pregnancies. The first case involved a 16-month-old pediatric patient with visceral leishmaniasis whose mother had traveled to endemic zones two years earlier [67]. The second case was a 15-month-old child with visceral leishmaniasis whose mother was on a farm in an endemic zone between 20 and 22 weeks of pregnancy [68].

Chronic visceral leishmaniasis has been linked to premature birth and materno-fetal deaths. [69] A histological analysis of the placenta and an aspirate of the lymphatic ganglion revealed the presence of thrombotic, vascular changes in the placenta of a fetus at five months of gestation in a mother that had been infected with leishmaniasis for two months [70]. Neonates carried to term from infected mothers have remained asymptomatic during the first weeks or months of life. However, Leishman bodies have ultimately been detected in the bone marrow, and anti-*Leishmania* antibodies have also been detected, corroborating the diagnosis of leishmaniasis [65, 69, 71].

Leishmaniasis can be accompanied by concomitant infections by organisms from similar genera. During the second trimester, a pregnant patient was initially treated for leishmaniasis and showed improvement at 30 days. The baby was born vaginally at 36 weeks without complications and weighed 1,700 grams. He was readmitted three days later for deterioration due to probable malaria and tuberculosis, but he did not show improvement following treatment. Amastigotes were detected in an aspirate of the lymphatic ganglion of the mother. In addition, IgG antibodies were detected in the baby; these antibodies were attributed to passive transplacental transfer of parasite-specific antibodies from the mother to the fetus, negating the need for treatment. He was admitted once more at seven months old for symptoms suggestive of *Plasmodium falciparum*, and he did not show improvement upon treatment. A bone marrow aspirate revealed *Leishmania*. However, despite treatment, the infant died. An autopsy revealed that the presence of abundant *Leishmania* parasites in the kidneys, spleen, thymus, bone marrow, liver, and lungs and *Candida* spp. in the respiratory tract [70].

Individuals, whether mother or offspring, in endemic zones can be infected for months or years prior to the onset of symptoms. For example, a woman visited an endemic zone and became pregnant two years later. She did not experience any symptoms during her pregnancy or postpartum while in the non-endemic zone nor was there evidence of the existence of the vector in the geographic area. While the mother remained asymptomatic, the infant exhibited symptoms of possible visceral leishmaniasis, which was confirmed by various laboratory tests [67].

There is evidence that cutaneous leishmaniasis is associated with perinatal health problems, as has been observed in Brazil, where women with *L. braziliensis*-mediated cutaneous leishmaniasis developed vegetative or atypical lesions at the 18th week of pregnancy. Of these patients, 10% delivered prematurely and the fetus died in another 10% of the cases. A biopsy of one of the fetuses revealed intense inflammatory exudates predominated by neutrophils, and parasites were detected by electrophoresis [72].

2.4.2. Congenital leishmaniasis in animals

In Brazil, a trial was performed with asymptomatic and symptomatic mixed-breed dogs that were infected with *L. donovani* and *L. infantum*. There were four dogs in each group, and the livers, spleens, lymph nodes, bone marrow, kidneys, and hearts of their offspring were analyzed by PCR for infection. The numbers of offspring obtained from symptomatic or asymptomatic mothers (26 vs. 27) were nearly identical. The placentas and the offspring were analyzed by PCR, and 13 of the 26 placentas and 9 of the 26 offspring of the symptomatic mothers were positive for the parasite, while 13 of the 27 placentas and 8 of the 27 offspring from the asymptomatic mothers were positive. Furthermore, it was noted that PCR was more sensitive for parasite detection in comparison to immunohistochemistry and hematoxylin and eosin staining [73]. Another study in Italy involved seven female dogs that had been diagnosed with leishmaniasis by serology, microscopy, and PCR. Two of the seven were treated with N-methylglucamine prior to pregnancy, and one of the seven was treated during pregnancy. The pups were examined between 3 and 30 days of age. The parasite was detected in 8 of the 31 pups in both groups, and only 2 of the 8 pups developed symptoms [74].

2.4.3. Experimental models of congenital transmission

In a murine model of visceral leishmaniasis, twenty 12-week -old female BALB/c mice were infected with *L. infantum*. They were mated 8 weeks later with healthy males, and the females were sacrificed at days 13 and 18 of gestation. The offspring were sectioned in half for PCR analysis. In 15 of the 20 pregnant mice, the parasite was detected by PCR in the spleen. In the offspring, 3 of the 88 placentas and 4 of the 88 pups tested positive for *Leishmania* by PCR [75]. In studies to determine vertical transmission of *Leishmania* in beagles, parasitemia was detected in the liver, spleen, and bone marrow of the offspring [63].

In experimental model in which hamsters were infected with 10^6 parasites/mL of *L. panamensis* during the first week of pregnancy, 24 of 93 (25.8%) of the offspring from infected mothers were PCR positive to *Leishmania*, 2 months after the birth [76]. Furthermore, mice infected with high inoculums of *L. mexicana* strain, known as cause of cutaneous leishmaniasis, showed that all female and their placentas were positive to PCR analysis, and revealed that the infection was present in 39 of 110 offspring of infected mothers, also fetal deaths and resorptions were observed [77]. Then is important to be aware to the fact that leishmaniasis could be transmitted transplacentally and causes fetal resorption, death, and reduction in offspring body weight.

2.5. Other factors related to substance abuse and work environment

2.5.1. Drug use

In cases of leishmaniasis infection due to fomites, such as sharp, contaminated objects, the most vulnerable population are illicit drug users. In a Spanish study of syringes used for recreational drug use, it was reported that 32-52% of the syringes were contaminated by *Leishmania*, as determined by PCR. Moreover, 3 different genotypes were identified in multiple samples, confirming that the individuals had shared syringes. Therefore, programs that limit the sharing of needles should decrease the infection rate among vulnerable individuals [78-79].

2.5.2. Work environment transmission

As described above, *Leishmania* spp. can be transmitted through fluids such as blood and by contact with animals or even contaminated objects. In all cases, there must be an entry route, which is usually a wound. In staffs dedicated to clinical, diagnostic or medical research, it is not uncommon to find reported cases of *Leishmania* infection, although many such likely go unrecognized [80]. Infections due to accidental exposure can be affected by a variety of factors, including kinematics (e.g., the path and characteristics of exposure and the amount of inoculum), parasite characteristics (e.g., pathogenicity, virulence, viability and infective dose) and host characteristics (e.g., immune status, barrier status and actions following the accident) [80]. However, the possibility of infection due to vector exposure in an endemic region should not be ruled out when performing questioning [81]. The first case of work-related leishmaniasis was reported in 1930, and to date, there have been 12 reported cases of *Leishmania* infection due to accidents at work; these have included 6 different *Leishmania* species, with *L. donovani* being implicated in half of the affected individuals. In these cases, the incubation period ranged

http://dx.doi.org/10.5772/57271

from 3 weeks to 8 months after the accident. Although the United States is not considered to be an endemic region, it has had more than half of reported leishmaniasis cases of laboratory transmission, with the parenteral route being the most frequent means of exposure, followed by animal bites, primarily from experimental animals. In one affected population, the average age of leishmaniasis cases due to work-related accidents was 30, and four of the affected individuals were students [80].

According to the CDC, the *Leishmania* parasite is considered to be a Biosafety Level 2 (BSL-2) organism, which implies that the individual transmission rate is moderate, and low in the case of a community. Therefore, *Leishmania* can cause disease in humans or animals without being considered a serious risk for laboratory staff. Although exposure can lead to serious infection, effective treatments are available and the risk is limited [82]. Potentially infectious parasites can be found in blood, tissues, exudates and infected arthropods, and they can be transmitted through wounds, micro-abrasions, accidental parenteral inoculation or transmission by arthropods [80]. Therefore, it is recommended that all staff having contact with potentially infectious material use protective equipment and that the handling of potentially infectious waste be carried out in accordance with appropriate regulations and good clinical/laboratory practices [80, 82]. In the case of staff with compromised immune systems, it is recommended that they avoid work with live organisms [82].

3. Conclusions

The *Leishmania* parasite can survive in a wide range of temperatures and pH conditions, which has allowed it to adapt to the diverse conditions encountered within different vector and host species. In recent years, transmission pathways other than those based on vector species have been described, including invasive procedures for therapeutic purposes, sexual practices, pregnancy, drug practices and work-related accidents among health/research staff members, all of which have led to an increase in the number of reported leishmaniasis cases. However, considering that the latency period of the parasite within the host can last up to one year, there are likely more infected individuals than those that have been reported. Because leishmaniasis is not considered to be a disease that can be transmitted between individuals without the intervention of a vector species, laboratory tests for the presence of these parasites to rule out prospective donors are not carried out prior to in most invasive therapeutic procedures. However, in the case of patients with immunodeficiency, the possibility of contracting the disease is significantly increased. Furthermore, during pregnancy, changes to the immune system can allow for the transmission of the parasite from the mother to the fetus. It should also be noted that maternal-fetal infection can also be of sexual origin. Among drug addicts, it was demonstrated that syringe sharing is a significant source of infection. Finally, in addition to populations exposed in endemic areas, staff working in the health or research sectors should also be considered as populations at risk of acquiring this disease.

Taken together, there is a clear need for the health system to reevaluate the global situation concerning leishmaniasis transmission and to implement strategies to reduce the exposure of individuals to *Leishmania* infections.

Acknowledgements

Financial support: The chapter was sponsored by Instituto Nacional de Perinatologia (212250-22701). Primary investigator: Dr. Norma Galindo-Sevilla.

Author details

Miroslava Avila-García, Javier Mancilla, Enrique Segura-Cervantes and Norma Galindo-Sevilla*

National Institute for Perinatology, Department of Infectious Diseases and Perinatal Immunology, Mexico City, Mexico

References

[1] Rosal Rabes Td, Baquero-Artigao F, García Miguel MJ. Leishmaniasis cutánea. Pediatría Atención Primaria. 2010;12:263-71.

[2] Kamhawi S. Phlebotomine sand flies and Leishmania parasites: friends or foes? Trends Parasitol. 2006;22:439-45.

[3] Huber-Lang M, Sarma JV, Zetoune FS, Rittirsch D, Neff TA, McGuire SR, et al. Generation of C5a in the absence of C3: a new complement activation pathway. Nat Med. 2006;12:682-7.

[4] Handman E. Cell biology of Leishmania. Adv Parasitol. 1999;44:1-39.

[5] Wheeler RJ, Gluenz E, Gull K. The cell cycle of Leishmania: morphogenetic events and their implications for parasite biology. Mol Microbiol. 2011;79:647-62.

[6] Warburg A, Schlein Y. The effect of post-bloodmeal nutrition of Phlebotomus papatasi on the transmission of Leishmania major. Am J Trop Med Hyg. 1986;35:926-30.

[7] Rogers ME, Ilg T, Nikolaev AV, Ferguson MA, Bates PA. Transmission of cutaneous leishmaniasis by sand flies is enhanced by regurgitation of fPPG. Nature. 2004;430:463-7.

[8] Kimblin N, Peters N, Debrabant A, Secundino N, Egen J, Lawyer P, et al. Quantification of the infectious dose of Leishmania major transmitted to the skin by single sand flies. Proc Natl Acad Sci U S A. 2008;105:10125-30.

[9] Lira R, Doherty M, Modi G, Sacks D. Evolution of lesion formation, parasitic load, immune response, and reservoir potential in C57BL/6 mice following high- and low-dose challenge with Leishmania major. Infect Immun. 2000;68:5176-82.

[10] Quiñones-Diaz L M-RJ, Avila-García M, Ortiz-Avalos J, Berrón A, Gonzalez S, Paredes Y, Galindo-Sevilla N. Effect of Ambient Temperature on the Clinical Manifestations of Experimental Diffuse Cutaneous Leishmaniasis in a Rodent Model. VECTOR-BORNE AND ZOONOTIC DISEASES. [Original Research Manuscript]. 2012;12.

[11] Coster LO. Parasitic infections in solid organ transplant recipients. Infect Dis Clin North Am. 2013;27:395-427.

[12] Miro JM, Blanes M, Norman F, Martin-Davila P. Infections in solid organ transplantation in special situations: HIV-infection and immigration. Enferm Infecc Microbiol Clin. 2012;30 Suppl 2:76-85.

[13] Basset D, Faraut F, Marty P, Dereure J, Rosenthal E, Mary C, et al. Visceral leishmaniasis in organ transplant recipients: 11 new cases and a review of the literature. Microbes Infect. 2005;7:1370-5.

[14] Oliveira CM, Oliveira ML, Andrade SC, Girao ES, Ponte CN, Mota MU, et al. Visceral leishmaniasis in renal transplant recipients: clinical aspects, diagnostic problems, and response to treatment. Transplant Proc. 2008;40:755-60.

[15] Oliveira RA, Silva LS, Carvalho VP, Coutinho AF, Pinheiro FG, Lima CG, et al. Visceral leishmaniasis after renal transplantation: report of 4 cases in northeastern Brazil. Transpl Infect Dis. 2008;10:364-8.

[16] Gontijo CM, Pacheco RS, Orefice F, Lasmar E, Silva ES, Melo MN. Concurrent cutaneous, visceral and ocular leishmaniasis caused by Leishmania (Viannia) braziliensis in a kidney transplant patient. Mem Inst Oswaldo Cruz. 2002;97:751-3.

[17] Antinori S, Cascio A, Parravicini C, Bianchi R, Corbellino M. Leishmaniasis among organ transplant recipients. Lancet Infect Dis. 2008;8:191-9.

[18] Barsoum RS. Parasitic infections in organ transplantation. Exp Clin Transplant. 2004;2:258-67.

[19] Frapier JM, Abraham B, Dereure J, Albat B. Fatal visceral leishmaniasis in a heart transplant recipient. J Heart Lung Transplant. 2001;20:912-3.

[20] Golino A, Duncan JM, Zeluff B, DePriest J, McAllister HA, Radovancevic B, et al. Leishmaniasis in a heart transplant patient. J Heart Lung Transplant. 1992;11:820-3.

[21] Iborra C, Caumes E, Carriere J, Cavelier-Balloy B, Danis M, Bricaire F. Mucosal leishmaniasis in a heart transplant recipient. Br J Dermatol. 1998;138:190-2.

[22] Larocca L, La Rosa R, Montineri A, Iacobello C, Brisolese V, Fatuzzo F, et al. Visceral leishmaniasis in an Italian heart recipient: first case report. J Heart Lung Transplant. 2007;26:1347-8.

[23] Zorio Grima E, Blanes Julia M, Martinez Ortiz de Urbina L, Almenar Bonet L, Peman Garcia J. [Persistent fever, pancytopenia and spleen enlargement in a heart transplant carrier as presentation of visceral leishmaniasis]. Rev Clin Esp. 2003;203:164-5.

[24] Morales P, Torres JJ, Salavert M, Peman J, Lacruz J, Sole A. Visceral leishmaniasis in lung transplantation. Transplant Proc. 2003;35:2001-3.

[25] Colomo Rodriguez N, De Adana Navas MS, Gonzalez Romero S, Gonzalez Molero I, Reguera Iglesias JM. [Visceral leishmaniasis in a type 1 diabetic patient with isolated pancreas transplant]. Endocrinol Nutr. 2011;58:375-7.

[26] Agteresch HJ, van 't Veer MB, Cornelissen JJ, Sluiters JF. Visceral leishmaniasis after allogeneic hematopoietic stem cell transplantation. Bone Marrow Transplant. 2007;40:391-3.

[27] Sirvent-von Bueltzingsloewen A, Marty P, Rosenthal E, Delaunay P, Allieri-Rosenthal A, Gratecos N, et al. Visceral leishmaniasis: a new opportunistic infection in hematopoietic stem-cell-transplanted patients. Bone Marrow Transplant. 2004;33:667-8.

[28] Chongo AG, ER. Leishmaniasis y transfusión. Artículo de revisión. Rev Mex Med Tran. 2010;3:5.

[29] Munoz P, Valerio M, Puga D, Bouza E. Parasitic infections in solid organ transplant recipients. Infect Dis Clin North Am. 2010;24:461-95.

[30] Veroux M, Corona D, Giuffrida G, Cacopardo B, Sinagra N, Tallarita T, et al. Visceral leishmaniasis in the early post-transplant period after kidney transplantation: clinical features and therapeutic management. Transpl Infect Dis. 2010;12:387-91.

[31] Berenguer J, Gomez-Campdera F, Padilla B, Rodriguez-Ferrero M, Anaya F, Moreno S, et al. Visceral leishmaniasis (Kala-Azar) in transplant recipients: case report and review. Transplantation. 1998;65:1401-4.

[32] Sagnelli C, Di Martino F, Coppola N, Crisci A, Sagnelli E. Acute liver failure: a rare clinical presentation of visceral leishmaniasis. New Microbiol. 2012;35:93-5.

[33] Cummins D, Amin S, Halil O, Chiodini PL, Hewitt PE, Radley-Smith R. Visceral leishmaniasis after cardiac surgery. Arch Dis Child. 1995;72:235-6.

[34] Dey A, Singh S. Transfusion transmitted leishmaniasis: a case report and review of literature. Indian J Med Microbiol. 2006;24:165-70.

[35] Mestra L, Lopez L, Robledo SM, Muskus CE, Nicholls RS, Velez ID. Transfusion-transmitted visceral leishmaniasis caused by Leishmania (Leishmania) mexicana in an immunocompromised patient: a case report. Transfusion. 2011;51:1919-23.

[36] Mathur P, Samantaray JC. The first probable case of platelet transfusion-transmitted visceral leishmaniasis. Transfus Med. 2004;14:319-21.

[37] Dey A, Singh S. Transfusion transmitted leishmaniasis: A case report and review of literature2006.

[38] Mpaka MA, Daniil Z, Kyriakou DS, Zakynthinos E. Septic shock due to visceral leishmaniasis, probably transmitted from blood transfusion. J Infect Dev Ctries. 2009;3:479-83.

[39] Magill AJ, Grogl M, Gasser RA, Jr., Sun W, Oster CN. Visceral infection caused by Leishmania tropica in veterans of Operation Desert Storm. N Engl J Med. 1993;328:1383-7.

[40] Grogl M, Daugirda JL, Hoover DL, Magill AJ, Berman JD. Survivability and infectivity of viscerotropic Leishmania tropica from Operation Desert Storm participants in human blood products maintained under blood bank conditions. Am J Trop Med Hyg. 1993;49:308-15.

[41] de Freitas E, Melo MN, da Costa-Val AP, Michalick MS. Transmission of Leishmania infantum via blood transfusion in dogs: potential for infection and importance of clinical factors. Vet Parasitol. 2006;137:159-67.

[42] Palatnik-de-Sousa CB, Paraguai-de-Souza E, Gomes EM, Soares-Machado FC, Luz KG, Borojevic R. Transmission of visceral leishmaniasis by blood transfusion in hamsters. Braz J Med Biol Res. 1996;29:1311-5.

[43] Paraguai de Souza E, Esteves Pereira AP, Machado FC, Melo MF, Souto-Padron T, Palatnik M, et al. Occurrence of Leishmania donovani parasitemia in plasma of infected hamsters. Acta Trop. 2001;80:69-75.

[44] Riera C, Fisa R, Udina M, Gallego M, Portus M. Detection of Leishmania infantum cryptic infection in asymptomatic blood donors living in an endemic area (Eivissa, Balearic Islands, Spain) by different diagnostic methods. Trans R Soc Trop Med Hyg. 2004;98:102-10.

[45] Scarlata F, Vitale F, Saporito L, Reale S, Vecchi VL, Giordano S, et al. Asymptomatic Leishmania infantum/chagasi infection in blood donors of western Sicily. Trans R Soc Trop Med Hyg. 2008;102:394-6.

[46] Colomba C, Saporito L, Polara VF, Barone T, Corrao A, Titone L. Serological screening for Leishmania infantum in asymptomatic blood donors living in an endemic area (Sicily, Italy). Transfus Apher Sci. 2005;33:311-4.

[47] Al-Said J, Pagaduan AC. Infection-free hemodialysis: can it be achieved? Saudi J Kidney Dis Transpl. 2009;20:677-80.

[48] Tong DS, Yang J, Xu GX, Shen GQ. [Serological investigation on Toxoplasma gondii infection in dialysis patients with renal insufficiency]. Zhongguo Xue Xi Chong Bing Fang Zhi Za Zhi. 2011;23:144, 53.

[49] Souza RM, de Oliveira IB, Paiva VC, Lima KC, dos Santos RP, de Almeida JB, et al. Presence of antibodies against Leishmania chagasi in haemodialysed patients. Trans R Soc Trop Med Hyg. 2009;103:749-51.

[50] Luz KG, da Silva VO, Gomes EM, Machado FC, Araujo MA, Fonseca HE, et al. Prevalence of anti-Leishmania donovani antibody among Brazilian blood donors and multiply transfused hemodialysis patients. Am J Trop Med Hyg. 1997;57:168-71.

[51] Mirzabeigi M, Farooq U, Baraniak S, Dowdy L, Ciancio G, Vincek V. Reactivation of dormant cutaneous Leishmania infection in a kidney transplant patient. J Cutan Pathol. 2006;33:701-4.

[52] Symmers WS. Leishmaniasis acquired by contagion: a case of marital infection in Britain. Lancet. 1960;1:127-32.

[53] Blickstein I, Dgani R, Lifschitz-Mercer B. Cutaneous leishmaniasis of the vulva. Int J Gynaecol Obstet. 1993;42:46-7.

[54] Cain C, Stone MS, Thieberg M, Wilson ME. Nonhealing genital ulcers. Cutaneous leishmaniasis. Arch Dermatol. 1994;130:1313, 5-6.

[55] Cabello I, Caraballo A, Millan Y. Leishmaniasis in the genital area. Rev Inst Med Trop Sao Paulo. 2002;44:105-7.

[56] Schubach A, Cuzzi-Maya T, Goncalves-Costa SC, Pirmez C, Oliveira-Neto MP. Leishmaniasis of glans penis. J Eur Acad Dermatol Venereol. 1998;10:226-8.

[57] Diniz SA, Melo MS, Borges AM, Bueno R, Reis BP, Tafuri WL, et al. Genital lesions associated with visceral leishmaniasis and shedding of Leishmania sp. in the semen of naturally infected dogs. Vet Pathol. 2005;42:650-8.

[58] Silva FL, Rodrigues AA, Rego IO, Santos RL, Oliveira RG, Silva TM, et al. Genital lesions and distribution of amastigotes in bitches naturally infected with Leishmania chagasi. Vet Parasitol. 2008;151:86-90.

[59] Rosen T, Brown TJ. Genital ulcers. Evaluation and treatment. Dermatol Clin. 1998;16:673-85.

[60] Gaskin AA, Schantz P, Jackson J, Birkenheuer A, Tomlinson L, Gramiccia M, et al. Visceral leishmaniasis in a New York foxhound kennel. J Vet Intern Med. 2002;16:34-44.

[61] Harris MP. Suspected transmission of leishmaniasis. Vet Rec. 1994;135:339.

[62] Silva FL, Oliveira RG, Silva TM, Xavier MN, Nascimento EF, Santos RL. Venereal transmission of canine visceral leishmaniasis. Vet Parasitol. 2009;160:55-9.

[63] Rosypal AC, Troy GC, Zajac AM, Frank G, Lindsay DS. Transplacental transmission of a North American isolate of Leishmania infantum in an experimentally infected beagle. J Parasitol. 2005;91:970-2.

[64] Mosby's Medical Dictionary. 8th ed: Elsevier; 2009.

[65] Low G, Cooke WE. A CONGENITAL CASE OF KALA-AZAR. The Lancet. [doi: 10.1016/S0140-6736(01)05214-X]. 1926;208:1209-11.

[66] Zinchuk A, Nadraga A. Congenital visceral leishmaniasis in Ukraine: case report. Ann Trop Paediatr. 2010;30:161-4.

[67] Meinecke CK, Schottelius J, Oskam L, Fleischer B. Congenital transmission of visceral leishmaniasis (Kala Azar) from an asymptomatic mother to her child. Pediatrics. 1999;104:e65.

[68] Bogdan C, Schonian G, Banuls AL, Hide M, Pratlong F, Lorenz E, et al. Visceral leishmaniasis in a German child who had never entered a known endemic area: case report and review of the literature. Clin Infect Dis. 2001;32:302-6.

[69] Figueiro-Filho EA, El Beitune P, Queiroz GT, Somensi RS, Morais NO, Dorval ME, et al. Visceral leishmaniasis and pregnancy: analysis of cases reported in a central-western region of Brazil. Arch Gynecol Obstet. 2008;278:13-6.

[70] Eltoum IA, Zijlstra EE, Ali MS, Ghalib HW, Satti MM, Eltoum B, et al. Congenital kala-azar and leishmaniasis in the placenta. Am J Trop Med Hyg. 1992;46:57-62.

[71] Nyakundi PM, Muigai R, Were JB, Oster CN, Gachihi GS, Kirigi G. Congenital visceral leishmaniasis: case report. Trans R Soc Trop Med Hyg. 1988;82:564.

[72] Morgan DJ, Guimaraes LH, Machado PR, D'Oliveira A, Jr., Almeida RP, Lago EL, et al. Cutaneous leishmaniasis during pregnancy: exuberant lesions and potential fetal complications. Clin Infect Dis. 2007;45:478-82.

[73] Pangrazio KK, Costa EA, Amarilla SP, Cino AG, Silva TM, Paixao TA, et al. Tissue distribution of Leishmania chagasi and lesions in transplacentally infected fetuses from symptomatic and asymptomatic naturally infected bitches. Vet Parasitol. 2009;165:327-31.

[74] Masucci M, De Majo M, Contarino RB, Borruto G, Vitale F, Pennisi MG. Canine leishmaniasis in the newborn puppy. Vet Res Commun. 2003;27 Suppl 1:771-4.

[75] Rosypal AC, Lindsay DS. Non-sand fly transmission of a North American isolate of Leishmania infantum in experimentally infected BALB/c mice. J Parasitol. 2005;91:1113-5.

[76] Osorio Y, Rodriguez LD, Bonilla DL, Peniche AG, Henao H, Saldarriaga O, et al. Congenital transmission of experimental leishmaniasis in a hamster model. Am J Trop Med Hyg. 2012;86:812-20.

[77] Avila-Garcia M, Mancilla-Ramirez J, Segura-Cervantes E, Farfan-Labonne B, Ramirez-Ramirez A, Galindo-Sevilla N. Transplacental Transmission of Cutaneous Leishmania mexicana Strain in BALB/c Mice. Am J Trop Med Hyg. 2013;89:354-8.

[78] Cruz I, Morales MA, Noguer I, Rodriguez A, Alvar J. Leishmania in discarded syringes from intravenous drug users. Lancet. 2002;359:1124-5.

[79] Pineda JA, Martin-Sanchez J, Macias J, Morillas F. Leishmania spp infection in injecting drug users. Lancet. 2002;360:950-1.

[80] Herwaldt BL. Laboratory-acquired parasitic infections from accidental exposures. Clin Microbiol Rev. 2001;14:659-88.

[81] Knobloch J, Demar M. Accidental Leishmania mexicana infection in an immunosuppressed laboratory technician. Trop Med Int Health. 1997;2:1152-5.

[82] Chosewood LC, Wilson DE, Centers for Disease Control and Prevention (U.S.), National Institutes of Health (U.S.). Biosafety in microbiological and biomedical laboratories. 5th ed. Washington, D.C.: U.S. Dept. of Health and Human Services, Public Health Service, Centers for Disease Control and Prevention, National Institutes of Health; 2009.

Chapter 3

Otorhinolaryngologic Manifestations in Leishmaniasis

Luiz Alberto Alves Mota and
Roberta Correia Ribeiro Ferreira de Miranda

Additional information is available at the end of the chapter

http://dx.doi.org/10.5772/57303

1. Introduction

Leishmaniasis is considered by the World Health Organization (WHO) as one of the five endemic infectious and parasitic diseases of greatest importance and as a world-wide public health problem [1]. It is an infectious disease that evolves chronically and is caused by a protozoon of the genus *Leishmania,* which may appear as a clinical form which is visceral, cutaneous, mucocutaneous, mucousal and rarely diffuse [2]. The term Leishmaniasis refers to the infection of vertebrate hosts *Leishmania,* which, like the other trypanosomatids of the order Kinetoplastida, characteristically present an extranuclear DNA in its cytoplasm in a mitochondrial organelle, the kinetoplast. This genus is characterized by having two ways of evolving during its biological cycle in host organisms: amastigote, which is an obligatory intracellular parasite in vertebrates, and promastigote, which develops in the digestive tube of invertebrate vectors or in axenic culture media [3].

In 1903, the agent of the disease was first described and separately by Leishman and Donovan. It is a protozoon identified in splenic tissue from two patients resident in India affected by a fatal disease [4]. It is primarily a zoonotic infection of wild animals, and more rarely pets, including marsupials, carnivores and even primates, with humans being accidental hosts.

All species of *Leishmania* are transmitted by the bite of female mosquitoes called phlebotominae of the genera *Lutzomyia* and *Phlebotomus,* this transmission being made by inoculation of promastigotes into the skin of the vertebrate host [5]. In larynegeal Leishmaniasis, contamination generally occurs starting with high lesions of the nasal cavities and oropharynx by contiguity. It is rare for parasites to be found inside the lesions [6].

The incubation period ranges from 2 weeks to several months [13]. Mucosal involvement is dependent on the combination of the virulence of the parasite and the immune cell response of the host. Within the population of infected individuals, 1-10% experience mucosal involvement [15]. Risk factors for the development of mucosal Leishmaniasis are: the presence of lesions above the pelvis, large skin ulcers and inadequate treatment of cutaneous Leishmaniasis [3].

For the diagnosis of mucosal Leishmaniasis, the clinical history and typical cutaneous scars have been considered as important clinical markers to corroborate the diagnosis of LM in patients with non-specific nasal/ oral granulomatous lesions [20].

In the Americas, pre-Colombus pottery, made by the Indians of Peru, has been found, dating from 400 to 900 AD. These show mutilations of lips and noses, characteristics of espundia, today known as muco-cutaneous leishmaniosis. Subsequently, through studies in paleomedicine, mummies with skin lesions and mucosas characteristic of Leishmaniasis were found [9]. Historical findings suggest that American Cutaneous Leishmaniasis (ACL) already affected the peoples of America before contact with Europeans and Africans. It is assumed that it may have originated in the western Amazon region during archeological times by means of human migrations and later ascended to the high jungle and then to the hot inter-Andean lands across the frontiers of Bolivia and of Peru with Brazil [5].

In the Old World (Asia, Africa and Europe) written accounts of the disease date from the first century AD. About two thousand years later, in 1903, the agent of the disease is described for the first time and separately by LEISHMAN and DONOVAN. The disease was visceral Leishmaniasis and its agent, the species now known as *Leishmania donovani* [4].

The first reference to American Tegumentary Leishmaniasis (ATL) in Brazil is in the document of the Religious Political-Geographical Pastoral 1827, quoted in Tello's book entitled "Antiguidad de la Syfilis en el Peru", where he recounts the journey of Friar Don Hipólito Sanches de Fayas y Quiros de Tabatinga (AM) to Peru, which crossed the regions of the Amazon basin [9]. In 1911, GASPAR VIANNA gave the parasite found by Lindenberg the name *Leishmania* brasiliensis, because he considered it morphologically different from *Leishmania* tropica. This characterized, from then on, the etiological agent of the disease being referred to as "Bauru ulcer", "angry angry" or "tapir-nose" [5].

In the 80s, the ATL was noted in 19 Federative Units (i.e. states), its geographical expansion being verified when, in 2003, autochthony was confirmed in all Brazilian states. It is seen to be widespread and, in some areas there is an intense concentration of cases, while in others, there are isolated cases [7]. The disease has been described in almost all American countries, from the extreme South of the United States to the North of Argentina, with the exception of Chile and Uruguay [22].

2. Epidemiology

Leishmaniasis is the second most common parasitic disease in the world, with an estimated 600,000 new cases per year [6]. It can also be considered an occupational disease, since it has affected workers in mining areas, geologists, scientific expeditions, military personnel in training [2]. It has been documented in several countries, with an estimated prevalence of 12 million worldwide [3]. More than 20 *Leishmania* species pathogenic to man have been described.

Until the 1990s, the classification of these species was based primarily on clinical and geographic criteria, taking into account on the one hand, the distinction between Old and New World, and, on the other, the clinical forms of the disease. This type of classification which has been progressively replaced by phylogenetic classification, is seen to be increasingly less tight and more superficial [4].

Leishmaniasis species are widely distributed and have been documented in Africa, Europe, Asia and America. In the Old World, *L. tropica, L. major* and *L. aethiopica*, which cause tegumentary Leishmaniasis, are identified as causal agents of the disease. In the Americas, several species of *Leishmania* are capable of causing tegumentary *Leishmaniasis*, such as *L. braziliensis (LVB), L. amazonensis, L. guianensis, L. pananmensis* and *L. Mexicana.*

The characterization of *Leishmania* species that was initially made, considering the behavior of the parasite in the vector, today has biochemical and imminological and molecular biology techniques, by isoenzyme analysis, reactivity with monoclonal antibodies and analysis of the DNA of kinetoplast [3]. In the Americas, 11 dermotropic species of *Leishmania* causing human disease are currently recognized and 8 species desrcibed as being only in animals [8].

It is in Brazil that the largest prevalence in the whole American continent is found, this being estimated as 65,000 new cases per year [6]. The coexistence is observed of a double epidemiological profile, expressed by the maintenance of cases coming from old foci or areas near them, and by the appearance of epidemic outbreaks associated with factors arising from the emergence of economic activities, such as mining, expansion of agricultural frontiers and extractivism, in environmental conditions that are highly favorable to the transmission of the disease [8].

A great number of the houses in recent population settlements are built very close to the edge of the forest and individuals are affected by the radius of action of these vectors that reach houses and are also attracted by several factors such as lighting, the presence of sinantropic animals such as Didelphis marsupialis, domestic animals and man himself [1]. Some species of rodents, marsupials, edentates and wild canids have already been recorded as hosts and possible natural reservoirs. The reservoir-parasite intersection is considered a complex system, insofar as it is multifactorial, unpredictable and dynamic, and forms a biological unit which can be in constant change as a result of the changes in the environment [8].

The disease occurs, more habitually, in the form of epidemic outbreaks. Thus, the degree of exposure of the individuals affected is related directly to agricultural population settlements which were planned or more often arise from occupation processes on the outskirts of a city, most of which are disorganized [1].

Initially, the reservoirs of the mosquito transmitter were in the wild or in rural areas, but the environmental transformations, provoked by the migratory process and by the increasing urbanization have been modifying this profile. The adaptation of the vectors to the new conditions enabled the disease to spread in the domiciliary and peri- domiciliary settings [5].

In several regions of the country, such as in the South and Southeast, intense environmental changes occurred due to anthropic action and agricultural and pastoral activities, which led to the near disappearance of cutaneous Leishmaniasis in the late 40s. However, from the 70s and 80s Leishmaniasis has reappeared in these regions, with a significant increase in the number of new cases arising from endemic areas [1]. Transmission classically was due to the bite of an insect, the so-called insect vector. This insect, also called a sandfly, belongs in the Old World to the genus Phlebotomus, and in the New World, to the genus Lutzomyia [4].

The first cases of ATL in America date from 1885 and in Brazil, the first report was in 1909. In the period 1985-1999, there were 388,155 auctothon cases in Brazil of ALT; from 1999 to 2003, 33,872 cases of ATL a year were registered [1]. In the period from 2000 to 2009, an average of 24,684 confirmed cases of Leishmaniasis was registered in Brazil the Information System for Notifiable Diseases (SINAN) [14]. In 2003, the regions with the highest prevalence of LTA were the North (14,200 cases) and the Northeast (8,005 cases) [5].

In Brazil, 23,399 confirmed cases of ATL were notified in 2009, of which 94.1% were new cases and 4.6% relapses. With respect to clinical manifestations, 93.7% of patients had the cutaneous clinical form and 6.2%, clinical mucosa. Of all patients, in 2009, only 73.5% [17, 23] were cured, 16 patients died due to ATL, and 122 died from other causes, noting that 21.2% there was no information on the evolution of 21.2% of the cases [14].

It is estimated that every year there are new cases in Brazil and the growth of this number is due in part to the emergence and growth of AIDS and deforestation areas [2]. It mostly affects young and adult males [16]. The greater number of cases of American Tegumentary Leishmaniasis among men and adults suggests extra-domiciliary transmission in the economically active population, while this occurrence among women, children and people with non-agricultural occupations suggests intra- and or peridomiciliary transmission.

The transmission of ATL in the Amazon presents a clear seasonal variation, it being more intense in the rainy season, when the temperature, solar radiation and evaporation are lower and humidity higher, thus favoring an increase in the density of the phlebotominae, including the species involved in the cycle of the disease [1]. In endemic areas, there may be significant percentages of children with the disease [16].

3. Etiological agents and vectors

In the Americas, 11 dermotropic species of *Leishmania* which cause the disease in humans are currently recognized and 8 species have been described as affecting only animals. However, in Brazil, 7 species, there being 6 of the subgenus *Viannia* and 1 of the subgenus *Leishmania,* have been identified. The three main species are: *Leishmania (Leishmania) amazonensis* - distributed throughout the primary and secondary forests of the Amazon (Amazonas, Pará, Rondônia, Tocantins and the southwest of Maranhão southwest), particularly in *igapó* and forest areas of the "swamp-forest" type. Its presence extends to the regions of the Northeast (Bahia), Southeast (Minas Gerais and São Paulo) and Midwest

(Goiás); *Leishmania (Viannia) guyanensi* - apparently limited to the north of the Amazon Basin (Amapá, Roraima, Amazonas and Pará) and extending to the Guianas. It is found mainly in *terra firme* forests in areas that do not flood during the rainy season; *Leishmania (Viannia) braziliensis* – is widely distributed, from the South of Pará to the Northeast, also reaching the center-south of the country and some areas of the Eastern Amazon East. In the Amazon, the infection is usually found in dry land areas.

As the subgenus *Viannia*, there are other species of *Leishmania* that have been recently described: *L. (V) lainsoni, L. (V) naiffi* with a few human cases in Pará; *L. (V) shawi*, with human cases found in Pará and Maranhão. More recently, the species *L. (V.) lainsoni, L. (V.) naiffi, L. (V.) lindenberg and L. (V.) shawi* were identified in states of the North and Northeast regions [8]. In areas of transmission of *L. braziliensis* concomitantly or after resolution of the cutaneous disease, about 3% of patients with cutaneous *Leishmania*sis will develop the mucosal form of the disease [3].

Mucosal Leishmaniasis (ML) is a form of tegumentary Leishmaniasis associated with *L. braziliensis, L. panamensis* and less frequently with *L. amazonensis* [11]. The vectors of ATL are insects known as phlebotominae, belonging to the order *Diptera, Psychodidae* family, sub-family *Phlebotominae*, genus *Lutzomyia*, popularly known, depending on the geographical location, as straw-mosquito straw, *tatuquira, birigui*, among others [8]. Generally not exceeding 0.5 cm in length, with long and spindly legs and a dense body follicles. A characteristic of theirs is a hopping flight and keeping their wings erect, unlike other dipteral [9]. The vectors are *Lutzomya anduzei, Lutzomyia whitmani* and *Lutzomyia umbratilis*, which is the main vector, which usually lands during the day on tree trunks and attacks people in large numbers, when disturbed [16]. It is usually brownish ("straw-mosquito"), only the females being adapted with the respective mouth part to prick the skin of vertebrates and suck blood.

The genus *Lutzomyia* is responsible for the transmission of Leishmaniasis in the Americas, and there are 350 species catalogued, which are distributed from the South of Canada to the North of Argentina. Of these, at least 200 occur in the Amazon basin. Very little is known of their breeding grounds, with immature forms being found in debris of rock crevices, caves, roots of the soil and of dead and damp leaves, and also in the forks of trees in animal burrows - ie in moist but not wet soil, and in debris rich in decaying organic matter [9].

4. Clinical state

Tegumentary Leishmaniasis is more common than the visceral disease and is characterized in its classical form by the presence of a well-bounded ulcer with raised edges. [17] ATL is an initial infection of the skin (its site of preferential location) from which it can undergo propagation or a secondary process which goes on to manifest itself in the mucosae of the upper airways [5]. The incubation period of the disease in humans is, on average, 2 months, it being possible for there to be shorter (two-week) periods and longer periods (of up to 2 years) [16].

The disease breaks out, in general, during the first five years that follow the appearance of the skin lesion, but may do so even a few decades after the primary cutaneous lesion, the scar from which can still be seen. However, in some patients the disease appears primarily in the mucosa membrane, without leaving traces on the skin. [2]. The most common manifestation is leishmaniotic ulcer: a single skin ulcer or only in small numbers, with raised edges, framed and the absence of local pain. Other morphological features can also be identified, such as: infiltrated plaque, tubercule, nodule and verrucous vegetating lesion. When the mucosa is injured, it can present an infiltrated erythema, granular or ulcerated aspect. In order of frequency, mucosal lesions are manifested mainly in the nose, hard palate, pharynx and larynx, which they can present themselves with an erythematous-infiltrated, granular, ulcerated or polypoid aspect with a roughly rounded surface [5].

Basically, it is possible to do the staging of the lesions that have occurred in the ATL by taking into consideration the time of onset, extent and spread of the lesion, and grouping them into: 1). Primary infections: which characterizes the primary accident (initial injury) or leishmaniotic cancer, found at the site of the bite, and after the incubation period (two weeks to one year), erythematous papules appear that progress to forming ulcers with serosanguinous crusts. 2) The onset of secondary Leishmaniasis ranges from one to three months after the primary infection, involving the skin, lymph nodes, lymphatic organs and mucosa and by contiguity, the mucous membranes of the nose, lips, eyelids and genitals are affected when the primary or secondary lesions settle near these regions. 3) Tertiary Leishmaniasis requires a longer period to appear, generally, five to ten years after the initial lesion and is characterized by the presence mainly of naso-oro-pharyngeal, laryngeal and ocular lesions, and it is in this period tertiary that the primary infection has already disappeared and the secondary one, in general, is still present [5]. The clinical presentation exhibits polymorphism and the spectrum of severity of the signs and symptoms is also variable, although there is a certain correspondence between the different clinical presentations and the different species of the parasite [7].

Mucosal Leishmaniasis appears under the following clinical forms: 1) Late –this is the most common form. Classically, it is associated with multiple or long-lasting skin lesions, spontaneous cures or insufficient CL treatments; 2) Of undetermined origin - when the ML is clinically isolated, it not being possible to detect any other evidence of prior CL; 3) Concomitant - when the mucosal lesion occurs at a distance, but at the same time as the active skin lesion (not contiguous to the natural orifices); 4) Contiguous – this occurs by direct propagation of the skin lesion, located next to natural orifices, to the mucosa of the aerodigestive tracts. The skin lesion may be in activity or healed at the time of diagnosis; 5) Primary – this occurs, possibly, by the bite of the vector in the mucosa or semimucosa of lips and genitals [7.8].

It is believed that untreated mucosal lesions are progressive, there being few reports of spontaneous cicatrizations of these lesions which, even if treated, may leave permanent sequelae [22]. There are several hypotheses that attempt to explain the predilection of the nasal mucosa: direct contact of the hand with the skin lesions and scratching one´s nose afterwards, the epithelium of the anterior part of the nasal cavities offer conditions to the location of Leishmanias and the lower temperature in the anterior area of the nasal septum, due to the presence of a current of inspiratory air. The transition zone between the squamous epithelia and the pseudostratified vibrating, in the anterior part of the nasal septum and the lower turbinate head, is the "*locus minoris resistentia*" to the Leishmaniasis process. However, the most

http://dx.doi.org/10.5772/57303

consistent hypothesis says that *Leishmania* requires lower temperatures for its growth. Thus, since the anterior area of the nasal septum is cooler due to the inspiratory airflow, there would be a predilection for proliferation of the parasites [13]. The association of low temperature with Leishmaniasis may, in part, be explained by the documentation *in vitro* that macrophages grown at 29°C are less able to destroy *Leishmania* than macrophages cultured at 33°C [3].

It occurs more often in males and at age bands usually higher than CL, which is probably due to its character of secondary complication [8]. The involvement of the nasal and/or mucosa is usually more severe and thus may cause sequelae and death [20].

The initial lesion is characterized by a whitish nodulation without ulceration which is usually observed in the cartaliginous septum (Kiesselbach's area), the floor and side wall, specifically on the head of the inferior turbinate. This impairment classified as stage I of the disease, represents a very early stage of inflammation and does not resemble, from the clinical standpoint, any other nasal disease. Subsequently, a fine granular lesion appears, characterized by superficial ulceration, documented at the anterior septum, inferior turbinates and floor of the nasal cavity (Stage II) [17]. At first, there is hyperemia and edema of the mucosa of the anterior septum, with the establishment of nodulations [3].

In Stage III, or the stage of deep ulceration, tissue reaction is more intense, with aberrant granulation tissue and infiltration of the mucosa, thus widening the nasal septum. There is sometimes edematous infiltration of the nasal pyramid itself. In this phase, hematic crusts can be observed on the septum, the inferior turbinates and the floor of the nasal cavities. These lesions are characterized by excessive fragility, as they bleed very easily when the mucosa is touched.

Clinically, the patient may complain of soreness at the level of the nasal pyramid, sanguinolent rhinorrhea and emission of hematic crusts. Nasal obstruction is a frequent symptom in this phase of the disease. From the external point of view, due to the inflammatory process that involves the cartilages and subcutaneous cell tissue and the very skin of the base of the nasal pyramid, the nose takes on the aspect known as tapir-nose.

Stage IV of the disease is characterized by the cartilaginous involvement of the anterior septum with necrosis and, sometimes, impairment of the columella. It is at this stage that perforation of the cartilaginous septum is established, also with marked infiltration of the posterior septum. In more advanced forms (Stage V), total destruction of the columella may occur and may drop, thus transforming the nasal cavity into a similar cloaca and sometimes there is perforation of the dorsum of the nasal pyramid [17]. For some researchers, the specific destruction of the nasal cartilage could also indicate an autoimmune reaction that would explain why some patients undergo severe tissue destruction and others only present mucosal involvement years later [21]. In some cases there may be total destruction of the anterior septum, only the entire columella remaining, with the nose being sealed. Extensive crusts of a hemorrhagic aspect or even resulting from the drying of mucous secretion caused by enlargement of the internal nasal structure can be observed as a consequence of the tissue injury, represented by the destruction of the cartilaginous septum and inferior turbinates. On this occasion, there is elimination of sanguinolent discharge and the presence of crusts is accentuated [17]. The patient's death usually occurs because of aspiration or respiratory failure [5].

The earliest signs and symptoms of mucosal Leishmaniasis are nasal obstruction, epistaxis and the establishment of granulomas in the anterior nasal septum. As the disease evolves, patients begin to present a leishmaniotic facies known as "tapir nose" due to edematous infiltration of the lining and supporting structures of the nose [3]. Lesions reach the cartilaginous nasal septum and may extend to the lateral wall and floor, the region of the palate, uvula, and less frequently, involvement of the pharynx, larynx, vocal cords and upper lip occur with varying degrees of infiltration, granulation and ulceration [17]. The infiltration of the soft palate reaches the proportions of a real tumor. The whole palate is changed: the uvula is reduced to a shapeless mass, with an irregular, vegetating surface. In the palatal vault, lobed prominences are formed, separating themselves by sinuous furrows and ulcerated erosions.

More rarely it can involve the gum and dental interstices, where voluminous and prominent granulations develop, and reach the upper lip. The tongue is usually spared [5]. The manifestations of the mucosal diseases include involvement of pillars and uvula with an increase in volume, hyperemia, roughness and superficial ulcers [12]. The pharynx is the second site of involvement when mucosal lesions caused by *L. braziliensis* set in. As in the nose, the lesion initially observed at the level of the mucosa of the pharynx takes on a lumpy aspect; however, here, there is a much more intense edematous infiltration, especially of the uvula and secondarily of the tonsillar pillars, extending also to the mucosa of the posterior pharyngeal wall.

The appearance can be observed at this stage of granulation tissue that is a little redundant intermingled with the lumpy aspect of the mucosa. The next stage is characterized by the appearance of abundant granulation tissue, which causes important tissue destruction, also involving the lymphoid tissue of Waldeyer's lymphatic ring at the level of tonsils. Areas with a tenuous fibrin layer mix in with the granulation tissue of a vegetating aspect.

Because of the intense tissue aggression, in the specific post-treatment healing process, the presence of abundant fibrous tissue, with the formation of true whitish cords can be documented. These completely deform the configuration of the anatomical structures of the velum of the palate and the posterior wall of the pharynx, leading to full stenosis in the communication of the oropharynx with the nasopharynx [3]. In the mouth, the hard palate is often involved, with dissemination of the process to the soft palate, uvula and pharynx. The proliferating infiltrative process can cause fusion of the uvula, pillars, lateral cords and posterior wall, causing obliteration of the nasopharynx. Deformity and narrowing of the lumen of the oropharynx may occur due to fibrosis of the tonsils [5].

Laryngeal mucosa is the 3rd site of election when mucosal Leishmaniasis sets in. As in the pharynx, the mucosal lesions present the same characteristics of finely granular tissue. There may be in situations of greater inflammation, the presence of granulation tissue with a vegetating aspect, covered at times with a tenuous fibrin layer, involving the mucosa that covers the cartilage of the epiglottis, extending to the mucosa of the structures of the laryngeal vestibule and vocal folds. At this stage, dysphonia characterized by a muffled voice is always present, which draws attention to the impairment of the organ [3]. Pharyngolaryngeal

http://dx.doi.org/10.5772/57303

involvement can be intense, to the point of causing dysphagia, dyspnea, dysphonia, odynophagia, and coughing [15]. The hypopharynx, larynx, epiglottis, arytenoid cartilages and the posterior commissure of the vocal cords are covered by a lesion with a vegetating aspect, which sometimes come to join up. These granulations often regress and eventually disappear, making the surface affected by a smooth and slightly whitish coloration.

There is generalized laryngeal inflammation particularly in the piriform sinuses. The vocal folds appear to be moving well, but phonation is weak and the muscular control of tension can be harmed by granulomatous formation and subsequent fibrosis. Even after successful treatment, the voice rarely returns to normal and the lumen of the larynx may be reduced [5]. Painful dysphagia in degrees of greater or lesser intensity prevents the normal feeding of the individual, with consequent impairment of general condition and, in very advanced cases, becoming cachexia. In post-treatment healing, the deformities that these cartilages present are very evident, such as fibrous tissue which is also whitish, thereby completely modifying the anatomy of the organ, except for a residual permanent dysphonia [3].

Complications include pneumonia due to aspiration, bacterial infections, secondary myiasis, cachexia due to difficulties in swallowing, laryngeal edema and asphyxiation, which may be lead on to the patient's death mainly due to respiratory failure and sepsis [5]. The presentation of the clinical form with lesions exclusive of mucosa of the larynx and trachea is relatively uncommon [2]. The ear is not usually affected in mucosal Leishmaniasis. However, the involvement of the mucosa of the nasopharynx leads to impairment of the pharyngeal orifice of the Eustachian tube, situated on its sidewall. A process of otitis media with effusion (secretory otitis media chronic) can be established in these cases.

The sensation of blocked ear, tinnitus and hearing loss are complaints in these cases [3]. Morbidity of the skin and ear cartilage occurs because it is a place of lower temperature, apt for the growth of *Leishmania*, besides being an area exposed to the inoculation of the vectors. The external ear commonly presents an increase in volume, ulcers with raised edges, sometimes covered with crusts, and may appear as an infiltrated plate, tubercule, vegetating warty nodule and lesion, on course in the end to mutilating the ear [5].

Mucosal Leishmaniasis can compromise the labial mucosa and gingival margin. This is a rarer manifestation of the disease [3]. The lesion in some individuals heals early, sometimes without seeking medical attention. Others remain for months with the lesion in activity and the healing process is slow. This phenomenon can be explained by the rapid or late establishment of a specific immune response which is effective in eliminating the parasite.

The cure of Leishmaniasis is not sterile. It has been possible to isolate viable parasites of ALT scars in individuals who have been cured for several years, a fact confirmed in experimental studies using an animal model. This phenomenon could thus explain the appearance of late relapses as well as the onset of the disease in immunocompromised patients, such as AIDS (Acquired Immunodeficiency Syndrome) [7].

5. Diagnosis

It is very hard to detect Leishmaniasis in the initial stage [15]. The long interval between the onset of symptoms and etiological diagnosis of the mucosal form of ATL may reflect the limitation of the training of most physicians in the proper approach to mucosal Leishmaniasis [2]. A laryngoscopy exam usually demonstrates an extensive inflammatory component, with erythema and edemas evident. The granulomatous aspect associated with the presence of ulcers is common, and may present purulent exudate. In the advanced disease, tissue destruction can be striking. As a protocol of etiological investigation on suspicion of granulomatous bodies that are difficult to access such as the larynx, laboratory tests and imaging should be requested, and should a diagnostic uncertainty be maintained, a biopsy of the lesions is recommended for histological study. If the appearance of the lesion suggests malignant neoplasm, research using noninvasive and invasive tests should occur simultaneously so as not to delay diagnosis [15].

The ENT examination associated with the Montenegro test remains the most important element for diagnosis, although it is usually of a presumptive character [20]. The encounter of *Leishmania* is the gold standard for the diagnosis of ATL [21]. The diagnosis can be confirmed by various tests: 1) Direct investigation of the parasite, which can be done by scraping the ulcerated surface or by compression of the slide on the wounded area of the lesion. The material is stained with Giemsa or Wright [2]. The direct parasitological examination is the procedure of first choice because it is faster, less expensive and easy to perform [16]. It gives good results in initial lesions, without associated bacterial infection [2], 2) Montenegro intradermoreaction: This translates the response of cell delayed hypersensitivity [16]. It consists of intradermal injection of 0.1 ml of antigen prepared from *Leishmania* promastigotes, with a reading after 48 hours. The test is considered positive that produces an induration of 5 mm or more. However, the positivity of the test indicates that the person has already been sensitized but is not necessarily a carrier of the disease [2]; 3) Histopathological examination of the tegumentary lesion [2]. The Biopsy can be performed with a "punch" of 4 mm in diameter, or a wedge, with the use of a scalpel. In ulcerated lesions, the whole edge of the whole lesion should be preferred, This, in general, shows a tumified and hyperemic aspect [16]; 4) Serology (indirect immunofluorescence or ELISA); they have good sensitivity but can give a reaction crossed with Chagas disease and visceral Leishmaniasis, this being the cause of false-positive results, thus reducing its specificity [2].

The most commonly used techniques for antibodies are: indirect immunofluorescence (IIF), counterimmunoelectrophoresis (CIE), ELISA and Western blot. The Western blot technique has a superior sensitivity to the other serologic techniques [70.6%), a sensibility of 70.3% and a precision of 72.7%. In the immunocompetents, the specificity and sensitivity are 100% [4]; 5) Immunohistochemical techniques (immunostaining with anti *Leishmania* antibodies); they permit evidence of the parasite in histological sections; 6) Method of culture: culture takes place in Novy-MacNeal-Nicolle medium from the biopsy or aspirate [4]. They are not practical for diagnosis, especially of *Leishmania brasiliensis*, since it does not grow easily in culture media; in addition, bacterial or fungal contamination often complicate this procedure [2]. Research can be done into *Leishmania* in other affected organs such as the spleen, liver and lymph node, and whenever there is a suspected diagnosis, into the pleural fluid, bronchoalveolar lavage, intestinal biopsy, skin, etc. Hepatic and spleen biopsies are used as a last resort due to the increased risk of potentially serious complications such as hemorrhaging [4].

Cases are confirmed according to the following criteria: 1) Residence, arrival in or moving away from the area with confirmation of transmission and presence of the parasite in direct and/or indirect parasitological exams; 2) Residence, arrival in or moving away from the area with confirmation of transmission and intradermoreaction of Montenegro (MRI) positive, 3) Residence, arrival in or moving away from the area with confirmation of transmission with other methods of positive diagnosis [19].

6. Differential diagnosis

The finding of symptoms and head and neck moles in patients with Leishmaniasis, paracoccidioidomycosis and leprosy underscore the need that they all undergo an ENT evaluation. In addition to these diseases, it would be an appropriate conduct to perform complete ENT examination in all patients with some form of granulomatous disease [11]. The differential diagnosis of laryngeal ATL is made with granulomatous lesions such as tuberculosis and paracoccidioidomycosis which have a predilection for the posterior portion of the larynx [2]. The diagnosis of paracoccidioidomycosis is characterized by erosion or exulceration in the oral mucosa, with a granulous base and the presence of stippled hemorrhage (Aguiar Puo's moriform stomatitis), regional lymph node and lung involvement [8]. Syphilitic laryngitis, which fortunately nowadays is rare and appears in the tertiary stage of syphilis may present diffuse infiltrate, which subsequently undergoes ulceration [2]. Tertiary syphilis can be confirmed by histopathological exam, and shows vascular lesions and plasma cell wealth, and VDRL may be positive [8].

Neoplastic lesions of the larynx are more localized and almost always there is a report of smoking and alcoholism in the medical history [2]. Epidermoid and basal cell carcinomas usually present themselves as hardened to palpation, and are confirmed by histopathological examination [8]. Histoplasmosis in its chronic disseminated form involves mucosa in 90%, and the upper airways are affected; the larynx is very adversely affected with infiltration and edema of the laryngeal vestibule, pink nodules on an infiltrated base and granulomatous ulcerations of a granulomatous depth partially covered by yellowish-white secretions that may lead to obstructive dyspnea, requiring a tracheostomy. Generally, in this form of presentation of histoplasmosis there will be alterations in the chest X-ray associated with pulmonary symptoms, which differentiates it from Leishmaniasis. Coccidioidomycosis of the larynx is very rare in our environment. Tracheobronchial amyloidosis with involvement of the larynx is very rare; however, it may present itself with pseudotumoral, bleeding, warty lesions, with a visual appearance similar to the case presented, which can lead to obstruction of the airways [2]. The differential diagnosis is made with rhinophyma, rhinosporidiosis, entomophthoromycosis, traumatic septal perforation or because of drug use, allergic rhinitis, sinusitis, sarcoidosis, Wegner's granulomatosis and other rarer diseases.

As for lymphomas, histopathological and immunohistochemical exams will help to conclude the diagnosis. In the case of rhinophyma, there is usually a history of rosacea (acne-like lesions and telangiectasias, of long evolution). In the differential diagnosis with rhinosporidiosis what are important are: the origin (Piauí, Maranhão), the history of possible exposure to the fungus in stagnant water and dams, the presence of polyps in the nasal and ocular mucous membranes, and upper respiratory tracts. Histopathological examination shows the microorganism (sporangia of 6 to 300μm). Lesions of entomophthoromycosis present a hardened or woody consistency to palpation and histopathological and mycological exams demonstrate the presence of hyphae and isolation of the fungus in cultur medium. In the differential diagnosis with leprosy, skin sensibility tests, testing of skin bacilli in the lymph of the pinna or lesions and histopathological examination will help confirm the diagnosis. The clinical history is essential when seeking information on personal or family atopy (allergic rhinitis, bronchitis, migraine), on traumatic perforation and use of drugs. Wegner's granulomatosis and sarcoidosis are rarer diseases, and sometimes difficult to confirm. Diagnosis may be aided by observation of the involvement of other organs such as the lungs and kidneys, it being stressed that the histopathology will contribute to the diagnosis [8].

7. Co-infection *Leishmania* and HIV

ATL can modify the progression of the disease due to HIV and immunosuppression caused by this virus facilitating progression of ATL [8]. Acquired immunodeficiency syndrome is caused by a retrovirus of the *Lentiviridae* family, HIV-1 and HIV-2. Those infected with the human immunodeficiency virus (HIV) progress to severe dysfunction of the immune system, as the CD4 + T lymphocytes, one of the major target cells of the virus, are being destroyed [19]. On destroying the immune system, the so-called "opportunistic infections" are manifested as this unfolds in which infections are included, namely infections by protozoa [4]. The assessment of the set of clinical manifestations of ATL in patients with HIV indicates that there is no definition of a clinical profile that may unarguably be associated with co-infection [8]. The exponential increase in the number of cases of co-infection of *Leishmania*/ HIV, especially in the late 1990s, has undergone modifications [4]. Unusual findings can be observed in co-infected patients, suchas, for example, finding *Leishmania spp* in intact skin, and overlying a Kaposi's sarcoma lesion, or *Herpes simplex* and *Herpes zoster* lesions. There may also be involvement of the gastrointestinal tract and the respiratory tract for the coinfection of ATL/AIDS [8]. The population of drug users who inject endovenously is the main group at risk of the co-infection of *Leishmania*/HIV in Southeast Europe, and form 72% of co-infected patients [4].

8. Prevention

Several thorough trials have been carried out on the production of anti- *Leishmania* vaccines: 1) "Leishmanization" has been used empirically since the distant past by people living in

http://dx.doi.org/10.5772/57303

endemic areas. This consists of scarification covered with virulent promastigotes of virulent to avoid the appearance of disfiguring lesions in exposed areas. 2) The association of BCG with dead *Leishmania* promastigotes. 3) Vaccines produced by molecular technology from DNA, probably the future of prophylaxis in infectious diseases in immunosuppressed patients [4].

9. Treatment

ENT activity is of primary importance [5]. The drug of first choice is the pentavalent antimonial one. With a view to standardizing the therapeutic regimen, WHO recommends that the dose of this antimonial be calculated in mg /SbV/ Kg day./ (SbV meaning a pentavalent antimonial).

There are two types of pentavalent antimonial that can be used, N-methylglucamine antimonate and sodium stibogluconate [10,16]. In all forms of mucosal involvement, the recommended dose is 20mg Sb+5/kg/day, for thirty consecutive days, preferably in a hospital environment. If healing is not complete within three months (twelve weeks) after treatment ends, the scheme should be repeated only once. Should there be no response, use one of the second choice drugs [16].

If there is no satisfactory response to the treatment with pentavalent antimony, the second choice drugs are amphotericin B and pentamidine isethionate. The injections must be made parenterally, intramuscularly (IM) or intravenously (IV), with rest after application. The IM may have the drawback of local pain. It is suggested, therefore, locations be alternated, the gluteal region being preferred.

In cases of malnourished patients with low muscle mass, and those with thrombocytopenia, the intravenous route should be given preference. This is the best route because it allows the application of large volumes without the inconvenience of local pain. The application should be slow (a minimum of 5 minutes), with a fine needle (gauge 25x7 or 25x8) and without needing to be diluted. To make it possible for rest after administration, it is generally advisable to apply the medication at the end of the day. It is worth noting that there is no difference between the IV and IM routes, with respect to the efficacy and safety of the drug [8].

The use of topical products such as paromomycin and imiquimod, associated or not with parenteral medication, have also presented preliminary satisfactory results, with cure rates ranging between 74% and 85% for the former drug, and 90% for the latter [9]. The imidazoquinoline, approved for the treatment of genital warts, [17] stimulates the Th1 response by increasing the production of TNF- α, IFN-γ and IL-12. *In vitro*, presents anti Leishmanial activity because it also stimulates the production of nitric oxide by macrophages, thus decreasing the number of parasites. Paromomycin is an antibiotic that inhibits the mitochondrial activity of *Leishmania*. rhGM-CSF is a glycoprotein that induces the growth of colonies of granulocytes and/or macrophages, by stimulating their phagocytic and metabolic functions. For this reason, it plays an important role in the immune response against intracellular pathogens. It has been used experimentally in the treatment of some inflammatory diseases as it has an inhibitory effect on TNF- α [18].

Local treatment of small lesions may not be necessary. Larger lesions may be treated with surgical excision, curettage or cryotherapy [13]. Secondary infection may occur in 54.2% of patients and the germ most frequently found is *Staphylococcus aureus* [21], which is why local care should be prescribed such as local cleansing with soap and water and if possible compresses with KMnO (potassium permanganate in a dilution of 1/5000ml) [8, 16].

The cure criterion is defined by the regression of all signs and confirmed by ENT examination, up to 6 months after completion of the treatment regimen. In the absence of the specialist, the clinician must be trained to perform, at least, anterior rhinoscopy and oroscopy. Where there is no clinician, the patient should be referred to the service that evaluates healing. The patient should return monthly for a consultation for 3 consecutive months after the end of the treatment regimen so that the clinical cure can be evaluated.

Once cured, the patient should be monitored every 2 months, until 12 months after completing treatment [8]. The control of ATL should be tackled in a comprehensive way, in five respects: epidemiological surveillance, measures of performance in the transmission chain, educational measures, administrative measures and vaccine [9]. To reduce the lethality of these diseases, what is above all necessary is early diagnosis and the timely treatment of cases [14].

The current challenges for ATL are: a) to increase investments in seeking drugs with better efficacy, safety, low cost, ease of administration and sustainability; b) to continue to be vigilant about the adverse effects of medication; c) to expand the health network for early diagnosis and adequate treatment of cases; d) to investigate and evaluate deaths; e) to implement surveillance actions in territorial units; f) to expand the activities of epidemiological surveillance [19].

Acknowledgements

Our thanks to the Teacher Roddy Kay for his dedication in translation of this chapter.

Author details

Luiz Alberto Alves Mota[1,2*] and Roberta Correia Ribeiro Ferreira de Miranda[3]

*Address all correspondence to: luizmota10@gmail.com

1 Faculty of Medical Sciences, Universidade de Pernambuco, Brasil

2 ENT service, Hospital Universitário Oswaldo Cruz, Brasil

3 Faculty of Medical Sciences, Universidade de Pernambuco, Brasil

References

[1] Guerra JAO, Barbosa MGV, Loureiro ACSP, Coelho CP, Rosa GG, Coelho LIACR. Leishmaniose tegumentar americana em crianças: aspectos epidemiológicos de casos atendidos em Manaus, Amazonas, Brasil. Cad. Saúde Pública, Rio de Janeiro. 2007, 23(9):2215-2223.

[2] Melo SMD, Todt Neto JC, Andrade LCF. Pseudo-hemoptise por leishmaniose. Jornal de Pneumologia. 1999, 25(6):347- 350.

[3] Lessa MM, Lessa HA, Castro TWN, Oliveira A, Scherifer A, Machado P, Carvalho EM. Leishmaniose mucosa: aspectos clínicos e epidemiológicos. Rev Bras Otorrinolaringol. 2007, 73(6):843-847.

[4] Catorze MGB. Leishmaniose e SIDA. Med. Cutan. Iber. Lat. Amer. 2005, 6:237-250.

[5] Neto FXP, Rodrigues AC, Silva LL, Palheta ACP, Rodrigues LG, Silva FA. Manifestações Otorrinolaringológicas Relacionadas à Leishmaniose Tegumentar Americana: Revisão de Literatura. Arq Int Otorrinolaringol./Intl Arch Otorhinolaryngol. 2008, 12(4):531-537.

[6] Silva L, Costa HO, Duprat AC, Bairão F, Della Nina M. Granulomatose laríngea. Avaliação e métodos diagnósticos e terapêuticos em 24 casos. ACTA ORL/ Técnicas em Otorrinolaringologia. 2007, 25(1):16-23.

[7] Ministério da Saúde do Brasil. Manual de Vigilância da Leishmaniose Tegumentar Americana. 2ª ed. Brasília; 2007, 1-30.

[8] Ministério da Saúde. Secretaria de Vigilância em Saúde. Leishmaniose Tegumentar Americana. Guia de Vigilância Epidemiológica; Caderno 11.

[9] Basano SA, Camargo LMA. Leishmaniose tegumentar americana: histórico, epidemiologia e perspectivas de controle. Rev Bras Epidemiol. 2004, 7(3):328-337.

[10] Secretaria Municipal de Saúde. Recomendações para o Manejo Clínico da Leishmaniose Tegumentar e Visceral. Belo Horizonte; 2007.

[11] Fornazieri MA, Yamaguti HY, Moreira JH, Takemoto LE, Navarro PL, Heshiki RE. Manifestações Otorrinolaringológicas Mais Comuns das Doenças Granulomatosas. Arq Int Otorrinolaringol./Intl Arch Otorhinolaryngol. 2008,12(3):362-365.

[12] Focaccia R, Veronesi R. Tratado de Infectologia. 3ª edição v.2 Atheneu, São Paulo, 1997.

[13] Gomes ACA, Dias EOS, Pita Neto IC, Bezerra TP. Leishmaniose muco-cutânea: relato de caso clínico Rev.Cirurgia e Traumatologia Buco-Maxilo-Facial. 2004, 4(4):223-228.

[14] Tratamento da Leishmaniose Visceral e Leishmaniose Tegumentar Americana no Brasil Epidemiol. Serv. Saúde, Brasília, 20(1):107-110, jan – mar 2011.

[15] Leishmaniose Laríngea. Arquivos Internacionais de Otorrinolaringologia. São Paulo - Brasil, v.16, n.4, p. 523-526, out – dez 2012.

[16] Ministério da Saúde. Gerência Técnica de Doenças Transmitidas por Vetores e Antropozoonoses. Coordenação de Vigilância Epidemiológica Centro Nacional de Epidemiologia. Manual de Controle da Leishmaniose Tegumentar Americana. Fundação Nacional de Saúde Brasília, 2000.

[17] Luiz Henrique Guimarães, et al. Aspectos clínicos da Leishmaniose tegumentar. Gaz. méd. Bahia 2005;75:1(Jan-Jun):66-74.

[18] Almeida OLS, Santos JB. Avanços no tratamento da leishmaniose tegumentar do novo mundo nos últimos dez anos: uma revisão sistemática da literatura. An Bras Dermatol. 2011;86(3):497-506.

[19] Penna GO, Domingues CMAS, Siqueira JB Jr, Elkhoury ANSM, Cechinel MP, Grossi MAF, et al. Doenças dermatológicas de notificação compulsória no Brasil. An Bras Dermatol. 2011;86(5):865-77.

[20] Diniz JLCP, Costa MOR, Gonçalves DU. Mucocutaneous Leishmaniasis: clinical markers in presumptive diagnosis. Brazilian Journal of Otorhinolaryngology 77 (3) Maio/Junho 2011;77(3):380-4.

[21] Silva MS, Sousa RT, Silva EB, Guerra JAO, Gomes NM, Santana RF, Mubarac RS. Primary lesion of Mucocutaneous Leishmaniasis simulating external otitis.

[22] Nunes CS, Yoshizawa JK, Oliveira RZ, Lima AP, Oliveira LZ, Lima MVN Leishmaniose mucosa: considerações epidemiológicas e de tratamento. Rev bras med fam comunidade. Florianópolis, 2011 Jan-Mar; 6(18): 52-56.

Chapter 4

Molecular Tools for Understanding Eco-Epidemiology, Diversity and Pathogenesis of *Leishmania* Parasites

Souheila Guerbouj, Imen Mkada–Driss and Ikram Guizani

Additional information is available at the end of the chapter

http://dx.doi.org/10.5772/57510

1. Introduction

Protozoan parasites of the genus *Leishmania* are responsible of a large variety of clinical manifestations ranging from self-healing cutaneous forms (CL), through mucocutaneous lesions (MCL), to lethal if untreated visceral disease (VL). Nevertheless, there is no absolute correlation between a particular clinical form and a causative species [1]. For instance, parasites of the *L. donovani* complex are generally responsible for VL cases in the Old and New World but can also cause CL. Another example is the *L. tropica* species, which causes a CL form but its association to VL cases was occasionally reported [2]. Identification of *Leishmania* parasites is a central issue to patients' management and to control. Leishmaniases have a worldwide distribution but only absent in the poles regions, and in Australia where in spite of presence of the parasites in Kangourous no human cases were described. According to the WHO, 350 million people are at risk, with a prevalence of 12 million and more than 98 countries affected [3]. More than twenty species are responsible for leishmaniasis in humans. However, *Leishmania* species present very similar morphologies in their flagellated, promastigote forms and their intracellular, amastigote forms which renders necessary the use of molecular or biochemical assays for their identification and characterization (see for review [4]).

The current identification and classification of *Leishmania* is still based on isoenzyme typing, using multilocus enzyme electrophoresis (MLEE) (reviewed in [5]). This approach has been widely used for the identification of *Leishmania,* but several limitations were reported. Most importantly, differences in electrophoretic profiles were shown to be due to heterozygosity at a single nucleotide position [6–8]. Molecular studies showed also that zymodemes included distinct DNA genotypes [7,9]. Consequently, other molecular studies do not always agree with the classification of *Leishmania* by MLEE. The other limitations of MLEE are that it requires bulk cultures of parasites, it is time-consuming, and it can be performed only in specialized laboratories. Therefore, alternative DNA based tools and assays are increasingly developed and used for effective investigation and characterization of the parasites.

Indeed, the diversity of *Leishmania* species, their vectors and their reservoir hosts is a main feature of leishmaniasis, so consequently the transmission cycles are very much dependent on the environment and are very prone to changes. So not only parasite identification is needed to establish etiology of the disease and understand the pathogeny, but knowledge of parasite diversity and its population structure is also needed for a better understanding of eco-epidemiology and its changing trends. For this purpose, molecular tools have been developed to allow differentiation of *Leishmania* parasites at species and strain levels within environmental or patients' samples.

Molecular tools are based mainly on the amplification and subsequent restriction fragment length polymorphism (PCR-RFLP) of several targets including repeated gene families and coding and non-coding regions, or the sequence analysis of the products. Recently multilocus sequence typing (MLST) and multilocus microsatellite typing (MLMT) were also developed for *Leishmania* DNA typing. Each of these molecular markers or tools has its specific discriminatory power, advantages and drawbacks.

2. Parasite identification

2.1. Differentiation at the genus level

This is based on the amplification of the kinetoplast minicircle DNA (kDNA, about 10000 copies per cell) or the variable sequences of the small subunit ribosomal DNA genes (SSU rDNA, 40–200 copies per cell) [10–13].

kDNA and SSU rDNA primers were initially designed for Trypanosomatids including *Leishmania, Sauroleishmania, Crithidia* and Trypanosomes. They allow identification of *Leishmania* parasites only at the generic and/ or subgeneric level. Both targets have also been used for the development of real-time PCR assays in order to determine parasite burden in clinical samples [14,15].

2.2. Differentiation at the species level

The ability to distinguish between *Leishmania* species is crucial for a correct diagnosis of the disease as well as for making decisions regarding treatment and control measures. This is especially useful in areas where several *Leishmania* species co-exist.

Numerous PCR approaches have been published based on different coding and non-coding regions in the *Leishmania* genome. Different targets have been used, including the ribosomal internal transcribed spacer (ITS) [12,16,17], the mini-exon genes [18,19], gp63 genes [20,21], hsp70 genes [22–24] and cysteine proteinase B gene sequences (cpB) [25,26].

http://dx.doi.org/10.5772/57510

2.2.1. Randomly amplified polymorphic DNA (RAPD) and anonymous markers

Randomly amplified polymorphic DNA (RAPD) technique is based on the PCR amplification of DNA fragments using only one short primer that was arbitrarily defined and thus could be applied to any organism without a prior knowledge on the genome [27]. Such primers correspond to decamers having 60-70 % GC content and no self-complementary ends, thus the number of primers that could be used is virtually unlimited. Only in few occasions, two primers were used for *Leishmania* DNA analysis [28]; primers longer than 10 mers like universal primers used in cloning technologies have been used in some instances [29–32]. A list of selected primers used for *Leishmania* characterization is reported on Table 1. The RAPD technique generates monomorphic or polymorphic banding patterns, analyzed upon electrophoresis on agarose gels (or other supports) like DNA fingerprints. Given the fact that in comparison studies absence of bands does not reflect absence of corresponding DNA fragment in the compared DNA [33,34], the analysis is based only on Jaccard (or equivalent) distance or Similarity index [33] that only takes into account the presence of bands. RAPD reaction is very sensitive to reaction conditions even when variations are minor. Relaxed conditions and particularly low annealing temperature underlie DNA amplification but concentration or batch (quality) of DNA, reaction component, additives, brand of DNA polymerase, thermocyclers impact size range, complexity and reproducibility of the amplification profiles [33,35]. Molecular mechanisms underlying *Leishmania* DNA amplification was proposed to be based mainly on DNA mutations occurring on potential priming sites, that seem to be in regions enriched for short repeated motives [34].

Potential of RAPD and a selection of 28 primers was assessed for the discrimination between members of the *Leishmania Viannia* sub-genus which have overlapping geographical distribution in Latin America and that were difficult to distinguish by the conventional PCR using the primers then available. The authors have identified primers able to distinguish the 4 species (*L. braziliensis, L. guyanensis, L. panamensis* and *L. peruviana*) in a pair wise way. They also addressed the reliability of the technique by developing a statistical measure of the variation range of Jaccard coefficient when comparing the parasites [33].

Primer	Nucleotide sequence 5'-3'	References	Primer	Nucleotide sequence 5'-3'	References
OPA-01	CAGGCCCTTC	[30,34,36,43,44]	OPR-16	CTCTGCGCGT	[38]
H4 (OPA-02)	TGCCGAGCTG	[31,41,46]	OPR-20	ACGGCAAGGA	[38]
C4 (OPA-04)	AATCGGGCTG	[41]	OPU-15	ACGGGCCAGT	[38]
A5, P8, (OPA-05)	AGGGGTCTTG	[31,38,41,48]	OPU-16	CTGCGCTGGA	[38]
A4, (OPA-07)	GAAACGGGTG	[30,31,36,41,43]	OPU-02	CTGAGGTCTC	[43]
OPA-08	GTGACGTAGG	[28,30,31,33]	ILO 509	TGGTCAGTGA	[42]
OPA-09	GGGTAACGCC	[31]	ILO 526	GCCGTCCGA	[42]
OPA-10	GTGATCGCAG	[28,30,31,36,38,43,48]	ILO 872	CCCGCCATCT	[42]
A12 (OPA-12)	TCGGCGATAG	[41]	ILO875	GTCCGTGAGC	[41,42]

Primer	Nucleotide sequence 5'-3'	References	Primer	Nucleotide sequence 5'-3'	References
A15 (OPA-15)	TTCCGAACCC	[41]	ILO 876	GGGACGTCTC	[42]
D10 (OPA-20)	GTTGCGATCC	[41]	ILO 878	GTCGCGGAG	[42]
D8 (OPA-16)	AGCCAGCGAA	[41]	A5, C5	CTCACGTAGG	[39,41]
OPB-01	GTTTCGCTCC	[30]	C6	CTGATCGCAG	[41]
C (OPB-04)	GGACTGGAGT	[28,33,43,44]	L2	CGGACGTCGC	[41]
B5 (OPB-05)	TGCGCCCTTC	[41]	H1	CGCGCCCGCT	[39,41]
B6 (OPB-06)	TGCTCTGCCC	[41]	L15996	CTCCACCATTAGCACCC AAAGC	[29,32]
OPB-07	GGTGACGCAG	[30,41]	λg11R	TTGACACCAGACCAACT GGTAAT	[29,32]
OPB-08	GTCCACACGG	[38,41]	M13a, M13	GTAAAACGACGGCCAG T	[30,33]
OPB-09	TGGGGGACTC	[30,33]	M13-40 F/ M13 (–40) a	GTTTTCCCAGTCACGAC	[29,30,32]
OPB-10	CTGCTGGGAC	[43,44]	M13/pUC	CGCCAGGGTTTTCCCAG TCACGA	[31]
OPB-12	CCTTGACGCA	[30,41]	P53-1	ACGACAGGGCTGGTTG CCCA	[32]
OPB-13	TTCCCCCGCT	[33,41]	PLiD2-9	CAAAAGTCCCCACCAA TCCC	[42]
OPB-15	GGAGGGTGTT	[30,43]	QG1	CCATTAGCACCCAAAG CAGACCTCACCCTGTGG AGC	[29,32]
A (OPB-18)	CCACAGCAGT	[28,30,33]	TA150	ATGCGATGAGTGGTTG AG	[41,42]
OPF-01	ACGGATCCTG	[38]	TA610	TCAACCGATTACAAACC A	[42]
OPF-10	GGAAGCTTGG	[43,44]	UMS	GGGGTTGGTGTA	[31,46]
OPF-13	GGCTGCAGAA	[38,43]	37	TGGATCCGGAATTTCGG CTTCACTAC	[42]
OPN-13	AGCGTCACTC	[38]	198	GCAGGACTGC	[41]
OPN-20	GGTGCTCCGT	[38]	233	CTATGCGCGC	[35]
OPR-13	GGACGACAAG	[38]	283	CGGCCACCGT	[35,48]
OPR-14	CAGGATTCCC	[38]	3301	TCGTAGCCAA	[30,33]
OPR-15	GGACAACGAG	[38,43,44]			

Name and sequence of the primers are reported on the table as described in the references. However, for the purpose of this work all the sequences were compared to lists provided by Operon Technologies (OP); primers thus identified are reported within brackets. Primers presenting discrepancies were not reported.

Table 1. Selection of primers used in RAPD analyses of *Leishmania* parasites generating polymorphic patterns.

http://dx.doi.org/10.5772/57510

We have used the RAPD technique to identify and discriminate Old World species using 57 strains from different hosts, countries and reservoirs. Six random primers were tested from which 3 allowed to distinguish *L. aethiopica, L. arabica, L. donovani, L. major, L. tropica and L. turanica* species. We have analyzed the RAPD profiles considering criteria of consistent presence of amplified bands at the same electrophoretic presence for strains/ isolates of the same species, and the discrimination between parasites belonging to different species. This constitutes a simpler way to results interpretation that emphasizes on presence of consistently amplified and discriminative bands within a profile to overcome lack of reliability of RAPD [36]. RAPD also allowed differentiating Old World *Leishmania* species from the often co-sympatric *Sauroleishmania* parasites [30,36].

Random amplification of polymorphic DNA has been also used alone or with other techniques to confirm taxonomic status of parasites, for instance putative natural hybrids such as *L. braziliensis/L. panamensis* hybrids isolated in Nicaragua [33] or *L. braziliensis* and *L. panamensis/ guyanensis* in Ecuador [37]. In another example, genetic analysis of *Leishmania* parasites in Ecuador with MLEE and RAPD questioned the separation of *L. panamensis* and *L. guyanensis* as distinct taxa as these tools failed to generate clearly distinct clusters of parasites [38].

The RAPD technique was also used to investigate genetic diversity within *Leishmania* species or complexes in diverse settings. Causal agents of visceral leishmaniasis belong to the *L. donovani* complex, which includes the species *L. donovani, L. infantum, L. chagasi* and *L. archibaldi* [39]; however, taxonomy within this complex is controversial considering for instance *L. infantum* as forming its own complex [40]. The RAPD technique has been used to investigate intraspecific diversity of the *L. donovani* complex, using an initial set of 43 random primers [41]. Like in other studies [36,42], some primers differentiated the *L. donovani* complex from the other Old World taxa. Seven distinguished within the complex, differentiating in the tested panel of DNAs, Mediterranean *L. infantum* from the other parasites of the complex. Strikingly, none of the primers distinguished *L. donovani, L. infantum* and *L. archibaldi* taxa. Geographical clustering was observed with 2 strong Indian and East African *L. donovani* groups and a third Mediterranean *L. infantum* group in support to a previous study using RAPD in addition to other DNA tools [39]. Distribution of other *L. infantum* in the dendrogram also supports the paraphyly of *L. infantum* [41].

L. infantum zymodeme MON-1 has a worldwide distribution and is responsible mainly for a form of VL. RAPD analysis contributed to describe heterogeneity within this zymodeme and to demonstrate its polyphyletic nature [43]. The RAPD technique also highlighted geographical structures of *L. infantum* in diverse settings. In [42] they have shown that 17 (out of 18) primers tested on 33 strains isolated from diverse hosts in various Spanish regions generated highly polymorphic RAPD patterns that grouped the parasites into two main clusters that included parasites from central–western region in one side and from eastern Spain in the other. This study in addition illustrated intra-zymodemic diversity and lack of correlation with the MLEE analysis conducted on these strains, the clinical or host origin of the parasites. In another example, 53 *L. infantum* isolates from VL cases and dogs originating from different endemic regions in Brazil were analyzed with 5 RAPD primers (also used in [43]), MLMT and SSR-PCR. RAPD analysis was shown to be the most appropriate to illustrate genetic diversity of the parasites. Interestingly, in spite of the homogenous genetic background the polymorphisms observed demonstrated correlation with geographical origin [44].

In Corte Pedra, North Eastern Brazil, *L. braziliensis* is causing different American Tegumentary Leishmaniasis (ATL) forms. Forty-five *L. braziliensis* strains isolated from patients having different ATL forms were shown to generate with 3 primers and 4 protocols, RAPD patterns having overall more than 80% fingerprint identity classifying the parasites into 5 clades. Significant distribution frequency of the different clinical forms along the clades was observed. The authors thus concluded on the suitability of the RAPD analysis of parasite strains' variability in Corte Pedra and that in such a spatially limited population geographical isolation precludes geographic sequestration as the mechanism for the observed genetic structures. In addition they assumed that infection with some *L. braziliensis* genotypes could be accompanied with different pathogenic mechanisms [28]. Other studies investigating *L. braziliensis* diversity in Brazil with other primers also highlighted contrasted diversity extent of parasites isolated from cutaneous leishmaniasis according to the transmission areas; parasites from Mato Grosso [32] or from Para [29] states were more diverse than the ones in Minas Gerais. These authors proposed that eco-epidemiology of the parasites in relation to environmental and geographical differences could explain in part such diversity patterns. Genetic diversity using intergenic region typing (ITSrDNA PCR-RFLP) and MLEE of *L. braziliensis* from diverse hosts and geographical origins in Brazil also illustrated occurrence of geographical clusters of parasites exerting different levels of variability; association of *L. braziliensis* to specific transmission cycles likely reflecting adaptation of different parasite clones to the vector (and diversity of) species involved in the transmission has been inferred [45].

The RAPD technique has also been used to investigate epidemiology of leishmaniases, characterizing clinical or field isolates in diverse settings. For instance, in India the increasing reports on drug resistance of the VL patients and the implication of *L. tropica* as a causal agent of VL, also hypothesized to be a potential reason for drug unresponsiveness [2], has prompted investigations of the causal agents of VL using various DNA tools. A first study for example characterized by MLEE and 8 RAPD primers 15 clinical isolates collected over 20 years from the eastern part of India from confirmed VL patients; this sample study comprised 1 PKDL and 6 antimony unresponsive cases. All parasites proved to be *L. donovani* [31]. Another study investigated with the same primers 9 other parasites isolated over the period 2006-2010 from hospital clinics in Kolkata from confirmed VL and a PKDL cases; one parasite was similar to *L. tropica* while the others were very close to *L. donovani* [46]. The association of *L. tropica* with the disease was further confirmed in another study using ITS, ITS1 and HP70 based assays [47]. In Iran, where cutaneous leishmaniasis is highly endemic, MLEE and kDNA were used to identify species of 565 parasites obtained from confirmed CL patients from the different provinces of the country during the 2002–2008 period [48]; this study associated *L. major* mainly to rural transmission and *L. tropica* to urban settings. RAPD using 3 primers allowed describing extensive genetic heterogeneity of a random selection of 65 *L. major* strains across the different transmission area and within the same foci.

In addition, RAPD technique constitutes a powerful alternative to the identification of PCR targets and markers. RAPD markers have been exploited for the design of species or complex specific PCR assays like for instance a PCR that only amplifies DNA of parasites of the *L. donovani* complex [34] or another that amplifies exclusively *L. braziliensis* [49]. Such markers proved to be highly informative as probes or as PCR targets [34].

Randomly amplified polymorphic DNA products were used to develop markers that were targeted to develop typing strategies. For example, RAPD products that were amplified consistently across tested DNAs with a combination of 2 primers have been selected and sequenced partially to design marker specific PCR primers. The resulting PCR products were then screened for single stranded conformation polymorphisms (SSCP) and subsequently confirmed by sequence analysis [50]. This sequence confirmed amplified region analysis (SCAR) approach was used to differentiate 29 *L. donovani* strains from Sudan, Kenya, India and China using 8 different markers. The study identified 19 unique multilocus genotypes and a correlation between genotypes and geographical origin; SCAR markers were considered as co-dominant for their ability to detect all possible allele combinations in a diploid organism and as a representative random sample of neutral genetic variation in natural populations thus constituting appropriate tools for population studies [50].

Alternatively, with the objective to identify markers and develop simple assays for the discrimination of viscerotropic parasites encountered in Africa, we have screened 5 Operon kits (100 primers) for reproducible profiles and a selection of 28 primers was then used to screen for DNA markers within a panel of viscerotropic parasites from different countries in Africa and India [51]. These primers organized the parasites according to their geographical origin in a similar way to other studies using RAPD or other types of tools [39,41]. Some of the differentially amplified RAPD bands obtained in our study were cloned and sequenced; their analysis with bioinformatics tools and comparison to their respective genomic sites in *L. infantum*, *L. donovani* and *L. major* genomes highlighted the markers' association with simple sequence repeats and microsatellites in non coding regions [51]. A selection of such markers in *L. archibaldi* was used to develop simple PCR assays differentiating viscerotropic parasites, some of which in a country–specific way [52].

Randomly amplified polymorphic DNA is highly suitable for analysis of cultured *Leishmania* promastigotes but of limited interest for analysis of patients or zoonotic samples due to sample contamination with host DNA. Its use could be however contemplated to characterize promastigotes at the isolation step given the technique does not require large amounts of DNA (20 ng or less). Another generally admitted drawback is the lack of reproducibility generated by complex reactions occurring under the relaxed reaction conditions, therefore inter-laboratory or inter-study comparison using the same primers appear difficult to achieve. Options to overcome this drawback were the prior selection of primers of interest, or the use of defined criteria for analysis as for example relying only on consistently observed bands within RAPD patterns to assign the parasites to taxonomic groups [36] or using statistical tools to assess significance of the range of distances evaluated [33]. Use of well–standardized protocols may also help overcoming such a drawback. Although simple and having potential for detecting variation where other techniques fail, other drawbacks of this technique could be that bands of equal electrophoretic mobility may not be homologous [34]; identification of allelic variants is also not possible in *Leishmania*. Yet, RAPD constitutes a powerful tool for the identification of markers and the design of PCR based assays [34, 49–52]. Diverse RAPD *Leishmania* studies reached conclusions that were confirmed by other tools or alternative studies making the RAPD approach still valuable.

2.2.2. Gp63 PCR-RFLP and sequencing analyses

Gp63 genes encode for the major metalloprotease of *Leishmania,* which is the most abundant surface glycoprotein found in promastigote and amastigote forms of the parasite. GP63 protein is encoded by a cluster of tandemly repeated genes, and has been identified as a virulence factor in several *Leishmania* species. Several groups have studied the potential of gp63 as a species discriminatory tool in *Leishmania.* Amplification of gp63 genes coupled with restriction analysis (PCR-RFLP) was applied to a large number of isolates belonging to 4 species of the subgenus *Viannia,* namely *L.* (*V.*) *braziliensis, L.* (*V.*) *peruviana, L.* (*V.*) *guyanensis* and *L.* (*V.*) *lainsoni* and allowed discrimination of all the species tested [20] (Table2).

Target	Primers sequences (5'–3')	Product size (bp)	Discrimination by		Refs
			PCR-RFLP	Seq.	
kDNA	(F) Pia1: ACGAGGTCAGCTCCACTCC	100	-	-	[11,13]
	(R) Pia2: CTGCAACGCCTGTGTCTACG		-	-	
	(F) Pia3: CGGCTTCGCACCATGCGGTG	260	-	-	
	(R) Pia4: ACATCCCTGCCCACATACGC		-	-	
	(F) K13A : GTGGGGGAGGGGCGTTCT	120			
	(R) K13B: ATTTTACACCAACCCCCAGTT				
	(F) RV1: CTTTTCTGGTCCCGCGGGTAGG	145			
	(R) RV2: CCACCTGGCCTATTTTACACCA				
SSU rDNA	(F) R221: GGTTCCTTTCCTGATTTACG (R) R332: GGCCGGTAAAGGCCGAATAG	603	+	+	[10]
Gp63	(F) TDM1: GTCTCCACCGCAGACCTCACGGA (R) TDM2: TGATGTAGCTGCCATTCACGAAG	1300	+	-	[20]
	(F) SG1: GTCTCCACCGAGGACCTCACCGA	1300	+	-	[21]
	(R) SG2: TGATGTAGCCGCCCTCCTCGAAG				
	(F) PDD1: TCGGTGAGGTCCTCGGTGGAGAC	1700	+	-	
	(R) PDD2: CTTCGAGGAGGGCGGCTACATCA				
	(F) C9F: GGCTCCCGACGTGAGTTA	1750	+	-	[58]
	(R) C1R: GGGCCCGGGCGACAGCAGCGATGACTG				

http://dx.doi.org/10.5772/57510

	(F) C10F: GGGAAGCTTACGTACAGCGTGCAGGTG (R) C1R: GGGCCCGGGCGACAGCAGCGATGACTG	1600, 2000 and 4500	+	-	
ITS	(F) LITSV: ACACTCAGGTCTGTAAAC (R) LITSR: CTGGATCATTTTCCGATG	1040 or 950–1100	+ +	+ +	[64,65,69]
ITS1	(F) IR1: GCTGTAGGTGAACCTGCAGCAGCTGGATCATT (R) IR2: GCGGGTAGTCCI'GCCAAACACTCAGGTCTG	1000–1200	+	-	[16]
	(F) LITSR: CTGGATCATTTTCCGATG (R) L5.8S: TGATACCACTTATCGCACTT	300–350	+	+	[12,13,61,65,82]
ITS2	(F) LGITSF2: GCATGCCATATTCTCAGTGTC (R) LGITSR2: GGCCAACGCGAAGTTGAATTC	372–450	-	+	[63]
	(F) L5.8SR: AAGTGCG-ATAAGTGGTA (R) LITSV: ACACTCAGGTCTGTAAAC	720	-	+	[65]
ITS1and part of ITS2	(F) LITS-MG: ATG GCC AAC GCG AAG TTG (R) LITSR: CTGGATCATTTTCCGATG	800	-	+	[69]
Hsp70	PCR-G : (F) HSP70sen: GACGGTGCCTGCCTACTTCAA (R) HSP70ant: CCGCCCATGCTCTGGTACATC	1422	+	-	[22,72]
	PCR-F : (F) F25: GGACGCCGGCACGATTKCT (R) R1310: CCTGGTTGTTGTTCAGCCACTC	1286	+	-	[73–75]
	PCR-N : (F) F25: GGACGCCGGCACGATTKCT (R) R617: CGAAGAAGTCCGATACGAGGGA	593	+	-	
	PCR-C : (F) F251: GACAACCGCCTCGTCACGTTC (R) R991: GTCGAACGTCACCTCGATCTGC	741	+	-	
	(F) HSP70sen: GACGGTGCCTGCCTACTTCAA (R) HSP70ant: CCGCCCATGCTCTGGTACATC	1422	-	+	[23]
	(F) HSP70-F335 CACGCTGTCGTCCGCGACG (R) HSP70-R429 AACAGGTCGCCGCACAGCTCC	113	-	+	
	(F) HSP70-2F CTGAACAAGAGCATCAACCC (R) HSP70-2R CTTGATCAGCGCCGTCATCAC	170	-	+	
	(F) HSP70-F893 GTTCGACCTGTCCGGCATCC (R) HSP70-R1005 GTGATCTGGTTGCGCTTGCC	130	-	+	
	PCR-F : (F) HSP70-F25: GGACGCCGGCACGATTKCT (R) HSP70-R1310: CCTGGTTGTTGTTCAGCCACTC	1286	-	+	[76]
	PCR-T : (F) HSP70-6F GTGCACGACGTGGTGCTGGTG (R) HSP70-R1310: CCTGGTTGTTGTTCAGCCACTC	766	-	+	
	PCR-N : (F) HSP70-F25: GGACGCCGGCACGATTKCT (R) HSP70-R617 CGAAGAAGTCCGATACGAGGGA	593	-	+	

	3'UTR : (F) 70-IR-D: CCAAGGTCGAGGAGGTCGACTA (R) 70-IR-M: ACGGGTAGGGGGAGGAAAGA	516–733	-	+	[77]
Mini-exon	(F) Fme: TATTGGTATGCGAAACTTCCG (R) Rme: GAAACTGATACTTATATAGCG	220–443	+	+	[19,13,78]
	(F) FME2: ACTTCCGGAACCTGTCTTCC (*Leishmania* subgenus) or ACTTCCGGGACCCGTCTTCC (*Viannia* subgenus) (R) ME2R: CAGAAACTGATACTTATATAGCGTTA	220–443	+	+	[82]
Cysteine protease B	intragenic region : (F) CPBFOR: CGAACTTCGAGCGCAACCT (R) CPBREV: CAGCCCAGGACCAAAGCAA	1079	+	-	[83,84]
	Intergenic region : (F) PIGS1A: CCTCATTGCTTTGGTCCTGG (R) PIGS2B: GGCGTGCCCACGTATATCGC	1600	+	-	
	cpbEF: (F) CGTGACGCCGGTGAAGAAT (R) CGTGCACTCGGCCGTCTT	702–741	-	-	[25,85]
	cpbEF: (F) CGTGACGCCGGTGAAGAAT (R) CGTGCACTCGGCCGTCTT	702–741	+	+	[26]
	Leishmania cpb: (F) LmcpbUNIF: ACGGTCTTAGCGTGCGAGTTGTG (R) LmcpbUNIR: CAAGGAGGTCCCCTCACGCG	1440	-	+	[85]
	L. major cpb (variant 1): (F) LmcpbUNIF: ACGGTCTTAGCGTGCGAGTTGTG (R) LmcpbR: TCGTGCAGCACATGTCGCTTG	1176	-	+	
	L. infantum cpb: (F) cpbEF For: CGTGACGCCGGTGAAGAAT (R) L. inf Rev: CGTTTCGTTGCTCGGGATCAT	325	-	-	
	L. tropica cpb: (F) LmcpbUNIF: ACGGTCTTAGCGTGCGAGTTGTG (R) Ltro Rev: ACAGGGCCGTCAGCCCGTGGC	600	-	-	
	L. infantum cpb: (F) infcpbE: GTCTTACCAGAGCGGAGTGCTACT (R) Inf2.1: ATAACCAGCCATTCGGTTTTG	278	-	-	[86]
	L. donovani cpb: (F) cpbF2.1: GCGGCGTGATGACCAGC (R) Do2.1: CAATAACCAGCCATTCGTTTTTA	309	-	-	
	(F) MATRAE2: GGCGATGGTGGAGCAGATGATCT		-	-	

(R) Ma4.1: CGGTTCTCGTAGCACACTTGTTG	99 (*L. major*)			
(R) Tr4.1: CTCCCCCGTTCGGAT	100 (*L. tropica*)			
(R) Ae2.1: AGTACGTGCACATCAGCACATGGG	154 (*L. aethiopica*)			
(F) V5F: GGTGATGTGCCCGAGTGCA (R) V10R: CGTGCACATCAGCACATGGG	564	-	-	
(F) CpbF: GTGCGTGCGGGTCGTGC (R) CpbR: AAAGCCCCGGACCAAAGCA	735	-	-	[87]

(F): Forward primer; (R): Reverse primer; Seq.: sequence analysis; Refs: references

Table 2. Overview of DNA targets, primers sequences, product sizes and the technique used to achieve discrimination of *Leishmania* taxa.

Gp63 PCR-RFLP tool was also used to characterize isolates representative of the *L. donovani* complex (*L. infantum, L. donovani, L. archibaldi* and *L. chagasi*), with special attention to Mediterranean *L. infantum* from different geographical origins, in addition to representative strains of Old World *Leishmania* (*L. major, L. tropica* and *L. aethiopica*) [21] (Table2). This allowed discrimination of the 4 species of the *L. donovani* complex, which were quite distinct from the outgroup. Within *L. infantum*, the parasites were found to be polymorphic showing a geographical structuring [21]. Sequences of the gp63 genes were explored in 33 strains of the *L. donovani* complex having different origins and zymodemes, in addition to reference strains of other Old World species [53]. Evolution of the gp63 multigene family was inferred to be under the influence of a mosaic or fragmental gene conversion mechanism. The sequences clustered according to the species, showing a concerted evolution of the different gene classes. Phylogenetic analyses confirmed the genetic diversity of the *L. donovani* complex, which showed that gp63 genes could provide the basis for rapid and reliable genotyping of strains in this complex [53].

Furthermore, still using gp63 coding sequences PCR-RFLP evaluated intra-specific polymorphism of *L. infantum* isolates in Tunisia [54]. In total, 22 *L. infantum* isolates responsible of visceral (14 isolates) and cutaneous (8 isolates) forms of leishmaniasis in Tunisia were analysed, in addition to reference isolates, representative of Old World complexes. The *Sal*I, *Hinc*II, *Bal*I and *Bsi*EI restriction enzymes were used in this intragenic gp63 PCR-RFLP analysis. Results showed profiles that allowed distinction of *L. infantum* from the other species belonging to the *L. donovani* complex (*L. donovani, L. archibaldi* and *L. chagasi*) but also from the Old World species *L. major, L. tropica* and *L. aethiopica*. Besides, polymorphic patterns were observed among *L. infantum* isolates that tend to be correlated to the clinical presentation of the disease; the phenetic analysis using a UPGMA clustering method (Phylip package) grouped all VL isolates together while most of the CL parasites clustered in a separate branch. Good bootstrapping values supported the clusters [54].

The gp63 PCR-RFLP method was applied to characterise parasites contained within the lesions of patients having cutaneous leishmaniasis, originating from areas in central Tunisia, known to be free of CL. This analysis confirmed assignment of the parasites to the *L. infantum* species, thus demonstrating the occurrence/emergence of sporadic cutaneous leishmaniasis (SCL) due to *L. infantum* in central Tunisia [55].

The gp63 PCR associated to RFLP analysis was also used to characterise transmitted *Leishmania* in Sudan. Patients that presented with uncommon cutaneous leishmaniasis, including one case with a *L. tropica* like-lesion, were confirmed, using this tool, to be infected by *L. major* [56]. In another study, *Leishmania* parasites from Sudanese patients having cutaneous ulcers were analyzed by gp63 PCR-RFLP and shown to belong to the *L. donovani* species [56]. This work allowed concluding that, in addition to *L. major, L. donovani* species can also be a major cause of CL in Sudan [57].

Another PCR-RFLP analysis of the gp63 intergenic region was also developed and tested on the *L. donovani* complex [58]. The markers generated robust and congruent phylogenies, identifying 5 genetic clusters within *L. donovani* complex. Furthermore, clusters strongly correlated with isoenzyme typing and some with geographical origin, which may be important for epidemiological and clinical studies [58].

Although the gp63 PCR RFLP technique has been successfully used for *Leishmania* discrimination at the species and strains levels, it presents several disadvantages. The fragment patterns obtained are sometimes vey complex and can be difficult to analyze and compare between laboratories. Also, partial restriction needs to be carefully evaluated as a potential source of artefacts. This technique depends therefore, on careful standardization and is recommended for comparative studies involving few strains rather than for large-scale epidemiological studies. Given the size of the sequences amplified (1.3Kb for the intragenic PCR) and the number of (GC rich) copies, the PCR assay requires good quality DNA and additives like DMSO [21] and thus a careful establishment step.

2.2.3. *ITS1 PCR–RFLP and ITS2 targets*

Ribosomal RNA (rRNA) genes are highly repetitive and conserved sequences. The ITS1 region is the sequence in between the 18S rRNA and 5.8S rRNA genes. It has enough conservation to serve as a PCR target but sufficient polymorphisms to facilitate species typing. ITS1 PCR has been developed in combination with an RFLP analysis (Table2) with different restriction enzymes (*Alu*I, *BstU*I, *EcoR*I, *Fsp*I, *Hae*III, *Hha*I, *Rsa*I, *Sau3A*I, *Sph*I and *Taq*I) [16]; *Hae*III is the mostly used restriction enzyme used for species identification. Indeed, ITS1 PCR–RFLP using *Hae*III is the most widely used assay for direct detection and identification of *Leishmania* species in the Old World.

It has been applied for the distinction of sympatric species, especially in the Mediterranean region [59,60]. However, representatives of the *L. donovani* complex (*L. donovani* and *L. infantum*) and also of the *L. braziliensis* complex (*L. braziliensis, L. guyanensis, L. panamensis, L. peruviana*) cannot be distinguished by this approach, even using a great variety of restriction enzymes [12]. This limitation can however be bypassed by sequencing of the ITS1 PCR product thus allowing for a clear separation of these species and also assignment of different strains [61].

Recently, real-time PCR product from the ITS1 region has been used in a high-resolution melt (HRM) analysis in order to identify and quantify Old World *Leishmania* species [62]. High resolution melt analysis is a molecular technique that uses a fluorescent intercalating dye to measure the rate of double stranded DNA dissociation consequent to an increase of temperature. The observed melting curve is characteristic of a particular DNA and depends on its sequence length, GC content, complementarity, and nearest neighbour thermodynamics. The dye is incorporated during the amplification; the DNA dissociation measures occur at the end of the PCR, which is performed in a dedicated thermocycler. The results are computerized and analyzed through a graphic output. When tested on 300 samples from human cases, reservoir hosts and sand flies, this approach distinguished all Old World *Leishmania* species causing human disease, except *L. donovani* from *L. infantum* [62].

The ITS2 region is located in between the 5.8S rRNA and LSU rRNA genes. It has been studied and found to be adequate for species identification. Indeed, generic PCR primers (LGITSF2/ LGITSR2) were designed to amplify this fragment from *Leishmania* spp. associated with human infection, using reference isolates [63] (Table 2). Substantial differences in the ITS2 region amplified by these primers followed by sequencing analysis, allowed detection of and discrimination among *Leishmania* species from the Old and New World [63]. The ITS2 PCR followed by DNA sequence analysis approach was validated on clinical specimens, which allowed identification of a total of 8 *Leishmania* species (*L. (V.) braziliensis, L. (V.) guyanensis, L. (V.) panamensis, L. (L.) mexicana, L. aethiopica, L. major, L. tropica and the L. donovani* complex) among 159 patients corresponding to U.S. civilians that had travel and immigration history to leishmaniasis endemic countries [63].

The ITS1 and ITS2 region have also been used to assess intra-specific DNA polymorphisms among *L. donovani* isolates from different geographical origins [64,65] (Table 2). Single-stranded conformation polymorphism (SSCP), and sequencing of the ITS regions were applied to clinical samples of *L. donovani* from Sudan and one from Kenya, one from India and one from China. Intra-specific variation in SSCP banding patterns was clearly observed in the ITS1 region and gave five different SSCP profiles; 3 profiles were detected among Sudan isolates and 2 ITS1-SSCP profiles were observed among the samples from Kenya, India, and China [65]. This corroborates the results of a previous study in which 11 polymorphic ITS1-SSCP patterns were identified among 63 clinical samples of *L. donovani* from eastern Sudan [64]. On the other hand, no variation was observed in the ITS2 region among the 63 studied cases from Sudan [64] and the study that analyzed the ITS2 locus among 23 Sudanese samples, showed again the same ITS2 SSCP pattern, with the exception of 1 isolate that had a different one [65].

When the species *L. tropica* was studied using ITS1 amplification and SSCP analysis, 14 SSCP profiles within 29 strains from different Old World geographical areas were found [66,67]. The *L. major* species was also investigated for DNA polymorphisms using ITS1 and ITS2 PCR amplification followed by SSCP analysis and sequencing [68]. Results revealed in total five genotypic variants among *L. major* isolates from Iran [68].

Recently, authors from Iran used primers LITSR and LITSV to amplify whole ITS region and found a double banded electrophoretic pattern in *L. tropica* species, while a sharp single band was observed for *L. infantum* and *L. major* isolates [69]. In order to explain how this two-band pattern occur in *L. tropica*, an *in silico* analysis of ITS sequences was conducted and showed the existence of two groups of sequences that differ by a 100bp gap, indicating existence of at least two alleles for ITS in ribosomal DNA. Thus, a specific reverse primer was developed (LITS-MG, Table 2) in order to amplify, with LITSR, sequences located just before the gap, which included ITS1 5.8S and a part of the ITS2 sequence. Amplification using LITS-MG/ LITSR primer set, followed by sequencing, allowed discriminating *L. tropica* from *L. infantum* or *L. major* [69].

Although PCR-RFLP of the ITS1 spacer is the most widely used assay for direct detection and identification of *Leishmania* species in the Old World, it has some limitations. Despite that all medically relevant *Leishmania* species can be distinguished by digesting the ITS1 PCR product with *Hae*III restriction enzyme, representatives of the *L. donovani* complex (*L. donovani* and *L. infantum*) or *L. braziliensis* complex (*L. braziliensis, L. guyanensis, L. panamensis* and *L. peruviana*) have almost identical RFLP patterns with a great variety of restriction enzymes and cannot be resolved further by this approach [12]. This problem can, however be solved partially by sequencing the ITS1 PCR product. Use of a highly resolutive agarose or SSCP analysis may be needed to resolve differences between some species or to investigate intra-specific polymorphism, respectively. ITS2 region has also served for species identification but the drawback of this approach is the need for DNA sequencing analysis. Sequencing or SSCP analysis may not be available in most laboratories in areas of endemicity.

2.2.4. hsp70 PCR–RFLP and sequencing

The 70kDa heat-shock proteins (HSP70) are encoded by genes that are highly conserved across prokaryotes and eukaryotes both in sequence and function. They have great importance as molecular chaperones in protein folding and transport [70]. Genes encoding cytoplasmic HSP70s were among the first kinetoplastid genes that were cloned and characterized because of their conserved nature [71]. HSP70 protein and its encoding gene have been widely used for phylogenetic and taxonomic studies of different parasites, including *Leishmania*.

The PCR-RFLP approach targeting hsp70 sequences has proven to be most useful for the differentiation between South American *Leishmania* species from the subgenus *Viannia* (Table2). Using the restriction enzyme *Hae*III to digest the amplified product, the produced RFLP patterns allowed discrimination between *L. guyanensis* species complex as well as for *L. lainsoni* and *L. shawi* [22,24]. However, *L. braziliensis* and *L. peruviana*, both belonging to the *L. braziliensis* complex, as well as *L. naiffi* showed an identical *Hae*III RFLP pattern. They can be distinguished by using other restriction endonucleases like *Mbo*I and *BstUI* [24]. The Hsp70 PCR-RFLP approach was extended for identification of Old World and additional New World species with an improved resolution within species complexes; in total 139 strains from 14 species were studied using *Hae*III, *Bcc*I, *Rsa*I, *Mlu*I, and *BsaHI* restriction enzymes [72]. Two subsequent digestions of the PCR products identified the species *L. infantum* and *L. donovani* (*Hae*III and *Mlu*I), *L. tropica* and *L. aethiopica* (*Hae*III and *BsaH*I), *L. braziliensis* and *L. peruviana* (*Hae*III and *Rsa*I), *L. guyanensis* and *L. panamensis* (*Hae*III and *Bcc*I); the first digestion using *Hae*III discriminates among the broad groups while the additional ones discriminate within these groups; the species *L. major, L. lainsoni* and *L. naiffi* had specific patterns with *Hae*III restriction enzyme, without need to use an additional digestion [72]. However, it was not possible to differentiate between the species *L. mexicana, L. amazonensis,* and *L. garnhami* [72].

In order to improve the sensitivity and specificity of the previously reported hsp70 PCR, alternative PCR primers and RFLPs were used [73] (Table2). Thus, three new PCR primer sets (PCR-F, PCR-N, and PCR-C) and their corresponding restriction scheme (RFLP-F, RFLP-N, and RFLP-C) were tested. The detection limit of the new PCRs was between 0.05 and 0.5 parasite genomes; they amplified clinical samples more efficiently, and were *Leishmania* specific. A specific discriminative power was found for each new RFLP analysis: in general species from the Old World (*L. major, L. tropica, L. aethiopica, L. donovani, L. infantum*) and from the New World (*L. infantum, L. lainsoni, L. peruviana, L. guyanensis, L. panamensis*) were well differentiated [73]. Discrimination of *L. guyanensis* and *L. panamensis* species, both belonging to the *L. guyanensis* complex is important for epidemiological purposes and has also consequences for the prognosis of the disease, since MCL, which is principally associated with *L. braziliensis*, can also be caused by other *L.* (*Viannia*) suspected species. Recently, an updated hsp70PCR RFLP protocol for RFLP-F and RFLP-N designed in [73] was published, with new restriction enzymes [74]. These new enzymes showed reduced cost and allowed better separation of some New World (sub)species [74].

Relevance of the hsp70 PCR-RFLP approach [72–74] is illustrated by a study that applied it on 89 clinical samples from a total of 73 Peruvian patients with either cutaneous or mucocutaneous leishmaniasis. The new PCRs were tested on tissue samples, lesion biopsies, aspirates, and scrapings. They showed an improved sensitivity both for genus detection and species typing and identified the species *L. braziliensis, L. peruviana* and *L. guyanensis* [75].

In addition to PCR-RFLP analysis, the hsp70 gene was also used in sequencing. Indeed, the 1380bp fragment of the coding region commonly used in RFLP analysis was sequenced in 43 isolates from different geographic origins for studying evolutionary relationships [23]. Fifty-two hsp70 sequences representing 17 species commonly causing leishmaniasis both in the New and Old World were analyzed. The authors found that the genus *Leishmania* formed a monophyletic group with three distinct subgenera *L. (Leishmania), L. (Viannia),* and *L. (Sauroleishmania).* The obtained phylogeny supported the eight species *L. (L.) donovani, L. (L.) major, L. (L.) tropica, L. (L.) mexicana, L. (V.) lainsoni, L. (V.) naiffi, L. (V.) guyanensis* and *L. (V.) braziliensis.* In some of the species, subspecies *L. (L.) donovani infantum, L. (V.) guyanensis panamensis,* and *L. (V.) braziliensis peruviana* were recognized [23]. Recently, sequencing of the hsp70 gene was useful for *Leishmania* species determination within clinical samples, overcoming need for parasite isolation [76]. The results obtained were in great agreement with those from multilocus enzyme electrophoresis [76].

The 3′-untranslated region (UTR) of hsp70-type I gene constitutes an alternative target for sequence analysis [77]. These authors who used it to analyse 24 strains representing 11 *Leishmania* species, found a remarkable degree of sequence conservation in this region, even between species of the subgenera *Leishmania* and *Viannia.* In addition, the presence of many microsatellites was a common feature of the 3′-UTR of HSP70-I genes in the *Leishmania* genus. Global sequence alignments and resulting dendrograms demonstrated usefulness of this particular region of hsp70 genes for species (or species complex) typing, improving the discrimination capacity of phylogenetic trees based on hsp70 coding sequences in case of some species (*L. donovani/L. infantum; L. tropica* and *L. aethiopica; L. braziliensis/L. peruviana; L. guyanensis/L. panamensis*) [77].

Using hsp70 gene in PCR followed by RFLP or sequence analysis presents many advantages. It is easily comparable across all *Leishmania* species worldwide and discriminates all relevant species in both subgenera *L. (Leishmania)* and *L. (Viannia)*. In addition, the approach has been optimized for direct amplification from clinical samples. However, systematic sequencing of the hsp70 gene for *Leishmania* identification purposes represents the major disadvantage of this approach, since this technique needs high-resource settings. For this, it was stated, "this method is especially suited for use in non-endemic infectious disease clinics dealing with relatively few cases on an annual basis, for which no fast high throughput diagnostic tests are needed" [76].

2.2.5. Mini-exon PCR-RFLP

The mini-exon genes are involved in the trans-splicing process of nuclear mRNA in kinetoplastid protozoa and are present as 100 to 200 tandemly repeated copies per nuclear genome. Mini-exon genes contain a highly conserved exon of 39 bp with a moderately variable transcribed intron region (55 to 101 bp) and a highly variable non-transcribed spacer sequence (51 to 341 bp). These genes were extensively used as a PCR target to identify and discriminate Old and New World *Leishmania* species [19,78]. This PCR assay amplified all the miniexon sequences in a single reaction (Table2). In addition, size variability of the amplification products allowed preliminary discrimination between the major complexes (Old and New World *Leishmania*, and New World *Viannia* complexes). After enzymatic restriction of the PCR product with *Hae*III or *Eae*I, a characteristic RFLP pattern is produced that depends on size variations in the polymorphic spacer regions as well as mutations in the recognition sites of the restriction enzymes. *Eae*I profiles were shown to be more informative than *Hae*III and allowed to distinguish between the most important Old World species, *L. major, L. tropica, L. aethiopica, L. infantum* and *L. donovani* [19,78]. However, with *Hae*III, species belonging to the *L. braziliensis* complex (*L. braziliensis* and *L. peruviana*) and to the *L. guyanensis* complex (*L. guyanensis* and *L. panamensis*) could be discriminated [19].

This genotyping method was successfully applied to naturally infected clinical samples for the differentiation of New and Old World *Leishmania* species and showed a high sensitivity and a robust and reliable species differentiation power [79]. Several other research groups have applied mini-exon PCR-RFLP method for identification and characterisation of *Leishmania* species, using various types of samples from different countries. In [80], they have analyzed microcapillary cultivated isolates from cutaneous and visceral cases in Turkey and identified the species *L. infantum* and *L. tropica* in CL cases, and *L. infantum* in VL ones. In Nepal, bone marrow aspirates from VL patients were analyzed by mini-exon PCR-RFLP and the parasites have been shown similar to the standard Indian strain of *L. donovani* and different from the Kenyan strain [81].

Recently, mini-exon PCR-RFLP was compared to the ITS1 PCR RFLP approach on a set of reference strains [82]. The ITS1 PCR proved to be slightly more sensitive and more practical than the mini-exon. Analysis using the ITS1 digested with *Hae*III allowed to distinguish most species but an additional digestion with *Cfo*I may be helpful in case of *L. mexicana*. However, using the mini-exon, sequencing was found to be the most practical approach as the mini-exon sequences add information since they are more polymorphic than the ITS1 sequences [82]. Therefore, the mini-exon genes were used for typing the species that belong to the *L. Viannia* subgenus, also known as *L. braziliensis* complex, which cannot be distinguished with the ITS1 [82].

2.2.6. *Cysteine protease B (cpb) based PCR and PCR RFLP*

Cpb genes are multicopy genes that encode for cathepsin L-like cysteine proteinase B (cpb), a major antigen of *Leishmania* parasites.

PCR RFLP assays targeting cpb genes and their non-coding inter-genic sequences were also developed and applied for characterization of strains from the *L. donovani* complex [83] (Table2). The following enzymes were used for intra-genic cpb PCR-RFLP: *Hinf*I, *Taa*I, *Hae*III, *Cfr*I, *Hpa*II, and *Sdu*I, and for inter-genic cpb PCR-RFLP: *Eam*1104I, *Nsp*I, *Hae*III, *Acy*I, and *Hae*II [83]. The discriminatory power of this assay was compared with that of PCR-RFLP analysis of the gp63 gene, and multilocus enzyme electrophoresis (MLEE). Restriction patterns of the cpb locus were polymorphic, but less so than gp63 patterns and presented differences with MLEE, supporting a different classification of parasites. The applicability of the developed cpb PCR RFLP approach also allowed direct genotyping of parasites in bone marrow aspirates and blood samples obtained from VL patients in Nepal [83]. This cpb PCR RFLP approach, in addition to a gp63 PCR-RFLP analysis, were applied to study 59 isolates of the *L. infantum* species obtained from different regions in Algeria, originating from various clinical forms and hosts, and assigned to different zymodemes [84]. Among the four analyzed zymodemes, 15 different genotypes were obtained. Also, cpb polymorphism showed two interesting trends: a possible relationship with the cutaneous origin of the isolates and an association with a West-East cline [84].

Different species–specific PCR assays were developed using these genes as target. PCR assays discriminating *L. donovani* from *L. infantum* were developed [25,26]. An *L. donovani* species-specific PCR primer pair amplifies a 317bp at the 3' end of cpb gene of *L. donovani* whereas it does not generate an amplicon for *L. infantum* [26]. Another PCR that was developed based on cysteine protease B genes differentiates *L. infantum* from *L. donovani* by their fragment length: a 741bp product (cpbF) characterized *L. donovani* strains, and a 702bp product (cpbE) *L. infantum* strains [25]. This primer pair more recently was tested, in addition to a newly designed one (cpbEF For/L.inf Rev, Table2), on 10 Tunisian *L. infantum* isolates. The amplification showed size polymorphism of cpbEF genes with either a 702bp or a 741bp product, even though the species *L. donovani* has never been described in Tunisia and the Mediterranean region [85].

Five species-specific PCR tests that can discriminate each of the Old World species: *L. infantum, L. donovani, L. tropica, L. aethiopica,* and *L. major* in cultured parasite isolates were also developed [86] (Table2). All the PCRs are based on the species-specific amplification of the cpb genes as each primer pair amplifies only one of the different cpb copies present in a particular species. In addition, the authors established the adaptation of 2 of these assays for oligochromatography detection, which is a rapid dipstick test for visualization of specific amplified *L. infantum* and *L. donovani* products. They concluded to the value of these assays for the identification of parasites *in vitro* but the assays were not shown sensitive enough to identify *Leishmania* parasites within clinical samples [86].

However, upon sequencing of the cpb- coding region in clinical isolates of *L. aethiopica*, specific PCR primers (V5F/V10R) were developed to differentiate this species from *L. tropica, L. major, L. donovani* and *L. infantum* by direct PCR (Table2). This cpb PCR proved to be sensitive enough to detect *L. aethiopica* from biopsy samples [87].

Recently, primers developed in [25] were used and new ones were designed, to set up three species-specific PCR assays based on the amplification of different copies and parts of the cpb genes (Table2) [85]. They allowed amplification of 1176bp, 600bp and 325bp fragments, thus discriminating between Old World Tunisian *L. major, L. tropica* and *L. infantum* species, respectively [85].

Multi-copy cpb genes have been recently used to develop a species–specific *L. infantum* LAMP assay (Loop-Mediated Isothermal reaction) for the diagnosis of canine leishmaniasis in Tunisia [88]. This isothermal nucleic acid amplification technique uses intrinsic properties of the enzyme (*Bst* DNA polymerase) for auto-strand displacement DNA synthesis to amplify large amounts of DNA within 30–60 minutes. The amplification reaction that is conducted at only one temperature does not require a thermocycler and takes profit of the intricate design of a set of six specific primers [89]. LAMP has emerged as a powerful tool for diagnostics and has been successfully developed for several protozoan parasitic diseases including leishmaniasis [90]. Use of cpb genes in the LAMP assay successfully allowed to detect the *L. infantum* DNA with a specific amplification, as no cross reaction was seen, with *L. major, L. tropica, L. turanica, L. aethiopica, L. tarentolae, L. gerbilli, Trypanosoma cruzi,* or human genomic DNA. In addition, LAMP assay showed a higher sensitivity when compared to conventional cpb based PCRs [88].

Cpb coding sequence and UTR targets have a proven and good potential to characterize or identify *Leishmania* species. Their antigenic nature makes them interesting to describe epidemiological features in some areas. However in spite of being multi-copy targets, sensitivity of their detection seem to be limited likely due to sequence variations underlying the primers used.

2.2.7. Cytochrome gene sequencing

Cytochromes are involved in the electron transport process of the mitochondrial respiratory chain. They are considered one of the most useful genes for taxonomy given their slow evolution rate. They were used for discrimination of *Leishmania* parasites as well as for exploring their phylogenetic relationships. Cytochrome oxidase II gene has been first analyzed for sequence variation in 22 *Leishmania* isolates representative of the *L. donovani* complex from different geographical origins [91]. Phylogenetic analysis produced maximum parsimony, neighbor joining and maximum likelihood trees that were congruent and showed two clades corresponding to the species *L. donovani* and *L. infantum*. Furthermore, the molecular haplotypes were concordant, in general, with the isoenzyme data of the complex [91]. Interestingly, *L. donovani* isolates from Sudan were shown to possess the most ancestral cytochrome oxidase II sequence with a single haplotype that was very close to that of *L. major* [91]. The data provided in this work allowed an approximate dating of the origin of the *L. donovani* complex to a period contemporary to or predating the spread of modern humans out of Africa [91].

Cytochrome b (*Cyt b*) gene has also been used to determine the nucleotide sequence from 13 human-infecting *Leishmania* species from the New and Old Worlds [92]. The phylogenetic relationships based on this gene, showed good agreement with the classification of Lainson & Shaw [93] except for the inclusion of *L. major* in the *L. tropica* complex and the placement of *L. tarentolae* in another genus [92]. The same group has further applied this method to other *Leishmania* species to construct a new phylogenic tree [94]. A total of 30 *Leishmania* and *Endotrypanum* WHO reference strains were analyzed. The phylogenic tree obtained showed mainly the exclusion of *L. major* from the *L. tropica* complex, the placement of *L. tarentolae* in the genus and location of *L. turanica* and *L. arabica* far from human pathogenic *Leishmania* strains [94].

Since that, *Cyt b* gene have been sequenced in several studies and was shown to be able to identify the *Leishmania* species, in Pakistan [95,96], in Colombia [97] and in China [98]. Furthermore, results of *Cyt b* gene sequencing of 69 cutaneous leishmaniasis cases in Pakistan showed that only *L. tropica* was found in highland areas and only *L. major* in lowland areas [96]. Importantly, among *L. major* samples analyzed, three types of *Cyt b* polymorphism were found, including 45 cases of type I, six of type II and one of type III [96]. The authors reported for the first time on the presence of polymorphisms in *L. major* (types I, II and III) based on species identification using *Cyt b* gene sequencing from clinical samples [96].

This target is a slow evolving DNA molecule and is thus considered as a good marker for phylogeny. Being located on the mitochondrial maxicercle, the copy number constitutes another advantage. Given demonstration of natural genetic exchange experimentally [99] and naturally [100], these targets known to have a monoparental transmission (also confirmed for *Leishmania*) could be ideal for genetic exchange analyses.

2.2.8. Other molecular tools

Several other molecular tools have also been used for identification and characterization of *Leishmania*. These include quantitative PCR, AFLP, LAMP assay and others.

In recent years, quantitative PCR methods based either on SYBR Green or TaqMan technology have been set up for the quantification of *Leishmania* in different types of biopsies from mice, dogs and also from human peripheral blood, targeting either single-copy or multi-copy sequences with high sensitivity and reproducibility [101–104]. In particular, quantitative real time PCR assays (qPCR) were developed to detect and rapidly differentiate *Leishmania* species and also to quantify parasites within clinical samples. Primers used recognized kinetoplast minicircle [105,106] and ribosomal DNA [107].

Amplified fragment length polymorphism (AFLP) has also been developed for *Leishmania* typing [108]. This technique essentially probes the entire genome at random, without prior sequence knowledge. Thus, it is ideally suited as a screening tool for molecular markers linked with biological and clinical traits. It is a PCR-based technique that uses restriction enzymes to digest DNA, followed by ligation of adapters to the ends of the restriction fragments, which will be then amplified using specific primers. The amplified fragments are separated and visualised on denaturing polyacrylamide gels, through autoradiography or fluorescence methodologies or using automated capillary sequencing instruments. AFLP was adapted to the *Leishmania* genome and validated on a panel of samples from the *L. donovani* complex. Results were highly congruent with previous analyses using multiple other molecular tests [109]. AFLPs are particularly useful for assessing genetic variation and genome mapping over other existing molecular techniques (reviewed in [110]).

Assays using alternative amplification technologies such as quantitative nucleic acid sequence-based amplification (QT-NASBA) based on amplification of 18S RNA or Loop mediated isothermal amplification (LAMP) targeting rRNA, kinetoplast DNA or a multigenic family were also tested on *Leishmania* infected samples. QT-NASBA yielded a sensitivity of 97.5% and a specificity of 100% when tested on skin biopsy samples from Old and New World CL patients [111]. A generic loop mediated isothermal amplification (LAMP) of reverse transcribed 18SRNA had a 83% sensitivity on blood samples of VL patients from Sudan and 98% sensitivity on skin biopsies of CL patients from Suriname [90]. An *L. donovani* specific LAMP was developed targeting kinetoplast minicircle DNA that had 80% sensitivity on 10 blood samples of VL patients from Bengladesh [112]. This assay evaluated on a larger number of patients (N=75) and 101 negative controls had 90% sensitivity and 100% specificity; these performances were found comparable to a nested PCR assay tested on the same samples [113]. An *L. infantum* specific LAMP assay, targeting the cysteine protease B multi copy gene was also recently developed [88]. This tool applied on detection of dog infection in Tunisia had a sensitivity of 54% and a specificity of 80%, a better performance than the one obtained with a Cpb PCR assay [88]. LAMP assays constitute promising tools for rapid and sensitive detection of *Leishmania* DNA, however for discrimination of *Leishmania* species and strains other tools may appear superior at this stage. Their main advantage remains the rapid delivery of results and the minimal equipment requirement.

3. Strain typing

3.1. Multilocus sequence typing (MLST)

Multilocus sequence typing (MLST) refers to analysis based on the DNA sequence of multiple gene targets. It is based on the comparison of partial sequences (usually 700 bp) of a defined set of housekeeping genes. Similarly to MLEE, alleles are scored as identical or not, regardless of how many different polymorphic loci they have. Strains sharing the same allele combina-

http://dx.doi.org/10.5772/57510

tions for the set of genes tested are referred to as sequence types. MLST is able to detect co-dominant single nucleotide polymorphisms (SNP) and although indels can complicate the analysis, they are extremely rare in protein-coding genes.

The first *Leishmania* complex that has been studied with MLST is the *L. donovani* complex. Two sets of 5 loci corresponding to genes coding for enzymes used in MLEE were studied: one set with asat, gpi, nh1, nh2 and pgd and the other one with icd, me, mpi, g6pdh, and fh [7,8]. Results were found to be largely in agreement with the results from MLEE although some key discrepancies were found and increased resolution was obtained. Thus silent SNPs were found that provide further resolution, such as a single SNP in gpi that distinguishes between strains of *L. infantum* [7]. However, SNPs responsible for amino acid changes were also found in genes coding for enzymes giving indistinguishable electrophoretic profiles, mainly in nh2, which had the same protein band for all *L. donovani* complex strains. MLST study contributed to better understanding of *L. donovani* complex phylogeny and taxonomical position of the species *L. infantum* and *L. donovani* [114]. It was a strong argument to question the position of *L. archibaldi* as a species [6] and existence of MLEE defined *L. infantum* in Sudan [8]. It also highlighted potential occurrence of genetic exchange among circulating parasites in East Africa [7,8].

MLST using 6 gene targets that are not associated with MLEE analysis (inorganic pyrophosphatase, spermidine synthase 1, hypoxanthine-guanine phosphoribosyl transferase, mitogen-activated protein kinase, RNA polymerase II largest sub-unit and adenylate kinase 2) have been used to characterize suspected *L. major/L. infantum* hybrids and representative co-endemic strains in Portugal [115]. Sequence analyses confirmed MLEE hybrid profiles and hybrid status with occurrence of heterozygous positions in the target genes that so far were not studied for their diversity within *Leishmania* species. In a more recent work, 2 of these genes and 5 others (Elongation initiation factor 2 alpha subunit, zinc binding dehydrogenase-like protein, translation initiation factor alpha subunit, nucleoside hydrolase-like protein and a hypothetical protein located on chromosome 31) were analyzed on a panel of 222 strains representative of 10 different species in 43 countries in Eurasia and Africa, corresponding to 110 zymodemes with the objective to study the genetic diversity of the genus *Leishmania*, improving our knowledge on the genetic structure and genomic evolution mechanisms of this genus [116]. Seven genetically robust clusters were obtained that overlapped with most of the biochemical taxonomy groups: clusters I, III, IV, V and VI included strains belonging to the MLEE-based species *L. aethiopica, L. arabica, L. turanica, L. gerbilli* and *L. major*, respectively and cluster II included the *L. tropica* and *L. killicki* strains; with the exception of the species that cause forms of visceral leishmaniasis (cluster VII that comprised strains from *L. donovani, L. infantum* and *L. archibaldi*) in line with the concept of species complex suggested for this group. No observations were made of interspecific recombination or genetic exchange between the different species but these strains were selected for the study as not resulting from a likely genetic exchange [116]. It is anticipated to observe more informative studies increasing the number of markers or the strains circulating within selected endemic areas notably that co-sympatry of multiple parasite species is a well-established feature in many endemic areas.

In the New World, four housekeeping genes (glucose-6-phosphate dehydrogenase (G6PD), 6-phosphogluconate dehydrogenase (6PGD), mannose phosphate isomerase (MPI) and isocitrate dehydrogenase (ICD)) were sequenced from 96 *Leishmania* (*Viannia*) strains that were chosen to be representative of the zymodeme and geographical species diversity of this subgenus, in South America, and in particular Brazil, in order to assess their discriminatory typing capacity and refine phylogeny of the *L.* (*Viannia*) species [117]. A large number of haplotypes were detected for each marker. Maximum parsimony-based haplotype networks showed separated clusters in each network, corresponding to strains of different species, congruent with the MLEE identification. Besides, NeighborNet formed by the concatenated sequences confirmed species-specific clusters. This analysis also suggested recombination occurring in *L. braziliensis* and *L. guyanensis*. However, using phylogenetic analysis, the species *L. lainsoni* and *L. naiffi* were shown to be the most divergent species and placed the *L. shawi* species in the *L. guyanensis* cluster, not as a distinct species. The authors also found the *L. braziliensis* strains to correspond to one widely geographically distributed clonal complex in Brazil and another restricted to one endemic area, in a region bordering Peru [117].

The main advantage of MLST is the possibility of generating genus-wide phylogenies, since MLST markers are co-dominant and are amenable for population and phylogenetic analyses. Also, given the high quality of sequence data, results can be easily compared between laboratories. Compared to MLEE, MLST does not necessarily require sterile culture of parasites. In addition, simultaneous typing of reference strains and sequencing can be done commercially without in-house specialized equipment. For those reasons, MLST is likely to become the gold standard basis for taxonomy and thus identification of *Leishmania*. One expected drawback could be the inherent limit of detection of nucleotide allelic diversity associated to direct sequencing of PCR products, which could be overcome by more lengthy analyses like cloning of parasites or PCR products. One consequence of this drawback is that MLST should not be considered as typing tool but an analysis tool. Another application could be diagnosis as recently new species-specific genetic polymorphisms were identified in the genes that confer the phenotypic variations in the MLEE assay [118]. Indeed, sequencing of the MPI and 6PGD genes was sufficient to differentiate among closely related species causing New World leishmaniasis, in Peru. The same group took advantage of these polymorphisms and designed a new real-time PCR assay based on FRET (fluorescence resonance energy transfer) technology and melting curve analysis using SYBR green. The assay was highly sensitive and correctly identified each of the five main species that cause tegumentary leishmaniasis in the New World, directly from clinical samples [119].

3.2. Multilocus microsatellite typing (MLMT)

Microsatellites are repeated motives of 1–6 nucleotide(s), which present allelic length variation. They mutate fast, therefore, 10–20 independent markers have to be analyzed for each strain owing to homoplasy. Microsatellite sequence variation results from the gain and loss of repeat units, which can easily be detected after amplification with specific primers annealing to their flanking regions. Then length polymorphisms are detected using PAGE, MetaPhor agarose gel electrophoresis or, preferably, automated capillary sequencers. A multilocus microsatellite profile is compiled for each sample from the fragment length measured for the microsatellite markers analyzed.

During the last years, microsatellite-based approaches have been developed for strain typing within the genus *Leishmania* to overcome the lack of discriminatory power of MLEE and other molecular tools. So far, microsatellite loci with high discriminatory power and suitable for characterizing closely related strains have been published for the *L. donovani/L. infantum* complex [120–122], *L. major* [123,124], *L. tropica* [125] and for species of the subgenus *L.* (*Viannia*) [126–128].

3.2.1. Subgenus L. Leishmania

3.2.1.1. L. donovani complex

Within the *L. donovani* complex, a set of 15 microsatellite markers have been applied to type strains of *L. donovani* and *L. infantum* isolated from the main endemic regions for VL (India, East Africa, Mediterranean region, Asia and South America) [129]. Six principal genetically distinct populations were identified: 2 populations of *L. infantum* from the Mediterranean area and South America comprising the MON-1 and non-MON-1 strains, respectively; 2 populations of *L. donovani* from Sudan and Ethiopia; 1 of *L. donovani* MON-2 from India; and 1 consisting of strains of *L. donovani* (MON-36, 37 and 38) from Kenya and India. These results corroborated the fragmentary data published in numerous studies using other genetic markers. Interestingly, the highest microsatellite diversity was observed for *L. infantum* from the Mediterranean basin and the lowest for *L. donovani* from India. Using 34 additional microsatellite sequences, analysis showed the homogeneity of *L. donovani* from the Indian subcontinent [130].

Different genetic groups of strains of *L. infantum* were also observed when strains from Algeria, Tunisia, the Palestinian Authority and Israel were subjected to MLMT. Microsatellite typing of strains belonging to zymodemes MON-1, MON-24 and MON-80 identified 3 different populations in Algeria and in Tunisia [131,132]. The MON-1 strains were assigned to 2 different populations one of which contained only local strains and the other local and European strains of MON-1. The non-MON-1 strains were always separated from the MON-1 ones. Gene flow was detected between the two MON-1 populations and the local MON-1 and the non-MON-1 populations, respectively [131,132]. *L. infantum* Israeli and Palestinian strains obtained from infected dogs and human cases showed 2 main populations genetically different from European populations, one of which is sub-divided in geographically distributed sub populations [133].

In Spain, *L. infantum* strains from a rural leishmaniasis-endemic area, from which 94 were obtained from dogs, 15 from sand flies, and 1 from a human visceral case, were MLMT studied [134]. Results showed existence of 17 genotypes that were detected using 10 microsatellite markers belonging to 3 different targets. They also showed the heterogeneous distribution of *L. infantum* species in hosts living in sympatric conditions.

Analysis of *L. infantum* strains having a New World origin by MLMT indicated that these strains were more similar to MON-1 and non-MON-1 sub-populations of *L. infantum* from southwest Europe, than to any other Old World sub-population [135] thus indicating that the parasite has been recently imported multiple times to the New World from southwest Europe.

Within the *L. donovani* complex, *L. donovani, L. infantum* and *L. archibaldi* strains from Sudan were studied by MLMT technique [6]. The authors found one single monophyletic *L. donovani* clade and argued that the isoenzyme differentiation of *L. donovani* and *L. infantum* in East Africa was misleading and that *L. archibaldi* is an invalid taxon [6].

Analysis of *L. donovani* strains from India, Bangladesh, Sri Lanka and Nepal showed that in Sri Lanka the causative agent of CL is most closely related to parasites causing VL in India [136] and that genetically homogeneous strains are circulating in the Indian subcontinent [130]. On the other hand, *L. donovani* strains belonging to the MON-37 zymodeme and originating from different geographical origins (India, Sri Lanka, Middle East, Cyprus and East Africa) were MLMT analyzed [9]. Zymodeme MON-37 was found to be paraphyletic, representing different genetic groups corresponding to their geographical origin and strains from Cyprus were clearly different from all others and could be autochthonous [9].

3.2.1.2. L. tropica

MLMT technique was also applied for *L. tropica* strain typing. Indeed, 117 strains from Asia and Africa were used and revealed 10 genetic groups, which were largely correlated to the geographical origin of the strains [125]. Different genetic groups were shown to co-exist in strains from the Middle East and Morocco. However, the authors postulated that recent spread of new genotypes has occurred recently in the Middle East and suspected an African origin of the *L. tropica* species [125].

3.2.1.3. L. major

Concerning *L. major*, 106 strains from Central Asia, Africa and the Middle East were analyzed using MLMT, based on 10 different microsatellite markers [124]. The study showed three main populations corresponding to the three geographical regions studied that were further subdivided into 2 sub-populations. Interestingly, the African and Middle Eastern populations seemed to be more genetically diversified than the Central Asian population [124].

3.2.2. Subgenus L. Viannia

Within the New World *L. Viannia* subgenus, the first MLMT studied species were *L. braziliensis* and *L. peruviana*. Fifty- nine analyzed Peruvian strains showed emergence of multiple *L. braziliensis/L. peruviana* hybrids [137]. Then, 124 *L. braziliensis* strains from Peru and Bolivia were investigated for their genetic polymorphism at 12 microsatellite loci [127,138]. A substantial genetic diversity with high levels of inbreeding, inconsistent with a strictly clonal reproduction was shown. Besides, a large genetic heterogeneity between populations within countries was described, which evidenced a strong population structure at a microgeographic scale [138].

In another study, polymorphisms of 30 strains of *L. braziliensis*, 21 strains of *L. guyanensis*, and 2 strains of *L. peruviana* from Brazil, Paraguay and Peru were analyzed at 15 independent microsatellite loci [128]. All strains except two *L. guyanensis* had individual MLMT types. In addition, three main clades were found, that consisted of one population of strains of *L.*

guyanensis only, another one with strains of *L. braziliensis* from Paraguay and Brazil, and the last one with strains of *L. braziliensis* and *L. peruviana* [128].

Recently, 28 strains of the main species of the *L. guyanensis* complex (*L. guyanensis* and *L. panamensis*), collected in Ecuador and Peru were investigated in an MLMT study, with 12 microsatellite markers [139]. An important heterozygote deficit was observed in these populations, similar to the previously reported results in *L. braziliensis* complex [138]. They further showed genetic polymorphism and geographical differentiation on the *L. guyanensis* complex [139].

All together, these studies confirmed that microsatellite markers constitute good tools for typing and population genetic studies of *Leishmania*. Their additional advantage resides in the possibility of their use directly in biological material without culturing of parasites [130,140]. Moreover, accurate, quality controlled microsatellite profiles could be stored in databases and compared between different laboratories.

4. *Leishmania* parasite evolution, genetics and genome analyses – Consequences and prospects

For many years *Leishmania* parasites have been considered to replicate clonally, without genetic exchange. Indeed, Tibayrenc proposed that clonal evolution in micropathogens be defined as restrained recombination on an evolutionary scale, with genetic exchange scarce enough to not break the prevalent pattern of clonal population structure (Reviewed in [141,142]). The two main manifestations of clonal evolution are strong linkage disequilibrium (LD) and wide-spread genetic clustering ("near-clading"). These authors hypothesized that this pattern is not mainly due to natural selection, but would originate chiefly from in-built genetic properties of pathogens, that would allow like for other microorganisms (viruses, bacteria, protozoan parasites) to keep a balance between clonality and recombination, which would help escape from recombinational load. This way, to face evolutionary challenges, pathogens would be equipped with "clonality/sexuality machinery" that would function as alternative allelic systems [141,142]. However, an accumulation of molecular evidence indicates that there are inter-specific [115,137,143–146] and intra-specific [132,138] hybrids among natural populations. Genetic exchange was finally demonstrated experimentally in 2009 [99]. In fact, double drug resistant *Leishmania* major hybrids were produced by co-infecting *Phlebotomus duboscqi* (a natural *L. major* vector) sand flies with two strains carrying different drug resistance markers. The nuclear genotypes were consistent with a Mendelian transmission leading to a heterozygous first generation progeny [99]. The anticipated continuity of these studies was to co-infect sand flies with transgenic *Leishmania* carrying two different markers that are fluorescent, in an attempt to visualize the recombination events microscopically [147]. In 2011, for the first time, using a fluorescent protein detection system to observe yellow hybrid promastigotes in *Phlebotomus perniciosus* and *Lutzomyia longipalpis* midguts, *L. donovani* hybrids were observed, 2 days post bloodmeal, and the morphological stages involved were found to be short procyclic promastigotes [100]. However, the parasites could not be recovered and propagated to confirm their hybrid genotypes [100]. Recently, the analysis of the mating competency of *L. major* strains have been expanded to include pairwise matings of multiple isolates bearing independent drug markers [148]. Also, the timing of the appearance of hybrids and their developmental stage associations within both natural (*Phlebotomus duboscqi*) and unnatural (*Lutzomyia longipalpis*) sand fly vectors was followed. Genotype analysis of a large number of progeny clones showed a chromosomal inheritance of both parental alleles at 4–6 unlinked nuclear loci, consistent with a meiotic process, and a uniparental inheritance of kinetoplast DNA [148]. A low frequency of nuclear loci showed only one parental allele, suggesting loss of heterozygosity, most likely arising from aneuploidy, which is common in *Leishmania*. In the natural vector, when comparing the timing of hybrid formation and the presence of developmental stages, the authors suggested that nectomonad promastigotes are the most likely mating competent forms, with hybrids emerging before the first appearance of metacyclic promastigotes [148].

MLMT analysis showed that recombination events are much more frequent in *Leishmania* than previously thought. Indeed, MLMT analysis of Bolivian and Peruvian *L. braziliensis* showed frequent sexual crosses of individuals from the same strain (inbreeding) [138]. The substantial heterozygote deficiency and extreme inbreeding found in this study is not consistent with a strictly clonal reproduction. The authors came to the conclusion that *Leishmania* parasites may alternate between clonal and sexual modes of reproduction, occurring most probably in the vector [138]. Sexual fusion may frequently take place between genetically related parasites or even within the same strain with occasional recombination events between individuals of different genotypes.

Also, *L. braziliensis/L. peruviana* hybrids were found to be quite common in a Peruvian focus where both species can occur sympatrically [137]. In the Old World, natural *L. infantum/L. major* hybrids were experimentally transmitted by *Ph. papatasi*, usually only competent to transmit *L. major* [149]. This suggests that hybrids may circulate using this sand fly vector and spread into new foci throughout the broad range of *Ph. papatasi* distribution.

The fact that *Leishmania* can undergo genetic exchange is potentially of profound epidemiological significance since this could facilitate the emergence and spread of new genotypes and phenotypic traits. Also, hybrid offspring might show a strong selective advantage relative to the parental strains. In [149], the authors have shown that natural hybrids could have enhanced transmission potential and a positively affected fitness.

New high-throughput sequencing technologies have opened the door for population genome analyses and genome-wide association studies. Genome of the *L. major* species was the first to be fully sequenced [150] followed by *L. infantum* and *L. braziliensis* [151]. Comparison of the three genomes revealed conservation of synteny and identified only 200 genes having a differential distribution between the three species. Such genes may encode for proteins implicated in host-pathogen interactions and parasite survival in the macrophage [151]. The species *L. mexicana* and *L. donovani* were subsequently sequenced [152,153] and the reference genomes for *L. major*, *L. infantum*, and *L. braziliensis* were refined [152]. This has allowed the identification of a remarkably low number of genes or paralog groups unique to each of the species *L. mexicana*, *L. major*, *L. infantum*, and *L. braziliensis* (2, 14, 19, and 67, respectively). Besides, *L. major* and *L. infantum* were found to have a surprisingly low number of predicted heterozygous SNPs compared with *L. braziliensis* and *L. mexicana*. Chromosome copy number also varied significantly between species, with nine supernumerary chromosomes in *L. infantum*, four in *L. mexicana*, two in *L. braziliensis*, and one in *L. major*. The authors also showed that gene duplication events occur more frequently on disomic chromosomes [152]. In addition to sequencing of an *L. donovani* reference genome, a recent study also included sequence analysis of a set of 16 related clinical lines, isolated from VL patients in Nepal and India, which also differ in their *in vitro* drug response [153]. Sequence comparisons with other *Leishmania* species and analysis of single-nucleotide diversity showed evidence of selection acting on different surface- and transport-related genes, including genes associated with drug resistance. Extensive variation in chromosome copy number between the analyzed lines was also shown. In association to drug resistance, they also showed structural variation, including gene dosage and copy number variation of a circular episome, present in all lines [153].

Genomic research on *Leishmania* is taking promising directions, mainly upon sequencing of the main pathogenic species [150–153] and also the non pathogenic *L. tarentolae* [154] which will enable to answer key questions on population genetics and ultimately unravel many important aspects related to drug resistance and virulence, which are especially relevant for control of the disease.

Novel genomics technologies are expected to bring more powerful tools to characterize the pathogens and particularly the infectious stages of *Leishmania* parasites. It will be particularly useful to fully characterize the parasites within the lesions/hosts in their microenvironment. While so far expression profiling relied mainly on microarray analysis which revealed only a limited number of differentially expressed genes across developmental stages [155], or species [156]. RNA sequencing technology seems very promising to highlight transcriptional events that are associated to parasite life cycle, infection or pathology. Previous studies have demonstrated a correlation between gene expression and gene copy number [157,158]. It was further hypothesized that "Increased gene copy number due to chromosome amplification may contribute to alterations in gene expression in response to environmental conditions in the host, providing a genetic basis for disease tropism" [152]. Other studies have also suggested that *Leishmania* parasites do not respond dynamically to host immune pressure, and that any influence of varying transcript levels on virulence and pathogenicity of the different *Leishmania* species is likely to result from the differential expression of conserved genes between species and/or the expression of a small number of genes that are differentially distributed between species [159].

Genome-wide multilocus genotyping in malaria research through novel sequencing technologies has allowed the identification of almost 47000 single nucleotide polymorphisms (SNPs) across the *Plasmodium* genome [160]. This allowed development of microarray–based platforms for screening more than 3000 SNPs that were successfully applied for population genetic analyses and genome-wide association studies in *P. falciparum* [161,162]. Similar studies still need to be developed for *Leishmania*.

5. Conclusion

Epidemiological, taxonomic and population genetic studies of *Leishmania* require good sampling methods and appropriate molecular markers that allow discrimination at different levels. Answering key epidemiological questions requires new or improved tools that allow discrimination of *Leishmania* parasites at different levels. The MLEE, considered as gold standard technique, needs cultured parasites and lacks discriminatory power. PCR assays are likely to replace isoenzyme analysis since they enable direct detection and identification of different *Leishmania* species in human and animal samples and also in infected sand flies. Many of the PCR assays described in the literature have proven useful in numerous field studies. However, they still need to be standardized and validated as diagnostic PCR assays and comparisons of the sensitivity and specificity parameters of the different approaches need also validation under routine conditions. In general, more than one assay is necessary to obtain fully satisfactory analysis of field samples. Given emergence context and changing eco-epidemiological trends, multiple tools will be needed to fully investigate the transmitted parasites.

At the strain level differentiation, MLMT has potential for being a gold standard, because on its principle it is expected to be reproducible and brings possibility of data storage and exchange. However, microsatellite markers are largely species-specific in *Leishmania* and different marker sets have to be used according to species. Such databases do not exist yet and data generation will need standardization. It may also require access to automated sequencers and good knowledge of population genetics programs. On the other hand MLST appears potentially as more powerful for phylogenetic and evolutionary studies although less discriminatory than MLMT. It is most probably this technique that will advantageously replace MLEE in the future. Some results showed that the same targets could be used across the *Leishmania* genus, which will enable comparisons of distances between the species but also of the degree of genetic diversity within species [163]. Here also it will require access to automated sequencers and adequate analytical programs. Cost of both approaches are relatively high and inherent limitations will be most likely overcome by the next generation sequencing approaches expected to gain momentum in a near future. *Leishmania* population genomics still needs to be developed and made accessible to researchers in disease endemic countries to best achieve its public health potential.

Parasite knowledge is so far built on strains obtained *in vitro*. Increasing interest in *Leishmania* parasite analyses will likely identify novel genotypes or organisms, a challenge for our current knowledge on parasite taxonomy and assays to identify and characterize parasites. Improving ways to enhance knowledge on parasites within samples remains a priority.

In spite of the increasing potential of sophisticated technologies and techniques, some disease endemic areas still need simple assays for eco-epidemiological investigations or diagnosis as well as capacity building in this highly relevant area to disease control.

Acknowledgements

Research on *Leishmania* Molecular diagnostics in our laboratory has received support from the Ministry of Higher Education and Scientific Research and Technology in Tunisia (BSP46, LR00SP04 & LR11IPT04) and from different international programs: EU–Avicenne (CT920013), STD3 (CT930253), INCO-DC (CT970256); TDR–RSG (ID890266), TDR–RTG (920781), TDR–PAG (A30380); MERC–NIAID–NIH (NO1AI45183); IAEA (TUN06–12; CRP15111); CRDF (TN1–7009–TP–09); AUF (PCSI 6319PS011).

Author details

Souheila Guerbouj, Imen Mkada–Driss and Ikram Guizani

Laboratoire d'Epidemiologie et d'Ecologie Parasitaire / Epidémiologie Moléculaire et Pathologie Expérimentale Appliquée (*Leishmania* Genomics and Genetics Program), Institut Pasteur de Tunis, Université Tunis el Manar, Tunisia

The number of references for this review has been restricted by space restraints. The authors apologize to the authors whose work was not cited in this review.

References

[1] Lainson R, Shaw JJ. New World leishmaniasis–the neotropical Leishmania species. In: Cox FEG, Kreier JP, Wakelin D, editors. Topley & Wilson's *Microbiology and Microbial Infections*. London: Arnold; 1998.

[2] Sacks DL, Kenney RT, Kreutzer RD, Jaffe CL, Gupta AK, Sharma MC, *et al.* Indian kala-azar caused by *Leishmania tropica. Lancet.* 1995 Apr 15;345(8955):959-61.

[3] Alvar J, Vélez ID, Bern C, Herrero M, Desjeux P, Cano J, et al.; WHO Leishmaniasis Control Team. Leishmaniasis worldwide and global estimates of its incidence. *PLoS One*. 2012;7(5):e35671.

[4] Guizani I, Mukhtar M, Alvar J, Ben Abderrazak S, Shaw J. (2011) Leishmaniases. In: Nriagu JO, editor. *Encyclopedia of Environmental Health,* volume 3, pp. 453–480. Burlington: Elsevier; 2011.

[5] Schönian G, Mauricio I, Gramiccia M, Cañavate C, Boelaert M, Dujardin JC. Leishmaniases in the Mediterranean in the era of molecular epidemiology. *Trends Parasitol.* 2008 Mar;24(3):135-42.

[6] Jamjoom MB, Ashford RW, Bates PA, Chance ML, Kemp SJ, Watts PC, *et al.* Leishmania donovani is the only cause of visceral leishmaniaisis in East Africa; previous de-

scriptions of L. infantum and "L. archibaldi" from this region are a consequence of convergent evolution in the isoenzyme data. *Parasitology*. 2004 Oct;129(Pt 4):399-409.

[7] Mauricio IL, Yeo M, Baghaei M, Doto D, Pratlong F, Zemanova E, *et al.* Towards multilocus sequence typing of the Leishmania donovani complex: resolving genotypes and haplotypes for five polymorphic metabolic enzymes (ASAT, GPI, NH1, NH2, PGD). *Int J Parasitol*. 2006 Jun;36(7):757-69.

[8] Zemanová E, Jirků M, Mauricio IL, Horák A, Miles MA, Lukes J. The Leishmania donovani complex: genotypes of five metabolic enzymes (ICD, ME, MPI, G6PDH, and FH), new targets for multilocus sequence typing. *Int J Parasitol*. 2007 Feb;37(2):149-60.

[9] Alam MZ, Haralambous C, Kuhls K, Gouzelou E, Sgouras D, Soteriadou K, *et al.* The paraphyletic composition of Leishmania donovani zymodeme MON-37 revealed by multilocus microsatellite typing. *Microbes Infect*. 2009 May-Jun;11(6-7):707-15.

[10] Van Eys GJ, Schoone GJ, Kroon NC, Ebeling SB. Sequence analysis of small subunit ribosomal RNA genes and its use for detection and identification of Leishmania parasites. *Mol Biochem Parasitol*. 1992 Mar;51(1):133-42.

[11] Lachaud L, Marchergui-Hammami S, Chabbert E, Dereure J, Dedet JP, Bastien P. Comparison of six PCR methods using peripheral blood for detection of canine visceral leishmaniasis. *J Clin Microbiol*. 2002 Jan;40(1):210-5.

[12] Schönian G, Nasereddin A, Dinse N, Schweynoch C, Schallig HD, Presber W, *et al.* PCR diagnosis and characterization of Leishmania in local and imported clinical samples. *Diagn Microbiol Infect Dis*. 2003 Sep;47(1):349-58.

[13] Bensoussan E, Nasereddin A, Jonas F, Schnur LF, Jaffe CL. Comparison of PCR assays for diagnosis of cutaneous leishmaniasis. *J Clin Microbiol*. 2006 Apr;44(4):1435-9.

[14] Nicolas L, Prina E, Lang T, Milon G. Real-time PCR for detection and quantitation of leishmania in mouse tissues. *J Clin Microbiol*. 2002 May;40(5):1666-9.

[15] Schulz A, Mellenthin K, Schönian G, Fleischer B, Drosten C. Detection, differentiation, and quantitation of pathogenic leishmania organisms by a fluorescence resonance energy transfer-based real-time PCR assay. *J Clin Microbiol*. 2003 Apr;41(4): 1529-35.

[16] Cupolillo E, Grimaldi Júnior G, Momen H, Beverley SM. Intergenic region typing (IRT): a rapid molecular approach to the characterization and evolution of Leishmania. *Mol Biochem Parasitol*. 1995 Jul;73(1-2):145-55.

[17] Nasereddin A, Bensoussan-Hermano E, Schönian G, Baneth G, Jaffe CL. Molecular diagnosis and species identification of Old World cutaneous leishmaniasis using a reverse line blot hybridization assay. *J Clin Microbiol*. 2008 Sep;46(9):2848-55.

[18] Harris E, Kropp G, Belli A, Rodriguez B, Agabian N. Single-step multiplex PCRassay for characterization of NewWorld Leishmania complexes. *J Clin Microbiol*. 1998 Jul; 36(7):1989-95.

[19] Marfurt J, Niederwieser I, Makia ND, Beck HP, Felger I. Diagnostic genotyping of Old and New World Leishmania species by PCR-RFLP. *Diagn Microbiol Infect Dis*. 2003 Jun;46(2):115-24.

[20] Victoir K, Bañuls AL, Arevalo J, Llanos-Cuentas A, Hamers R, Noël S, *et al*. The gp63 gene locus, a target for genetic characterization of Leishmania belonging to subgenus Viannia. *Parasitology*. 1998 Jul;117(Pt 1):1-13.

[21] Guerbouj S, Victoir K, Guizani I, Seridi N, Nuwayri-Salti N, Belkaid M, *et al*. Gp63 gene polymorphism and population structure of Leishmania donovani complex: influence of the host selection pressure? *Parasitology*. 2001 Jan;122(Pt 1):25-35.

[22] Garcia L, Kindt A, Bermudez H, Llanos-Cuentas A, De Doncker S, Arevalo J, *et al*. Culture-independent species typing of neotropical Leishmania for clinical validation of a PCR-based assay targeting heat shock protein 70 genes. *J Clin Microbiol*. 2004 May;42(5):2294-7.

[23] Fraga J, Montalvo AM, De Doncker S, Dujardin JC, Van der Auwera G. Phylogeny of Leishmania species based on the heat-shock protein 70 gene. *Infect Genet Evol*. 2010 Mar;10(2):238-45.

[24] Da Silva LA, de Sousa Cdos S, da Graça GC, Porrozzi R, Cupolillo E. Sequence analysis and PCR-RFLP profiling of the hsp70 gene as a valuable tool for identifying Leishmania species associated with human leishmaniasis in Brazil. *Infect Genet Evol*. 2010 Jan;10(1):77-83.

[25] Hide M, Bañuls AL. Species-specific PCR assay for L. infantum/L. donovani discrimination. *Acta Trop*. 2006 Dec;100(3):241-5.

[26] Oshaghi MA, Ravasan NM, Hide M, Javadian EA, Rassi Y, Sedaghat MM, *et al*. Development of species-specific PCR and PCR-restriction fragment length polymorphism assays for L.infantum/L. donovani discrimination. *Exp Parasitol*. 2009 May; 122(1):61-5.

[27] Williams JG, Kubelik AR, Livak KJ, Rafalski JA, Tingey SV. DNA polymorphisms amplified by arbitrary primers are useful as genetic markers. *Nucleic Acids Res*. 1990 Nov 25;18(22):6531-5.

[28] Schriefer AL, Góes-Neto A, Guimarães LH, Carvalho LP, Almeida RP, *et al*. Multiclonal Leishmania braziliensis population structure and its clinical implication in a region of endemicity for American tegumentary leishmaniasis. *Infect Immun*. 2004 Jan; 72(1):508-14.

[29] Gomes RF, Macedo AM, Pena SD, Melo MN. Leishmania (Viannia) braziliensis: genetic relationships between strains isolated from different areas of Brazil as revealed by DNA fingerprinting and RAPD. *Exp Parasitol.* 1995 Jun;80(4):681-7.

[30] Motazedian H, Noyes H, Maingon R. Leishmania and Sauroleishmania: the use of random amplified polymorphic DNA for the identification of parasites from vertebrates and invertebrates. *Exp Parasitol.* 1996 Jun;83(1):150-4.

[31] Manna M, Majumder HK, Sundar S, Bhaduri AN. The molecular characterization of clinical isolates from Indian Kala-azar patients by MLEE and RAPD-PCR. *Med Sci Monit.* 2005 Jul;11(7):BR220-7.

[32] Carvalho Mde L, de Andrade AS, Fontes CJ, Hueb M, de Oliveira Silva S, Melo MN. Leishmania (Viannia) braziliensis is the prevalent species infecting patients with tegumentary leishmaniasis from Mato Grosso State, Brazil. *Acta Trop.* 2006 Jul;98(3): 277-85.

[33] Noyes HA, Belli AA, Maingon R. Appraisal of various random amplified polymorphic DNA-polymerase chain reaction primers for Leishmania identification. *Am J Trop Med Hyg.* 1996 Jul;55(1):98-105.

[34] Hanafi R, Barhoumi M, Ali SB, Guizani I. Molecular analyses of Old World Leishmania RAPD markers and development of a PCR assay selective for parasites of the L. donovani species Complex. *Exp Parasitol.* 2001 Jun;98(2):90-9.

[35] Diakou A, Dovas CI. Optimization of random-amplified polymorphic DNA producing amplicons up to 8500 bp and revealing intraspecies polymorphism in Leishmania infantum isolates. *Anal Biochem.* 2001 Jan 15;288(2):195-200.

[36] Guizani I, Dellagi K, Ismaïl RB. Random amplified polymorphic DNA technique for identification and differentiation of Old World Leishmania species. *Am J Trop Med Hyg.* 2002 Feb;66(2):152-6.

[37] Bañuls AL, Guerrini F, Le Pont F, Barrera C, Espinel I, Guderian R, *et al.* Evidence for hybridization by multilocus enzyme electrophoresis and random amplified polymorphic DNA between Leishmania braziliensis and Leishmania panamemsis/ guyanensis in Ecuador. *J Eukaryot Microbiol.* 1997 Sep-Oct;44(5):408-11.

[38] Bañuls AL, Jonquieres R, Guerrini F, Le Pont F, Barrera C, Espinel I, *et al.* Genetic analysis of Leishmania parasites in Ecuador : are Leishmania (Viannia) panamensis and Leishmania (V.) guyanensis distinct taxa ? *Am J Trop Med Hyg.* 1999 Nov;61(5): 838-45.

[39] Mauricio IL, Howard MK, Stothard JR, Miles MA. Genomic diversity in the Leishmania donovani complex. *Parasitology.* 1999 Sep;119 (Pt 3):237-46.

[40] Rioux JA, Lanotte G, Serres E, Pratlong F, Bastien P, Perieres J. Taxonomy of Leishmania. Use of isoenzymes. Suggestions for a new classification. *Ann Parasitol Hum Comp.* 1990;65(3):111-25.

[41] Zemanová E, Jirků M, Mauricio IL, Miles MA, Lukes J. Genetic polymorphism within the Leishmania donovani complex: correlation with geographic origin. *Am J Trop Med Hyg*. 2004 Jun;70(6):613-7.

[42] Toledo A, Martín-Sánchez J, Pesson B, Sanchiz-Marín C, Morillas-Márquez F. Genetic variability within the species Leishmania infantum by RAPD. A lack of correlation with zymodeme structure. *Mol Biochem Parasitol*. 2002 Feb;119(2):257-64.

[43] Hide M, Bañuls AL, Tibayrenc M. Genetic heterogeneity and phylogenetic status of Leishmania (Leishmania) infantum zymodeme MON-1: epidemiological implications. *Parasitology*. 2001 Nov;123(Pt 5):425-32.

[44] Segatto M, Ribeiro LS, Costa DL, Costa CH, Oliveira MR, Carvalho SF, *et al*. Genetic diversity of Leishmania infantum field populations from Brazil. *Mem Inst Oswaldo Cruz*. 2012 Feb;107(1):39-47.

[45] Cupolillo E, Brahim LR, Toaldo CB, de Oliveira-Neto MP, de Brito ME, Falqueto A, *et al*. Genetic polymorphism and molecular epidemiology of Leishmania (Viannia) braziliensis from different hosts and geographic areas in Brazil. *J Clin Microbiol*. 2003 Jul; 41(7):3126-32.

[46] Khanra S, Bandopadhyay SK, Chakraborty P, Datta S, Mondal D, Chatterjee M, *et al*. Characterization of the recent clinical isolates of Indian Kala-azar patients by RAPD-PCR method. *J Parasit Dis*. 2011 Oct;35(2):116-22.

[47] Khanra S, Datta S, Mondal D, Saha P, Bandopadhyay SK, Roy S, *et al*. RFLPs of ITS, ITS1 and hsp70 amplicons and sequencing of ITS1 of recent clinical isolates of Kala-azar from India and Bangladesh confirms the association of L. tropica with the disease. *Acta Trop*. 2012 Dec;124(3):229-34.

[48] Mahmoudzadeh-Niknam H, Ajdary S, Riazi-Rad F, Mirzadegan E, Rezaeian A, Khaze V, *et al*. Molecular epidemiology of cutaneous leishmaniasis and heterogeneity of Leishmania major strains in Iran. *Trop Med Int Health*. 2012 Nov;17(11):1335-44.

[49] Martinez E, Alonso V, Quispe A, Thomas MC, Alonso R, Piñero JE, González AC, Ortega A, Valladares B. RAPD method useful for distinguishing Leishmania species: design of specific primers for L. braziliensis. *Parasitology*. 2003 Dec;127(Pt 6):513-7.

[50] Lewin S, Schönian G, El Tai N, Oskam L, Bastien P, Presber W. Strain typing in Leishmania donovani by using sequence-confirmed amplified region analysis. *Int J Parasitol*. 2002 Sep;32(10):1267-76.

[51] Mkada-Driss I, Lahmadi R, Chakroun AS, Talbi C, Elamin EM, Cupollilo E, *et al*. Screening and characterization of RAPD polymorphic markers in viscerotropic Leishmania parasites. In preparation.

[52] Mkada-Driss I, Talbi C, Elamin EM, Lahmadi R, Bakhiet S, Fathallah-Mili A, *et al*. Simple DNA assays for molecular epidemiology of visceral leishmaniasis in Africa:

development and evaluation of species and countries specific PCR assays. In preparation.

[53] Mauricio IL, Gaunt MW, Stothard JR, Miles MA. Glycoprotein 63 (gp63) genes show gene conversion and reveal the evolution of Old World Leishmania. *Int J Parasitol.* 2007 Apr;37(5):565-76.

[54] Guerbouj S, Chamekh L, Jlassi M, Jbir R, Guizani I. Genetic polymorphism of Tunisian Leishmania infantum species by restriction analysis of PCR amplified gp63 and PSA2 coding genes. Personal communication.

[55] BenSaid M, Guerbouj S, Saghrouni F, Fathallah-Mili A, Guizani I. Occurrence of Leishmania infantum cutaneous leishmaniasis in central Tunisia. *Trans R Soc Trop Med Hyg.* 2006 Jun;100(6):521-6.

[56] Elamin EM, Guerbouj S, Musa AM, Guizani I, Khalil EA, Mukhtar MM, *et al.* Uncommon clinical presentations of cutaneous leishmaniasis in Sudan. *Trans R Soc Trop Med Hyg.* 2005 Nov;99(11):803-8.

[57] Elamin EM, Guizani I, Guerbouj S, Gramiccia M, El Hassan AM, Di Muccio T, *et al.* Identification of Leishmania donovani as a cause of cutaneous leishmaniasis in Sudan. *Trans R Soc Trop Med Hyg.* 2008 Jan;102(1):54-7.

[58] Mauricio IL, Gaunt MW, Stothard JR, Miles MA. Genetic typing and phylogeny of the Leishmania donovani complex by restriction analysis of PCR amplified gp63 intergenic regions. *Parasitology.* 2001 Apr;122(Pt 4):393-403.

[59] Al-Jawabreh A, Schnur LF, Nasereddin A, Schwenkenbecher JM, Abdeen Z, Barghuthy F, *et al.* The recent emergence of Leishmania tropica in Jericho (A'riha) and its environs, a classical focus of L. major. *Trop Med Int Health.* 2004 Jul;9(7):812-6.

[60] Rhajaoui M, Nasereddin A, Fellah H, Azmi K, Amarir F, Al-Jawabreh A, *et al.* New clinico-epidemiologic profile of cutaneous leishmaniasis, Morocco. *Emerg Infect Dis.* 2007 Sep;13(9):1358-60.

[61] Kuhls K, Mauricio IL, Pratlong F, Presber W, Schönian G. Analysis of ribosomal DNA internal transcribed spacer sequences of the Leishmania donovani complex. *Microbes Infect.* 2005 Aug-Sep;7(11-12):1224-34.

[62] Talmi-Frank D, Nasereddin A, Schnur LF, Schönian G, Töz SO, Jaffe CL, *et al.* Detection and identification of Old World Leishmania by high resolution melt analysis. *PLoS Negl Trop Dis.* 2010 Jan 12;4(1):e581.

[63] De Almeida ME, Steurer FJ, Koru O, Herwaldt BL, Pieniazek NJ, da Silva AJ. Identification of Leishmania spp. by molecular amplification and DNA sequencing analysis of a fragment of rRNA internal transcribed spacer 2. *J Clin Microbiol.* 2011 Sep;49(9): 3143-9.

[64] El Tai NO, Osman OF, el Fari M, Presber W, Schönian G. Genetic heterogeneity of ribosomal internal transcribed spacer in clinical samples of Leishmania donovani

spotted on filter paper as revealed by single-strand conformation polymorphisms and sequencing. *Trans R Soc Trop Med Hyg.* 2000 Sep-Oct;94(5):575-9.

[65] El Tai NO, El Fari M, Mauricio I, Miles MA, Oskam L, El Safi SH, *et al.* Leishmania donovani: intra-specific polymorphisms of Sudanese isolates revealed by PCR-based analyses and DNA sequencing. *Exp Parasitol.* 2001 Jan;97(1):35-44.

[66] Schönian G, Schnur L, el Fari M, Oskam L, Kolesnikov AA, Sokolowska-Köhler W, *et al.* Genetic heterogeneity in the species Leishmania tropica revealed by different PCR-based methods. *Trans R Soc Trop Med Hyg.* 2001 Mar-Apr;95(2):217-24.

[67] Schönian G, El Fari M, Lewin S, Schweynoch C, Presber W. Molecular epidemiology and population genetics in Leishmania. *Med Microbiol Immunol.* 2001 Nov;190(1-2): 61-3.

[68] Tashakori M, Kuhls K, Al-Jawabreh A, Mauricio IL, Schönian G, Farajnia S, *et al.* Leishmania major: genetic heterogeneity of Iranian isolates by single-strand conformation polymorphism and sequence analysis of ribosomal DNA internal transcribed spacer. *Acta Trop.* 2006 Apr;98(1):52-8.

[69] Ghatee M, Sharifi I, Mirhendi H, Kanannejad Z, Hatam G. Investigation of Double-Band Electrophoretic Pattern of ITS-rDNA Region in Iranian Isolates of Leishmania tropica. *Iran J Parasitol.* 2013 Apr;8(2):264-72.

[70] Hartl FU, Hayer-Hartl M. Molecular chaperones in the cytosol: from nascent chain to folded protein. *Science.* 2002 Mar 8;295(5561):1852-8.

[71] Folgueira C, Requena JM. A postgenomic view of the heat shock proteins in kinetoplastids. *FEMS Microbiol Rev.* 2007 Jul;31(4):359-77.

[72] Montalvo AM, Fraga J, Monzote L, Montano I, De Doncker S, Dujardin JC, *et al.* Heat-shock protein 70 PCR-RFLP: a universal simple tool for *Leishmania* species discrimination in the New and Old World. *Parasitology.* 2010 Jul;137(8):1159-68.

[73] Montalvo AM, Fraga J, Maes I, Dujardin JC, Van der Auwera G. Three new sensitive and specific heat-shock protein 70 PCRs for global *Leishmania* species identification. *Eur J Clin Microbiol Infect Dis.* 2012 Jul;31(7):1453-61.

[74] Fraga J, Montalvo AM, Maes L, Dujardin JC, Van der Auwera G. HindII and SduI digests of heat-shock protein 70 PCR for *Leishmania* typing. *Diagn Microbiol Infect Dis.* 2013 Nov;77(3):245-7.

[75] Fraga J, Veland N, Montalvo AM, Praet N, Boggild AK, Valencia BM, *et al.* Accurate and rapid species typing from cutaneous and mucocutaneous leishmaniasis lesions of the New World. *Diagn Microbiol Infect Dis.* 2012 Oct;74(2):142-50.

[76] Van der Auwera G, Maes I, De Doncker S, Ravel C, Cnops L, Van Esbroeck M, *et al.* Heat-shock protein 70 gene sequencing for *Leishmania* species typing in European tropical infectious disease clinics. *Euro Surveill.* 2013 Jul 25;18(30):20543.

[77] Requena JM, Chicharro C, García L, Parrado R, Puerta CJ, Cañavate C. Sequence analysis of the 3'-untranslated region of HSP70 (type I) genes in the genus *Leishmania*: its usefulness as a molecular marker for species identification. *Parasit Vectors*. 2012 Apr 28;5:87.

[78] Serin MS, Waki K, Chang KP, Aslan G, Direkel S, Otag F, *et al.* Consistence of miniexon polymerase chain reaction–restriction fragment length polymorphism and single-copy gene sequence analyses in discriminating Leishmania genotypes. *Diagn Microbiol Infect Dis*. 2007 Mar;57(3):295-9.

[79] Marfurt J, Nasereddin A, Niederwieser I, Jaffe CL, Beck HP, Felger I. Identification and differentiation of Leishmania species in clinical samples by PCR amplification of the miniexon sequence and subsequent restriction fragment length polymorphism analysis. *J Clin Microbiol*. 2003 Jul;41(7):3147-53.

[80] Serin MS, Daglioglu K, Bagirova M, Allahverdiyev A, Uzun S, Vural Z, *et al.* Rapid diagnosis and genotyping of Leishmania isolates from cutaneous and visceral leishmaniasis by microcapillary cultivation and polymerase chain reaction-restriction fragment length polymorphism of miniexon region. *Diagn Microbiol Infect Dis*. 2005 Nov;53(3):209-14.

[81] Pandey K, Yanagi T, Pandey BD, Mallik AK, Sherchand JB, Kanbara H. Characterization of Leishmania isolates from Nepalese patients with visceral leishmaniasis. *Parasitol Res*. 2007 May;100(6):1361-9.

[82] Roelfsema JH, Nozari N, Herremans T, Kortbeek LM, Pinelli E. Evaluation and improvement of two PCR targets in molecular typing of clinical samples of Leishmania patients. *Exp Parasitol*. 2011 Jan;127(1):36-41.

[83] Quispe Tintaya KW, Ying X, Dedet JP, Rijal S, De Bolle X, Dujardin JC. Antigen genes for molecular epidemiology of leishmaniasis: polymorphism of cysteine proteinase B and surface metalloprotease glycoprotein 63 in the Leishmania donovani complex. *J Infect Dis*. 2004 Mar 15;189(6):1035-43.

[84] Seridi N, Belkaid M, Quispe-Tintaya W, Zidane C, Dujardin JC. Application of PCR-RFLP for the exploration of the molecular diversity of Leishmania infantum in Algeria. *Trans R Soc Trop Med Hyg*. 2008 Jun;102(6):556-63.

[85] Chaouch M, Fathallah-Mili A, Driss M, Lahmadi R, Ayari C, Guizani I, *et al.* Identification of Tunisian Leishmania spp. by PCR amplification of cysteine proteinase B (cpb) genes and phylogenetic analysis. *Acta Trop*. 2013 Mar;125(3):357-65.

[86] Laurent T, Van der Auwera G, Hide M, Mertens P, Quispe-Tintaya W, Deborggraeve S, *et al.* Identification of Old World Leishmania spp. by specific polymerase chain reaction amplification of cysteine proteinase B genes and rapid dipstick detection. *Diagn Microbiol Infect Dis*. 2009 Feb;63(2):173-81.

[87] Kuru T, Janusz N, Gadisa E, Gedamu L, Aseffa A. Leishmania aethiopica: development of specific and sensitive PCR diagnostic test. *Exp Parasitol*. 2011 Aug;128(4): 391-5.

[88] Chaouch M, Mhadhbi M, Adams ER, Schoone GJ, Limam S, Gharbi Z, *et al*. Development and evaluation of a loop-mediated isothermal amplification assay for rapid detection of Leishmania infantum in canine leishmaniasis based on cysteine protease B genes. *Vet Parasitol*. 2013 Nov 15;198(1-2):78-84.

[89] Notomi T, Okayama H, Masubuchi H, Yonekawa T, Watanabe K, Amino N, *et al*. Loop-mediated isothermal amplification of DNA. *Nucleic Acids Res*. 2000 Jun 15;28(12):E63.

[90] Adams ER, Schoone GJ, Ageed AF, Safi SE, Schallig HD. Development of a reverse transcriptase loopo-mediated isothermal amplification (LAMP) assay for the sensitive detection of Leishmania parasites in clinical samples. *Am J Trop Med Hyg*. 2010 Apr;82(4):591-6.

[91] Ibrahim ME, Barker DC. The origin and evolution of the Leishmania donovani complex as inferred from a mitochondrial cytochrome oxidase II gene sequence. *Infect Genet Evol*. 2001 Jul;1(1):61-8.

[92] Luyo-Acero GE, Uezato H, Oshiro M, Takei K, Kariya K, Katakura K, *et al*. Sequence variation of the cytochrome b gene of various human infecting members of the genus Leishmania and their phylogeny. *Parasitology*. 2004 May;128(Pt 5):483-91.

[93] Lainson R, Shaw JJ. Evolution, classification and geographical distribution. In: Peters W, Killick-Kendrick R, editors. The Leishmaniasis in Biology and Medicine. Vol. I *Biology and Epidemiology*. Orlando, USA: Orlando Academic Press; 1987.

[94] Asato Y, Oshiro M, Myint CK, Yamamoto Y, Kato H, Marco JD, *et al*. Phylogenic analysis of the genus Leishmania by cytochrome b gene sequencing. *Exp Parasitol*. 2009 Apr;121(4):352-61.

[95] Marco JD, Bhutto AM, Soomro FR, Baloch JH, Barroso PA, Kato H, *et al*. Multilocus enzyme electrophoresis and cytochrome B gene sequencing-based identification of Leishmania isolates from different foci of cutaneous leishmaniasis in Pakistan. *Am J Trop Med Hyg*. 2006 Aug;75(2):261-6.

[96] Myint CK, Asato Y, Yamamoto Y, Kato H, Bhutto AM, Soomro FR, *et al*. Polymorphisms of cytochrome b gene in Leishmania parasites and their relation to types of cutaneous leishmaniasis lesions in Pakistan. *J Dermatol*. 2008 Feb;35(2):76-85.

[97] Martínez LP, Rebollo JA, Luna AL, Cochero S, Bejarano EE. Molecular identification of the parasites causing cutaneous leishmaniasis on the Caribbean coast of Colombia. *Parasitol Res*. 2010 Feb;106(3):647-52.

[98] Yang BB, Chen DL, Chen JP, Liao L, Hu XS, Xu JN. Analysis of kinetoplast cytochrome b gene of 16 Leishmania isolates from different foci of China: different spe-

cies of Leishmania in China and their phylogenetic inference. *Parasit Vectors*. 2013 Feb 5;6:32.

[99] Akopyants NS, Kimblin N, Secundino N, Patrick R, Peters N, Lawyer P, *et al.* Demonstration of genetic exchange during cyclical development of Leishmania in the sand fly vector. *Science* 2009 Apr 10;324(5924):265-8.

[100] Sadlova J, Yeo M, Seblova V, Lewis MD, Mauricio I, Volf P, *et al.* Visualisation of Leishmania donovani fluorescent hybrids during early stage development in the sand fly vector. *PLoS One*. 2011;6(5):e19851.

[101] Lombardo G, Pennisi MG, Lupo T, Migliazzo A, Caprì A, Solano-Gallego L. Detection of Leishmania infantum DNA by real-time PCR in canine oral and conjunctival swabs and comparison with other diagnostic techniques. *Vet Parasitol*. 2012 Feb 28;184(1):10-7.

[102] Da Silva RN, Amorim AC, Brandão RM, de Andrade HM, Yokoo M, Ribeiro ML, *et al.* Real-time PCR in clinical practice: a powerful tool for evaluating Leishmania chagasi loads in naturally infected dogs. *Ann Trop Med Parasitol*. 2010 Mar;104(2):137-43.

[103] De Paiva Cavalcanti M, Felinto de Brito ME, de Souza WV, de Miranda Gomes Y, Abath FG. The development of a real-time PCR assay for the quantification of Leishmania infantum DNA in canine blood. *Vet J*. 2009 Nov;182(2):356-8.

[104] Antinori S, Calattini S, Piolini R, Longhi E, Bestetti G, Cascio A, *et al.* Is real-time polymerase chain reaction (PCR) more useful than a conventional PCR for the clinical management of leishmaniasis? *Am J Trop Med Hyg*. 2009 Jul;81(1):46-51.

[105] Weirather JL, Jeronimo SM, Gautam S, Sundar S, Kang M, Kurtz MA, *et al.* Serial quantitative PCR assay for detection, species discrimination, and quantification of Leishmania spp. in human samples. *J Clin Microbiol*. 2011 Nov;49(11):3892-904.

[106] Jara M, Adaui V, Valencia BM, Martinez D, Alba M, Castrillon C, *et al.* Real-time PCR assay for detection and quantification of Leishmania (Viannia) organisms in skin and mucosal lesions: exploratory study of parasite load and clinical parameters. *J Clin Microbiol*. 2013 Jun;51(6):1826-33.

[107] De Paiva Cavalcanti M, Dantas-Torres F, da Cunha Gonçalves de Albuquerque S, Silva de Morais RC, de Brito ME, Otranto D, *et al.* Quantitative real time PCR assays for the detection of Leishmania (Viannia) braziliensis in animals and humans. *Mol Cell Probes*. 2013 Jun-Aug;27(3-4):122-8.

[108] Kumar A, Boggula VR, Misra P, Sundar S, Shasany AK, Dube A. Amplified fragment length polymorphism (AFLP) analysis is useful for distinguishing Leishmania species of visceral and cutaneous forms. *Acta Trop*. 2010 Feb;113(2):202-6.

[109] Odiwuor S, Vuylsteke M, De Doncker S, Maes I, Mbuchi M, Dujardin JC, *et al.* Leishmania AFLP: paving the way towards improved molecular assays and markers of diversity. *Infect Genet Evol*. 2011 Jul;11(5):960-7.

[110] Kumar A, Misra P, Dube A. Amplified fragment length polymorphism: an adept technique for genome mapping, genetic differentiation, and intraspecific variation in protozoan parasites. *Parasitol Res.* 2013 Feb;112(2):457-66.

[111] Van der Meide WF, Schoone GJ, Faber WR, Zeegelaar JE, de Vries HJ, Ozbel Y, *et al.* Quantitative nucleic acid sequence-based assay as a new molecular tool for detection and quantification of Leishmania parasites in skin biopsy samples. *J Clin Microbiol.* 2005 Nov;43(11):5560-6.

[112] Takagi H, Itoh M, Islam MZ, Razzaque A, Ekram AR, Hashighuchi Y, *et al.* Sensitive, specific, and rapid detection of Leishmania donovani DNA by loop-mediated isothermal amplification. *Am J Trop Med Hyg.* 2009 Oct;81(4):578-82.

[113] Khan MG, Bhaskar KR, Salam MA, Akther T, Pluschke G, Mondal D. Diagnostic accuracy of loop-mediated isothermal amplification (LAMP) for detection of Leishmania DNA in buffy coat from visceral leishmaniasis patients. *Parasit Vectors.* 2012 Dec 3;5:280.

[114] Lukes J, Mauricio IL, Schönian G, Dujardin JC, Soteriadou K, Dedet JP, *et al.* Evolutionary and geographical history of the Leishmania donovani complex with a revision of current taxonomy. *Proc Natl Acad Sci U S A.* 2007 May 29;104(22):9375-80.

[115] Ravel C, Cortes S, Pratlong F, Morio F, Dedet JP, Campino L. First report of genetic hybrids between two very divergent Leishmania species: Leishmania infantum and Leishmania major. *Int J Parasitol.* 2006 Nov;36(13):1383-8.

[116] El Baidouri F, Diancourt L, Berry V, Chevenet F, Pratlong F, Marty P, *et al.* Genetic structure and evolution of the Leishmania genus in Africa and Eurasia: what does MLSA tell us. *PLoS Negl Trop Dis.* 2013 Jun 13;7(6):e2255.

[117] Boité MC, Mauricio IL, Miles MA, Cupolillo E. New insights on taxonomy, phylogeny and population genetics of Leishmania (Viannia) parasites based on multilocus sequence analysis. *PLoS Negl Trop Dis.* 2012;6(11):e1888.

[118] Tsukayama P, Lucas C, Bacon DJ. Typing of four genetic loci discriminates among closely related species of New World Leishmania. *Int J Parasitol.* 2009 Feb;39(3): 355-62.

[119] Tsukayama P, Núñez JH, De Los Santos M, Soberón V, Lucas CM, Matlashewski G, *et al.* A FRET-based real-time PCR assay to identify the main causal agents of New World tegumentary leishmaniasis. *PLoS Negl Trop Dis.* 2013;7(1):e1956.

[120] Bulle B, Millon L, Bart JM, Gállego M, Gambarelli F, Portús M, *et al.* Practical approach for typing strains of Leishmania infantum by microsatellite analysis. *J Clin Microbiol.* 2002 Sep;40(9):3391-7.

[121] Jamjoom MB, Ashford RW, Bates PA, Kemp SJ, Noyes HA. Towards a standard battery of microsatellite markers for the analysis of the Leishmania donovani complex. *Ann Trop Med Parasitol.* 2002 Apr;96(3):265-70.

[122] Ochsenreither S, Kuhls K, Schaar M, Presber W, Schönian G. Multilocus microsatellite typing as a new tool for discrimination of Leishmania infantum MON-1 strains. *J Clin Microbiol.* 2006 Feb;44(2):495-503.

[123] Jamjoom MB, Ashford RW, Bates PA, Kemp SJ, Noyes HA. Polymorphic microsatellite repeats are not conserved between Leishmania donovani and Leishmania major. *Molecular Ecology Notes.* 2002 June;2(2):104–6.

[124] Al-Jawabreh A, Diezmann S, Müller M, Wirth T, Schnur LF, Strelkova MV, *et al.* Identification of geographically distributed subpopulations of Leishmania (Leishmania) major by microsatellite analysis. *BMC Evol Biol.* 2008 Jun 24;8:183.

[125] Schwenkenbecher JM, Wirth T, Schnur LF, Jaffe CL, Schallig H, Al-Jawabreh A, *et al.* Microsatellite analysis reveals genetic structure of Leishmania tropica. *Int J Parasitol.* 2006 Feb;36(2):237-46.

[126] Russell R, Iribar MP, Lambson B, Brewster S, Blackwell JM, Dye C, *et al.* Intra and inter-specific microsatellite variation in the Leishmania subgenus Viannia. *Mol Biochem Parasitol.* 1999 Sep 20;103(1):71-7.

[127] Rougeron V, Waleckx E, Hide M, DE Meeûs T, Arevalo J, Llanos-Cuentas A, *et al.* PERMANENT GENETIC RESOURCES: A set of 12 microsatellite loci for genetic studies of Leishmania braziliensis. *Mol Ecol Resour.* 2008 Mar;8(2):351-3.

[128] Oddone R, Schweynoch C, Schönian G, de Sousa Cdos S, Cupolillo E, Espinosa D, *et al.* Development of a multilocus microsatellite typing approach for discriminating strains of Leishmania (Viannia) species. *J Clin Microbiol.* 2009 Sep;47(9):2818-25.

[129] Kuhls K, Keilonat L, Ochsenreither S, Schaar M, Schweynoch C, Presber W, *et al.* Multilocus microsatellite typing (MLMT) reveals genetically isolated populations between and within the main endemic regions of visceral leishmaniasis. *Microbes Infect.* 2007 Mar;9(3):334-43.

[130] Alam MZ, Kuhls K, Schweynoch C, Sundar S, Rijal S, Shamsuzzaman AK, *et al.* Multilocus microsatellite typing (MLMT) reveals genetic homogeneity of Leishmania donovani strains in the Indian subcontinent. *Infect Genet Evol.* 2009 Jan;9(1):24-31.

[131] Seridi N, Amro A, Kuhls K, Belkaid M, Zidane C, Al-Jawabreh A, *et al.* Genetic polymorphism of Algerian Leishmania infantum strains revealed by multilocus microsatellite analysis. *Microbes Infect.* 2008 Oct;10(12-13):1309-15.

[132] Chargui N, Amro A, Haouas N, Schönian G, Babba H, Schmidt S, *et al.* Population structure of Tunisian Leishmania infantum and evidence for the existence of hybrids and gene flow between genetically different populations. *Int J Parasitol.* 2009 Jun; 39(7):801-11.

[133] Amro A, Schönian G, Al-Sharabati MB, Azmi K, Nasereddin A, Abdeen Z, *et al.* Population genetics of Leishmania infantum in Israel and the Palestinian Authority through microsatellite analysis. *Microbes Infect.* 2009 Apr;11(4):484-92.

[134] Montoya L, Gállego M, Gavignet B, Piarroux R, Rioux JA, Portús M, *et al.* Application of microsatellite genotyping to the study of a restricted Leishmania infantum focus: different genotype compositions in isolates from dogs and sand flies. *Am J Trop Med Hyg*. 2007 May;76(5):888-95.

[135] Kuhls K, Alam MZ, Cupolillo E, Ferreira GE, Mauricio IL, Oddone R, *et al.* Comparative microsatellite typing of new world leishmania infantum reveals low heterogeneity among populations and its recent old world origin. *PLoS Negl Trop Dis*. 2011 Jun; 5(6):e1155.

[136] Siriwardana HV, Noyes HA, Beeching NJ, Chance ML, Karunaweera ND, Bates PA. Leishmania donovani and cutaneous leishmaniasis, Sri Lanka. *Emerg Infect Dis*. 2007 Mar;13(3):476-8.

[137] Nolder D, Roncal N, Davies CR, Llanos-Cuentas A, Miles MA. Multiple hybrid genotypes of Leishmania (Viannia) in a focus of mucocutaneous leishmaniasis. *Am J Trop Med Hyg*. 2007 Mar;76(3):573-8.

[138] Rougeron V, De Meeûs T, Hide M, Waleckx E, Bermudez H, Arevalo J, *et al.* Extreme inbreeding in Leishmania braziliensis. *Proc Natl Acad Sci U S A*. 2009 Jun 23;106(25): 10224-9.

[139] Rougeron V, De Meeûs T, Hide M, Waleckx E, Dereure J, Arevalo J, *et al.* A battery of 12 microsatellite markers for genetic analysis of the Leishmania (Viannia) guyanensis complex. *Parasitology*. 2010 Nov;137(13):1879-84.

[140] Alam MZ, Kovalenko DA, Kuhls K, Nasyrova RM, Ponomareva VI, Fatullaeva AA, *et al.* Identification of the agent causing visceral leishmaniasis in Uzbeki and Tajiki foci by analysing parasite DNA extracted from patients' Giemsa-stained tissue preparations. *Parasitology*. 2009 Aug;136(9):981-6.

[141] Tibayrenc M, Ayala FJ. Reproductive clonality of pathogens: a perspective on pathogenic viruses, bacteria, fungi, and parasitic protozoa. *Proc Natl Acad Sci U S A*. 2012 Nov 27;109(48):E3305-13.

[142] Tibayrenc M, Ayala FJ. How clonal are Trypanosoma and Leishmania? *Trends Parasitol*. 2013 Jun;29(6):264-9.

[143] Delgado O, Cupolillo E, Bonfante-Garrido R, Silva S, Belfort E, Grimaldi Júnior G, *et al.* Cutaneous leishmaniasis in Venezuela caused by infection with a new hybrid between Leishmania (Viannia) braziliensis and L. (V.) guyanensis. *Mem Inst Oswaldo Cruz*. 1997 Sep-Oct;92(5):581-2.

[144] Dujardin JC, Banuls AL, Llanos-Cuentas A, Alvarez E, DeDoncker S, Jacquet D, *et al.* Putative Leishmania hybrids in the Eastern Andean valley of Huanuco, Peru. *Acta Trop*. 1995 Aug;59(4):293-307.

[145] Belli AA, Miles MA, Kelly JM. A putative Leishmania panamensis/Leishmania braziliensis hybrid is a causative agent of human cutaneous leishmaniasis in Nicaragua. *Parasitology*. 1994 Nov;109 (Pt 4):435-42.

[146] Kelly JM, Law JM, Chapman CJ, Van Eys GJ, Evans DA. Evidence of genetic recombination in Leishmania. *Mol Biochem Parasitol*. 1991 Jun;46(2):253-63.

[147] Miles MA, Yeo M, Mauricio IL. Genetics. Leishmania exploit sex. *Science*. 2009 Apr 10;324(5924):187-9.

[148] Inbar E, Akopyants NS, Charmoy M, Romano A, Lawyer P, Elnaiem DE, *et al*. The mating competence of geographically diverse Leishmania major strains in their natural and unnatural sand fly vectors. *PLoS Genet*. 2013 Jul;9(7):e1003672.

[149] Volf P, Benkova I, Myskova J, Sadlova J, Campino L, Ravel C. Increased transmission potential of Leishmania major/Leishmania infantum hybrids. *Int J Parasitol*. 2007 May;37(6):589-93.

[150] Ivens AC, Peacock CS, Worthey EA, Murphy L, Aggarwal G, Berriman M, *et al*. The genome of the kinetoplastid parasite, Leishmania major. *Science*. 2005 Jul 15;309(5733):436-42.

[151] Peacock CS, Seeger K, Harris D, Murphy L, Ruiz JC, Quail MA, *et al*. Comparative genomic analysis of three Leishmania species that cause diverse human disease. *Nat Genet*. 2007 Jul;39(7):839-47.

[152] Rogers MB, Hilley JD, Dickens NJ, Wilkes J, Bates PA, Depledge DP, *et al*. Chromosome and gene copy number variation allow major structural change between species and strains of Leishmania. *Genome Res*. 2011 Dec;21(12):2129-42.

[153] Downing T, Imamura H, Decuypere S, Clark TG, Coombs GH, Cotton JA, *et al*. Whole genome sequencing of multiple Leishmania donovani clinical isolates provides insights into population structure and mechanisms of drug resistance. *Genome Res*. 2011 Dec;21(12):2143-56.

[154] Raymond F, Boisvert S, Roy G, Ritt JF, Légaré D, Isnard A, *et al*. Genome sequencing of the lizard parasite Leishmania tarentolae reveals loss of genes associated to the intracellular stage of human pathogenic species. *Nucleic Acids Res*. 2012 Feb;40(3): 1131-47.

[155] Srividya G, Duncan R, Sharma P, Raju BV, Nakhasi HL, Salotra P. Transcriptome analysis during the process of in vitro differentiation of Leishmania donovani using genomic microarrays. *Parasitology*. 2007 Oct;134(Pt 11):1527-39.

[156] Rochette A, Raymond F, Ubeda JM, Smith M, Messier N, Boisvert S, *et al*. Genome-wide gene expression profiling analysis of Leishmania major and Leishmania infantum developmental stages reveals substantial differences between the two species. *BMC Genomics*. 2008 May 29;9:255.

[157] Ubeda JM, Légaré D, Raymond F, Ouameur AA, Boisvert S, Rigault P, *et al.* Modulation of gene expression in drug resistant Leishmania is associated with gene amplification, gene deletion and chromosome aneuploidy. *Genome Biol.* 2008;9(7):R115.

[158] Leprohon P, Légaré D, Raymond F, Madore E, Hardiman G, Corbeil J, *et al.* Gene expression modulation is associated with gene amplification, supernumerary chromosomes and chromosome loss in antimony-resistant Leishmania infantum. *Nucleic Acids Res.* 2009 Apr;37(5):1387-99.

[159] Depledge DP, Evans KJ, Ivens AC, Aziz N, Maroof A, Kaye PM, *et al.* Comparative expression profiling of Leishmania: modulation in gene expression between species and in different host genetic backgrounds. *PLoS Negl Trop Dis.* 2009 Jul 7;3(7):e476.

[160] Volkman SK, Sabeti PC, DeCaprio D, Neafsey DE, Schaffner SF, Milner DA Jr, *et al.* A genome-wide map of diversity in Plasmodium falciparum. *Nat Genet.* 2007 Jan;39(1): 113-9.

[161] Neafsey DE, Schaffner SF, Volkman SK, Park D, Montgomery P, Milner DA Jr, *et al.* Genome-wide SNP genotyping highlights the role of natural selection in Plasmodium falciparum population divergence. *Genome Biol.* 2008;9(12):R171.

[162] Mu J, Myers RA, Jiang H, Liu S, Ricklefs S, Waisberg M, *et al.* Plasmodium falciparum genome-wide scans for positive selection, recombination hot spots and resistance to antimalarial drugs. *Nat Genet.* 2010 Mar;42(3):268-71.

[163] Miles MA, Llewellyn MS, Lewis MD, Yeo M, Baleela R, Fitzpatrick S, *et al.* The molecular epidemiology and phylogeography of Trypanosoma cruzi and parallel research on Leishmania: looking back and to the future. *Parasitology.* 2009 Oct;136(12): 1509-28.

Chapter 5

Geographical and Environmental Variables of Leishmaniasis Transmission

Roqueline A.G.M.F. Aversi-Ferreira,
Jucimária Dantas Galvão, Sylla Figueredo da Silva,
Giovanna Felipe Cavalcante,
Ediana Vasconcelos da Silva, Naina Bhatia-Dey and
Tales Alexandre Aversi-Ferreira

Additional information is available at the end of the chapter

http://dx.doi.org/10.5772/57546

1. Introduction

Leishmaniasis, an infectious disease is not contagious. It belongs to the group of tropical neglected diseases [1, 2] that are ignored as priority in terms of eradication. It is estimated to be the ninth largest cause of disease among infected individuals [3, 4] ; it can cause intense epidemics that are primarily associated with the nutritional and the migratory factors [5, 6].

Most likely leishmaniasis originated in East Africa, however, it has been reported in ancient Egypt and in Christian Nubian approximately 4,000 B.C. In fact, it appears that Egyptians got the disease in the trade, as Egyptian Nile Valley is not a niche to sand flies [7]. Currently it has been reported in more than 80 countries, primarily in the developing countries in 4 continents, reaching indices around 500,000 new cases/year, with relatively higher incidence in India, Bangladesh, Nepal, Sudan and Brazil; approximately 200 million people have been estimated to get the exposure to the risk of its transmission [8].

Protozoan *Leishmania*, a unicellular flagellate, is the root cause of the disease; the parasite is transmitted to humans via female sand flies and manifests into two main forms: visceral [LV], and tegumentary [LT], the later divides into cutaneous [LC] and mucocutaneous [LMC] sub forms [7] (figure 1). Leishmaniasis has different clinical forms depending on the parasite, immune responses of the infected individuals and additional still unknown factors. Indeed, studies on leishmaniasis could be focused on both unknown and known factors to eradicate this disease.

The LV, also known as Kala-azar (Indian name), black fever or DumDum fever, is the most severe form of leishmaniasis (figure 1) caused by *Leishmania donovani* and *Leishmania infantum* (*Leishmania infantum chagasis*, a subspecies typical of Brazil), both protozoans belonging to the same family, *Trypanossomatidae*. These species have different geographical distribution: *Leishmania infantum* is typical of South America, Europe and Northern Africa, while *Leishmania donovani* is commonly found in Eastern Africa.

LV is a chronic and systemic disease characterized by anemia, mucosal ulcers, fever, hepatomegaly and splenomegaly, lymphadenopathy, pancytopenia, weight loss, weakness and, eventually death due to lack of treatment [9].

The most common form of leishmaniasis in the world is LC, it can progress to other forms and is caused by about 20 different species of *Leishmania*; it is known with various different names, such as Aleppo boil, Chiclero ulcer, Bauru's ulcer, Bay sore, Biskra button, Lahore sore, Oriental sore, Pian bois, Uta and leishmaniasis tropica.

LMC produces destructive and disfiguring lesions in the body, especially in the face (figure 1), they are primarily caused by *Leishmania braziliensis* and rarely by *Leishmania aethiopica*.

Regardless of the type of leishmaniasis this disease is transmitted through the bite of the female sand flies and the geographical distribution of this disease is directly associated with the habitat of its vector. Phlebotomine sand flies primarily inhabit hot and wet tropical regions with regular pluvial index [10], however, sometimes they also inhabit the dry and hot places; therefore, the environmental and geographical niches of this vector that are associated with its natural vertebrate hosts are determinants of the disease transmission.

The association of the vector with natural reservoir became a propitious factor towards keeping an endemic status for leishmaniasis. In fact, there are many natural reservoirs such as canine, avian (chicken), bovine, equine, caprine, ovine, swine and feline [11-14] ; all of them inhabit the same regions as Phlebotomine.

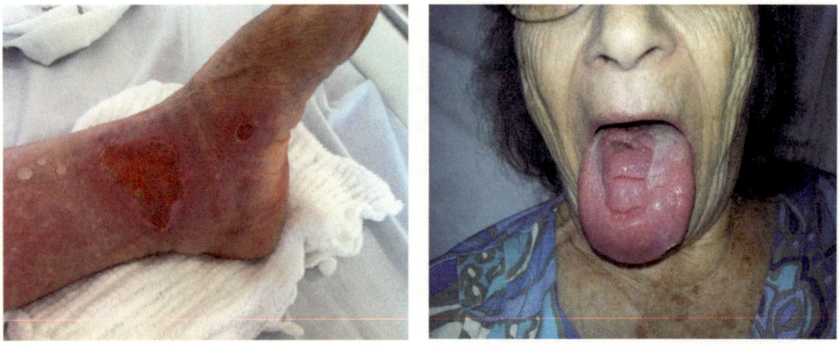

Figure 1. Clinical features of *cutaneous leishmaniasis* (left), and *mucocutaneous leishmaniasis* (right).

http://dx.doi.org/10.5772/57546

In addition, an important factor associated with leishmaniasis occurrence is the canine leishmaniasis (figure 2), a zoonosis that indirectly indicates the prevalence of this disease in humans at a specific site.

Indeed, leishmaniasis is associated with the tropical and the equatorial zones, poor sanitary conditions and surveillance in the areas where the parasites and the vectors are close to the reservoir and the humans, therefore, the most important point to understand the cause of epidemic and the transmission of the disease is the knowledge on the geographical and the environmental variables. Nevertheless, both these variables will be considered here into two categories: the worldwide and the regional.

In the geographic terms, the worldwide variables represent the geographic area where the vector has its niches and where the climate is favorable to its development. However, there are places and the environmental factors that are relatively propitious to the transmission of leishmaniasis than other factors such as higher population of the sand flies; these are considered.as the regional variables that would be accountable for the frequency of the disease.

In the environmental terms, the worldwide variables indicate the global climate and the associated landscape; however, the anthropomorphic factors and the climate peculiarities in a specific region represent the regional variables.

This chapter will present the worldwide and the regional aspects of geographical and environmental variables associated with leishmaniasis transmission.

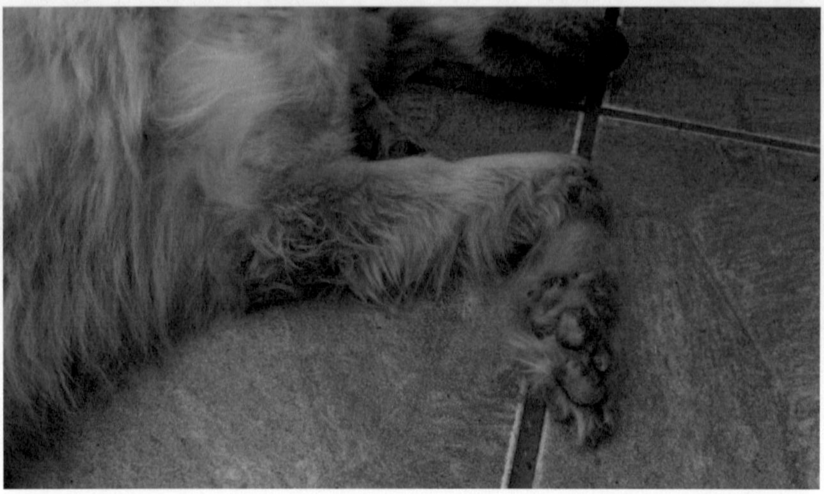

Figure 2. A photographic representation of a dog displaying clinical symptoms of canine leishmaniasis.

2. Materials and methods

The goal of this chapter is to collect the information from an extensive literature using the followings electronic databases: MEDLINE, Plos, PubMed, LILACS, CAPES periodic, Open Journal System, Scielo and Google Academic. The descriptors used were: *leishmaniasis, leishmaniasis visceral, leishmaniasis cutaneous, leishmaniasis mucocutaneous, Phlebotomine, the sand flies, the geographical aspects of leishmaniasis* and the *environmental aspects of leishmaniasis.*

2.1. Inclusion criteria

Indexed papers published in the last 20 years; classic indexed papers on more ancient and severe areas. Some textbooks have also been used to elaborate this chapter.

2.2. Exclusion criteria

Papers that did not mention the main ideas used in this chapter and the texts with the same contents as the most recent papers used here.

3. Geographical variables

3.1. Worldwide variables

In the terms of biosphere, geographical variables of leishmaniasis transmission are associated with tropical zone as well as hot and the wet climates with regular pluvial index [10]. The countries that are underdeveloped as well as the developing countries show the highest incidence of leishmaniasis transmission (figures 3 and 4).

Indeed, both human LV and LC follow the geographical distribution of the insect vector (see [15]); it is found globally between tropics but has also been detected in some regions with relatively rigorous winter such as in France [16], Portugal, Russia and China [3].

Based on the information available since past ten years, in Africa, the data on reported cases of LV are sparse and the reported cases in sub-Saharan African region are scarce (table 1); Nigeria had just one reported case within this period [3]. However, in Eastern African countries, LV is endemic and the reported cases have increased above predicted expectation in the last 20 years [9]. The countries with the most infections are Sudan [17, 18], Ethiopia [2, 9], South Sudan [3], Somalia, Uganda, Kenya [9] and Eritrea [3] (table 1, figures 3 and 4).

As for LC, Sub-Saharan region (figures 3 and 4) showed elevated number of the reported cases than cases for LV, i.e., 154 cases of LC in comparison to 1 case of LV; whereas the countries with higher number of LC cases are Cameroon and Nigeria respectively. In Eastern Africa, interestingly, Eritrea is the country with the lowest cases of LV and the highest cases of LC, while other countries in this region have no reported cases in the past ten years (table 1). In general, in African subcontinent, the number of reported cases of LV is much higher than those of LC, i.e., 8,571 of LV in comparison to 204 of LC.

http://dx.doi.org/10.5772/57546

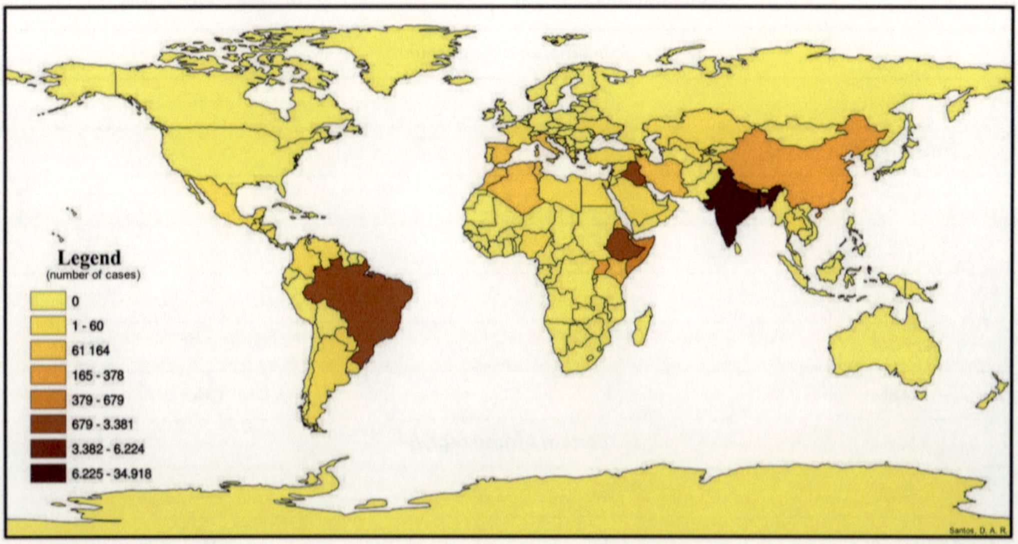

Figure 3. World LV distribution in the last 10 years.

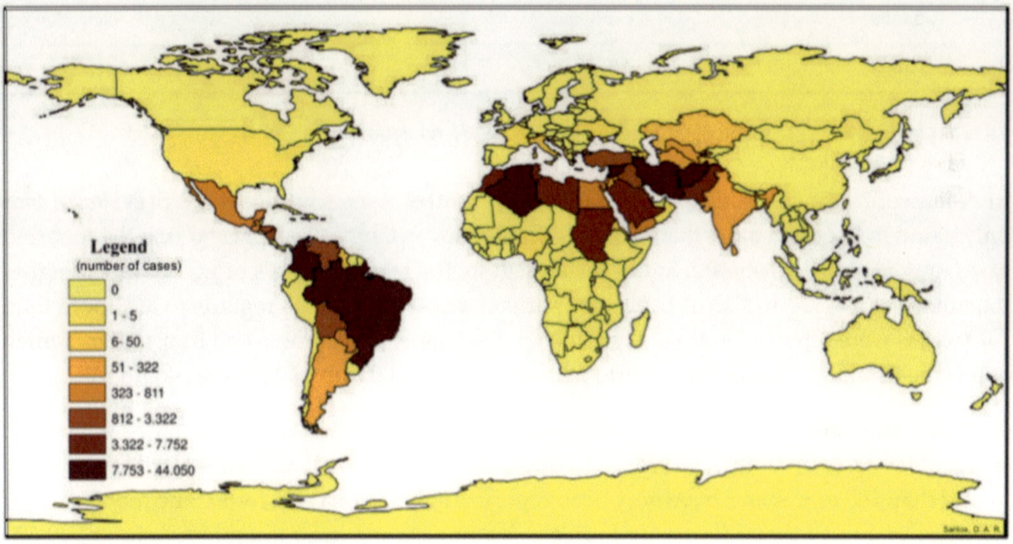

Figure 4. World LC distribution in the last 10 years.

Reported cases in Africa		
	Visceral leishmaniasis	**Cutaneous leishmaniasis**
	Sub-Saharan African region	
Cameroon	0	55
Cote d'Ivore	0	1
Ghana	0	27
Mali	0	58
Nigeria	1	5
Senegal	0	8
Total	**1**	**154**
	Eastern African region	
Eritrea	100	50
Ethiopia	1860	0
Kenya	145	0
Somalia	679	0
Sudan	3742	0
South Sudan	1756	0
Uganda	288	0
Total	**8570**	**50**

Table 1. Geographical distribution of LV and LC in Africa based on reference [3].

In Asian subcontinent from the Middle East to Central Asia, significant LV prevalence was only found in Iraq with more than 1,000 reported cases; in China, Georgia and Iran the reported cases ranged at little over 100. In this Asian region, the reported cases of LC are much higher than those of LV, i.e., 61,015 of LC in comparison to 2,497 of LV. As regards to LC, more than 1,000 cases were reported in Iran, Afghanistan, Pakistan, Saudi Arabia and Iraq; and in Yemen and Uzbekistan the number of reported cases was over 100 (table 2) (figures 4 and 5).

In Indian subcontinent [3, 20] and in Southwestern Asia [3, 21], there are more than 1,000 reported LV cases in countries like India, Bangladesh and Nepal; in this same territory LC cases higher than 100 in number have only been reported in Sri Lanka and India. The reported total LV cases are higher than LC cases in Indian Subcontinent and in Southeastern Asia, i.e., 42,623 of LV in comparison to 478 of LC (table 2, figures 4 and 5).

In Asia, overall number of the reported LC cases is higher than those of LV cases, i.e., 61,493 of LC while 45,120 of LV.

Reported cases in Asia		
	Visceral leishmaniasis	**Cutaneous leishmaniasis**
	Middle East to Central Asia	
Afghanistan	0	22620
Armenia	7	0
Azerbaijan	28	17
China	378	0
Georgia	164	5
Iran	149	24630
Iraq	1711	1655
Kazakhstan	1	15
Oman	1	5
Pakistan	0	7752
Saudi Arabia	34	3445
Tajikistan	15	25
Turkmenistan	0	99
Ukraine	2	2
Uzbekistan	7	142
Yemen	0	603
Total	**2497**	**61015**
	Indian Subcontinent and Southeastern Asia	
Bangladesh	6224	0
Bhutan	2	0
India	34918	156
Nepal	1477	0
Sri Lanka	0	322
Thailand	2	0
Total	**42623**	**478**

Table 2. Geographical distribution of LV and LC in Asia based on reference [3].

In the Mediterranean region, countries with more than 100 reported LV cases are Morocco, Italy, Spain, Albania and Algeria; for LC, the countries with more than 1,000 reported cases are Algeria, Syria, Tunisia, Libya, Morocco and Turkey (table 3, figures 3 and 4). Israel, Egypt, Jordan and Palestine are on lower tier of LC prevalence, in these countries, over 100 LC cases have been reported (table 3, figures 3 and 4). Thus in this region, overall number of the reported

LC cases is much higher than LV cases, i.e., 85,886 of LC in comparison to 874 of LV in the last ten years.

Reported cases in the Mediterranean region		
	Visceral leishmaniasis	**Cutaneous leishmaniasis**
Albania	114	6
Algeria	111	44050
Bosnia and Herzegovina	2	0
Bulgaria	7	0
Croatia	5	2
Cyprus	2	1
Egypt	1	471
France	18	2
Greece	42	3
Israel	2	579
Italy	134	49
Jordan	0	227
Libya	3	3540
Macedonia	7	0
Malta	2	0
Montenegro	3	0
Morocco	152	3430
Palestine	5	218
Portugal	15	0
Spain	117	0
Syria	14	22882
Tunisia	89	7631
Turkey	29	2465
Total	**874**	**85556**

Table 3. Geographical distribution of LV and LC in the Mediterranean region based on reference [3].

In Latina America, the number of LV cases have increased in northern Argentina [22], in areas bordering Brazil and Paraguay, in Colombia [23], in Venezuela [24] as well as in North America [25] ; recently one case has been recorded in Uruguay as well [19] (table 4).

http://dx.doi.org/10.5772/57546

Brazil is the only country in the Americas with over 1,000 reported cases of LV, in other countries the reported cases of LV are lower than 100 (table 4). In contrast, LC is relatively widespread with 10 countries that have over 1,000 reported cases, these are Brazil, Colombia, Peru, Nicaragua, Bolivia, Venezuela, Panama, Ecuador, Costa Rica and Honduras in descending order of prevalence. Additionally, 5 countries show over 100 reported cases, they are Mexico, Guatemala, Paraguay, Argentina and French Guyana respectively (table 4).

An interesting aspect in the Americas is the inclusion of the United States in the world scenario with 42 reported cases of LC [25].

The overall number of the reported cases of LC is much higher than those of LV, i.e., 66,983of LC in comparison to only 3,668 of LV in the American subcontinent.

Specifically in Brazil, and mostly in other developing countries, leishmaniasis was restricted to rural areas; however, currently the disease has advanced to other regions and has reached urban peripheries [26-28]. This demonstrates that the urbanization process is one of the major factors for the scattering of leishmaniasis.

	Reported cases in America	
	Visceral leishmaniasis	**Cutaneous leishmaniasis**
Argentina	8	261
Bolivia	0	2647
Brazil	3481	26008
Colombia	60	17420
Costa Rica	0	1249
Ecuador	0	1724
French Guyana	0	233
Guatemala	15	684
Guyana	0	16
Honduras	6	1159
Mexico	7	811
Nicaragua	3	3222
Panama	0	2188
Paraguay	48	431
Peru	0	6405
Suriname	0	3
Venezuela	40	2480
Uruguay	1	0
United States	0	42
Total	**3668**	**66983**

Table 4. Geographical distribution of LV and LC in the Americas, based on references [3], [19] and [25].

The geographical distribution of leishmaniasis in the world appears to be changing, firstly, the variation of global climate [25, 29] could be increasing the area of Phlebotomine niches; and secondly, the globalization of economy increases the migration of the people among countries thereby increasing the contact of people with Phlebotomine niche where leishmaniasis is either incipient or non-existent. The former hypothesis could be explained by the growing economy in BRIC countries, such as Brazil, Russia, India and China; among these India and Brazil are endemic to leishmaniasis.

Nowadays, the geographical distribution of leishmaniasis is similar for LC and LV in the continents; however, differences exist among the countries. Indeed, approximately 57% of countries studied here showed both LC and LV. Nevertheless, in the last ten years the number of the reported LV cases in the world is approximately 58,413 with 77.2% in Asia. In contrast, the number of the reported LC cases in the world is approximately 214,082 with almost 40% of those in the Mediterranean region.

In fact, the reported LC cases are much higher than those reported for LV. A possible explanation for this scenario is the number of LC parasites, there are over 20 parasites causing LC whereas only just few parasites cause LV. Although there are only few sand fly species that are vectors for both LV and LC, both conditions have the same kind of reservoir hosts [30].

The above problems that have emerged from studying the worldwide geographical distribution must be resolved with the collaborative prevention measures by the countries where leishmaniasis is endemic; such cumulative force would lead to the global solutions to eradicate this disease.

3.2. Regional variables

Regional variables represent areas of the countries where the probability of existence of leishmaniasis has increased. In fact, there are internal regions in different countries such as the rural zone and the urban periphery where the incidence of leishmaniasis has increased (figure 6). A plausible explanation for such increase is the higher density of Phlebotomine and natural reservoir hosts of the parasites inhabiting these areas; these areas in the developing countries are infused with poverty where people live and work close to the forests or the woodlands.

In the developing countries, leishmaniasis was a rural disease, however, it was found to be associated with the growing urbanization. This disease began to develop in the urban periphery in Brazil and it was noted around 1970s [31]. A probably explanation of such spreading is the internal migration of the people from the rural zone to the urban areas [30].

People that arrive from the rural zones to the urban areas usually have limited and scant financial resources and therefore, they inhabit the periphery of the towns that are regions with the woodland and he forest remnants; they are basically inter topical zones. Such city periphery is a risk zone for the dissemination of leishmaniasis since here the contact among humans, Phlebotomine and their hosts is maximized. Indeed, some reservoir hosts are used as the pets and others are raised in peridomicile to feed these people.

http://dx.doi.org/10.5772/57546

This regional geographical distribution of leishmaniasis incidence must be analyzed by public health agencies to identify and verify the risk zone for leishmaniasis. Additional studies are also required to identify all the causative factors; specifically the data on Phlebotomine niches, presence of natural reservoir hosts of *Leishmania* and the sanitary quality of the habitat for the people are of utmost importance.

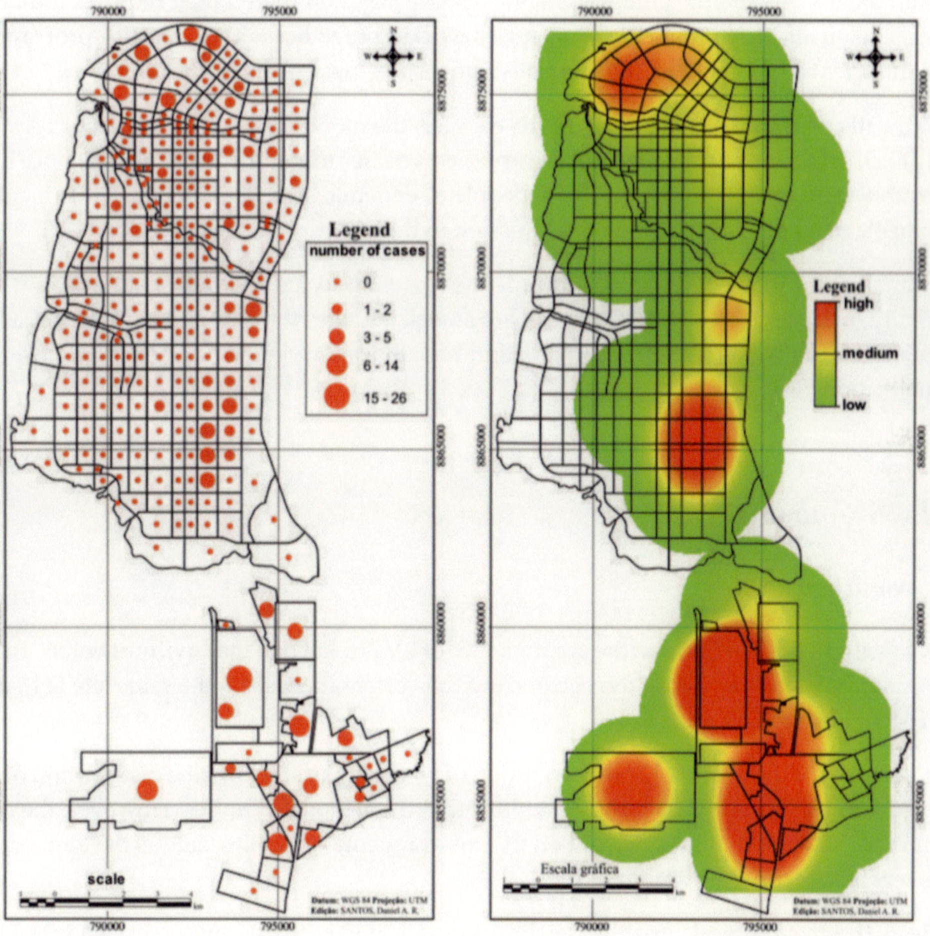

Figure 5. The map of city of Palmas, northern Brazil, is shown. On the left the dots represent reported cases fo leishmaniasis in this municipality from 2007 to 2012. The Kernel map of the same locality is demonstrated on the right, where darker/stronger color indicates the higher number of cases. The bigger dots (left) and the dark color distribution (right) are present in periphery of the town, that is closest to the forest.

Briefly, the geographical areas of leishmaniasis dissemination are the rural zones and the urban peripheries.

In geographical and regional terms the best way to start the fight against this disease, is the construction of a risk map for each municipality where leishmaniasis is endemic; it will indicate the points where the eradication effort should be focused. Such approach would include the elimination of Phlebotomine along with the complete removal and killing of the natural reservoir hosts of *Leishmania* from the population. We shall not address these specific problems in this chapter, however, georeferencing studies using adequate maps such as Kernel maps (figure 5), utilizing the new technologies for geographical representation along with spatial analysis of databases [32] appear to be the principle strategies to combat leishmaniasis.

Leishmaniasis is a complex multi-systemic disease [33], and therefore, it requires multidisciplinary team effort of public health agencies working together with the health professionals and the scientists to generate the most positive results towards its eradication.

Specifically as regards to the topic of this chapter, the monitoring of the reported cases from the data is an important tool on the geographical variables to control leishmaniasis since it may spread by the internal migration of the people to endemic areas and increasing its incidence due to elevated person-to-person transmission in the crowded living conditions [32].

The analysis of the geographical region is the first step to monitor leishmaniasis, however, majority of causes for endemic outbreak are associated with the natural environment as well as man-made factors such as the human migration, the deforestation, the urbanization and the malnutrition [34].

4. Environmental variables

4.1. World variables

It is a well-established fact that the maintenance of LV is related to the environmental variables favoring the presence of both the vectors and the vertebrate hosts at the same site [24], and it can occur also for LC.

It is known that the geographical distribution of leishmaniasis follows the distribution of sand fly niches, this fact is observed worldwide and in the regional analyses. However, the distribution of the sand flies is dependent on the environmental variables such as the temperature, the vegetation, and the humidity.

Indeed, the geographical variables are directly associated with the environmental variables in the biosphere and are inter-dependent. The geographical distribution of leishmaniasis generally occurs in the tropical and the equatorial regions, where warm and rainy weather prevails [10, 35, 36] favoring Phlebotomine reproduction [37, 38].

In fact, the analysis of the planet temperature map compared to the maps of reported cases of leishmaniasis (figures 4 and 5) demonstrates that these regions are parallel (figure 7).

In general, leishmaniasis is primarily present in the tropics, however, its incidence is increasing in other areas as well, and most likely this increase is associated with the global climate changes [25].

http://dx.doi.org/10.5772/57546

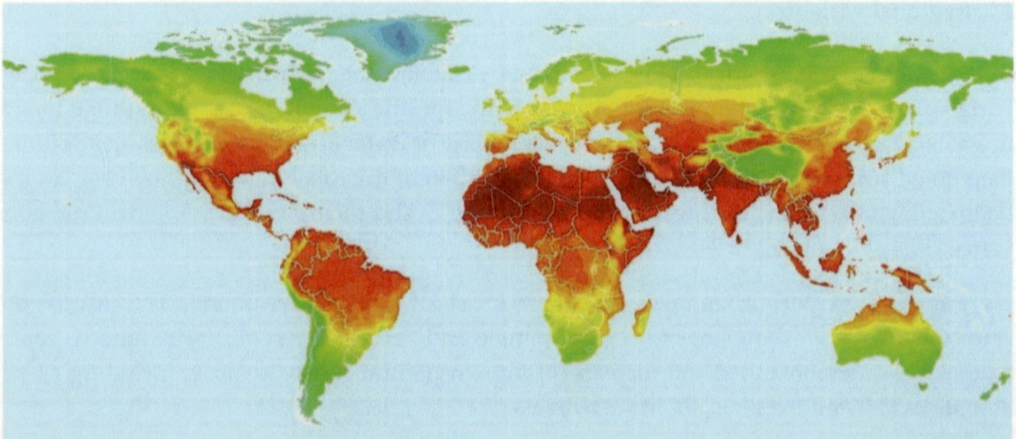

Figure 6. World temperature map where darker colors indicate higher temperatures

The world climate changes are implicated with physical consequences [21] as well as with the alterations of the vector niches and the reservoir species for the infectious diseases [21, 25].

According to Gonzalez *et al* [25], leishmaniasis is expanding to northern United States from Mexico and Texas, where it is considered autochthonous, primarily due to the increase in the niches of the sandflies associated with the reservoir hosts to *Leishmania*; however, other associated reasons could be dog importation [30] and the increase in human migration and/or travel in the recent years.

The movement of people occurs from countries where leishmaniasis is endemic to countries where climate is temperate. The people move from the temperate areas to the tropical and the equatorial climates, particularly for the holidays, sometimes they carry their dogs and other pets [30].

Climate is not the only factor associated with the vector niches, the vegetation also has some impact. In fact, in some regions, the climate indicates the existence of certain kind of vegetation, i.e., it is usual to think of the tropical forest in the tropical climate and the equatorial forest in the equatorial climate, however, it is possible to find desert, savanna, Cerrado (Brazilian savanna) and Atlantic forest in the same regions where the tropical and the equatorial climates prevail.

Phlebotomine prefers the forest areas, but, interestingly, it can also be found in open and urban areas [35].

In summary, the world environmental variables linked to Phlebotomine niche exist mainly in Latina America and some parts of Africa and Asia. The hot and the wet climates are associated with the forest and the woodlands areas; however, some species prefer open and the dry areas. In all these regions, it is possible to find some kind of host to *Leishmania*, nevertheless, the density of sand flies in some areas depends on the regional environmental variables.

4.2. Regional variables

In terms of the geographical and the regional variables, the main factor for the scattering leishmaniasis is the presence of Phlebotomine in the specific areas. In fact, since sandflies breed in soil or litter, they are dependent on the availability of water and the dampness. In addition, their small size enables them to live in various different microhabitats [36], however, an in-depth analysis detailing the breeding sites of sand flies and their larval development remains scarce [15].

Nevertheless, the peri-urban areas are important risk factors for leishmaniasis transmission since they maintain the niches for Phlebotomine and natural reservoir hosts. Indeed, some studies have demonstrated the increase of known natural reservoir hosts including *Galus domesticus* [39] and the pigs [40] in such areas.

In relation to the local environment, the urban periphery is frequently inhabited by poor populations, they are forced to live far from downtown and these habitats grow as the people arrive there from the rural areas. This is a common case in the poor and developing countries. Such lesser-developed areas are comprised of the forests or the woodlands and become a favorable place to increase contact of sandflies with the people as well as domestic and wild reservoir hosts of leishmaniasis.

At the same time, this population has limited access to basic sanitation and sewage treatment, and therefore, it generates exclusionary urbanization [41].

In fact, the deforestation linked to unplanned urbanization seems to be the cause of peak incidence of leishmaniasis in some regions [32]. Urbanization parameters associated with the growing cities and the deforestation areas generate ecological changes [41] that could modify the forest flora; this in turn generates trunks of dead trees thereby increasing the amount of decomposed organic material as well as the microorganisms on the ground that positively affect Phlebotomine cycle [38, 42-45].

These findings justify that in the peri-urban areas there is increase in number of the infected people carrying leishmaniasis and other infectious diseases that are dependent on the vector transmission, the people in those areas get higher exposure to vectors and reservoir hosts.

The reservoir hosts to *Leishmania* are the rodents, the marsupials, the monkeys, wild canines [30], the domestic dogs, chickens, the cattle, the equine, the caprine, the bovine, the swine and the feline species [11-14, 30], they all inhabit the areas populated with the sand flies.

Indeed, the presence of the swine species in the peridomicile is an important risk of the contamination [40], and the contamination has also been found associated with the presence of chickens as wild predators that are potential wild reservoirs hosts of *Leishmania* and *feed* on them, thereby intensifying the parasite cycle to the human and the canine populations [39].

The life cycle of Leishmania is mainly associated with the ecological factors in the rural or the peridomicile areas that harbor the sand fly niches and the reservoir hosts with human habitation (figure 7).

http://dx.doi.org/10.5772/57546

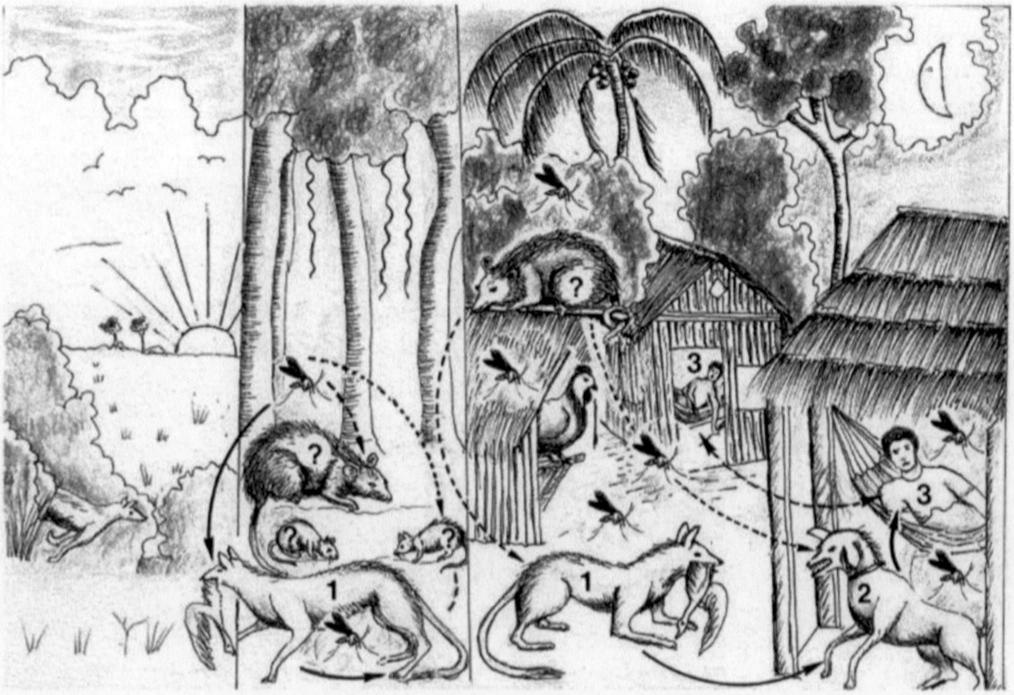

Figure 7. Scheme showing the life cycle of sandflies, reservoir hosts and humans, based on [46].

The human knowledge about leishmaniasis is not complete; many factors are still unknown or only partially known. Nevertheless, the current knowledge on this disease is adequate to develop accurate eradication strategies for the government and the public to work together developing specific protections with control of Phlebotomine by using insecticides, by removing organic material in the peridomicile areas [47, 48] and exterminating the contaminated reservoir hosts.

5. Conclusions

The aim of this chapter was simply to put together the collected information about the geographical and the environmental variables of leishmaniasis transmission. Leishmaniasis transmission is dependent on the association of contaminated sandflies with the reservoir hosts of *Leishmania* and the humans. In geographical terms association is favored in inter tropical regions, where the environmental factors such as the warm and the wet climate and certain types of the forest vegetation are predominant. In regional terms, the vicinity of the forest remnants or the woodland in the respective local periphery increases the density of sandflies thereby creating favorable conditions for the propagation of *Leishmania* life-cycle and its exposure to the people inhabiting that area.

Accurate and adequate public health policies and the proper dissemination of relevant information to the populations living in the endemic areas along with the severe control and the surveillance would be helpful in eliminating the contamination of humans and reservoir hosts by sandflies.

Author details

Roqueline A.G.M.F. Aversi-Ferreira[1,2,4], Jucimária Dantas Galvão[2,3], Sylla Figueredo da Silva[2,3], Giovanna Felipe Cavalcante[2], Ediana Vasconcelos da Silva[2,3], Naina Bhatia-Dey[1] and Tales Alexandre Aversi-Ferreira[1,2,3]

1 Department of Anatomy, Howard University, Washington, DC, USA

2 LABINECOP, Federal University of Tocantins, Palmas, state of Tocantins, Brazil

3 Graduate Program in Health Sciences, Federal University of Tocantins, Palmas, state of Tocantins, Brazil

4 Graduate Program in Animal Biology, University of Brasilia, Brasilia, DF, Brazil

References

[1] Feitosa MM, Ikeda FA, Luvizotto MCR, Perri SHV. Aspectos clínicos de cães com leishmaniose visceral no município de Araçatuba São Paulo (Brasil). Clínica Veterinária 2000; 2836-4.

[2] Custodio E, Gadisa E, Sordo L, Cruz I, Moreno J, Nieto J, Chicharro C, Aseffa A, Abraham Z, Hailu T, Canãvate C. Factors Associated with Leishmania Asymptomatic Infection: Results from a Cross-Sectional Survey in Highland Northern Ethiopia. PLOS Neglected Tropical Diseases 2012; 9(6) e1813.

[3] Alvar J, Velez ID, Bern C, Herrero M, Desjeux P, Cano J, Jannin J, Den Boer M. Leishmaniasis Worldwide and Global Estimates of Its Incidence. PLOS One 2012; 5(7) e35671.

[4] Hotez PJ, Molyneaux DH, Fenwick A, Ottesen E, Ehrlich, Sachs SE, Sachs, JD. Incorporating a rapid impact package for neglected tropical disease with programs for HIV/AIDS, tuberculosis and Malaria. Plos Med. 2006; 5(3) e102.

[5] Silva, ES, Roscoe EH, Arruda, LQ. Leishmaniose visceral canina: estudo clínico-epidemiológico e diagnóstico. Revista Brasileira de Medicina Veterinária 2001; 23(3) 111-16.

[6] Marins, JRP. Leishmaniose Visceral: uma doença em expansão: 15ª Reunião de Pesquisa Aplicada em Leishmaniose. Centro Educacional e Administrativo da Universidade Federal do Triângulo Mineiro, Uberaba, Brasil. 2011.

[7] Zink RA, Spigelman M, Schraut, B Greenblatt CL, Nerlich AG, Donoghue, HD. Leishmaniasis in Ancient Egypt and Upper Nubia. Emerg Infect Dis. 2006; 12(10) 1616-17.

[8] WHO (World Health Organization). Leishmaniasis: Burden of Disease. Geneva: World Health Organization 2013.

[9] Kolaczinski JH, Reithinger R, Dagemlider TW, Ocheng A, Kasimiro J, Kabatereine N, Brooker S. Risk factors of visceral leishmaniasis in East Africa: a case-control study in Pokot territory of Kenya and Uganda. International Journal of Epidemiology 2008; 2(37) 344-52.

[10] Rebelo JMM, Oliveira ST, Silva FS, Barros VLL, Costa JML. Sandflies (diptera:psychodidae) of the Amazonia of Maranhao v. seasonal occurrence in ancient colonization area and endemic for cutaneous leismaniasis. Rev Brasil Biol. 2001; 1(61) 107-15.

[11] Aguiar GM, Medeiros WM, De Marco TS, Santos SC, Gambardella S. Ecologia dos flebotomíneos da Serra do Mar, Itaguaí, Estado do Rio de Janeiro, Brasil. I - A fauna. flebotomínica e prevalência pelo local e tipo de captura (Diptera, Psychodidae, Phlebotominae). Caderno de Saúde Pública 1996; 2(12) 195-06.

[12] Domingos MF, Carreri-Bruno GC, Ciaravolo RMC, Galati EAB, Wanderley DMV, Corrêa FMA. Leishmaniose tegumentar americana: flebotomíneos de área de transmissão, no município de Pedro de Toledo, região sul do Estado de São Paulo, Brasil. Revista Sociedade Brasileira de Medicina Tropical 1998; 31(5) 425-32.

[13] Freitas JS, Santana RG, Melo SR. Levantamento dos casos de leishmaniose registrados no município de Jussara, Paraná, Brasil. Arquivo Ciências Saúde Unipar 2006; 1(10) 23-7.

[14] Moraes-Silva E, Antunes FR, Rodrigues MS, Silva FJ, Dias-Lima AG, Lemos-de-Sousa V, Alcantara AC, Reis EAG, NakataniM, Badaró R, Reis MG, Pontes-de-Carvalho L, Frankeb CR. Domestic swine in a visceral leishmaniasis endemic area produce antibodies against multiple *Leishmania infantum* antigens but apparently resist to *L. infantum* infection. Acta Tropica. 2006; 98176-82.

[15] Feliciangeli MD. Natural breeding places of phlebotomine sandflies. Med Vet Entomol. 2004; 18(4) 71-80.

[16] Hartemink N, Vanwambeke SO, Heesterbeek H, Rogers D, Morley, Pesson B, Davies C, Mahamdallie S, Ready P. PLoS ONE 2011; 8(6) e20817.

[17] Thomson MC,Elnaiem DA, Ashford RW, Connor SJ. Towards a kalaazar risk map for Sudan: mapping the potential distribution of *Phlebotomus orientalis* using digital data

of environmental variables. Tropical Medicine and International Health.1999; 4105-13.

[18] Elnaiem DE, Schorscher J, Bendall A, Obsmer V, Osman ME, Mekkawi AM, Connor SJ, Ashford RW, Thomson MC. Risc mapping of visceral leishmaniasis: the role of local variation in rainfall and altitude on the presence and incidence of kala-azar in eastern Sudan. Am J Trop Med Hyg. 2003; 68(1) 10-7.

[19] Salomón OD, Basmajdian Y, Fernández MS, Santini MS. *Lutzomyia longipalpis*in Uruguay: the first report and the potential of visceral leishmaniasis transmission. Mem Inst Oswaldo Cruz. 2011; 106(3) 381-382.

[20] Bhunia GS, Chatterjee N, Kumar V, Siddiqui NA, MandalR, Das P, Kesari S. Delimitation of kala-azar risk areas in the district of Vaishali in Bihar (India) using a geo-environmental approach. Mem Inst Oswaldo Cruz. 2012; 107(5) 609-20.

[21] Cross ER, Hyams KC. The potential effect of global warming on the geographic and seasonal distribution of *Phlebotomus papatasi* in Southwest Asia. Environment Health Perspectives 1996; 7(104) 724-27.

[22] Santini MS, Salamón OD, Acardi SA, Sandoval EA, Tartaglino L. *Lutzomyia longipalpis* behavior and control at an urban visceral leishmaniasis focus in Argentina. Rev Inst Med Trop. 2010; 52(4) 187-91.

[23] King RJ, Campbell-Lendrum DH, Daview CR. Predicting Geographic Variation in Cutaneous leishmaniasis, Colombia. Emerging Infectious Diseases 2004; 4(10) 598-07.

[24] Feliciangeli MD, Delgado O, Suarez B, Bravo A. *Leishmania* and sand flies: proximity to woodland as a risk factor for infection in a rural focus of visceral leishmaniasis in west central Venezuela. Tropical Medicine and International Health 2006; 12(2) 1785-91.

[25] Gonzales C, Wang O, Strutz SE, Gonzalez-Salazar C, Sanchez-Cordeiro V, Sarkar S. Climate change and risk of leishmaniasis in North America: predicitions from ecological niche models of vector and reservoir species. Plos Neglected Tropical Diseases 2010; 1(4) e585.

[26] Monteiro EM, Silva JCF, Costa RT, Costa DC, Barata RA, Paula EV, Machado-Coelho GLL, Rocha MF, Fortes-Dias CL, Dias ES. Leishmaniose Visceral: Estudo de Flebotomíneos e Infecção canina em Montes Claros. Revista Sociedade Brasileira de Medicina Tropical 2005; 2(38) 147-52.

[27] Sangioni LA, Gebara CMS, Aragão GM, Bezerra CAA, Almeida CC. Busca ativa de casos de leishmaniose cutânea em humanos e cães em area periférica do município de Campo Mourão - PR, Brasil. Ciência Rural 2007; 5(37) 1492-94.

[28] Zanzarini PD, Santos DR, Santos AR, Oliveira O, Poiani LP, Lonardoni MVC, Teodoro U, Silveira TGV. Leishmaniose tegumentar Americana canina em municípios do norte do Estado do Paraná, Brasil. Caderno de Saúde Pública 2005; 6(21) 1957-61.

[29] Barcellos C,Monteiro AMV, Corvalán C,Gurgel HC, Carvalho MS, Artaxo P, Hacon S,RagoniV. Mudançasclimáticas e ambientais e as doenças infecciosas: cenários e incertezas para o Brasil. Epidemiologia e Serviços de Saúde 2009; 3(18) 285-04.

[30] Ready PD. Leishmaniasis emergence and climate change. Rev Sci Tech Off Int Epiz. 2008; 2(27) 399-12.

[31] Cerbino Neto J, Werneck GL, Costa CHN. Factors associated with the incidence of urban visceral leishmaniasis: an ecological study in Teresina, Piauí state, Brazil. Caderno Saúde Pública. 2009; 7(25) 1543-51.

[32] Mott KE, Nuttal I, Desjeux P, Cattand P. New geographical approaches to control of some parasitic zoonoses. Bull World Health Organ. 1995; 2(73) 247-57.

[33] Nieto P, Malone JB, Bavia ME. Ecological niche modeling for visceral leishmaniasis in the state of Bahia, Brazil, using genetic algorithm for rule-set prediction and growing degree day-water budget analysis. Geospat Health. 2006; 1(1) 115-26.

[34] Desjeux P. The increase in risk factors for leishmaniasis worldwide. Transactions of the Royal Society of Tropical Medicine and Hygiene 2001; 3(95) 239-43.

[35] Oliveira EF, Silva EA, Fernandes CES, Paranhos Filho AC, Gamarra RM, Ribeiro AA, Brazil RP, Oliveira AG. Biotic factors and occurrence of *Lutzomya longipalpis* in endemic area of visceral leishmaniasis, Mato Grosso do Sul, Brazil. Mem Inst Oswaldo Cruz. 2012; 3(107) 396-401.

[36] Lewis DJ. Plebotomid Sandflies. Bull World Health Organ.1971; 44(4)535–51.

[37] Guerra JAO, Onety AC, Santos SL, Santos FGC, Talhari S, Paes MG. Situação da Leishmaniose em Manaus na última década. Revista Sociedade Brasileira de Medicina Tropical 2001; 34 Suppl244.

[38] Dias-Lima AG, Castéllon EG, Sherlock I. Flebotomíneos (*Diptera: Psychodidae*) de uma floresta primária de terra firme da estação experimental de silvicultura tropical, estado do amazonas, Brasil. Acta Amazônica 2003; 2(33) 303-16.

[39] Alexander B, Carvalho RL, Mccallum H, Pereira MH.Role of the domestic chicken (*Gallus gallus*) in the epidemiology of urban visceral leishmaniasis in Brazil. Emerging Infectious Diseases 2002; 12(8) 1480-85.

[40] Barboza DCPM, Gomes Neto CMB,Leal DC, Bittencourt DVV, Carneiro AJB, Souza BMPS, Oliveira LS, Julião FS, Souza VMM, Franke CR. Estudo de coorte em áreas de risco para leishmaniose visceral canina, em municípios da Região Metropolitana de Salvador, Bahia, Brasil. Revista Brasileira de Saúde e Produção Animal 2006; 2(7) 152-63.

[41] Kran FS, Ferreira FPM. Qualidade de Vida naCidade de Palmas TO: uma Análise Através de Indicadores Habitacionais e Ambientais Urbanos. Ambiente e Sociedade 2006; 2(9) 123-41.

[42] Rutledge LC, Ellenwood DA. Production of Phlebotomine sandflies on the open forest floor in Panama: The species complement. EnvEntomol. 1975; 471-7.

[43] Hanson WJ. The immature stages of the subfamily Phlebotominae in Panama (Diptera: Psychodidae). PhD thesis.University of Kansas; 1968.

[44] Geoffroy B, Dedet JP, Lebbe J, Esterre P, Trape JF. Note sur les relations des vecteurs de leishmaniose avec les essences forestieres en Guyane Française. Ann Parasitol Hum Com. 1986; 61(4) 491-05.

[45] Cabanillas MRS, CastellónEG. Distribution of sandflies (*Diptera: Psychodidae*) on Treetrunks in a Non-flooded area of the Ducke Forest Reserve, Manaus, AM, Brazil. Memórias do Instituto Oswaldo Cruz 1999; 94(3) 289-96.

[46] Apostila UFPE 2013.http://www.ufpe.br/biolmol/Leishmanioses-Apostila_on_line/infogerais.htm.

[47] Teodoro U, Vicent LSF, Lima EM, Misuta NM, Silveira TGV, Ferreira MEMCF. American cutaneous leishmaniasis: phlebotominae of the area of transmission in the North of Paraná, Brazil. Revista de Saúde Pública 1991;2(25) 129-33.

[48] Teodoro U, Thomaz-Soccol V, Kühl JB, Santos DR, Santos ES, Santos AR, Abbas M, Dias AC. Reorganization and cleaness of peridomiciliar area to control sand flies (Diptera, Pschodidae, Phlebotominae) in South Brazil. Arquivos Brasileiros de BiologiaTecnológica 2004; 2(47) 205-12.

Chapter 6

The Geospatial Approach on Eco-Epidemiological Studies of Leishmaniasis

João Carlos Araujo Carreira,
Mônica de Avelar Figueiredo Mafra Magalhães and
Alba Valéria Machado da Silva

Additional information is available at the end of the chapter

http://dx.doi.org/10.5772/57210

1. Introduction

1.1. Leishmaniasis

Leishmaniasis is a vector-borne disease transmitted by numerous sand fly species caused by obligate intracellular parasitic protozoa of the genus Leishmania. It can infect besides the man, a wide range of sylvatic and domestic mammal hosts producing either tegumentar or visceral lesions.

The life of *Leishmania* get going, when phlebotomine sand flies, mostly *Lutzomyia* in the New Word and *Phlebotomus* in the Old Wold, become infected during the blood meal, by ingesting infected mononuclear phagocytic cells. The amastigotes in the gut of sand flies, differentiates into promastigotes and multiply. In the *Viannia* subgenus the parasites develop in the hindgut of the vectors while in the *Leishmania* subgenus, the growth occurs in the midgut. In the insect's gut several promastigotes differentiate into metacyclic forms and migrate to the proboscis.

The parasites are transmitted by the bite of infected female of phlebotomine sand flies during the blood meal when the insects inject from their proboscis, the metacyclic promastigotes. Those forms are capable to survive inside the phagolysosomes of macrophages and other types of mononuclear phagocytic cells. Once inside of the cells, promastigotes differentiate into amastigotes, a stage that is associated mammal tissues. The amastigotes multiply by simple division and continue to infect other mononuclear phagocytic cells (Figure 1).

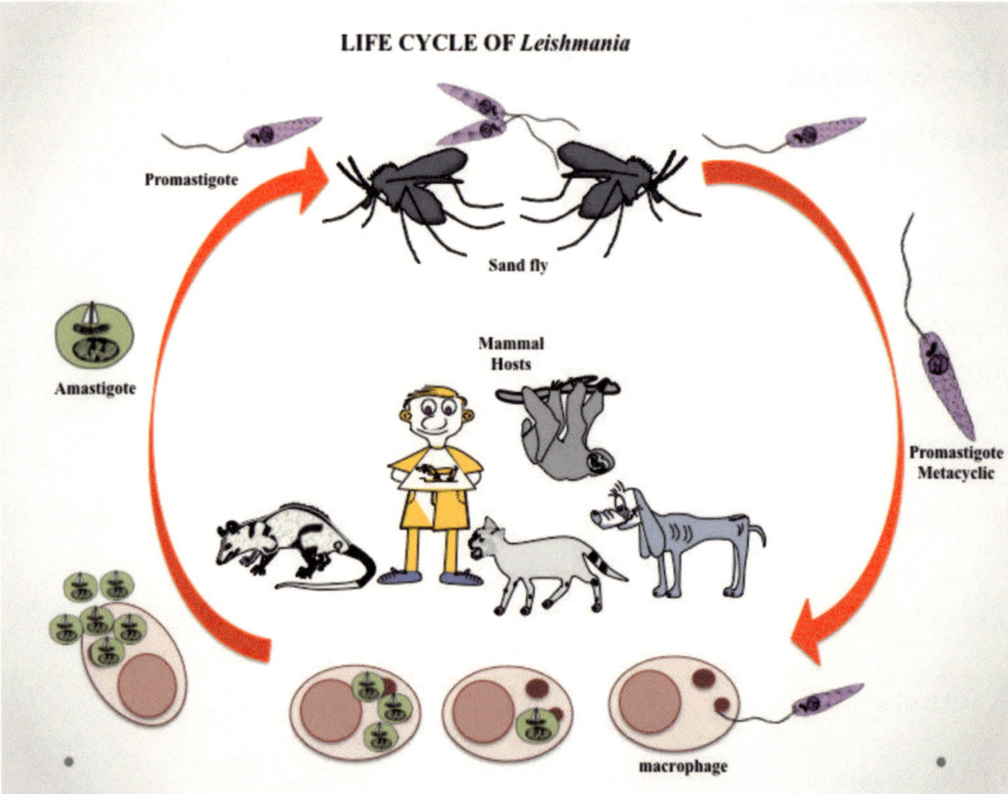

Figure 1. Life cycle of *Leishmania.*

Depending on the parasite and host species in addition to numerous factors related to the hosts' genetic background, the progress of the infection might be influenced, determining if the patient will become symptomatic or sick, eventually resulting in cutaneous or visceral leishmaniasis.

The geographical distribution of leishmaniasis includes 88 countries and almost 350 million of peoples live in these areas where the disease has been considered one of the most severe problem of public health. The majority of the countries affected are in the tropics and sub-tropics, consequently leishmaniasis covers a wide range from rain forests in Central and South America to deserts in West Asia [1,2] (Table 1 and 2).

Depending on the eco-epidemiological conditions, the leishmaniasis can present sylvatic or domestic transmission cycles (Figure 2). Among the most important factors composing those conditions, we could mention the environmental characteristics (biotic and abiotic factors) as well as the parasite, vector and host species involved.

The sylvatic cycles are quite ancient; they have been molded for millions of years before the emergence of man, through co evolutionary relationships among the parasite, vectors and

http://dx.doi.org/10.5772/57210

SPECIES	CLINICAL FORMS	REGION	VECTOR	HOST
Leishmania major	Cutaneous	Asia, Africa	*Phlebotomus papatasi*	Human, rodents
Leishmania tropica	Cutaneous	Europe, Asia, Africa	*P.sergenti*	Human, dogs, rock-hyraxes
Leishmania aethiopica	Cutaneous, mucocutaneous	Africa	*P. longipes, P. pedifer*	Human, hyracoids
Leishmania infantum	Visceral	Europe, Asia, Africa	*P. perniciosus, P. ariasi*	Human, dogs, sylvatic canids
Leishmania donovani	Visceral, PKDL	Asia, Africa	*P. argentipes, P. orientalis*	Human
Leishmania siamensis	Visceral	Europe, Asia, and North America	?	Human, horse, cows

Table 1. The main species of *Leishmania* from the Old World: with the correspondent clinical forms, regions of occurrence, vectors and mammal hosts. (? - Not known).

SPECIES	CLINICAL FORMS	REGION	VECTOR	HOST
L (V) braziliensis	Cutaneous, mucocutaneous	South and Central America	*Nyssomyia intermedia, N. whitmani, Migonemyia migonei*	Human, terrestrial rodents, marsupials, equines, dogs, cats
L (V) peruviana	Cutaneous	South America	*Lutzomyia peruensis, L. verrucarum*	Human, dogs, rodents* opossums*
L (V) guyanensis	Cutaneous	South America	*L. umbratilis*	Human, sloth, anteater, rodents, opossums
L (V) panamensis	Cutaneous	South and Central America	*L. panamensis, L. trapidoi*	Human, sloth, arboreal animals, monkeys, rodents, hunting dogs
L (L) mexicana	Cutaneous, diffuse cutaneous	South, Central and North America	*L. olmeca*	Human, forest rodents
L (L) amazonensis	Cutaneous, diffuse cutaneous	South America	*L. flaviscutellata, L. panamensis*	Human, forest rodents, marsupials, fox
L (L) pifanoi	Cutaneous, diffuse cutaneous	South America (Venezuela)	*L. flaviscutellata* *	Human, Rodents?
L (L) venezuelensis	Cutaneous	South America (Venezuela)	*L. olmeca* *	Human, domestic cats, rodents?
L (L) infantum	Visceral	South, Central and North America	*L. longipalpis, L. cruzi, L. evansi*	Human, sylvatic canids and felids, opossums, dogs

Table 2. The main species of *Leishmania* from the New World: with the correspondent clinical forms, regions of occurrence, vectors and mammal hosts. (*- Putative).

mammal hosts. Mammal reservoirs and insect vectors have been continuously maintaining the parasites in equilibrium without human involvement.

In our time sylvatic cycles are restricted to wild places where disease outbreaks can eventually occur when people make incursions or settlements in those areas.

Concerning to domestic cycle an intra-domiciliary type (figure 2) of transmission is characteristic and the principal components for the disease establishment and maintenance, are the occurrence of vectors with the capacity of domiciliary human landing/biting, besides humans and domestic animals as mammal hosts [2].

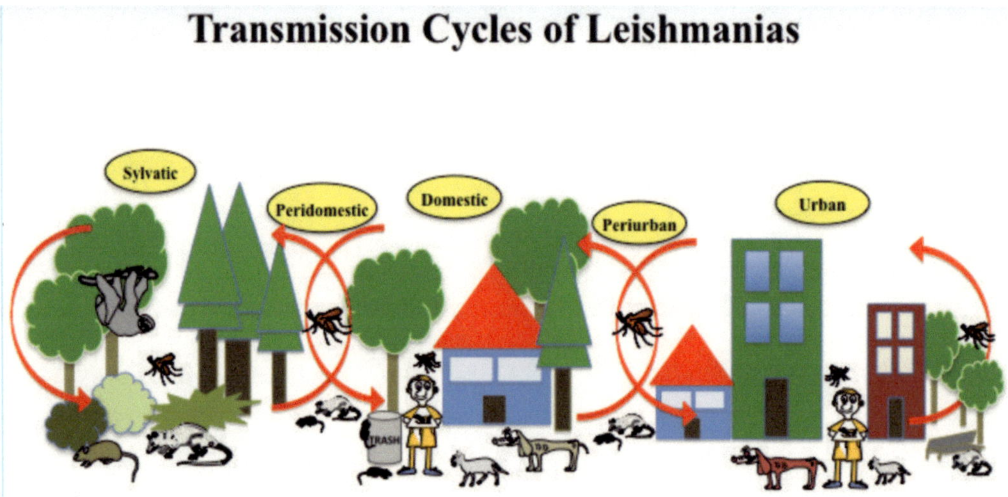

Figure 2. Schematic drawing: eco-epidemiological picture of transmission cycles of Leishmanias.

The earliest steps for the origin of domestic cycles of leishmaniasis probably started around 12.000 years ago, when the ancient human populations began to practice sedentary agriculture and also have introduced domestic animals and livestock causing drastic alterations on the natural habitats.

As a result of such environmental modifications, a large avoidance of the sylvatic animals occurred from the surroundings of human habitations; that together with the insertion of new potential mammal hosts gave rise to a progressive adaptation process in some populations of sylvatic vectors toward a domiciliary behavior. Then little by little certain sand flies populations adopted some introduced species as their new feeding sources [2-4].

In our time, after thousands of years of interaction with domestic mammals as hosts, some vectors hosts species that originally were totally sylvatic, have evolved to exist even in great urban areas, permitting the transmission of the parasite and its maintenance practically restricted to the participation of domestic and/or synanthropic hosts, sand fly and the man [5-7].

http://dx.doi.org/10.5772/57210

So, actually the eco-epidemiological picture of leishmaniasis could be represented as a complex puzzle where each piece is formed by the interaction of a parasite species with their correlated hosts and vectors, in a determined habitat. Nevertheless, it should not be considered as a static process because the occurrence of other parasite species, besides the action of the temporal component they can play a very important role, by influencing the whole process making it possible the occurrence of a variety of transmission patterns that sometimes may result in disease.

Considering the several difficulties to elaborate Leismaniasis control plans, probably the most significant is the high complexity of eco-epidemiological features of the disease. They are greatly influenced by the wide distribution of the parasites, the existence of a large variety of vector species in addition to the pressure of local environmental factors affecting the populations of human hosts, vectors and reservoirs [3-4,8].

The leishmaniasis control measures in use, including spraying to eliminate the adult forms of the vector, diagnosis and treatment of human patients and elimination of seropositive dogs, have failed in preventing new epidemics [9,10].

Therefore, a spatial and temporal approach to analyze endemic foci of the disease could be very a useful method to understand the dynamic of transmission [11,12].

1.2. Methods

Geographic information systems (GIS) and remote sensing (RS) are important tools that comprise computational systems, which permit to map and analyze environmental factors related to the spatial and temporal distribution environmental components that affect the distribution of diseases [12]. The availability of climatic, geological and phytographic digital data and the accessibility of GIS software also have permitted the implementation of several epidemiological studies in relation to ecological factors and disease prediction, as well as have been providing evidences that its use is indispensable before the elaboration of control plans [5, 11,12].

As examples of GIS software we could mention: ArcGis, TerraView, TerraHidro, Gvsig, etc.

The Remote Sensing is also an important data resource for presentation of vegetation, land cover and land use as well as the categorization of the habitats and population density of insect vectors, parasite and reservoir hosts [12,13].

An important feature available in GIS methodology consists of Kernel's method. It is considered a new class of pattern analysis algorithms also utilized in GIS, which can operate on a wide-ranging types of data and relationships. Correlation, factor, cluster and discriminant analysis are just some of the types of pattern analysis tasks that can be performed on data as diverse as sequences, text, images, graphs and of course vectors. The method provides also a natural way to merge and integrate different types of data [5,14].

Kernel density estimators belong to a class of estimators called *non-parametric* density estimators. In comparison to parametric estimators where the estimator has a fixed functional form (structure) and the parameters of this function are the only information we need to store, Non-parametric estimators have no fixed structure and depend upon all the data points to reach an estimate [15].

Differently from conventional histograms where it is necessary to sub-divide the whole data in equal intervals and also to determine the end point of each interval, producing a not smooth representation. On the kernel method those problems can be minimized by the production of a kind of smooth histogram [15] (Figure 3).

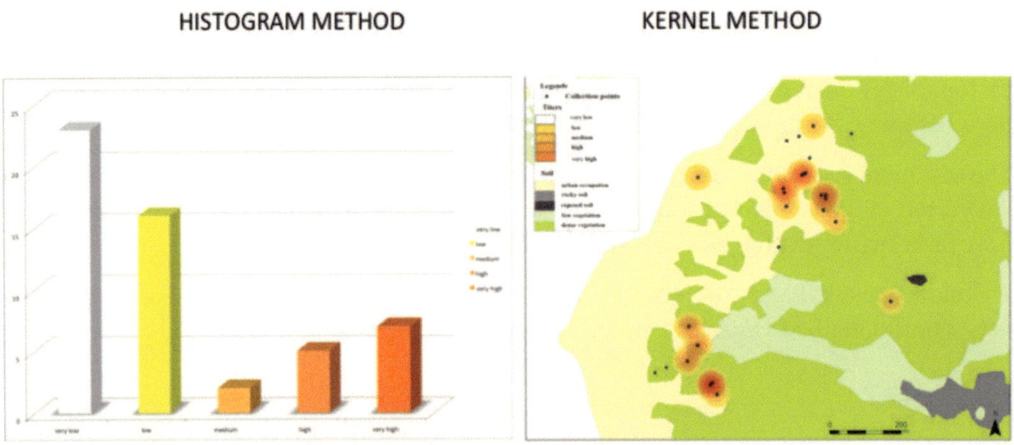

Figure 3. Depiction of doghouses geo-referenced and canine leishmaniasis cases in function of serological titers, represented by histograms and Kernel method (ArcGis).

Other attributes of GIS methodology very useful to the study epidemiology of leishmaniasis is the possibility to create digital maps after performing cluster analysis on the populations of vectors and mammal hosts, including the man; and also to represent circumscribed areas in the same maps, indicating potential regions of vector flight or putative hosts' home ranges [11,14,16] (Figure 4 and 5).

Clustering is a method also applied in GIS, and comprises a common technique for statistical data analysis used in many fields, including machine learning, data mining, pattern recognition image analysis and bioinformatics.

So, the use of new technologies based on eco-epidemiological indicators is essential on the identification of circumstances that impair the spread and maintenance of the disease and certainly could be used to set priorities for implementing disease control measures, thus reducing operational costs and increasing their effectiveness.

In conclusion, the notorious difficulty in controlling the transmission of leishmaniasis, a disease caused by a parasitic protozoa described at 1903 and that still persists currently showing a re-emerging pattern in some places, indicates that such parasites have been developing a great number of evolutionary advantages and despite all the efforts of scientists an effective control was not achieved yet. It is important to remember that those organisms

http://dx.doi.org/10.5772/57210

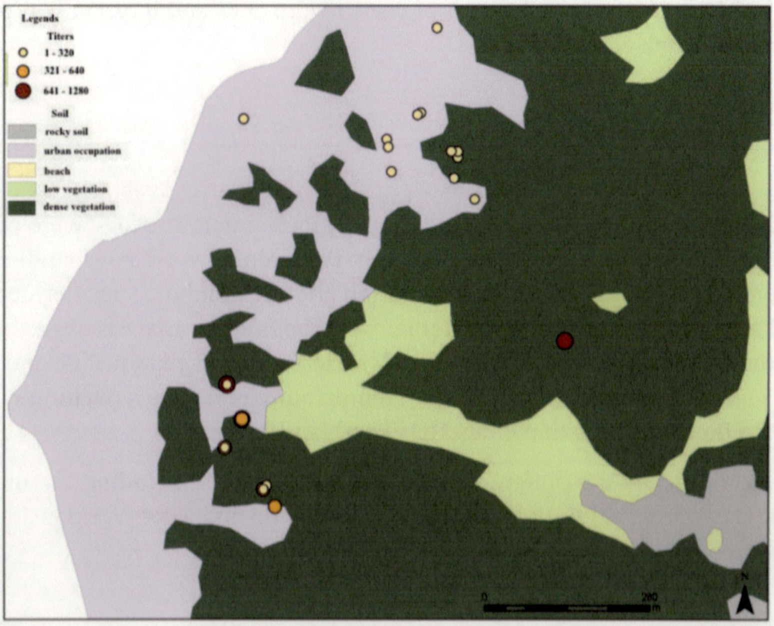

Figure 4. Vegetation, land cover and land use patterns and general distribution of canine leishmaniasis cases, with the respective serological titers, from an endemic focus in Brazil (ArcGis).

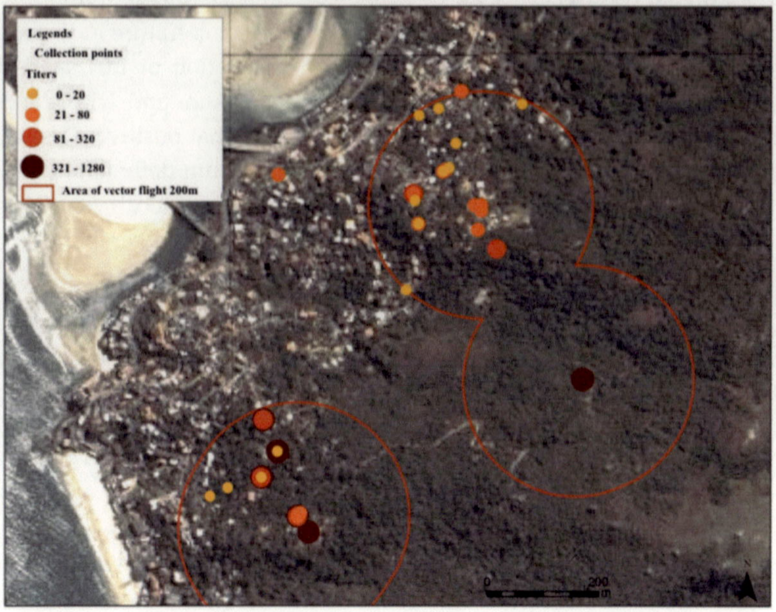

Figure 5. Visual interpretation of an aerial mosaic of photographs from an endemic focus in Brazil, showing the area of influence of the vector flight and the general distribution of canine *Leishmania* infections in addition to the serological titers (source: website of the Pereira Passos Institute http://www.armazemdedados.rio.rj.gov.br/).

have been dwelling on earth for millions of years before of us and it certainly represents that they have skills we not elucidated yet.

2. Overview

The first studies on leishmaniasis utilizing the geoprocessing technology were carried out in the 90s. After that, several groups from different parts of the world have studied important epidemiological aspects of this disease through the integration of results obtained from serological techniques, biological characteristics and population analysis of vectors and hosts with environmental factors such as: elevation, temperature parameters, mean monthly precipitation, relative humidity, land surface temperature parameters (including amplitude), normalized-difference vegetation index NDVI and land cover.

In the following section we presented a chronological review including the more relevant papers, originated from studies achieved in the Old World and New World, using the above-mentioned approach.

3. Leishmaniasis in the Old World

Elnaiem 1998 [17] in Sudan, investigating the importance of the effect of environmental data (obtained from digital records collected by satellites), such as: rainfall, minimum and maximum temperatures, soil class, vegetation and land-surface-temperature indices, on a population of *Phlebotomus orientalis*, observed a significant association of this sand fly with the presence of the tree species *Acacia seyal* and *Balanites aegyptiaca* and with the black cotton (vertisolic) soils of eastern Sudan. The authors also showed that positive sites were found to have significantly higher annual mean maximum and minimum daily temperatures and the annual mean maximum normalized-difference vegetation index (NDVI) value was also found to be significantly higher in these in comparison with those places where no *P. orientalis* were found.

Bern et al 2005 [18] studied the spatial patterns and risk factors for anthroponotic visceral leishmaniasis in Bangladesh. Integrating the GIS approach with data related to history, active case detection, and serologic screening, from residents had kala-azar, they observed that the risk was highest for persons 3–45 years of age, and no significant difference by sex. Considering the age-adjusted multivariable models, 3 factors were identified: proximity to a previous kala-azar patient, bed net use in summer and cattle per 1,000 m2. The authors observed no difference by income, education, or occupation; land ownership or other assets; housing materials and condition; or keeping goats or chickens inside bedrooms. The results confirmed a strong clustering occurrence and suggested that insecticide-treated nets could be effective in preventing kala-azar.

In this study, the households were mapped by a GPS and the data were processed into ArcGis. Through the GIS data, distances were determined from the household to the closest kala-azar

http://dx.doi.org/10.5772/57210

cases in the previous year. Kernel density estimation was used to estimate cattle per 1,000 m^2 in order to calculate the effect of cows, oxen or calves on the kala-azar risk for nearby residents.

Ryan et al 2006 [19], studying visceral leishmaniasis in Kenya, used *Leishmania*-specific antibodies to estimate the seroprevalence and GIS and spatial clustering techniques to study the presence of spatial clusters in two villages. In only one of the villages, significant associations among seropositivity and house construction, age, and proximity to domestic animal enclosures were found. In the same place, a significant spatial cluster of VL was found and the spatial distribution of cases in the two villages was different with respect to risk factors, such as presence of domestic animals. The authors suggested that disease control efforts could be focused on elimination of sand fly habitat, placement of domestic animal enclosures, and targeted use of insecticides.

Sudhakar et al., 2006 [20] in a study carried out in India, analyzed in Silicon graphic image processing system, using ERDAS software, some data obtained from a remote sensing satellite.

The GIS functions were applied to quantify the remotely sensed landscape proportions of 5 km^2 buffer in determined places of high occurrence of sand flies in endemic and nonendemic areas. Through the combination of remote sensing (RS) and geographical information system (GIS) they developed landscape predictors of sand fly abundance an indicator of human vector contact and as a measure of risk prone areas.

It was indicated, that the environmental factors such as type and density of settlements, proximity to these with that of water bodies, marshy areas with succulent weed cover and also crops of high succulent in nature like sugarcane, bananas coupled with local prevailing conditions had definitely interactive influencing effect of vector density and also incidents of vector borne diseases.

Rossi et al 2007 [21] in Southern Italy, applied GIS and SR to analyze the distribution of the *Leishmania infantum-Phlebotomus perniciosus* parasite-vector system in relation to environmental features of two opposite sides (coastal and Apennine) of an area of intense transmission of human and canine leishmaniasis.

The cumulative density, a term determined by the authors as the number of specimens/m2 of sticky trap/two nights, of this vector species was related as significantly more abundant in the coastal side. The authors suggested that the predominance of green vegetated environments in the coastal side, in contrast with the predominance of urban environment in the Apennine side, could be responsible for the different *P. perniciosus* densities between the areas.

Ready 2010 [22] reported that climate change could affect leishmaniasis distribution, by the effect of temperature on parasite development in insect vector, or because of the effect of environmental variation on the range and seasonal abundances of the sand fly species.

He also suggested that bio-climate zones and their vegetation indicators vary regionally, and continuing climate change could alter the patterns of land cover and land use. Thus, the GIS-based spatial modeling of the Emerging Diseases in a changing European Environment was providing analysis of alterations in climate and land cover and their effects on sand flies.

Bhunia et al 2010 [23] in India, through satellite imagery complemented with a GIS database, estimated parameters such as altitude, temperature, humidity, rainfall and the normalized difference vegetation index (NDVI) for correlation with the distribution of Kala-azar. They observed that the highest prevalence was below 150 m of altitude with very few cases located above the 300 m level and a low NDVI value ranges correlated with a high occurrence of the disease. They also showed, that most of the cases occurred in non-vegetative areas or low density vegetation zones highlighting that the low density vegetation zones were significant for the *P. argentipes* vector distribution in the disturbed areas.

Khanal et al 2010 [24] in Nepal, merged results from a serological test made in humans and domestic animals with GIS technology to evaluate the exposure to *L. donovani* on two populations in a recent focus of visceral leishmaniasis (VL). They used a Poisson regression model to evaluate the risk of infection in humans associated with seropositive animals in the proximities of the household. It was also demonstrated that seropositive animals and humans were spatially clustered and the presence of positive goats, past VL cases and the proximity to a forest island increased the risk of occurrence of seropositivity in humans. The authors also suggested that goats might play some role in the distribution of *L. donovani,* in the VL focus studied.

Bhattarai et al 2010 [25] also in Nepal, with the purpose of determining possible reasons for persistence of VL during inter-epidemic periods, they mapped cases *Leishmania* infections among apparently healthy persons and animals in an area of active VL transmission. The results of a bivariate K-function analysis showed the occurrence of spatial clustering of *Leishmania* spp.–positive persons and domestic animals, addition the investigation through classification tree, determined that the proximity of *Leishmania* spp.–positive goats ranked as the first risk factor for *Leishmania* infection among persons.

Salahi-Moghaddam et al 2010 [26] in Iran performed a serological study on a population of dogs from an endemic area.

No significant correlation between topographic conditions and the prevalence of positive cases was observed after regression analysis. Nevertheless, positive correlations were found in relation to the amount of rainfall, between infected dogs with high titers (≥1/640) and the number of days with temperatures below 0 °C during one year. The same correlation was observed when they were considered past meteorological records, conversely the humidity showed an inversely correlated with the *Leishmania* infections.

The authors suggested that in mapped areas the prevailing low temperatures could represent an important factor influencing the distribution of leishmaniasis.

More recently, Bhunia et al 2013 [27] in India, assumed that the utilization of GIS and RS technologies on the control of VL dates back to the late 2000s and those control programs have mostly focused on mapping prevalence and association of *Phlebotomus argentipes* habitats, predicting transmission risk in relation to ecological transformation.

Besides, the authors proposed that the multiplicity of satellite and sensors technics offer relevant data to assembly spatial, spectral and temporal scales. They also argued about the advantages of remotely sensed imagery technology in studies in sand fly ecology and vector-borne diseases, by the generation of a proper household breeding documentation at higher spatial resolution.

4. Leishmaniasis in the New World

One of the first works, carried out in the New World that have exploited SR- satellite imagery technology on an epidemiological survey with American Cutaneous Leishmaniasis, was presented by Miranda et al 1996 [28] in Brazil. In that study, the data were plotted on a TM-LANDSAT image a color composition of bands 3, 4 and 5 (see supplementary information on table 3,4 and 5) that were considered useful to identify the relevant vegetation (shrubs and trees) within the boundaries of the studied areas and in their neighborhood about 250 meters from the perimeter of each area. It was suggested, the use of means qualified as presenting a larger view of a geographical area, composed the advantages of remote satellite sensing to study this endemic foci.

Lima et al 2002 [29] also in Brazil, studied the geographical distribution of notified human TL cases and correlated with the occurrence of the remaining vegetation and water streams, through satellite monitoring (LANDSAT level 4).

They observed that the geographical distribution of cases displayed a higher concentration in the northern and western regions of the studied area and a close relationship between TL and modified native forest areas, gallery forest areas or the remnants of both.

Landsat 4-5 Thematic Mapper (TM) and Landsat 7 Enhanced Thematic Mapper Plus (ETM+)		
Band	**Wavelength**	**Attributes**
Band 1 - blue	0.45-0.52	Bathymetric mapping, differentiating soil from vegetation and deciduous from coniferous vegetation
Band 2 - green	0.52-0.60	Highlights peak vegetation, useful for assessing plant vigor
Band 3 - red	0.63-0.69	Distinguish vegetation slopes
Band 4 - Near Infrared	0.77-0.90	Accentuates biomass content and coastlines
Band 5 - Short-wave Infrared	1.55-1.75	Categorizes wetness matter of soil and vegetation; permeates thin clouds
Band 6 - Thermal Infrared	10.40-12.50	Thermal mapping and predictable soil wetness
Band 7 - Short-wave Infrared	2.09-2.35	Hydrothermally transformed rocks related to mineral deposits
Band 8 - Panchromatic (Landsat 7 only)	.52-.90	15 meter resolution, sharper image definition

Table 3. Parameters utilized on Landsat 4-5 Thematic Mapper (TM) and Landsat 7 Enhanced Thematic Mapper Plus (ETM+) methodologies (based on the data obtained from the website http://landsat.usgs.gov).

Landsat 8 Operational Land Imager (OLI) and Thermal Infrared Sensor (TIRS)		
Band	**Wavelength**	**Attributes**
Band 1 – coastal aerosol	0.43-0.45	coastal and aerosol analyzes
Band 2 – blue	0.45-0.51	Bathymetric mapping, characterizing soil from vegetation and deciduous from coniferous vegetation
Band 3 - green	0.53-0.59	Highlights peak vegetation, which is functional for plant vigor assessing
Band 4 - red	0.64-0.67	Distinguishes vegetation slopes
Band 5 - Near Infrared (NIR)	085.-0.88	Highlights biomass and coastlines
Band 6 - Short-wave Infrared (SWIR) 1	1.57-1.65	Distinguishes wetness content of soil and vegetation; infiltrates thin clouds
Band 7 - Short-wave Infrared (SWIR) 2	2.11-2.29	Enriched wetness content of soil and vegetation and thin cloud infiltration
Band 8 - Panchromatic	.50-.68	15 meter resolution, intense image definition
Band 9 – Cirrus	1.36 -1.38	Increased detection of cirrus cloud pollution
Band 10 – TIRS 1	10.60 – 11.19	100 meter resolution, thermal mapping and predictable soil wetness
Band 11 – TIRS 2	11.5-12.51	100 meter resolution, enhanced thermal mapping and predictable soil wetness

Table 4. Parameters utilized on Landsat 8 Operational Land Imager (OLI) and Thermal Infrared Sensor (TIRS) methodologies (based on the data obtained from the website http://landsat.usgs.gov).

Landsat Multi Spectral Scanner (MSS)			
Landsat MSS 1, 2,3 Spectral Bands	**Landsat MSS 4,5 Spectral Bands**	**Wavelength**	**Attributes**
Band 4 - green	**Band 1 - green**	0.5-0.6	Sediment-laden water, delimits areas of shallow water
Band 5 - red	**Band 2 - red**	0.6-0.7	Cultural features
Band 6 - Near Infrared	**Band 3 - Near Infrared**	0.7-0.8	Vegetation boundary between land and water, and natural features of landscape
Band 7 - Near Infrared	**Band 4 - Near Infrared**	0.8-1.1	Infiltrates atmospheric cloud over best, highlights vegetation, boundary between land and water, and natural features of landscape

Table 5. Parameters utilized on Landsat Multi Spectral Scanner (MSS) method (based on the data obtained from the website http://landsat.usgs.gov).

Peterson et al 2004 [30] investigates the potential of ecological niche modeling techniques for interpolating into unsampled areas in order to understand the geographic distributions of vector species. They used multiple subsamples from accessible distributional points to analyze the question of how much sampling is needed to assemble a suitable distributional interpretation for vector species.

The Genetic algorithm for rule-set prediction (GARP) was utilized for modeling the ecological niches. The authors inferred that GARP associates ecological characteristics of known occurrence points to those randomly sampled from the rest of the study region, pursuing the development of a series of decision rules that can best summarize those factors related with the presence of species.

They also demonstrated that moderate sampling densities at sample sizes that possibly could characterize many epidemiological studies, including the distributions of vector or reservoir were sufficient to produce excellent briefs of the geographic distributions of species permits development of geographic predictions for poorly known species to promote the knowledge about geographic aspects of disease systems.

Carneiro et al 2004 [31] in Brazil, used geo-technologies including satellite images, as normalized difference vegetation index (NDVI), in the collection and analysis of epidemiological data from an LV endemic area. It was observed that, the power of specific variable such as: demographic density, age, occurrence of sand flies, contaminated dogs, and human living in specific area, as well as the practical value of using NDVI values to identify risk areas.

Salomón et al 2006 [32] in Argentine, utilized the RS to study the spatial distribution of Phlebotominae associated with a focus of tegumentary leishmaniasis. Satellite images were used to estimate the influence of the maximal and minimal flow of a river present on the area of study, on the transmission of the disease. The probable correlation with the gallery forest was also rated.

The images were obtained from LANDSAT 5 TM and 7 ETM, they were georreferenced using satellite ephemeris and the nearest-neighbor method. The Band 5 was also used to discriminate areas covered by the river, and the neighboring the land uncovered of vegetation trough visual identification.

The authors concluded that the fishing spots were significantly overflowed during the transmission peak because the spatial restricted flood could concentrate vectors, reservoirs, and humans in high places.

They also suggested through both spatial distribution of vectors and remote sensing data the higher transmission risk in the area it is still related with the gallery forest, despite of the urban influence.

Margonari et al 2006 [5] in Brazil, applied the GIS methodology integrated with demographic, socio-economic and environmental data to study some aspects of the epidemiology of a visceral leishmaniasis focus.

It was observed that among biogeographic parameters such as: altitude, area of vegetation influence, hydrographic, and areas of poverty, only altitude showed to influence emergence of leishmaniasis because most canine and human cases of leishmaniasis cases were localized between 780 and 880 m above the sea level and at these same altitudes, a large number of phlebotomine sand flies were collected.

Nieto et al 2006 [33] also in Brazil, used models developed within a GIS employing Genetic Algorithm Rule-Set Prediction (GARP) and the growing degree day (GDD)-water budget (WB) concept to predict the distribution and potential risk of visceral leishmaniasis (VL).

It was described a high and moderate prevalence sites for VL were significantly related to areas of high and moderate risk prediction. Indeed the area expected by the GARP model, hinged on the number of pixels that overlapped among eleven annual model years and the quantity of potential generations per year that could be completed by the *Lu. longipalpis-L. chagasi* system by GDD-WB analysis.

In both the GARP and the GDD-WB prediction models suggested that the highest VL risk was characterized by a semi-arid and hot climate (Caatinga), but the risk in the interior forest and the Cerrado was lower and the coastal forest was predicted as a low-risk area due to the unsuitable conditions for the vector and VL transmission.

Neto et al 2009 [34] in Brazil, applied GIS and SR to examine factors associated with the incidence of urban VL. They observed that the annual incidence rates were related to socioeconomic and demographic indicators as well as the vegetation index.

The highest incidence occurred in the peripheral areas of the city and areas with high population growth and abundant vegetation. On the other hand the percentage of households with piped water was inversely associated with the disease incidence.

The authors conclude that spatial distribution of the disease in the area was heterogeneous, and the incidence was associated with the peripheral neighborhoods fullest vegetation cover, considered subject to anthropic action.

Shimabukuro et al 2010 [35] in Brazil, utilized GIS and SR to study the geographical distribution of American cutaneous leishmaniasis and its phlebotomine vectors and generate risk maps. They observed that generally, the sand fly vector species evaluated have presented unique and heterogeneous distributions, although often overlapped. Numerous sand fly species were highly localized, while the others were much more largely spread.

The authors emphasized the complexity and geographical pattern of ACL transmission in the region.

Valderrama-Ardila et al 2010 [36] in Colombia, evaluate through spatial analysis, the environmental risk factors for CL. The applicant predictor variables were land use, elevation, and climatic (mean temperature and precipitation).

They observed that incidence of the disease was higher in townships with mean temperatures in the middle of the county's range. The frequency was independently associated with forest or shrubs and lower population density. The coverage of forest or shrub have not presented main changes over time.

The results confirmed the effect of weather and land use in leishmaniasis transmission.

Silva et al 2011 [14] in Brazil, studied a dog population from an endemic focus of LV. Through GIS and SR and applying kernel density estimator with Gaussian function and smooth kernel of 100 m radius, they observed local variations related to infection the incidence and distribution of serological titers, i.e. high titers were noted close to areas with preserved vegetation, while low titers were more frequent in areas where people kept chickens.

The authors conclude that the environment plays an important role in generating relatively protected areas within larger endemic regions, but it could also contribute to the creation of hotspots with clusters of comparatively high serological titers indicating a high level of transmission compared with neighboring areas.

Cluster analysis of the serological titers in dogs in the study area showed a non-random distribution, demonstrating that the patterns of transmission of canine VL can undergo local alterations, producing hotspots where the risk of infection was very high compared to neighboring areas.

It was suggested the possibility to predict the specific places of high-risk VL transmission within an endemic area through the mapping of canine serological titers.

Almeida et al 2011 [37] in Brazil, used spatial analysis to identify regions at highest risk of VL in an urban area. They showed from kernel ratios results, that peripheral census tracts were the most heavily affected. The spatial analysis showed that local clusters of high incidence of VL could change their locations depending on the time, suggesting that the pattern of VL is not static, and the disease may occasionally spread to other areas.

The authors also observed a spatial correlation between VL rates and all socioeconomic and demographic indicators evaluated, such as: 1) illiteracy rate; 2) children less than five years of age as a percentage of the total population; 3) mean income of heads-of-households; 4) percentage of permanent private households connected to the water supply; 5) percentage of households with regular garbage collection; and 6) percentage of permanent private households connected to the sewage system.

Foley et al 2012 [38], created a very useful tool that comprises a new map service within VectorMap (www.vectormap.org). Using the words of the authors, "It allows free public online access to global sand fly, tick and mosquito collection records and habitat suitability models, given the short home range of sand flies, combining remote sensing and collection point data, offering a powerful insight into the environmental determinants of sand fly distribution.

Sand fly Map uses Microsoft Silverlight and ESRI's ArcGIS Server 10 software platform to present disease vector data and relevant remote sensing layers in an online geographical information system format. Users can view the locations of past vector collections and the results of models that predict the geographic extent of individual species. Collection records are searchable and downloadable, and Excel collection forms with drop down lists, and Excel charts to country, are available for data contributors to map and quality control their data.

Sand fly Map makes accessible, and adds value to, the results of past sand fly collecting efforts. It is detailed the workflow for entering occurrence data from the literature to Sand fly Map, using an example for sand flies from South America.

The proper use of a global positioning system (GPS) device and a detailed text description of the locality are encouraged to minimize this uncertainty [39]. The calculation of spatial uncertainty, for example for Martins et al [40], allows data to be matched to appropriate resolution remote sensing data, for modeling or other spatial analyses".

Saraiva et al 2012 [41] in Brazil, utilizing GIS methodology associated with serological tests, studied a VL focus. They described the occurrence of serologically positive dogs was spread out throughout all geographical area. The places of concentration of serologically positive dogs appeared both in risk areas and outside them.

Overlaying the map of the human and canines cases with factors traditionally related to VL as vegetation, hydrography, and areas of poverty, it was not possible identify a spatial correlation between them, which demonstrates that in urban areas there are still unknown parameters.

Souza et al 2012 [42] in Brazil, carried out a space-time analysis of AVL cases in humans. They conclude by the time series analysis, a positive tendency over the period analyzed, completing that the disease was clustered in the Southwest side of area of study, suggesting it could require special attention with regard to control and prevention measures.

Finally, González et al 2013 [43] in Colombia, have surveyed the spatial distribution of two vector species of *L. infantum*, after predicting its future dispersal into climate change situations to establish the potential dissemination of the disease. They used ecological niche models through the Maxent software and 13 Worldclim bioclimatic coverages. Through predictions for the pessimistic CSIRO A2 scenario, was calculated the higher increase in temperature in function of non-emission reduction, and by the optimistic Hadley B2 Scenario, was predicted the minimum increase in temperature.

Concerning the climate change projections, they observed an overall reduction in the spatial distribution of the two vector species, progressing a shift in the vertical distribution for one species and restricting the other to certain regions at the sea level.

The authors predicted an outcome for VL vectors in Colombia and suggested that Changes in spatial distribution patterns could be affecting local abundances due to climatic pressures on vector populations thus reducing the incidence of human cases.

4. Conclusion

In conclusion, the employment of a geospatial approach to interpret eco-epidemiological phenomena related to vector borne diseases have been used for some groups in significant studies. The possibilities of use of that very effective tool, considering the advances on computational knowledge and the possibilities of accessing information at a global level, make this technology indispensable to make a broad analysis objecting the optimizing of planning control campaigns.

http://dx.doi.org/10.5772/57210

Author details

João Carlos Araujo Carreira[1*], Mônica de Avelar Figueiredo Mafra Magalhães[2] and Alba Valéria Machado da Silva[3]

*Address all correspondence to: carreira@ioc.fiocruz.br; jcacarreira@gmail.com

1 Núcleo IOC- Jacarepaguá/Fundação Oswaldo Cruz, Rio de Janeiro, Brazil

2 Laboratório de Geoprocessamento, Fundação Oswaldo Cruz, Rio de Janeiro, Brazil

3 Laboratório de Bioquímica de Proteínas e Peptídeos, Fundação Oswaldo Cruz, Rio de Janeiro, Brazil

References

[1] TDR for research on diseases of poverty. http://www.who.int/tdr/research/ntd/leishmaniasis (accessed 04/03/2013).

[2] Lainson R, Rangel E. *Lutzomyia longipalpis* and the ecoepidemiology of American visceral leishmaniasis, with particular reference to Brazil – A review. Memórias do Instituto Oswaldo Cruz 2005; 100: 811-827.

[3] Ashford RW. The Leishmaniasis as emerging and reemerging zoonoses. International Journal for Parasitology 2000; 30: 1269-1281.

[4] Maia-Elkhoury ANS, Alves WA, Sousa-Gomes ML, Sena JM, Luna EA. Visceral leishmaniasis in Brazil: trends and challenges. Cad Saúde Pública 2008; 24: 2941-2947.

[5] Margonari C, Freitas CR, Ribeiro RC, Moura ACM, Timbó M, Gripp AH, Pessanha JE, Dias ES. Epidemiology of visceral leishmaniasis through spatial analysis, in Belo Horizonte municipality, state of Minas Gerais, Brazil. Memórias do Instituto Oswaldo Cruz 2006; 101: 31-38.

[6] Silva, AVM, Paula AA, Pereira DP, Brazil RP, Carreira JCA. Canine Leishmaniasis in Brazil: Serological Follow-Up of a Dog Population in an Endemic Area of American Visceral Leishmaniasis. Journal Parasitology Research 2009; 2009: 1-6.

[7] Carreira JCA, Silva AVM, Pereira DP, Brazil RP. Natural infection of *Didelphis aurita* (Mammalia: Marsupialia) with *Leishmania infantum* in Brazil. Parasites & Vectors 2012; 5:111 - 116.

[8] Cabrera MAA, De Paula AA, Camacho LAB, Marzochi CA, Aguiar GM, Xavier SC, Da Silva AVM, Jansen AM. Canine Visceral Leishmaniasis in Barra de Guaratiba, Rio de Janeiro, Brazil: assessment of some risk factors. Revista do Instituto de Medicina Tropical de São Paulo 2003; 45: 79-83.

[9] Ministério da Saúde. Brasil: Editora MS. Manual de Vigilância e Controle da Leishmaniose Visceral; 2003.

[10] Palatnik-de-Souza CB, Dos Santos WR, França-Silva JC, Da Costa RT, Reis AB, Palatnik M, Mayrink W, Genaro O. Impact of canine control on the epidemiology of canine and human visceral leishmaniasis in Brazil. American Journal of Tropical Medicine and Hygiene 2001; 65: 510-517.

[11] Bavia ME, Carneiro DDMT, Costa Gurgel H, Madureira Filho C, Rodrigues Barbosa MG. Remote Sensing and Geographic Information Systems and risk of American Visceral Leishmaniasis in Bahia, Brazil. Parassitologia 2005; 47: 165-169.

[12] Beck LR, Lobitz BM, Wood BL. Remote sensing and human health: new sensors and new opportunities. Emerging Infectious Diseases 2000; 6: 217-226.

[13] Zhou XN, Lv S, Yang GJ, Kristensen TK, Bergquist R, Utzinger J, Malone JB. Spatial epidemiology in zoonotic parasitic diseases: insights gainedat the 1st International Symposium on Geospatial Health in Lijiang, China, 2007. Parasites & Vectors 2009; 2:10-26.

[14] Silva AVM, Magalhães MAFM, Brazil RP, Carreira JCA. Ecological study and risk mapping of leishmaniasis in an endemic area of Brazil based on a geographical information systems approach. Geospatial Health 2011; 6 (1) 33-40.

[15] Shawe-Taylor J, Cristianini N. Kernel Methods for Pattern Analysis. Cambridge University Press; 2004.

[16] Elnaiem DA, Schorscher J, Bendall A, Obsomer V, Osman ME, Mekkawi AM, Connor SJ, Ashford RW, Thomson CM. Risk mapping of visceral leishmaniasis: the role of local variation in rainfall and altitude on the presence and incidence of kala-azar in Eastern Sudan. American Journal of Tropical Medicine and Hygiene 2003; 68: 10-17.

[17] Elnaiem DA, Connor SJ, Thomson MC, Hassan MM, Hassan HK, Aboud MA, Ashford RW. Environmental determinants of the distribution of *Phlebotomus orientalis* in Sudan. Annals of Tropical Medicine and Parasitology 1998; 92(8) 877-887.

[18] Bern C, Hightower AW, Chowdhury R, Ali M, Amann J, Wagatsuma Y, Haque R, Kurkjian K, Vaz LE, Begum M, Akter T, Cetre-Sossah CB, Ahluwalia IB, Dotson E, Secor WE, Breiman RF, Maguire JH. Risk Factors for Kala-Azar in Bangladesh. Emerging Infectious Diseases 2005; 11 (5) 655- 662.

[19] Ryan JR, Mbui J, Rashid JR, Wasunna MK, Kirigi G, Magiri C, Kinoti D, Ngumbi PM, Martin SK, Odera SO, Hochberg LP, Bautista CT, Chan AS. Spatial clustering and epidemiological aspects of Visceral Leishmaniasis in two endemic villages, Baringo District, Kenya. American Journal of Tropical Medicine and Hygiene 2006; 74(2) 308-317.

[20] Sudhakar S, Srinivas T, Palit A, Kar SK, Battacharya SK. Mapping of risk prone areas of kala-azar (Visceral leishmaniasis) in parts of Bihar state, India: an RS and GIS approach. Journal of Vector Borne Diseases 2006; 43: 115-122.

[21] Rossi E, Rinaldi L, Musella V, Veneziano V, Carbone S, Gradoni L, Cringoli G, Maroli. Mapping the main Leishmania phlebotomine vector in the endemic focus of the Mt. Vesuvius in southern Italy. Geospatial Health 2007; 2: 191-198.

[22] Ready PD. Leishmaniasis emergence in Europe. EuroSurveillance 2010; 15(10) 1-11.

[23] Bhunia GS, Kesari S, Jeyaram A, Kumar V, Das P. Influence of topography on the endemicity of Kala-azar: a study based on remote sensing and geographical information system. Geospatial Health 2010; 4(2) 155-165.

[24] Khanal B, Picado A, Bhattarai NR, Auwera GVD, Das ML, Ostyn B, Davies CR, Boelaert M, Dujardin JC, Rijal S. Spatial analysis of *Leishmania donovani* exposure in humans and domestic animals in a recent kala azar focus in Nepal. Parasitology 2010; 137: 1597-1603.

[25] Bhattarai NR, Auwera GV, Rijal S, Picado A, Speybroeck N, Khanal B, Doncker S, Das ML, Ostyn B, Davies C, Coosemans M, Berkvens D, Boelaert M, Dujardin JC. Domestic animals and Epidemiology of Visceral Leishmaniasis, Nepal. Emerging Infectious Diseases 2010; 16(2) 231- 237.

[26] Salahi-Moghaddam A, Mohebali M, Moshfae A, Habibi M, Zarei Z. Ecological study and risk mapping of visceral leishmaniasis in an endemic area of Iran based on a geographical information systems approach. Geospatial Health 2010; 5(1) 71-77.

[27] Bhunia GS, Kesari S, Chatteerjee N, Kumar V, Das P. The Burden of Visceral Leishmaniasis in India: Challenges in Using Remote Sensing and GIS to Understand and Control. Infectious Diseases 2013; 2013: 1-14.

[28] Miranda C, Massa JL, Marques CCA. Analysis of the occurrence of American Cutaneous Leishmaniasis in Brazil by remote sensing satellite imagery. Revista de Saúde Pública 1996; 30 (5) 433-437.

[29] Lima AP, Minelli L, Teodoro U, Comunello E. Tegumentary leishmaniasis distribution by satellite remote sensing imagery, in Paraná State, Brazil. Anais Brasileiros de Dermatologia 2002; 77(7) 681-692.

[30] Peterson AT, Pereira RS, Neves VFC. Using epidemiological survey data to infer geographic distributions of leishmaniasis vector species. Revista da Sociedade Brasileira de Medicina Tropical 2004; 37: 10-14.

[31] Carneiro DDMT, Bavia ME, Rocha WJSF, Lobão JSB, Oliveira CMFJB, Silva CEP, Barbosa MGR, Rios RB. Identificação de áreas de risco para Leishmaniose Visceral Americana, através de estudos epidemiológicos e sensoriamento remote orbital, em Feira de Santana, Bahia, Brasil (2000-2002). Revista Baiana de Saúde Pública 2004; 28(1) 19-32.

[32] Salomón OD, Orellano PW, Lamfri M, Scavuzzo M, Dri L, Farace MI, Quintana DO. Phlebotominae spatial distribution asssociated with a focus of tegumentary leishmaniasis in Las Lomitas, Formosa, Argentina, 2002. Memórias do Instituto Oswaldo Cruz 2006; 101(3) 295-299.

[33] Nieto P, Malone JB, Bavia ME. Ecological niche modeling for visceral leishmaniasis in the state of Bahia, Brazil, using genetic algorithm for rule-set prediction and growing degree day-water budget analysis. Geospatial Health 2006; 1:115-126.

[34] Neto JC, Werneck GL, Costa CHN. Factors associated with the incidence of urban visceral leishmaniasis: an ecological study in Teresina, Piauí State, Brazil. Cadernos de Saúde Pública 2009; 25(7) 1543-1551.

[35] Shimabukuro PHF, Silva TRR, Fonseca FOR, Baton LA, Galati EAB. Geographical distribution of American cutaneous leishmaniasis and its phlebotomine vectors (Diptera: Psychodidae) in the state of São Paulo, Brazil. Parasites & Vectors 2010; 3:121-133.

[36] Valderrama-Ardila C, Alexander N, Ferro C, Cadena H, Marin D, Holford TR, Munstermann LE, Ocampo CB. Environmental Risk Factors for the Incidence of American Cutaneous Leishmaniasis in a Sub-Andean Zone of Colombia (Chaparral, Tolima). American Journal of Tropical Medicine and Hygiene 2010; 82(2) 243-250.

[37] Almeida AS, Medronho RA, Werneck GL. Identification of Risk Areas for Visceral Leishmaniasis in Teresina, Piaui State, Brazil. American Journal of Tropical Medicine and Hygiene 2011; 84(5) 681-687.

[38] Foley DH, Wilkerson RC, Dornak LL, Pecor DB, Nyari AS, Rueda LM, Long LS, Richardson JH. Sand flyMap: leveraging spatial data on sand fly vector distribution for disease risk assessments. Geospatial Health 2012; 6(3) S25-S30.

[39] Foley DH, Wilkerson RC, Rueda LM. Importance of the "what", "when", and "where" of mosquito collection events. Journal of Medical Entomology 2009; 46: 717-722.

[40] Martins AV, Williams P, Falcao AL. American sand flies (Diptera: Psychodidae, Phlebotominae). Academia Brasileira de Ciencias, Rio de Janeiro; 1978.

[41] Saraiva L, Leite CG, Carvalho LOA, Filho JDA, Menezes FC, Fiuza VOP. Information System and Geographic Information System Tools in the Data Analyses of the Control Program for Visceral Leishmaniases from 2006 to 2010 in the Sanitary District of Venda Nova, Belo Horizonte, Minas Gerais, Brazil. Journal Tropical Medicine 2012; 2012: 1-10.

[42] Souza VAF, Cortez LRPB, Dias RA, Amaku M, Neto JSF, Kuroda RBS, Ferreira F. Space-time cluster analysis of American visceral leishmaniasis in Bauru, São Paulo State, Brazil. Cadernos de Saúde Pública 2012; 28(10) 1949-1964.

[43] González C, Paz A, Ferro C. Predicted altitudinal shifts and reduced spatial distribution of *Leishmania infantum* vector species under climate change scenarios in Colombia. Acta Tropica 2013; In Press.

Chapter 7

Conflict Leishmaniasis

David M. Claborn

Additional information is available at the end of the chapter

http://dx.doi.org/10.5772/57262

1. Introduction

Conflict and war can have obvious and profound effects on the transmission and severity of infectious diseases. Although poverty is often listed as the most important external influence on disease rates, the impacts of war and conflict are also important and can lead not only to damaged public health infrastructure, displaced populations and disrupted habitats of zoonotic reservoirs and vectors, but also to the economic perturbations that increase poverty rates within affected populations [1]. Sedentary rural populations are particularly vulnerable to the disruptions of conflict due to their limited ability to adapt after the destruction or confiscation of their crops and arable land [2]. After initial losses, limited access to seeds, tools or draft animals also leads to a vicious cycle of decreasing production, resulting in increased starvation and decreased health status. This is complicated even further by dysfunctional distribution caused by lack of transportation and fuel, damaged roadways, road blocks and local violence. Malnutrition is the inevitable result of these disruptions to the food security of affected populations. Children under the age of five are the most vulnerable to nutritional deficits and thus they frequently suffer disproportionately from the effects of violence and conflict. Pregnant and breast-feeding women are also vulnerable to the effects of disrupted food supplies due to their increased nutritional needs. Increases in malnutrition in turn lead to compromised immune systems, leaving individuals susceptible to many conflict-associated infectious diseases.

Populations that are impacted by violence are often forced or choose to leave their traditional family homes to migrate to a safer environment. Public health workers have known for many years that displaced populations are particularly vulnerable to epidemics of infectious disease [3]. This increased vulnerability can be due to a variety of factors including compromised immune systems as a result of malnutrition, decreased sanitation, insufficient housing or protection from disease vectors, exposure to regional diseases to which immigrants have little or no immunity, and other factors. Thus conflict and poverty are related, and can work synergistically to increase disease risks in affected populations, especially those that are displaced.

Conflict can also increase disease risk in populations of warfighters (referred to as "soldiers" here even though it is acknowledged that not all warfighters are soldiers). Soldiers often deploy to regions that are endemic for diseases to which they have no previous exposure. As a result of their lack of exposures, the soldiers are often immunologically naïve to the endemic diseases of the areas to which they deploy, rendering them vulnerable to outbreaks of exotic diseases. Although modern militaries often have sophisticated immunization programs, there are no effective vaccines for many diseases of military importance, including malaria, dengue and leishmaniasis. In such situations, the soldiers must rely on other means of protection including strictly enforced hygiene, anti-vector measures, chemoprophylaxis and personal protection such as mosquito netting and repellents. Disease risk to soldiers is especially high during the initial stages of a conflict when the soldiers may live in rudimentary shelters that provide inadequate protection from vectors, vermin and the elements. Food safety, good water quality, and adequate general hygiene are particularly difficult to maintain during this phase of the conflict. As the conflict ages, the soldiers often acquire better housing and protection from the environmental hazards; however, the protracted stresses associated with war fighting, accompanied by more mundane factors such as boredom and separation from families, can also contribute to immune system dysfunctions and increased disease transmission.

Paradoxically, the impact that conflict-associated diseases have on militaries can improve the success of programs to lower the risk of acquiring those diseases. This observation does not imply in any way that wars are beneficial to public health, but only that the efforts that militaries put toward protecting their troops can improve treatment and prevention of those same diseases in other environments free of conflict or war. For instance, the impact of malaria during WWI and the need to acquire more dependable supplies of the anti-malarial quinine stimulated efforts by the U.S. military to develop cheaper synthetic substitutes like meparene and chloroquine. Similarly, the military's use of insecticidal chemicals such as DDT and BHC served as models for subsequent successful civilian programs to control the disease vectors of malaria and dengue. Also, effective vaccines are often developed initially in response to military need. Finally, one of the most effective repellents used as a personal protective measure against mosquitoes and other vectors, N,N-diethy-meta-toluamide or DEET, was developed by the U.S. Army in large part as a result of its experiences with malaria and other vector-borne diseases during WWII [4]. Such developments are direct results of the attention to the disease during military operations in endemic areas, as well as the medical and scientific expertise and relatively large sums of money available to develop disease interventions for the population of soldiers.

Many of these general conclusions about the impact of conflict on disease rates have particular significance to the disease leishmaniasis. This chapter provides a review of conflict leishmaniasis, especially as related to two events: (a) the civil war in Sudan and, (b) recent conflicts in the Middle East involving the militaries of the U.S. and its allies.

http://dx.doi.org/10.5772/57262

1.1. General background on the disease and its vector

Leishmaniasis is a result of a parasitic infection by any of several species of the protozoan *Leishmania.* The parasite genus is somewhat catholic in distribution, infecting up to 12 million people on all continents except Australia and Antarctica [5]. Parasites have been identified in Australia but, to date, have not infected humans, only kangaroos and wallabies [6]. The disease manifests in a variety of pathologies depending on the species of parasite and perhaps other factors, with effects ranging from mild scarring to severe disfiguration to death [7]. Localized cutaneous leishmaniasis usually affects body parts that are typically uncovered such as the face and hands. An initial papule lesion often develops into a circumscribed ulcer that may elicit little pain or itching. However, secondary infections are common. Many smaller lesions of the cutaneous form will self-heal, providing incomplete immunity for the person to further infections with the same parasite species; however, multiple lesions may occur. Diffuse cutaneous leishmaniasis may occur when lesions disseminate and this form of the disease often resembles lepromatous leprosy.

A more severe form of the disease usually associated with infections in the New World is mucocutaneous leishmaniasis. This infection often develops in the nasal septum and can result in severe mutilation of the lip, gums, tonsils, pharynx and palate. Damage may be severe enough to cause death through malnutrition and acute respiratory pneumonia.

The most severe form of the disease is visceral leishmaniasis, or kala-azar. This form is usually fatal if left untreated and most deaths from this disease are due to the visceral form. Victims progress through fevers, malaise, and weight loss that are associated with anemia, hepatomegaly and spleenomegaly. Secondary bacterial infections are also common and may lead to tuberculosis, pneumonia or diarrhea; these conditions contribute to the high mortality associated with this form of leishmaniasis.

The *Leishmania* parasites spend part of their development cycles in a variety of reservoirs depending on parasite species. For example, for *L. infantum,* a cause of visceral leishmaniasis, researchers believe the reservoirs are domestic dogs, jackals, foxes and perhaps certain rodents. Conversely, humans are considered to be the reservoir for another parasite associated with visceral leishmaniasis in China, *L. donovani.* [5, 8]. More complete reviews of the various forms of the disease are found in other chapters of this book.

Leishmaniasis is a vector-borne disease and the primary means of transmission from reservoir to host is via the phebotomine sand fly, though there have been reports of transmission by blood transfusion [9]. Common names associated with this insect can be misleading because they are known as 'straw mosquitoes' in some parts of their range even though they are not mosquitoes. Also, non-vector insects, such as certain midges, are sometimes known as sand flies so it is important to understand the difference between this vector and other insects. The phlebotomine sand fly is a small, delicate insect which typically flies in short hops close to the surface of the ground. Knowledge about the larval development sites is incomplete so attempts to control the disease through larval control have been frustrating. The adult sand flies are usually less than 3.5 mm in length and are covered with dense "hairs". When at rest they hold their wings in a characteristic "V" shape over their backs. Only the female sand fly takes a blood meal as the blood is essential to complete the development of egg batches. Like the male, her primary source of nutrition is carbohydrates from plant juices. The acquisition of the *Leishmania* parasite, then, is incidental to taking blood meals. The sand flies usually feed at night or in the early evening. In the New World, they are mostly encountered near forested environments, often being found near particular types of trees or tree buttresses. However, in the Old World, they are mostly associated with rodent burrows in dry or desert environments. Unlike mosquitoes, the larvae do not develop in water, though they do require a moist, warm environment in which to grow. This explains their association with rodent burrows as this environment provides the organic matter needed for nutrition of the growing larvae as well as a degree of protection from extremes in heat and moisture.

There are no vaccines or chemoprophylactic drugs to prevent leishmaniasis, so any focus on the prevention of the disease is usually associated with preventing the bite of an infective sand fly. Such efforts are obviously impeded when the public health infrastructure is disrupted, including during times of conflict.

2. Literature review

2.1. Civil War in Sudan

The civil war in Sudan that occurred between 1983 and 2005 is often called the Second Sudanese Civil War. It was fought primarily between the central government and a rebel group called the Sudan People's Liberation Army. The causes of the conflict were complex and multiple, having been attributed to ethnic and religious differences between the mostly Moslem north and the non-Moslem south. However, other causes may have also played some role including a long history of internecine strife and colonial reorganization that ignored that history. Whatever, the cause, there is little doubt that nearly two million people died as a result of the war, primarily as a result of violence, famine and disease. The Sudan Civil War had a large impact on civilian populations that were displaced from their traditional homelands and subsequently forced to transit rugged, dangerous environments in search of safer places.

A few years prior to the beginning of the Sudan Civil War, a series of floods occurred in a large stretch of the Western Upper Nile Province which probably contributed to the subsequent epidemic of visceral leishmaniasis. The floods destroyed a large part of the forest in the region and the regrowth of the forest provided what has been described as optimum habitat for the development of the sand fly vector population, supposedly the larval stage of the insect [10]. This proposed initial cause for the introduction of the disease agent and the subsequent epidemic was likely exacerbated greatly by the civil war which displaced large groups of people, many of whom transited the regrowing acacia forests which sheltered the increased vector populations of *Phlebotomus orientalis*, the presumed vector. DeBeer and co-authors described the impact with the following words:

"The continuous civil war has destabilized the agricultural activities, nomadic movements and health services in this region. Likewise, transportation of food from the north and

http://dx.doi.org/10.5772/57262

implementation of health care measures including control of malaria and VL [visceral leishmaniasis] were interrupted. The implication of those deficiencies was clearly reflected in the severe malnutrition signs in the population studied. The combination of these factors may have also contributed in this VL outbreak. Previous studies have shown that VL can be latent for very long periods, acquiring an overt clinical form after exposure to stresses such as malnutrition." [11].

Analysis of the epidemic at that point indicated that of the patients reporting to clinics for a variety of symptoms, 44% had clinical symptoms of VL. As is usual for this disease, males were more likely to be infected probably due to occupational exposures, but younger children and women also exhibited high rates of infection. Subsequent analysis of the epidemic suggested remarkably high death rates among the population of the western Upper Nile Province. The number of deaths between 1984 and1994 was estimated at 100,000 people, which was about a third of the population in that region [12]. Although *Medicin Sans Frontiers* (MSF) provided a free and effective antimonial treatment, access to the MSF clinics was limited by tribal and military conflict in the region. Eventually, MSF was forced to evacuate due to the threat of attack, greatly reducing the opportunities for local populations to receive effective treatment. Another study of the epidemic estimated the death rate at approximately 38-57% [13]

The Middle East and nearby regions have also experienced mass movement of populations and growth of refugee populations due to military conflict and civil disruptions; these disruptions also appear to have contributed to increased rates of cutaneous leishmaniasis transmission. However, increased disease rates are not always among refugee populations displaced by conflict. For instance, prevalence of cutaneous leishmaniasis, usually *L. major*, among the general civilian population of Israel is estimated at about 3/100,000, but in the population of Israeli soldiers, the rates may be as high as 196/100,000. This remarkable difference is thought to be the result of exposures during exercises in the desert and the soldiers' practice of resting on top of raised animal burrows where both the rodent reservoir and the sand fly vector are abundant [14]. More typically, perhaps, rates of infantile visceral leishmaniasis in the West Bank have reportedly increased due to the re-emergence of the golden jackal as a reservoir in the region.

Leishmaniasis is also endemic to the Khyber Pakhtunkhwa region of Pakistan where a conflict with insurgents has been continuing for several years. Cutaneous leishmaniasis is common among soldiers there, though more common in those from certain regions of the country, especially central Punjab. The reason for the higher rates in these Punjab soldiers is not known, but some have speculated that it is due to the lack of immunity among these soldiers due their lack of exposure in their home district [15].

Conversely, cutaneous leishmaniasis is very much endemic to Syria and the recent civil war in that region appears to have contributed to increased transmission in that country. The number of cases on an annual basis averages about 22,000; however, the conflict appears to be increasing disease transmission in some of the rural areas. Some small towns are reporting infection rates as high as 25%. These rates are being reported in new ways; so-called "doctor-activists" are using social media to document and warn of disease outbreaks in various parts of Syria. In one case, 125 out of 450 students in a local school were infected as reported through the social media [16]. The reliability of such reports has not, as yet, been documented.

Thus, conflict in regions endemic for leishmaniasis appears to affect disease transmission rates and occurrence. The increase in disease rates can be linked to population displacement, compromised infrastructure like housing, and disruption of healthcare and public health services. Efforts to provide effective treatment of disease victims are often impeded by local violence and lack of transportation.

2.2. Western military experience with leishmaniasis in the Middle East

There were thousands of cases of leishmaniasis among American and European soldiers during WWII with most of them originating in the Middle East, so it was no surprise that the disease would become an issue when coalition forces returned to the Arabian peninsula in 1990 for Operations Desert Shield and Desert Storm (aka the Gulf War or the First Gulf War). There were 20 cases of cutaneous leishmaniasis reported among American soldiers, but medical personnel were surprised by the emergence of viscerotropic *L. tropica,* a species of the parasite that usually elicited cutaneous disease. There were 12 cases of viscerotropic leishmaniasis among Americans and this development started a search for new methods of diagnosis and treatment of the disease [5]. It should be noted that the American military actually had quite a bit of experience with leishmaniasis in another setting, that is, Central America; however, the disease ecology, vector biology and the parasite species were very different in that region as compared to those in the Middle East. One of the repercussions of these infections was that veterans of the campaign were barred from donating blood for many months after deployment. However, the extent of the outbreak among American soldiers was limited, due in part to the timing of the operation and the areas in which most of the troops were housed during the buildup stages prior to the short war. In addition, all of the services established extensive preventive medicine programs that utilized topical repellents, clothing treatments, vector control and public education to reduce the risk to military personnel deployed to the region. (Toward full disclosure, the author was a U.S. Navy medical entomologist stationed with a Marine Corps unit in eastern Saudi Arabia during that conflict.)

When the U.S. military returned to the region in large numbers in 2003 for Operation Iraqi Freedom, military units almost immediately experienced an outbreak of cutaneous leishmaniasis. In early 2004, over 500 cases had been diagnosed among American servicemen. Concurrently, two cases of visceral leishmaniasis were diagnosed in Americans deployed to Afghanistan [17]. By late November of the same year, nearly 1200 cases had been reported [18]. The extent of this early outbreak was attributed to high levels of exposure to the vector during the early, mobile stages of the war. Soldiers often slept outside or in relatively primitive housing, mostly tentage. With time, better tents or relatively permanent buildings with insect-excluding screens, even air conditioning, provided much better protection and led directly to decreased disease rates. Also, vector control efforts were increased and improved as units settled into semi-permanent cantonment areas. Particularly important to improvement in the efficacy of vector control was field research on the biology of the local vector and the efficacy of different potential control methods.

http://dx.doi.org/10.5772/57262

Both disease prevention and disease treatment benefited from the increased attention paid to leishmaniasis by military medical authorities as a result of the conflict in Iraq. Early in the conflict, military medical personnel sought to define appropriate treatments and, given the possibility that cutaneous lesions might heal without treatment, to provide standardized guidelines on the decision to treat or not to treat [19]. Treatment of Old World cutaneous leishmaniasis was considered justified if lesions were present on the face, ears or other cosmetically sensitive areas, if the lesions persisted for many months, if the lesions spread over the fingers, the wrist, the elbow or other joints, or if lesions occurred on the hands or feet where the risk of secondary infection was increased. Treatment was also justified if there was evidence of dissemination or if sores occurred on a patient with an impaired immune system. At that stage in the conflict, treatment for Old World cutaneous leishmaniasis included the following:

1. curettage, or removal of all inflamed tissues;
2. cryotherapy using liquid nitrogen;
3. local heat therapy;
4. treatment with topical creams, some including paromomycin or SNAP (S-nitro-N-acetypenicillamine);
5. intralesional injection of pentavalent antimony'
6. various oral medications; and others.

Medical authorities in the U.S. military identified a need for improved treatment of leishmaniasis, noting the "optimal treatment for the localized infection has not been identified." [20]. Noting that the parasite was thermosenstive, the researchers compared a heat therapy technique to a standard treatment of intravenous sodium stibogluconate for treatment of cutaneous *L. major* infections. They noted similar rates of cure between both but also noted the patients treated with thermal treatments exhibited fewer toxic side effects. Many other alternative therapies and short-course treatments were investigated.

Also subsequent to military experience with leishmaniasis was concern regarding the infection of the blood supply with viable parasites. After Operations Desert Shield and Desert Storm, researchers with the Walter Reed Institute of Research investigated the survivability of *Leishmania* parasites under blood bank storage conditions, concluding that *L. tropica* and *L. dovovani* were a risk to the blood supply for at least 25 days post-donation [21]. As a result of these and other findings, military veterans of Desert Shield and Desert Storm were banned from donating blood for several months. The military experience with *Leishmania* parasites, as well as more recent transfusion-associated transmission, have brought greater attention to this issue and have led to more research on methods to detect and eliminate contamination of blood bank products. In Spain, a country endemic for leishmaniasis, it was noted that there was no suitable screening test to identify the parasite in donor blood and that the only preventive measure available to prevent transfusion of viable parasites was the donor selection criteria; however, some research on methods to inactivate the parasites was underway [22].

A great deal of knowledge about preventing leishmaniasis has become available as a result of military experience with the disease. In an exhaustive series of papers on the importance, biology and control of the vector, Coleman and co-authors identified several issues that were directly applied to control of leishmaniasis in Iraq [23, 24, 25]. Important findings in this series included:

1. Air conditioning reduced the number of sand flies inside a tent by up to 83%;

2. Sand flies in the region were more active in early evening during cooler months, but changed during warmer months to peak activity in the middle of the night;

3. Lights could be used to improve the effectiveness of various traps for surveillance of the vector;

4. PCR techniques could be utilized to identify the probable vector of leishmaniasis for a given region.

These and other practical findings enabled military preventive medicine personnel to establish an effective leishmaniasis control program based on improved housing, targeted use of pesticides, expanded use of repellents, public education and effective vector surveillance. Many elements of this and similar programs have been implemented in the civilian environment and in other militaries, sometimes with mixed effects. One part of the U.S. Army's personal protection regimen that is heavily emphasized is the use of permethrin-treated uniforms. The permethrin serves as a contact irritant and has been shown to be effective against many vectors. In one such study in Iran, soldiers were placed in leishmaniasis-endemic areas either with or without permethrin-treated uniforms and forbidden to use topical repellents. There was not a statistical difference in the rate of disease incidence between the two groups, leading the researchers to conclude that permethrin-treated uniforms were not effective for prevention of cutaneous leishmaniasis [26]. This finding is not surprising given that permethrin is not a spatial repellent and would not be effective in preventing the sand flies from biting on exposed skin. Conversely, Egyptian and U.S. Navy researchers tested commonly used insecticides on cotton duck and vinyl military tent surfaces for efficacy against sand flies, noting that insecticides on vinyl surfaces exhibited lower toxicities to the flies as well as shorter periods of efficacy [27].

The practical findings from the entomological research that was initiated because of the war in Iraq have been applied in endemic areas, especially after disasters and inside refugee camps. These environments resemble those of military campaigns in that large numbers of people are subjected to the elements while residing in emergency housing (tents) that is often less than adequate.

3. Conclusions

Conflicts often result in significant displacements of large populations, both civilian and military. These displacements and the accompanying violence often lead to breakdowns in infection control in medical care facilities, disruption of public health and disease control programs, reduced access to populations in need, and greater exposure to vectors and environmental hazards [28]. All of these issues have application to the disease leishmaniasis. Public health and clinical workers in endemic areas should be aware of the increased risk of disease in the conflict environment, whether that conflict be a civil war, internecine strife, or a declared international conflict.

Of utmost importance in such environments is the establishment of effective disease surveillance, especially among the vulnerable population of impoverished or displaced persons. Surveillance systems are notoriously weak in conflict environments [28]. As a result, detection and reporting of outbreaks and epidemics are often delayed or even non-existent. This may be due to the absence of laboratory facilities or the lack of expertise required to collect, process and identify specimens. Vector surveillance programs can also be important in identifying locales where disease transmission risk is particularly high, but lack of access to the populations at risk and to the surrounding environment may prevent any meaningful surveillance. The data from such surveillance programs are essential to the allocation of limited resources for control of several diseases associated with disrupted environments, including leishmaniasis, but if such allocation is impossible due to the conflict, the options for disease control are very limited.

It is well-known that many military forces voluntarily implement public health assistance for conflict-affected population. In addition, the militaries may spend a great deal of time researching effective prevention and treatment of disease among their own soldier population. These efforts often have application outside the originally military funding the research. Although certain benefits can be realized from increased awareness of disease effects as a result of foreign military presence in an endemic locale, in most instances it would be difficult to contend that the local populations see benefits in public health and disease control as a result of conflict. These general remarks have particular application to the disease called leishmaniasis.

Author details

David M. Claborn

Master of Public Health Program, College of Health and Human Services, Missouri State University, Springfield, MO, USA

References

[1] Hotez PJ. The four horsemen of the apocalypse: tropical medicine in the fight against plague, death, famine and war. Am J Trop Med Hgy 2012 87:3-10.

[2] Perrin P. War and Public Health: A Handbook. International Committee of the Red Cross. Geneva, Switzerland. 2011 446 pp.

[3] Watson JT, Gayer M, Connally MA. Epidemics and natural disasters. Emerging Infectious Diseases 2007 13(1): 1-5.

[4] Kitchen LW, Laurence KL, Coleman RE. The role of the United States military in the development of vector control products, including insect repellents, insecticides and bed nets. J Vector Ecology 2009 34(1): 50-61.

[5] Kenner JR, Aronson NE, Benson PM. The United States military and leishmaniasis. Adv Mil Dermatology 1999 17(1): 77- 92.

[6] PROMED. Leishmaniasis, Cutaneous-Australia, New Vector. 2010-12-28. Archive Number 20101228.4571.

[7] Claborn, DM. The biology and control of leishmaniasis vectors. J Global Inf Dis 2010 2(2): 44-51.

[8] Coleman RE, Burkett DA, Putnam JL, Sherwood V, Caci JF, Jennings BT, Hochberg LP, Spadling SL, Rotwton ED, Blount K, Ploch J, Hopkins G, Raymond JW, O'Guinn ML, Lee JS, Weina PJ. Impact of Phlebotomine sand flies on U.S. military operation at Tallil Air Base, Iraq: 1. Background, military situation and development of a "leishmaniasis control program." J Med Entomol 2006 43(4): 647-662.

[9] PROMED. Leishmaniasis-Columbia: Blood transfusion. 10 Mar 2011. Archive number: 20110323.0914.

[10] Ashford RW, Thompson MC. Visceral leishmaniasis in Sudan: A delayed development disaster. Annals Trop Med Parasitol 1991 85:571-572.

[11] De Beer P, El Harith A, Deng LL, Semiao-Santos SJ, Chantal B, Groothest MV. A killing disease epidemic among displaced Sudanese population identified as visceral leishmaniasis. Am J Trop Med Hyg 1991 90:283-289.

[12] Collin SM, Coleman PG, Retmeiher K, Davidson RN. Unseen kala-azar deaths in south Sudan (1999-2002. Trop Med International Hel 2006 11:509-512.

[13] Seaman J. Mercer AJ, Dondop S. The epidemic of visceral leishmaniasis in western Upper Nile, Southern Sudan: Course and impact from 1984-1994. Int J of Epidem 1996 25:862-871.

[14] Jacobson R. Leishmaniasis in an era of conflict in the Middle East. Vectorborne Zoonotic Dis 2011 11(3): 247-258.

[15] Ul Bari A, Hasshim R, Mahmood K, Muhammed I, Shahbaz N, Tariq KM. Clinical-epidemiological pattern of cutaneous leishmaniasis in armed forces personnel fighting war against terrorism in Khyber Pahtunkhwa and Fata regions. J Pakistan Assoc Dermatologists 2011 21: 10-15.

[16] Al Assad S. War diseases revealed by the social media: massive leishmaniasis outbreak in the Syrian Spring. Parasites and Vectors 2013 6:94.

[17] Aronson NE. Leishmaniasis in relation to service in Iraq/Afghanistan, U.S. Armed Forces, 2001-2006. Med Surv Monthly Rep, U.S. Army Center for Health Promotion and Preventive Medicine 2007 4(1): 2-5.

[18] Lay, JC. Leishmaniasis among U.S. Armed Forces, January 2003-November 2004. Med Surv Monthly Rep, U.S. Army Center for Health Promotion and Preventive Medicine 2004 10:2-5

[19] Weina PF, Neafie RC, Wortmann G, Polhemus M, NE Aronson. Old World leishmaniasis: An emerging infection among deployed U.S. military and civilian workers. Clin Inf Dis 2004 39:1674-80.

[20] Aronson, NE, Hummer KD, Gasser FA, Jr., Oster CN, Benson PM. A randomized controlled trial of local health therapy versus intravenous sodium stibogluconate for the treatment of cutaneous Leishmania major infection. PLoS Neglected Trop Dis 2010 4(3):e628. Doi: 10.1371/journal.pntd.0000628.

[21] Grogi M, Daugirda JL, Hoover DL, Magill AJ, Berman JD. Survivability and infectivity of viscerotropic Leishmania tropica from Operation Desert Storm participants in human blood products maintained under blood bank conditions. Am J Trop Med Hyg 1993 49(3): 308-315.

[22] Jimenez-Marc, T. C Riera, R Fisa, E Girona-Llobera, M Sedeno, RP Goodrich, A Pujol, C Gullen, J Muncunill. The utility of pathogen inactivation technology: a real-life example of Leishmania infantum inactivation in platelets from a donor with an asymptomatic infection. Blood Transfusion 2012 10(4):536-541.

[23] Coleman, RE, Burkett DA, Sherwood V, Caci J, Spradling S, Jennings BT, Rowton E, Gilmore W, Blount K, White CE, Putnam PL. Impact of phelbotomine sand flies on U.S. military operation at Tallil air base, Iraq: 2. Temporal and geographic distribution of sand flies. J Med Entomol 2007 44(1): 29-41.

[24] Burkett DA, Knight R, Dennett JA, Sherwood V, Rowton E, Coleman RE. Impact of phlebotomine sand flies on U.S. military operations at Tallil Air Base, Iraq: 3. Evaluation of surveillance devices for the collection of adult sand flies. J Med Entomol 2007 44(2): 381-384.

[25] Coleman RE, Hochberg LP, Swanson KI, Lee JS, McAvin JC, Moulton JK, Edition DO, Greoebner JL, O'Guinn ML, Putnam JL. Impact of phlebotomine sand flies on U.S. military operations at Tallil Air Base, Iraq: 4. Detection and identification lf Leishmania parasites in sand flies. J Med Entomol 2007 46(3): 649-663.

[26] Asilian, A. Sadeghinia A, Shariati F, Jome I. Efficacy of permethrin-impregnated uniforms in the prevention of cutaneous leishmaniasis in Iranian soldiers. J Clinical Pharm Therapeutics 2003 28: 175-178.

[27] Zayed AB, Hoel DF, Tageldin RA, Furman BD, Hogsette JA, Bernier UR. 2013. Efficacy and duration of three residual insecticides on cotton duck and vinyl tent surfaces

for control of the sand fly Phlebotomus papatasi (Diptera: Psychodidae). U.S. Army Med Dep J Apr-Jun pp. 66-72.

[28] Gayer M, Legros D, Formenty P, Connoly MA. Conflict and emerging infectious diseases. Emerging Inf Dis 2006 13: 1-10.

Section 2

Diagnosis of Leishmaniasis

Chapter 8

Molecular Diagnosis of Leishmaniasis, Species Identification and Phylogenetic Analysis

Constantina N. Tsokana, Labrini V. Athanasiou, George Valiakos, Vassiliki Spyrou, Katerina Manolakou and Charalambos Billinis

Additional information is available at the end of the chapter

http://dx.doi.org/10.5772/57448

1. Introduction

Leishmaniases are vector-borne infections caused by protozoa of genus *Leishmania*, affecting various mammals, mainly carnivores and humans. Clinical patent disease is relatively easy to be diagnosed and laboratory-confirmed by direct detection of the parasite in clinical samples. However, in subclinical cases detection of the causative agent is possible by highly sensitive diagnostic techniques such as molecular assays. Different molecular methods have been developed and evaluated including multilocus enzyme electrophoresis, conventional polymerase chain reaction (PCR) based assays, quantitative Real Time PCR as well as simplified PCR methods.

More than 30 *Leishmania* species have been recognized, of which 20 are considered infective for humans and animals. The ability to distinguish between *Leishmania* species is crucial for differentiation of various forms of disease (visceral, cutaneous, mucocutaneus) at least in humans in order to establish correct diagnosis and prognosis of the disease as well as to support decision-making regarding application of the appropriate treatment protocols.

Available tools for species identification and phylogenetic analysis include DNA sequencing analysis, restriction fragment length polymorphism (RFLP) analysis, and PCR-fingerprinting techniques as well as novel methods such as multilocus sequence typing (MLST) and multilocus microsatellite typing (MLMT). MLST is regarded as the most powerful phylogenetic approach and will be a better alternative to Multilocus Enzyme Electrophoresis (MLEE) in the future. Various studies showed that the same target genomic regions can be used to compare distances among species but also to evaluate genetic diversity within species.

This review aims to critically present current molecular approaches for leishmaniasis diagnosis, species identification and phylogenetic analysis.

2. Molecular diagnosis

PCR is being used for the diagnosis of parasitic diseases, including leishmaniasis. PCR is considered to be the most sensitive and specific technique among the methods applied so far for the direct detection and identification of the causative agent. The procedure is rapid and can be applied to a variety of clinical samples. Regarding the efficacy of the assay, it depends on the target selected for amplification (conserved or variable target region), the number of the target copies, the extraction technique used, the biological sample tested and the PCR protocol adapted or developed [1,2].

The PCR-based assays are advantageous over immunological techniques such as enzyme linked immunosorbent assay (ELISA) and immunofluorescence antibody test (IFAT) as host species specific reagents are not required. The increased PCR sensitivity over serology for the detection of infection is of great interest in certain cases such as in patients with cutaneous, muco-cutaneous leishmaniasis (CL or MCL) and the immunocompromised ones (e.g. coinfected with HIV, under chemotherapy etc). The former have low or no concentrations of antibodies against *Leishmania* due to the localized character of the disease while the latter present limited antibody production both resulting in negative serological tests [3]. In particular, in chronic CL patients, who constitute the greater diagnostic challenge due to their low parasite density, PCR assays for the detection of *Leishmania* DNA presented 100% sensitivity. Moreover, the fact that antibodies remain detectable for years after successful treatment makes the application of PCR a necessity[4].

PCR has been also proved to be valuable in the diagnosis of post-kala-azar dermal leishmaniasis (PKDL) [5]. Additionally, the detection of parasite DNA has been shown to be a useful prognostic marker for the disease relapse or the development of PKDL even after successful treatment outcome. [6]. Furthermore, persistent infection has been found in apparently healed scars from MCL patients [7], the presence of *Leishmania braziliensis* was reported in patients previously treated by immunotherapy or patients being at different stages of treatment and in subjects who had never presented clinical manifestations but they had lived in endemic areas and migrated to nonendemic regions [8].

Moreover, several studies reported that PCR detects parasitaemia a few weeks before the appearance of clinical manifestations. The detection of asymptomatic infected humans contributes to the prevention of the sand fly infection and the transfusion-transmitted kala-azar especially for the patients that require multiple transfusions, at least in endemic areas [3,9].

Regarding canine leishmaniasis, PCR assays constitute useful tools in cases of clinically healthy dogs which harbour infection but may never develop clinical disease. As the PCR positive results indicate infection, these assays could contribute to the prevention of the importation of infected clinically healthy dogs to nonendemic areas where infection may spread via local sand fly vectors and the transmission via blood transfusion [10]. Finally, the parasite detection is crucial in case of negative results obtained by serology. This discrepancy may be attributed

http://dx.doi.org/10.5772/57448

to the gap between infection and seroconversion, the transient presence of specific antibodies and the possibility for some infected dogs never to be seroconverted. In contrast, false positive results may be obtained due to the existence of anti-*Leishmania* antibodies for a considerable time after convalescence [11]. On the other hand, a positive PCR result in asymptomatic dogs cannot support decision-making regarding treatment as the parasite DNA may be present for a long time after the parasite has been cleared while also a single negative PCR result in a clinically suspected dog cannot rule out infection. Along with the need for PCR assays simplification, there is also a demand for standardization and optimization due to the lack of a universal PCR assay for the diagnosis of leishmaniasis [12]. Most laboratories perform "in-house" PCR assays using different primer pairs, DNA targets and PCR protocols [13].

A variety of clinical samples have been used for the detection of *Leishmania* DNA such as whole blood, buffy coat, bone marrow, lymph node, spleen, conjunctival swabs [14,15] and other biological samples such liver, lung, heart, penis, vagina, testis, semen, uterus, placenta, kidney, intestine, milk and urine [16] and more recently nasal, ear and oral swabs [17,18]. Bone marrow, lymph node, spleen and skin are the tissues presenting the highest sensitivity for the diagnosis of canine leishmaniasis [11,19]. The same holds true for the non invasive sampling techniques using conjunctival swabs [15,17]. Whole blood, buffy coat, urine and the other biological samples mentioned above have been shown to be less sensitive.

Several target sequences and different PCR protocols have been described for the detection of *Leishmania* DNA. The most frequently used amplification targets are the Kinetoplast DNA minicircle (kDNA) [20–25] and the small subunit ribosomal RNA (SSU rRNA) [26–29]. There are various gene targets which are also commonly used such as the ribosomal internal transcriped spacer (ITS) [15,30–34], the mini-exon gene (spliced leader) [32,35–40] and a repetitive genomic sequence [41,42].

It is worth mentioning that variable and sometimes conflicting results have been reported by several studies evaluating PCR using different target sequences in different host tissues. These results have been mostly obtained from asymptomatic infected hosts and they may vary depending on the sampling technique, storage method and the PCR protocol employed [1]. Some indicative studies evaluating the most frequently used PCR targets in different tissues are summarized in Table 1.

Target	PCR product size (bp)	Tissue tested	Sensitivity %	Specificity %	References
kDNA	120,297,790,792	WB,BM	68.8-100	100	[21] [22] [24] [25]
ssurRNA	358, 603	WB,BM	72.2-97	100	[27] [43][29] [28]
ITS1	300-350	BM,WB,SB,SS,DS,CS,CB,SA	68-100	100	[44] [33] [30] [32] [31]
Mini-exon	378-450	BM,WB,SB,LA,DB,GB	53.8-89.7	100	[37] [38] [35] [32]

BM: Bone marrow, WB: whole blood, SB: Skin biopsy, SS: Skin scrapings, DS: Dermal smear, SA: Skin aspirates LA: Lesion aspirates CS: Conjunctival swab, CB: Cultured biopsies, DB: Duodenal biopsy, GB: Gastric biopsy

Table 1. Evaluation of the most frequently used PCR targets in different tissues

Real time PCR (or quantitative PCR-qPCR), a molecular technique which has revolutionized the pathogen diagnosis, is considered to be the future reference method for molecular diagnosis. In recent years, qPCR assays based either on SYBR Green or TaqMan chemistries have been developed and evaluated for the detection, quantification and even species differentiation of *Leishmania spp* in a variety of clinical samples showing high sensitivity and reproducibility [45,46]. qPCR is considered to be a helpful tool for *Leishmania* diagnosis, monitoring during therapy, development of new drugs and diagnostic tools, comparison of drug efficacy or prophylactic schemes, and for epidemiological studies. Regarding diagnosis of leishmaniasis, the kinetic study of parasitemia in the immunocompromised hosts, the diagnosis of relapses and the quantification of the low parasitic load in asymptomatic patients are of great interest [47].

qPCR is highly sensitive especially at the lower parasite loads [48,49], specific and reproducible offering the ability to monitor therapy and to prevent relapses. The applications mentioned above make qPCR an attractive alternative to conventional PCR in routine diagnosis [47,49]. Some of the studies carried out so far and their findings regarding the detection threshold, sensitivity and specificity are summarized in Table 2.

Target	Tissue tested	Detection threshold	Sensitivity %	Specificity %	References
kDNA	BM, WB	0.001 p/ r			[50]
kDNA	WB	0.07 p/ r	100	83.33	[51]
kDNA	BM, WB, LN, CS, S, L, LU,K, BC	0.03 p/ r			[52]
kDNA	WB	0.004 p/ r			[53]
TRYP	BS		98.7	59.8	[54]
ITS1	WB, SB, S	0.25 p/s			[55]

BM: Bone marrow, WB: whole blood, SB: Skin biopsy, CS: Conjunctival swab, LN: Lymph node, S: Spleen, L: Liver, LU: Lung, K: Kidney, BC: Buffy coat, BS: Biopsy specimen, p/r:parasites/reaction, p/s: parasite/sample TRYP: tryparedoxin peroxidase gene

Table 2. Detection threshold, sensitivity and specificity of qPCR using various targets in different tissues

Given that PCR is restricted to well equiped laboratory settings, and that there is a need for simplification of the PCR assay and a demand for standardization and optimization [56], the described tools below may represent a good alternative for rapid and simple diagnosis of leishmaniasis in endemic areas and epidemiological studies [12,57].

Quantitative nucleic acid sequence-based amplification (QT-NASBA) has proven to be a very sensitive and specific assay in diagnostic microbiology which is based on the amplification of single-stranded RNA sequences. In fact, this technique detects RNA in a background of DNA [13]. Several QT-NASBA assays have been developed for the detection of *Leishmania* parasites including QT-NASBA combined with electro-chemiluminescence (ECL) [57,58] and QT-NASBA combined with oligochromatographic technology (OC) [12,59] for the detection of NASBA products. The QT-NASBA assays developed, are commonly based on amplification

http://dx.doi.org/10.5772/57448

of single-stranded 18S ribosomal RNA sequences [12,57,58,60,61]. This target is considered to be highly efficient for the diagnosis of leishmaniasis as each parasite contains a large number of copies of the 18SrRNA gene [62] while also the cytoplasm is assumed to contain approximately 104 rRNA copies [62]. Moreover the target is present in all *Leishmania* species and it does not vary between different species allowing high sensitivity and quantification of all species in a similar manner [12,57,58]. However, this target shows high similarity with the 18S rRNA gene sequence of *Endotrypanum, Crithidia, Wallaceina*, and *Leptomonas* organisms which may result in false positive results especially in the case of immunocompromised patients [12]. The fact that NASBA detects RNA, makes it a molecular tool of great importance for the measurement of viable parasites. As a consequence, its application makes possible the assessment of the efficacy of drug therapies, the prediction of treatment outcome and the monitoring of the emergence of drug resistance. As it is well known, the DNA is still detected for a long time after parasite death, thus making RNA a preferable amplification target for the demonstration of parasite viability [13,56,58]. Moreover, when targeting RNA, the starting number of the template molecules is much higher resulting in increased assay sensitivity and decreased sample volume required [56]. The latter, makes also QT-NASBA a highly sensitive assay as it is able to detect very low target levels on clinical samples.

Loop-mediated isothermal amplification (LAMP), a novel method of DNA amplification under isothermal condition [63], has been developed to detect *Trypanosoma spp, Plasmodium spp, Mycobacterium spp and Filaria spp* [64]. Recently a reverse transcriptase step has been developed to specifically amplify RNA so as to amplify RNA viruses such as HIV and avian influenza viruses and to increase the assay sensitivity [65]. The recently developed LAMP seems to be a promising diagnostic tool. The results obtained from several studies are encouraging as this assay is much faster than conventional or nested PCR, it may be applied in field conditions, it shows high specificity and sensitivity [63,64,66–69].

In the context of a generalized effort for simplification of the parasite detection, assays including PCR-ELISA and PCR-OC have been developed and evaluated. Several studies reported that PCR-ELISA showed high sensitivity. In a study, PCR-ELISA in blood samples from HIV negative VL patients was evaluated and presented higher sensitivity (83.9% and 73.2%) and specificity (100% and 87.2%) than conventional PCR [70]. Other investigators have also evaluated the use of the assay in blood samples from HIV co-infected VL patients and PCR-ELISA found to be highly sensitive [23,71,72]. Basiye et al, reported that PCR-OC is highly sensitive for *Leishmania* diagnosis on blood samples from VL patients (sensitivity 96,4% and specificity 88.8%) compared to NASBA-OC which was shown to be more specific (specificity 100%) [60]. In another study the repeatability and reproducibility of the assay was studied and found to be 95.9% and 98.1% in purified nucleic acid specimens and 87.1% and 91.7% in blood specimens spiked with parasites respectively [73].

3. Species identification

The species identification is useful in areas with various sympatric *Leishmania* species such as the southern Mediterranean Basin where CL is caused by *L. major, L. tropica* or *L.infantum* and South America where CL may be caused by *L.mexicana* and *L.amazonensis* as well as the species of the subgenus *L.(Viannia).* Regarding the areas where only one species is considered to be responsible for the disease, the species identification is an important tool for the differentiation between *Leishmania* species and lower trypanosomatids related to the monoxenous parasites of insects of the genera *Leptomonas* or *Herpetomonas* which are also considered to cause VL in Southern Europe, South America and in the Indian subcontinent. As far as it concerns the non-endemic areas, they seem to be at risk for parasite importation due to the increasing international travel and population migration [74].

In recent years, there has been great scientific interest in the development of molecular tools, based on PCR or other amplification techniques, for *Leishmania* parasites identification at species and even strain level. The molecular tools used, range from amplification and subsequent RFLP or DNA sequence analysis of multicopy targets or multigene families, including coding and non-coding regions, and PCR-fingerprinting techniques to the recently developed MLST and MLMT with different discriminatory power, sensitivity and specificity while also each one has its specific advantages and drawbacks [74]. Additionally, in most cases, the level of polymorphism found with coding or repeated non-coding PCR-amplified sequences is not refined enough to distinguish between closely related strains while application of MLST and MLMT approaches may reveal important strain polymorphisms.

PCR assays amplifying the conserved region of kinetoplast minicircle DNA or SSU rDNA have been shown to be the most sensitive, but they are able to identify *Leishmania* parasites only to the generic and/or subgeneric level [34,35,41,62]. However, the kDNA PCR-RFLP assay has been used as a molecular marker for *Leishmania* identification at strain level and found to be discriminative between closely related organisms such as *L.infantum* MON-1. In this case, PCR-RFLP of whole minicircle DNA, a highly polymorphic assay, has been applied for differentiation between recrudescence and re-infection [75,76] and for *L.infantum* strain typing [77]. However, the interpretation of the RFLP patterns is difficult as well as the comparison of the results obtained between laboratories [74,77].

The targets used for species identification include the ribosomal internal transcribed spacer (ITS) [34,78,79]; the mini-exon gene [38,39]; repetitive nuclear DNA sequences [80]; the glucose-6-phosphate dehydrogenase gene [81]; gp63 genes [82]; hsp70 genes[83,84]; cytochrome b gene [85], 7SL RNA gene sequences [86].

Other PCR-based approaches used for *Leishmania* parasites identification at strain level include the sequences of cysteine protease B (cpb) gene [87–90], the gp63 [87,91], the ITS1 [33,92–94], the mini-exon [95] and the kinetoplast minicircles [76,96–99].

The digestion of ITS1 PCR product with the restriction enzyme HaeIII can distinguish all medically relevant *Leishmania* species. However, almost identical RFLP patterns arise for the representatives of the *L. donovani* complex *(L. donovani* and *L.infantum)* or *L. braziliensis* complex (*L. braziliensis, L. guyanensis, L. panamensis, L. peruviana* etc.) with a great variety of restriction enzymes [34]. According to Schönian et al, in such a case, the sequencing of the ITS1 PCR product will allow the species differentiation [74]. Nasereddin et al developed a simple reverse line blot hybridization (RLB) assay based on ITS1 sequences, which could distinguish all Old World *Leishmania* species, even *L. donovani* from *L.infantum*. This approach was found to be highly sensitive, approximately 10- to100-fold more sensitive than ITS1 PCR while the results obtained were comparable to those found by kDNA PCR [79]. Moreover, Talmi-Frank et al, described a new application of high resolution melt (HRM) analysis of a real time PCR product from the ITS1 region in samples from human, reservoir hosts and sand flies for rapid detection, quantification and speciation of Old World *Leishmania* species. In this assay, different characteristic high resolution melt analysis patterns were exhibited by *L.major, L.tropica, L. aethiopica,* and *L.infantum* making this approach able to distinguish all Old World *Leishmania* species causing human disease, except *L. donovani* from *L.infantum* [55]. Recently, an alternative technique, PCR-fluorescent fragment length analysis (PCR-FFL), has been developed by Tomás-Pérez et al, for use in *Leishmania* while its use has been reported previously for species identification in Trypanosoma [100,101]. In this study the fluorescently tagged primers used, were designed in the rRNA fragment ITS1 and 7SL region. The amplified fragments were digested and their sizes were determined by an automated DNA sequencer. PCR-FFL was found to be accurate and more sensitive than PCR-RFLP analysis [101].

Regarding the hsp70 PCR-RFLP approach, it is considered to be useful for the *L.(Viannia)* species discrimination while its sensitivity is poor for *L.(Leishmania)* species. Diagnostic RFLP patterns for the *L.guyanensis* species complex as well as for *L. lainsoni* and *L. shawi* are produced after restriction with the enzyme HaeIII [84,102]. However, this assay was not able to discriminate between *L. braziliensis* and *L. peruviana* as well as *L. naiffi,* requiring a second restriction enzyme for the differentiation [102] while also *L. guyanensis* and *L. panamensis* both belonging to the *L. guyanensis* complex share identical RFLP pattern [83]. The discrimination of the species mentioned above is of great significance due to the fact that even if *L. braziliensis* is considered to be the main causative agent of MCL [103] other *L.(Viannia)* species are also suspected of causing MCL. Additionally, a differential response to antimonial treatment has been documented [104–106]. This assay was suggested to be applicable on clinical samples [107,108].

Montalvo et al, extended the use of the hsp70 PCR-RFLP for identification of Old World and additional New World species and improved resolution within New World species complexes [108]. Recently, they developed an adequate and flexible toolbox which consists of one improved and three new PCR approaches based on hsp70 target amplification and subsequent RFLP, able to diagnose and identify the most medically relevant New and Old World *Leishmania* species. The new PCR variants were highly sensitive and specific and they presented improved amplification efficiency in clinical samples compared to hsp70 PCR described previously by Garcia et al [84]. The choice of the most suitable PCR among the four described, depends on factors like the origin of infection, the sympatry of species, the imported versus endemic pathology, the clinical presentation and the clinical sample [109].

Fernandes et al first developed a PCR approach based on mini-exon gene [36] which was later adapted by Mauricio et al. In this study the mini-exon PCR-RFLP was compared with ITS1 PCR-RFLP. Both targets were shown to be able to identify the strains studied but mini-exon was found to be more polymorphic than ITS1 whereas neither ITS1 nor mini -exon produced as many robust groups as gp63 based restriction analyses published before [91,95]. Marfurt et al also developed a mini-exon PCR-RFLP assay [39]. The pair of primers deriving from the conserved region was able to amplify DNA from Old and New World *Leishmania* species while the diversity detected in the non transcribed spacers represented an informative phylogenetic marker. The digestion of the PCR products with one or two different restriction enzymes resulted in species-specific patterns allowing the species differentiation. Thus, they designed a mini-exon PCR-RFLP genotyping scheme, using different restriction enzymes. However, a single EaeI digest was informative enough for the speciation needed in clinical setting [39]. Furthermore, the repetitive character of this template made it highly sensitive even when applied to clinical samples [38]. On the other hand, when Bensoussan et al compared three PCR assays (kDNA,ITS1 and mini-exon used as targets) found that mini-exon presented the lowest sensitivity (53.8%) and suggested that this discrepancy may be attributed to the examination of stored clinical samples collected on filter papers instead of fresh samples, the extraction or the purification technique [110]. Rocha et al also adapted the PCR approach of Fernades et al and compared four PCR assays (kDNA and mini-exon used as targets) for the evaluation of New World *Leishmania* strains typing. Species belonging to the subgenus *Leishmania* were not amplified with the mini-exon target and the author suggested that this difference probably resulted from intraspecific variation [111]. Recently, in another study, ITS1 and mini-exon targets were compared with 18SrRNA in terms of sensitivity and discriminatory power in clinical samples, under routine laboratory settings. A new pair of primers for mini-exon target was designed due to the inability of the previous published primers to amplify the target in all clinical samples while also the protocol was slightly modified in order to achieve better diagnostic sensitivity. However, ITS1 was found to be more sensitive and practical than mini-exon. In contrast, mini-exon was again more polymorphic and revealed a great discriminatory power in *L.(Viannia)* subgenus [32].

The *L.donovani* complex is the causative agent of visceral leishmaniasis, the most severe form of the disease. The discrimination between the representatives of *L.donovani* complex, *L.infantum* and *L.donovani*, is important as they are morphologically indistinguishable while also they are associated with different epidemiology, ecology and pathology as *L.donovani* is anthroponotic and *L.infantum* is anthropozoonotic. Moreover, there are not discriminative markers to identify certain strains which status is questioned. Thus, the development of molecular tools capable of identifying diagnostic markers and allowing a better understanding of phylogenetic relationships is of great importance. In a study a PCR assay based on cysteine proteinase B (cpb) was developed which was able to differentiate between the two species. The cathepsin-1 proteases CPB which belong to the papain-like superfamily, clan CA and family C1, play an important role in the host protein destruction and evasion of the host immune response [88,112]. CPB enzymes are encoded by a tandem array located in a single locus. Mundodi et al, have compared a *L. donovani* strain and a *L.chagasi*(syn *L.infantum*) strain and revealed at least five tandemly arranged genes [113]. Hide and Banuls, used the last repeats of the cluster (cpbE for *L.infantum* and cpbF for *L.donovani*) and designed a PCR assay able to differentiate the two species by their fragment length as *L.donovani* strains were characterized by a 741-bp product and *L.infantum* strains by a 702-bp product. This PCR assay did not generate amplification for other *Leishmania* species nor trypanosomatids. Although sensitive and specific in cultured parasites, the assay is not sensitive enough for diagnosis on clinical samples [88]. The fact that the species discrimination is based on 39 bp difference in PCR product may cause problems in species identification when using normal agarose gel electrophoresis and where both species are not available for comparison. Thus, another cpb PCR assay was developed with subsequent digestion with DraIII which cuts the 741-bp amplicon of *L.donovani* into 400 and 341 bp and a PCR using a species-specific primer pair capable of amplifying a 317 bp of *L. donovani* whereas it did not amplify *L.infantum* [89]. Two cpb PCR-RFLP and one fluorogenic PCR assay for the molecular typing of *L.donovani* complex have been also developed and it was reported that the assays described were valid and informative for *Leishmania* typing in clinical samples [90,114]. Furthermore, a multilocus approach, using new and previously reported targets including cpb genes, was applied to neotropical isolates (*L.braziliensis, L.peruviana, L.guyanensis, L.lainsoni and L. amazonensis*) and was shown to be a highly robust method of distinguishing different strains [87].

Real-time PCR is considered to be a useful, sensitive, accurate and rapid tool for detection, quantification and even genetic characterization of *Leishmania* parasites. A LightCycler RT-PCR assay based on fluorescence melting curve analysis of PCR products generated from the minicircles of kDNA was developed. This assay was able to detect and differentiate four Old World *Leishmania* species (*L. major* was differentiated from *L. donovani* and from *L.tropica* and *L.infantum*) [45]. In another study, a qPCR based on glucosephosphate isomerase (GPI) gene was able to discriminate between subgenus *Viannia* and the complexes *L.mexicana, L.donovani/ infantum* and *L.major* [115]. A qPCR based on glucose-6-phosphate dehydrogenase (g6pd) using either SYBR-Green or TaqMan probes has also been described. This assay was able to differentiate *L.braziliensis* from other *L. (Viannia)* species and from those of *L.(Leishmania)* [116]. Weirather et al used a set of primers and probes for serial qPCR assays based on kDNA which was able to detect and differentiate *Leishmania* species in clinical samples due to different melt temperature of the amplicon or by observing the presence or absence of some amplicons [117]. Recently, tryparedoxine peroxidase gene was used as amplification target in a qPCR assay able to identify Old-World *Leishmania* species causing CL [54]. An alternative 18S rDNA based qPCR using fluorescence resonance energy transfer probes (FRET) was able to discriminate the *L.donovani* complex, the *L.brasiliensis* complex, and species other than these based on the distinct melting temperature obtained [46]. Finally, a new qPCR assay based on FRET technology and melting curve analysis was designed based on mannose phosphate isomerase (MPI) and 6-phosphogluconate dehydrogenase (6PGD) genes which found to be highly sensitive and discriminative for the five species of *Leishmania* being evaluated (*L.braziliensis, L.panamensis, L.guyanensis, L.peruviana* and *L.lainsoni*) [118].

MLEE, the technique which is regarded as the 'gold standard' for the identification of *Leishmania* parasites to species and subspecific levels and for genetic diversity studies, has been widely used since its introduction [119]. MLEE detects different alleles of housekeeping genes indirectly by scoring the electrophoretic mobility of the enzymes they encode. The nucleotide differences in the genes encoding the enzymes are reflected by their mobility differences. Thus, the parasites are identified by their enzymatic profile and are grouped in taxonomic units termed zymodemes, each one of whom consists of all the strains showing exactly the same profiles for all the enzymatic systems under study. Distinct combinations of isoenzyme mobilities for up to 15 enzymes have been assigned zymodeme numbers (MON-1–MON-274) [120].

However, this molecular method presents several disadvantages including the need for mass culture of *Leishmania* parasites and large amount of protein, it is timeconsuming, labour-intensive, costly and technically demanding. It is also worth mentioning that the MLEE methods used in Europe and in South America are based on different enzyme panels and cannot be compared directly [74,93,119]. As far as it concerns its discriminatory power, it is considered to be poor due to its inability to detect nucleotide substitutions that do not change the amino acid composition and changes in the amino acid composition that does not modify the electrophoretic mobility. The discriminatory power of MLEE for classifications below species level is limited. For instance, the *L.infantum* zymodeme MON-1, the causative agent of the majority of visceral leishmaniasis cases around the Mediterranean basin and South America, has been shown to be genetically heterogeneous and polyphyletic with molecular markers presenting higher resolution level [121,122]. Moreover, other molecular studies do not always agree with the classification of *Leishmania* parasites by MLEE. For instance, the differentiation between the representatives of *L.donovani* complex, *L.donovani* and *L.infantum,* is based on only one enzymatic system (glutamate–oxaloacetate transaminase-GOT) making the species distinction poor. In fact, the zymodeme MON-30 which was regarded as *L.infantum,* has recently shown to be *L.donovani* [123,124]. Furthermore, the existence of *L.archibaldi* as a distinct species belonging to *L.donovani* complex was supported by MLEE but it was not in agreement with the results of many different molecular markers [125] while also *L.killicki* was not confirmed to be a separate species [94,126] and *L.donovani* zymodeme MON-37 was assigned to strains of different genetic background [74,120,127]. However, the codominant character of this molecular tool is advantageous as it is able to identify heterozygous profiles and thus potential hybrids while also if the proteins are highly polymeric, the distinction can be made between a heterozygous profile and a mixed infection [120].

Randomly Amplified Polymorphic DNA (RAPD), a simple process, distinct from the PCR, based in the amplification of genomic DNA with short oligonucleotides of arbitrary nucleotide sequence used as primers, has been also applied for *Leishmania spp*. The primers are designed and used for the detection of polymorphisms without relying on prior knowledge of the DNA sequence to be amplified [128]. From the advent of RAPD technique [128,129] numerous studies, only a few of them can be cited here, have been published reporting the use of RAPD as a molecular tool for *Leishmania* species identification and strain characterization. RAPD has been used for the investigation of the genomic diversity of *L.braziliensis* strains [130,131], *L.major* isolates [132], *L.donovani* complex [124,133,134] and *L.infantum* [77,121,135]. Regarding the use of RAPD in species identification, it has been applied for the differentiation between the species *L.braziliensis, L.mexicana, L.infantum, L.tropica, L.chagasi, L.amazonensis and L.major* [136], the identification and differentiation of Old World species at complex level [137] and recently for the characterization of clinical isolates responsible for kala-azar in India [138]. The main disadvantages of this technique are the need for parasite culture due to the use of non *Leishmania* specific primers and the poor reproducibility of the assay. Moreover, the bands of equal electrophoretic mobility may not be homologous and it is impossible to distinguish homozygous from heterozygous genotypes at specific loci because it is difficult to recognize allelic variants of randomly amplified polymorphic DNA markers in the absence of crossing data [74,120]

PCR hybridization is one of the first molecular methods for species identification and genotyping. DNA probes have been designed for *Leishmania* species identification. The most common target used for *Leishmania spp* identification is kDNA. DNA probes targeting kDNA have been applied for *L.major* [139], *L.infantum* [140], *L.aethiopica* [141], *L.mexicana* and *L.braziliensis* [142], and *L.mexicana, L.donovani* and *L.braziliensis* complexes [143]. Other specific probes developed include a cDNA probe, designed from a repetitive degenerate sequence isolated from *L.donovani,* which specifically hybridized only with isolates of the *L.donovani* complex [144] and two probes, the pDK10 and the pDK20, which were able to differentiate between the Old World *Leishmania* species belonging to *L.donovani* complex and between all Old World *Leishmania* species respectively [145,146]. DNA probes generated from mini-exon genes have also been developed [147]. Other probes developed so far include a *L.braziliensis* specific probe [148] and *L.guyanensis* specific one [149].

MLEE has been recently modified in a direct sequencing allele detection method at each locus, called MLST. Partial sequences of approximately 700 bp in size, belonging to a defined set of housekeeping genes, are directly compared; the alleles are scored as identical or not and the same allele combinations are referred as sequence types. Alternatively, data analysis by sequencing of the alleles may be implemented. This technique was first used for bacterial pathogens whereas in *Leishmania,* steps have been taken to develop a MLST system [150]. The *L. donovani* complex has been studied by 2 sets of 5 loci for genes coding for enzymes used in MLEE [151,152]. These 10 targets in combination should be a complete MLST system for application in *L. donovani* complex. These studies showed that results from MLST are in agreement with results from MLEE whereas some discrepancies were found and MLST presented higher resolution level such as a silent Single Nucleotide Polymorphism (SNP) in gpi that distinguishes between strains of *L.infantum* [151]. Moreover, SNPs resulting in amino acid changes were also found in genes coding for enzymes giving indistinguishable electrophoretic profiles such as in nh2, which has the same protein band size for all *L.donovani* complex strains. These authors reported that MLST could be applied directly to clinical samples or to small-volume cultures. Furthermore, it can be used to detect recombination indirectly and for population genetics studies [151]. Tsukayama et al investigated the intraspecific and interspecific variation in the coding sequences of four enzymes (gpi, mdh, mpi and 6pgd), used in the MLEE typing method, in order to identify SNPs able to discriminate among closely related species. The assay was applied to clinical samples and successfully identified the species of *Leishmania* responsible for the clinical disease [153]. However, the analysis did not include sufficient diversity of strains for each species [74]. Recently, in another study a combination of the previous published enzyme-coding genes (fh, g6pdh, icd, mpi and pgd) was used so as to differentiate the Chinese *Leishmania* isolates and to investigate their phylogenetic relationships [154]. MLST is likely to become the gold standard basis for taxonomy and identification of *Leishmania.*

MLMT is based on the amplification of microsatellites sequences, tandem repeats of a simple nucleotide motif, 1-6 nucleotides, which are distributed abundantly in the eukaryotic and prokaryotic genomes and may reveal important strain polymorphisms. These markers are very useful for studying genetic variation between closely related organisms. Length polymorphisms in microsatellites sequences result from gain and loss of single repeat units which can be detected after amplification with specific to their flanking regions primers. MLMT approaches developed so far for *Leishmania spp*, make use of sets of 14–20 unlinked microsatellite loci. Microsatellite loci with high discriminatory power and being suitable for characterizing closely related strains have been published for the *L.donovani* complex [155–158], *L.donovani* strains [127] *L.major* [159], *L.tropica* [126,160] and for species of the subgenus *L. (Viannia)* [161]. Moreover, as the genetic diversity of *L.infantum* strains has been the subject of intense interest, several studies used MLMT approaches for the evaluation of the genomic variation in *L.infantum* strains [122,135]. It is worth mentioning that when MLMT was compared with other molecular markers for strain typing of *L.infantum*, the results obtained with kDNA PCR-RFLP were comparable to MLMT. kDNA and MLMT presented the highest discriminatory power especially for the MON-1 strains discrimination and appeared to be the most adequate for strain fingerprinting. However, MLMT is advantageous over kDNA PCR-RFLP because of its better reproducibility and feasibility of inter-lab comparisons and the co-dominant character of the markers used, making MLMT suitable for population genetic studies [77]. MLMT is suitable for high-throughput analysis and the data obtained are reproducible and exchangeable between laboratories. Moreover, accurate, quality controlled microsatellite profiles can be stored in databases and compared between different laboratories. In contrast to MLEE, selection does not seem to act on polymorphisms in microsatellite length while also the codominant nature of these markers permits the detection of the allelic variants. MLMT can be used directly on biological samples without prior culture of the parasite. DNA extracted from specimens spotted on filter paper or glass slides or from old Giemsa stained microscope slides was successfully applied in MLMT approaches [155]. It is recommended to use a panel of 10–20 unlinked microsatellite markers in all studies for nearly every species because microsatellite sequences are prone to homoplasy. Additionally, polymorphic repeats are not conserved between different species of *Leishmania* [74,122,157].

4. Phylogenetic analysis

Phylogenetics is the study of evolutionary relationships among various groups of organisms (e.g., species or populations). Their relatedness is evaluated through morphological and molecular sequencing data. This analysis leads to a hypothesis about the evolutionary history of taxonomic groups, their phylogeny. Regarding evolution, it is considered to be a branching process. Populations are altered with time and may split into separate branches, hybridize or be eliminated. The order in which evolutionary events are assumed to have occurred is revealed and may be visualized in a phylogenetic tree.

As mentioned before, MLEE is still regarded as the reference technique for the identification of *Leishmania* species and subspecies. The data obtained from MLEE were analyzed by phenetic and cladistic techniques and led to the construction of the first phylogenetic tree of the genus *Leishmania* [162]. The latter, revealed the monophyletic origin of the genus *Leishmania* and its subdivision into two subgenera, the *L.(Leishmania)* and the *L.(Viannia)* subgenus. *L.(Leishmania)* included the Old World species and *L.mexicana* and complexes from the New World. *L. (Viannia)* subgenus was composed from the other New World species. As *Sauroleishmania* was considered to be a separate genus, the lizard species were not included in these studies. MLEE has been applied to a great variety and amount of isolates in comparison to other molecular methods in the past 25 years, resulting in the current classification system [93,162]. Phylogenetics based on different molecular methods, has confirmed the previous suggested taxonomy of the genus *Leishmania* by MLEE. However, the existence of a larger number of species has been proposed.

PCR-based methods with subsequent RFLP or DNA sequence analysis of multicopy targets or multigene families, to the recently developed MLST and MLMT, have been applied for the identification of the *Leishmania* species being responsible for the disease and for epidemiological studies in different endemic regions, as well as for taxonomic, phylogenetic, and population genetic studies. These tools except from their enhanced sensitivity they are also able to distinguish *Leishmania* parasites at species and intraspecies level. As for phylogenetic studies, the sequence analysis of single-copy gene targets is preferred while also the recombination and the different mutation rates between lineages make the use of one gene less suitable for the phylogenic analysis of the Trypanosomatidae or its subgroups[163].

Several DNA targets have been used to reveal the phylogeny of the *Leishmania* genus including single-copy genes encoding the catalytic polypeptide of DNA polymerase a (polA), the largest subunit of RNA polymerase II (rpoIILS) [164] and 7SL RNA [86], the ITS [165,166], the N-acetylglucosamine-1-phosphate transferase (NAGT) gene [167], the mitochondrial cytochrome b gene (cytb) [168], and most recently, sequences of the hsp70 subfamily [83]. Sequence analysis of these targets led to the conclusion that the subgenera L. (*Leishmania*) and *L. (Viannia)* constitute distinct monophyletic clades and that species of the Old and New World are segregated within the *L. (Leishmania)* subgenus. *Sauroleishmania* species branched off between the *L.(Leishmania)* and *L.(Viannia)* subgenera as an independent taxon suggesting that lizard *Leishmania* might be derived from mammalian parasites [164] and that they should be regarded as a subgenus of *Leishmania* rather than an independent genus [99]. However, the fact that RNA and DNA polymerase genes presented higher evolution rate in the lizard *Leishmania* than in the mammalian *Leishmania* species set into question the exact taxonomic position of lizard parasites [164].

In another study, Cupolillo et al. based on various molecular criteria, suggested the division of the genus *Leishmania* into two sections, *Euleishmania* and *Paraleishmania. Euleishmania* consisted of the subgenera *L.(Leishmania), L.(Sauroleishmania), and L.(Viannia). Paraleishmania* included *L. hertigi, L.deanei, L.colombiensis, L.equatorensis, L.herreri,* and strains of *Endotrypanum*. In the latter section, the parasites of hystricomorph rodents, *L.hertigi* and *L.deanei* and the remaining species that are mainly parasites of sloths were genetically different while strains of *Endotrypanum* formed a paraphyletic group [169].

More recently Fraga et al. analyzed the phylogeny of the genus *Leishmania* based on the hsp70 gene. In this study the isolates and strains used, were of different geographic origins. The resulting phylogeny supported that the monophyletic genus *Leishmania* consisted of three distinct subgenera, the *L.(Leishmania), L.(Viannia), and L.(Sauroleishmania).* The obtained phylogeny supported the following eight species: *L.donovani, L.major, L.tropica, L.mexicana, L.lainsoni, L.naiffi, L.guyanensis* and *L.braziliensis*. In some of these species, subspecies were recognized including *L.donovani infantum, L.guyanensis panamensis, and L.braziliensis peruvi-*

ana. The so far recognized species *L.aethiopica, L.garnhami, and L.amazonensis* did not form monophyletic clusters [83].

Several discrepancies were reported for the taxonomic status of species obtained by MLEE compared to DNA based sequences. It is worth mentioning that the existence of *L.chagasi* and *L. archibaldi* as distinct species, was not supported by any molecular analyses as *L.chagasi* cannot be distinguished from strains of *L.infantum* and should therefore be regarded as South American strains of *L.infantum* [170,171] whereas *L. archibaldi* is not a valid species [125,159]. Numerous molecular studies did not even support the monophyly of the two remaining species, *L.donovani* and *L.infantum* [83,164,168]. Therefore, it was proposed that *L.donovani* is the only species of the *L.donovani* complex [83] while *L.donovani infantum* was recognized as subspecies. Regarding other geographically defined genetic groups within *L.donovani*, it was suggested that they could be delimited. Furthermore, the status of *L.killicki* has been debated. MLEE analysis supported the classification of *L.killicki* as a separate species while other molecular methods proposed that it was identical to *L.tropica* [94,126,168]. At the same time, *L.tropica* clusters to a single branch with *L.aethiopica*, making it difficult to be distinguished by the most of the DNA-based phylogenies [83,86,168]. It was suggested that they may represent different subspecies of the species *L.tropica* which is however needed to be investigated with a larger number of strains. Another discrepancy concerns the existence of the *L.mexicana* complex species. The strains of *L.mexicana* and *L.amazonensis* species are overpresented in DNA based phylogenies while only one *L. garnhami* strain was analysed in the hsp70 trees. In the latter study, none of these species could be distinguished as a monophyletic clade and *L.mexicana* was the only recognized species [83]. These results are in agreement with previous published studies [164,172,173] whereas they are in contrast to others [86,165,168]. Thus, the *L.mexicana* complex should be investigated, including *L.venezuelensis* and *L.aristidesi* strains, in order to evaluate the species and subspecies constituting this complex. The same holds true for the *L.braziliensis* complex species. Several molecular phylogenies including hsp70, RAPD and MLEE, supported the distinction of *L.peruviana* from other strains of *L.braziliensis* [83,174] and it was recognized as a subspecies in the *L.braziliensis* complex. However, this classification was questioned by a study using monoclonal antibodies [175] and another one analyzing the microsatellite variation [161] which suggested that strains of *L.peruviana* were grouped together with strains of *L.braziliensis* from Peru and from the Acre State, a Brazilian region bordering Peru. The use of a sufficiently large number of strains from different areas of distribution is needed so as the taxonomic status of the repsesentatives of the *L.braziliensis* complex to be evaluated. Moreover, in different phylogenetic trees, strains of *L.guyanensis* and *L.panamensis* formed a monophyletic cluster which was then divided into two monophyletic subclusters. Thus, the existence of two subspecies within the species *L.guyanensis* was proposed. A possible explanation for these discrepancies reported in different studies regarding the taxonomic status of both *L.peruviana* and *L.panamensis*, is the application of different molecular markers and the analysis of different strains.

Several molecular methods including MLEE [93], PCR-RFLP of ITSrDNA [78] and PCR-RFLP and sequence analysis of the hsp70 gene [102], were also suggested the inclusion of *L.shawi* in the *L. guyanensis* group. The same applies for *L.naiffi* whereas *L.lainsoni* was confirmed to be the most divergent species inside the *L.(Viannia)* subgenus [83,102].

Noyes et al. (2002) identified a parasite isolated from human cutaneous lesions. Both stains were analysed by MLEE and found to be identical to each other and distantly related to all other *Leishmania* species. The application of other molecular methods revealed a low support for both its position basal to all *Euleishmania* and its clustering with *L.enriettii*. Thus, it was suggested that this strain may cluster with *L.*(*Leishmania*) or *L.(Viannia)* or form a novel clade within the *Euleishmania* either with or without *L.enriettii* [176]. Recently *Leishmania* species isolated from clinical samples from immunocompetent and immunosuppressed patients in Thailand [177,178] and a focal CL outbreak in Ghana [179] were identified and named as *L.siamensis*. Furthermore, novel *Leishmania* species, genetically indistinguishable, were isolated from kangaroos, wallaroos, and wallabies, living in captivity in the Northern Territory of Australia, a region that was considered free of *Leishmania* parasites [180]. Additionally, autochthonous cases of CL in German and Swiss horses and in a Swiss cow could not be classified neither as Old World nor New World *Leishmania* species while they were found to be most closely related to *L.siamensis* [181,182]. Finally, two new *L.(Viannia)* species were described and named *L.lindenbergi* [183] and *L.utingensis*. The last one was represented by only one sample isolated from a *Lutzomyia tuberculata* sand fly. Although the sequence analysis of single-copy gene targets has shown to be informative, the use of several independent genes displaying different evolutionary histories is preferable [184]. Such genes have applied in MLST and provided new insights on taxonomy and evolutionary history of *Leishmania*. MLST is currently considered the most powerful phylogenetic approach, it has been shown to have high discriminatory power, reproducibility and transportability of results between laboratories. Thus far, there are 10 published MLST targets available for the *L.donovani* complex [151,152], most of which are also applicable to other Old World *Leishmania* [185] and 4 targets for the sub-genus *Leishmania (Viannia)* [153]. This should form a complete MLST system applicable to *Leishmania* parasites.

5. Conclusion

Molecular methods have revolutionised the diagnosis of leishmaniasis. A variety of target sequences has been used and evaluated in different clinical samples of parasite hosts. Regarding PCR based assays, they were found to be rapid, sensitive and discriminative at species or even strain level. However the diagnosis of leishmaniasis remains a scientific challenge. There is a gap between the scientific advances, diagnostics and management of *Leishmania* infections in the field which should be decreased and an urgent need for standardization, optimization and simplification of PCR based applications. In this context, there is a generalized effort to make these assays available mainly in endemic areas around the world which will have an impact in disease control.

The great scientific interest for species identification may be attributed to its significance in prompt diagnosis and prognosis of the disease, decision making regarding treatment and control measures. Despite the abundance of the studies carried out and the molecular markers used so far, the species discrimination is still tough in several closely related species. Thus, molecular tools with high discriminatory power are currently under development, optimization and evaluation.

Many molecular tools have been used for the *Leishmania* phylogeny and the definition of its taxonomy. However, evaluation of the phylogenetic relationships of *Leishmania* species is not an easy task. Moreover, there is a need for simplification of the classification and a meaningful nomenclature of *Leishmania* genus particularly for the clinicians.

Acknowledgements

This research has been co-financed by the European Union (European Social Fund – ESF) and Greek national funds through the Operational Program "Education and Lifelong Learning" of the National Strategic Reference Framework (NSRF) - Research Funding Program: THALES. Investing in knowledge society through the European Social Fund

Author details

Constantina N. Tsokana[1], Labrini V. Athanasiou[2*], George Valiakos[1], Vassiliki Spyrou[3], Katerina Manolakou[4] and Charalambos Billinis[1]

*Address all correspondence to: lathan@vet.uth.gr

1 Department of Microbiology and Parasitology, Faculty of Veterinary Medicine, University of Thessaly, Karditsa, Greece

2 Department of Medicine, Faculty of Veterinary Medicine, University of Thessaly, Karditsa, Greece

3 Department of Animal Production, Technological Education Institute of Larissa, Greece

4 Department of Animal Husbandry and Nutrition, Faculty of Veterinary Medicine, University of Thessaly, Karditsa, Greece

References

[1] Baneth G, Aroch I. Canine leishmaniasis: a diagnostic and clinical challenge. Veterinary Journal (London, England: 1997) 2008;175:14–5.

[2] Cortes S, Rolão N, Ramada J, Campino L. PCR as a rapid and sensitive tool in the diagnosis of human and canine leishmaniasis using *Leishmania donovani* s.l.-specific kinetoplastid primers. Transactions of the Royal Society of Tropical Medicine and Hygiene 2004;98:12–7.

[3] Singh S. New developments in diagnosis of leishmaniasis. The Indian Journal of Medical Research 2006;123:311–30.

[4] De Almeida Silva L, Romero HD, Prata A, Costa RT, Nascimento E, Carvalho SFG, et al. Immunologic tests in patients after clinical cure of visceral leishmaniasis. The American Journal of Tropical Medicine and Hygiene

[5] Osman OF, Oskam L, Kroon NC, Schoone GJ, Khalil ET, El-Hassan AM, et al. Use of PCR for diagnosis of post-kala-azar dermal leishmaniasis. Journal of Clinical Microbiology 1998;36:1621–4.

[6] Osman OF, Oskam L, Zijlstra EE, el-Hassan AM, el-Naeim DA, Kager PA. Use of the polymerase chain reaction to assess the success of visceral leishmaniasis treatment. Transactions of the Royal Society of Tropical Medicine and Hygiene

[7] Schubach A, Marzochi MC, Cuzzi-Maya T, Oliveira AV, Araujo ML, Oliveira AL, et al. Cutaneous scars in American tegumentary leishmaniasis patients: a site of *Leishmania* (Viannia) braziliensis persistence and viability eleven years after antimonial therapy and clinical cure. The American Journal of Tropical Medicine and Hygiene 1998;58:824–7.

[8] Guevara P, Ramírez JL, Rojas E, Scorza JV, González N, Añez N. *Leishmania braziliensis* in blood 30 years after cure. Lancet 1993;341:1341.

[9] Martín-Sánchez J, Pineda JA, Morillas-Márquez F, García-García JA, Acedo C, Macías J. Detection of *Leishmania infantum* kinetoplast DNA in peripheral blood from asymptomatic individuals at risk for parenterally transmitted infections: relationship between polymerase chain reaction results and other *Leishmania* infection markers. The American Journal of Tropical Medicine and Hygiene 2004;70:545–8.

[10] Solano-Gallego L, Koutinas A, Miró G, Cardoso L, Pennisi MG, Ferrer L, et al. Directions for the diagnosis, clinical staging, treatment and prevention of canine leishmaniosis. Veterinary Parasitology 2009;165:1–18.

[11] Maia C, Ramada J, Cristóvão JM, Gonçalves L, Campino L. Diagnosis of canine leishmaniasis: conventional and molecular techniques using different tissues. Veterinary Journal (London, England: 1997) 2009;179:142–4.

[12] Deborggraeve S, Laurent T, Espinosa D, Van der Auwera G, Mbuchi M, Wasunna M, et al. A simplified and standardized polymerase chain reaction format for the diagnosis of leishmaniasis. The Journal of Infectious Diseases 2008;198:1565–72.

[13] Schallig HDFH, Oskam L. Molecular biological applications in the diagnosis and control of leishmaniasis and parasite identification. Tropical Medicine & International Health TM IH 2002;7:641–51.

[14] Ferreira S de A, Ituassu LT, de Melo MN, de Andrade ASR. Evaluation of the conjunctival swab for canine visceral leishmaniasis diagnosis by PCR-hybridization in Minas Gerais State, Brazil. Veterinary Parasitology 2008;152:257–63.

[15] Strauss-Ayali D, Jaffe CL, Burshtain O, Gonen L, Baneth G. Polymerase chain reaction using noninvasively obtained samples, for the detection of *Leishmania infantum* DNA in dogs. The Journal of Infectious Diseases 2004;189:1729–33.

[16] Maia C, Campino L. Methods for diagnosis of canine leishmaniasis and immune response to infection. Veterinary Parasitology 2008;158:274–87.

[17] Ferreira S de A, Almeida GG, Silva S de O, Vogas GP, Fujiwara RT, de Andrade ASR, et al. Nasal, oral and ear swabs for canine visceral leishmaniasis diagnosis: new practical approaches for detection of *Leishmania infantum* DNA. PLoS Neglected Tropical Diseases 2013;7:e2150.

[18] Lombardo G, Pennisi MG, Lupo T, Migliazzo A, Caprì A, Solano-Gallego L. Detection of *Leishmania infantum* DNA by real-time PCR in canine oral and conjunctival swabs and comparison with other diagnostic techniques. Veterinary Parasitology 2012;184:10–7.

[19] Manna L, Reale S, Vitale F, Picillo E, Pavone LM, Gravino AE. Real-time PCR assay in *Leishmania*-infected dogs treated with meglumine antimoniate and allopurinol. Veterinary Journal (London, England: 1997) 2008;177:279–82.

[20] Andresen K, Gasim S, Elhassan AM, Khalil EA, Barker DC, Theander TG, et al. Diagnosis of visceral leishmaniasis by the polymerase chain reaction using blood, bone marrow and lymph node samples from patients from the Sudan. Tropical Medicine & International Health TM IH 1997;2:440–4.

[21] Da Silva ES, Gontijo CMF, Pacheco R da S, Brazil RP. Diagnosis of human visceral leishmaniasis by PCR using blood samples spotted on filter paper.Genetics and Molecular Research GMR 2004;3:251–7.

[22] Hu XS, Yang WT, Lu HG, Yan HP, Cheng JP, Ma Y, et al. Sequencing a specific kinetoplast DNA fragment of *Leishmania donovani* for polymerase chain reaction amplification in diagnosis of leishmaniasis in bone marrow and blood samples. The Journal of Parasitology 2000;86:822–6.

[23] Martín-Sánchez J, Pineda JA, Andreu-Lopez M, Delgado J, Macías J, De La Rosa R, et al. The high sensitivity of a PCR-ELISA in the diagnosis of cutaneous and visceral leishmaniasis caused by *Leishmania infantum*. Annals of Tropical Medicine and Parasitology 2002;96:669–77.

[24] Pal S, Aggarwal G, Haldar A, Majumdar A, Majumdar HK, Duttagupta S. Diagnosis of symptomatic kala-azar by polymerase chain reaction using patient's blood. Medi-

cal Science Monitor: International Medical Journal of Experimental and Clinical Research 2004;10:MT1–5.

[25] Salotra P, Sreenivas G, Pogue GP, Lee N, Nakhasi HL, Ramesh V, et al. Development of a species-specific PCR assay for detection of *Leishmania donovani* in clinical samples from patients with kala-azar and post-kala-azar dermal leishmaniasis. Journal of Clinical Microbiology 2001;39:849–54.

[26] Cruz I, Chicharro C, Nieto J, Bailo B, Canavate C, Figueras M-C, et al. Comparison of New Diagnostic Tools for Management of Pediatric Mediterranean Visceral Leishmaniasis. Journal of Clinical Microbiology 2006;44:2343–7.

[27] Cruz I, Cañavate C, Rubio JM, Morales MA, Chicharro C, Laguna F, et al. A nested polymerase chain reaction (Ln-PCR) for diagnosing and monitoring *Leishmania infantum* infection in patients co-infected with human immunodeficiency virus. Transactions of the Royal Society of Tropical Medicine and Hygiene 2002;96 Suppl 1:S185–189.

[28] Lachaud L, Dereure J, Chabbert E, Reynes J, Mauboussin JM, Oziol E, et al. Optimized PCR using patient blood samples for diagnosis and follow-up of visceral leishmaniasis, with special reference to AIDS patients. Journal of Clinical Microbiology 2000;38:236–40.

[29] Mathis A, Deplazes P. PCR and in vitro cultivation for detection of *Leishmania* spp. in diagnostic samples from humans and dogs. Journal of Clinical Microbiology 1995;33:1145–9.

[30] Azmi K, Nasereddin A, Ereqat S, Schnur L, Schonian G, Abdeen Z. Methods incorporating a polymerase chain reaction and restriction fragment length polymorphism and their use as a "gold standard" in diagnosing Old World cutaneous leishmaniasis.Diagnostic Microbiology and Infectious Disease 2011;71:151–5.

[31] Leite RS, Ferreira S de A, Ituassu LT, de Melo MN, de Andrade ASR. PCR diagnosis of visceral leishmaniasis in asymptomatic dogs using conjunctival swab samples. Veterinary Parasitology 2010;170:201–6.

[32] Roelfsema JH, Nozari N, Herremans T, Kortbeek LM, Pinelli E. Evaluation and improvement of two PCR targets in molecular typing of clinical samples of *Leishmania* patients. Experimental Parasitology 2011;127:36–41.

[33] Rotureau B, Ravel C, Couppie P, Pratlong F, Nacher M, Dedet J-P, et al. Use of PCR-Restriction Fragment Length Polymorphism Analysis To Identify the Main New World *Leishmania* Species and Analyze Their Taxonomic Properties and Polymorphism by Application of the Assay to Clinical Samples. Journal of Clinical Microbiology 2006;44:459–67.

[34] Schönian G, Nasereddin A, Dinse N, Schweynoch C, Schallig HDF., Presber W, et al. PCR diagnosis and characterization of *Leishmania* in local and imported clinical samples.Diagnostic Microbiology and Infectious Disease 2003;47:349–58.

[35] Bensoussan E, Nasereddin A, Jonas F, Schnur LF, Jaffe CL. Comparison of PCR Assays for Diagnosis of Cutaneous Leishmaniasis. Journal of Clinical Microbiology 2006;44:1435–9.

[36] Fernandes O, Murthy VK, Kurath U, Degrave WM, Campbell DA. Mini-exon gene variation in human pathogenic *Leishmania* species. Molecular and Biochemical Parasitology 1994;66:261–71.

[37] Katakura K, Kawazu S, Naya T, Nagakura K, Ito M, Aikawa M, et al. Diagnosis of kala-azar by nested PCR based on amplification of the *Leishmania* mini-exon gene. Journal of Clinical Microbiology 1998;36:2173–7.

[38] Marfurt J, Nasereddin A, Niederwieser I, Jaffe CL, Beck H-P, Felger I. Identification and Differentiation of *Leishmania* Species in Clinical Samples by PCR Amplification of the Miniexon Sequence and Subsequent Restriction Fragment Length Polymorphism Analysis. Journal of Clinical Microbiology 2003;41:3147–53.

[39] Marfurt J, Niederwieser I, Makia ND, Beck H-P, Felger I. Diagnostic genotyping of Old and New World *Leishmania* species by PCR-RFLP.Diagnostic Microbiology and Infectious Disease 2003;46:115–24.

[40] Serin MS, Waki K, Chang K-P, Aslan G, Direkel S, Otag F, et al. Consistence of mini-exon polymerase chain reaction–restriction fragment length polymorphism and single-copy gene sequence analyses in discriminating *Leishmania* genotypes.Diagnostic Microbiology and Infectious Disease 2007;57:295–9.

[41] Lachaud L, Marchergui-Hammami S, Chabbert E, Dereure J, Dedet JP, Bastien P. Comparison of Six PCR Methods Using Peripheral Blood for Detection of Canine Visceral Leishmaniasis. Journal of Clinical Microbiology 2002;40:210–5.

[42] Minodier P, Piarroux R, Gambarelli F, Joblet C, Dumon H. Rapid identification of causative species in patients with Old World leishmaniasis. Journal of Clinical Microbiology 1997;35:2551–5.

[43] Cruz I, Chicharro C, Nieto J, Bailo B, Canavate C, Figueras M-C, et al. Comparison of New Diagnostic Tools for Management of Pediatric Mediterranean Visceral Leishmaniasis. Journal of Clinical Microbiology 2006;44:2343–7.

[44] Schönian G, Nasereddin A, Dinse N, Schweynoch C, Schallig HDF., Presber W, et al. PCR diagnosis and characterization of *Leishmania* in local and imported clinical samples.Diagnostic Microbiology and Infectious Disease 2003;47:349–58.

[45] Nicolas L, Milon G, Prina E. Rapid differentiation of Old World *Leishmania* species by LightCycler polymerase chain reaction and melting curve analysis. Journal of Microbiological Methods 2002;51:295–9.

[46] Schulz A, Mellenthin K, Schonian G, Fleischer B, Drosten C. Detection, Differentiation, and Quantitation of Pathogenic *Leishmania* Organisms by a Fluorescence Resonance Energy Transfer-Based Real-Time PCR Assay. Journal of Clinical Microbiology 2003;41:1529–35.

[47] Paiva-Cavalcanti M, Regis-da-Silva C, Gomes Y. Comparison of real-time PCR and conventional PCR for detection of *Leishmania (Leishmania infantum)* infection: a mini-review. Journal of Venomous Animals and Toxins Including Tropical Diseases 2010;16:537–42.

[48] Mary C, Faraut F, Lascombe L, Dumon H. Quantification of *Leishmania infantum* DNA by a Real-Time PCR Assay with High Sensitivity. Journal of Clinical Microbiology 2004;42:5249–55.

[49] Vitale F, Reale S, Vitale M, Petrotta E, Torina A, Caracappa S. TaqMan-based detection of *Leishmania infantum* DNA using canine samples. Annals of the New York Academy of Sciences 2004;1026:139–43.

[50] Francino O, Altet L, Sánchez-Robert E, Rodriguez A, Solano-Gallego L, Alberola J, et al. Advantages of real-time PCR assay for diagnosis and monitoring of canine leishmaniosis. Veterinary Parasitology 2006;137:214–21.

[51] De Paiva Cavalcanti M, Felinto de Brito ME, de Souza WV, de Miranda Gomes Y, Abath FGC. The development of a real-time PCR assay for the quantification of *Leishmania infantum* DNA in canine blood. Veterinary Journal (London, England: 1997) 2009;182:356–8.

[52] Galletti E, Bonilauri P, Bardasi L, Fontana MC, Ramini M, Renzi M, et al. Development of a minor groove binding probe based real-time PCR for the diagnosis and quantification of *Leishmania infantum* in dog specimens. Research in Veterinary Science 2011;91:243–5.

[53] Abbasi I, Aramin S, Hailu A, Shiferaw W, Kassahun A, Belay S, et al. Evaluation of PCR procedures for detecting and quantifying *Leishmania donovani* DNA in large numbers of dried human blood samples from a visceral leishmaniasis focus in Northern Ethiopia. BMC Infectious Diseases 2013;13:153.

[54] Khosravi S, Hejazi SH, Hashemzadeh M, Eslami G, Darani HY. Molecular diagnosis of Old World leishmaniasis: real-time PCR based on tryparedoxin peroxidase gene for the detection and identification of *Leishmania* spp. Journal of Vector Borne Diseases 2012;49:15–8.

[55] Talmi-Frank D, Nasereddin A, Schnur LF, Schönian G, Töz SO, Jaffe CL, et al. Detection and identification of old world *Leishmania* by high resolution melt analysis. PLoS Neglected Tropical Diseases 2010;4:e581.

[56] Reithinger R, Dujardin J-C. Molecular Diagnosis of Leishmaniasis: Current Status and Future Applications. Journal of Clinical Microbiology 2006;45:21–5.

[57] Van der Meide W, Guerra J, Schoone G, Farenhorst M, Coelho L, Faber W, et al. Comparison between quantitative nucleic acid sequence-based amplification, real-time reverse transcriptase PCR, and real-time PCR for quantification of *Leishmania* parasites. Journal of Clinical Microbiology 2008;46:73–8.

[58] Van der Meide WF, Schoone GJ, Faber WR, Zeegelaar JE, de Vries HJC, Ozbel Y, et al. Quantitative nucleic acid sequence-based assay as a new molecular tool for detection and quantification of *Leishmania* parasites in skin biopsy samples. Journal of Clinical Microbiology 2005;43:5560–6.

[59] Mugasa CM, Laurent T, Schoone GJ, Basiye FL, Saad AA, El Safi S, et al. Simplified molecular detection of *Leishmania* parasites in various clinical samples from patients with leishmaniasis. Parasites & Vectors 2010;3:13.

[60] Basiye FL, Mbuchi M, Magiri C, Kirigi G, Deborggraeve S, Schoone GJ, et al. Sensitivity and specificity of the *Leishmania* OligoC-TesT and NASBA-oligochromatography for diagnosis of visceral leishmaniasis in Kenya. Tropical Medicine & International Health TM IH 2010;15:806–10.

[61] Saad AA, Ahmed NG, Osman OS, Al-Basheer AA, Hamad A, Deborggraeve S, et al. Diagnostic Accuracy of the *Leishmania* OligoC-TesT and NASBA-Oligochromatography for Diagnosis of Leishmaniasis in Sudan. PLoS Neglected Tropical Diseases 2010;4:e776.

[62] Van Eys GJ, Schoone GJ, Kroon NC, Ebeling SB. Sequence analysis of small subunit ribosomal RNA genes and its use for detection and identification of *Leishmania* parasites. Molecular and Biochemical Parasitology 1992;51:133–42.

[63] Notomi T, Okayama H, Masubuchi H, Yonekawa T, Watanabe K, Amino N, et al. Loop-mediated isothermal amplification of DNA.Nucleic Acids Research 2000;28:E63.

[64] Khan MGM, Bhaskar KRH, Salam MA, Akther T, Pluschke G, Mondal D. Diagnostic accuracy of loop-mediated isothermal amplification (LAMP) for detection of *Leishmania* DNA in buffy coat from visceral leishmaniasis patients. Parasites & Vectors 2012;5:280.

[65] Adams ER, Schoone GJ, Ageed AF, Safi SE, Schallig HDFH. Development of a reverse transcriptase loop-mediated isothermal amplification (LAMP) assay for the sensitive detection of *Leishmania* parasites in clinical samples. The American Journal of Tropical Medicine and Hygiene 2010;82:591–6.

[66] Mori Y, Notomi T. Loop-mediated isothermal amplification (LAMP): a rapid, accurate, and cost-effective diagnostic method for infectious diseases. Journal of Infection and Chemotherapy: Official Journal of the Japan Society of Chemotherapy 2009;15:62–9.

[67] Nagamine K, Hase T, Notomi T. Accelerated reaction by loop-mediated isothermal amplification using loop primers. Molecular and Cellular Probes 2002;16:223–9.

[68] Takagi H, Itoh M, Islam MZ, Razzaque A, Ekram ARMS, Hashighuchi Y, et al. Sensitive, specific, and rapid detection of *Leishmania donovani* DNA by loop-mediated isothermal amplification. The American Journal of Tropical Medicine and Hygiene 2009;81:578–82.

[69] Verma S, Avishek K, Sharma V, Negi NS, Ramesh V, Salotra P. Application of loop-mediated isothermal amplification assay for the sensitive and rapid diagnosis of visceral leishmaniasis and post-kala-azar dermal leishmaniasis. Diagnostic Microbiology and Infectious Disease 2013;75:390–5.

[70] De Doncker S, Hutse V, Abdellati S, Rijal S, Singh Karki BM, Decuypere S, et al. A new PCR-ELISA for diagnosis of visceral leishmaniasis in blood of HIV-negative subjects. Transactions of the Royal Society of Tropical Medicine and Hygiene 2005;99:25–31.

[71] Costa JM, Durand R, Deniau M, Rivollet D, Izri M, Houin R, et al. PCR enzyme-linked immunosorbent assay for diagnosis of leishmaniasis in human immunodeficiency virus-infected patients. Journal of Clinical Microbiology 1996;34:1831–3.

[72] Martin-Sanchez J, Lopez-Lopez MC, Acedo-Sanchez C, Castro-Fajardo JJ, Pineda JA, Morillas-Marquez F. Diagnosis of infections with *Leishmania infantum* using PCR-ELISA. Parasitology 2001;122:607–15.

[73] Mugasa CM, Deborggraeve S, Schoone GJ, Laurent T, Leeflang MM, Ekangu RA, et al. Accordance and concordance of PCR and NASBA followed by oligochromatography for the molecular diagnosis of Trypanosoma brucei and *Leishmania*. Tropical Medicine & International Health TM IH 2010;15:800–5.

[74] SchöNian G, Kuhls K, Mauricio IL. Molecular approaches for a better understanding of the epidemiology and population genetics of *Leishmania*. Parasitology 2010;138:405–25.

[75] Morales MA, Cruz I, Rubio JM, Chicharro C, Cañavate C, Laguna F, et al. Relapses versus reinfections in patients coinfected with *Leishmania infantum* and human immunodeficiency virus type 1. The Journal of Infectious Diseases 2002;185:1533–7.

[76] Morales MA, Chicharro C, Ares M, Cañavate C, Barker DC, Alvar J. Molecular tracking of infections by *Leishmania infantum*. Transactions of the Royal Society of Tropical Medicine and Hygiene 2001;95:104–7.

[77] Botilde Y, Laurent T, Quispe Tintaya W, Chicharro C, Cañavate C, Cruz I, et al. Comparison of molecular markers for strain typing of *Leishmania infantum*.Infection, Genetics and Evolution: Journal of Molecular Epidemiology and Evolutionary Genetics in Infectious Diseases 2006;6:440–6.

[78] Cupolillo E, Grimaldi Júnior G, Momen H, Beverley SM. Intergenic region typing (IRT): a rapid molecular approach to the characterization and evolution of *Leishmania*. Molecular and Biochemical Parasitology 1995;73:145–55.

[79] Nasereddin A, Bensoussan-Hermano E, Schönian G, Baneth G, Jaffe CL. Molecular diagnosis of Old World cutaneous leishmaniasis and species identification by use of a reverse line blot hybridization assay. Journal of Clinical Microbiology 2008;46:2848–55.

[80] Piarroux R, Azaiez R, Lossi AM, Reynier P, Muscatelli F, Gambarelli F, et al. Isolation and characterization of a repetitive DNA sequence from *Leishmania infantum*: development of a visceral leishmaniasis polymerase chain reaction. The American Journal of Tropical Medicine and Hygiene 1993;49:364–9.

[81] Castilho TM, Shaw JJ, Floeter-Winter LM. New PCR assay using glucose-6-phosphate dehydrogenase for identification of *Leishmania* species. Journal of Clinical Microbiology 2003;41:540–6.

[82] Victoir K, Bañuls AL, Arevalo J, Llanos-Cuentas A, Hamers R, Noël S, et al. The gp63 gene locus, a target for genetic characterization of *Leishmania* belonging to subgenus Viannia. Parasitology 1998;117 (Pt 1):1–13.

[83] Fraga J, Montalvo AM, De Doncker S, Dujardin J-C, Van der Auwera G. Phylogeny of *Leishmania* species based on the heat-shock protein 70 gene. Infection, Genetics and Evolution 2010;10:238–45.

[84] Garcia L, Kindt A, Bermudez H, Llanos-Cuentas A, De Doncker S, Arevalo J, et al. Culture-Independent Species Typing of Neotropical *Leishmania* for Clinical Validation of a PCR-Based Assay Targeting Heat Shock Protein 70 Genes. Journal of Clinical Microbiology 2004;42:2294–7.

[85] Kato H, Uezato H, Katakura K, Calvopiña M, Marco JD, Barroso PA, et al. Detection and identification of *Leishmania* species within naturally infected sand flies in the andean areas of ecuador by a polymerase chain reaction. The American Journal of Tropical Medicine and Hygiene 2005;72:87–93.

[86] Zelazny AM, Fedorko DP, Li L, Neva FA, Fischer SH. Evaluation of 7SL RNA gene sequences for the identification of *Leishmania* spp. The American Journal of Tropical Medicine and Hygiene 2005;72:415–20.

[87] Garcia AL, Kindt A, Quispe-Tintaya KW, Bermudez H, Llanos A, Arevalo J, et al. American tegumentary leishmaniasis: antigen-gene polymorphism, taxonomy and clinical pleomorphism.Infection, Genetics and Evolution: Journal of Molecular Epidemiology and Evolutionary Genetics in Infectious Diseases 2005;5:109–16.

[88] Hide M, Bañuls A-L. Species-specific PCR assay for L. infantum/L. donovani discrimination. Acta Tropica 2006;100:241–5.

[89] Oshaghi MA, Ravasan NM, Hide M, Javadian E-A, Rassi Y, Sedaghat MM, et al. Development of species-specific PCR and PCR-restriction fragment length polymor-

phism assays for L.infantum/L.donovani discrimination. Experimental Parasitology 2009;122:61–5.

[90] Quispe-Tintaya KW, Laurent T, Decuypere S, Hide M, Bañuls A-L, De Doncker S, et al. Fluorogenic assay for molecular typing of the *Leishmania donovani* complex: taxonomic and clinical applications. The Journal of Infectious Diseases 2005;192:685–92.

[91] Mauricio IL, Gaunt MW, Stothard JR, Miles MA. Genetic typing and phylogeny of the *Leishmania donovani* complex by restriction analysis of PCR amplified gp63 intergenic regions. Parasitology 2001;122:393–403.

[92] Cupolillo E, Brahim LR, Toaldo CB, de Oliveira-Neto MP, de Brito MEF, Falqueto A, et al. Genetic Polymorphism and Molecular Epidemiology of *Leishmania (Viannia) braziliensis* from Different Hosts and Geographic Areas in Brazil. Journal of Clinical Microbiology 2003;41:3126–32.

[93] Cupolillo E, Grimaldi G Jr, Momen H. A general classification of New World *Leishmania* using numerical zymotaxonomy. The American Journal of Tropical Medicine and Hygiene 1994;50:296–311.

[94] Schönian G, Schnur L, el Fari M, Oskam L, Kolesnikov AA, Sokolowska-Köhler W, et al. Genetic heterogeneity in the species *Leishmania tropica* revealed by different PCR-based methods. Transactions of the Royal Society of Tropical Medicine and Hygiene 2001;95:217–24.

[95] Mauricio IL, Stothard JR, Miles MA. *Leishmania donovani* complex: genotyping with the ribosomal internal transcribed spacer and the mini-exon. Parasitology 2004;128:263–7.

[96] Chicharro C, Morales MA, Serra T, Ares M, Salas A, Alvar J. Molecular epidemiology of *Leishmania infantum* on the island of Majorca: a comparison of phenotypic and genotypic tools. Transactions of the Royal Society of Tropical Medicine and Hygiene 2002;96 Suppl 1:S93–99.

[97] Cortes S, Mauricio I, Almeida A, Cristovão JM, Pratlong F, Dedet JP, et al. Application of kDNA as a molecular marker to analyse *Leishmania infantum* diversity in Portugal. Parasitology International 2006;55:277–83.

[98] Laurent T, Rijal S, Yardley V, Croft S, De Doncker S, Decuypere S, et al. Epidemiological dynamics of antimonial resistance in *Leishmania donovani*: genotyping reveals a polyclonal population structure among naturally-resistant clinical isolates from Nepal.Infection, Genetics and Evolution: Journal of Molecular Epidemiology and Evolutionary Genetics in Infectious Diseases 2007;7:206–12.

[99] Noyes HA, Reyburn H, Bailey JW, Smith D. A nested-PCR-based schizodeme method for identifying *Leishmania* kinetoplast minicircle classes directly from clinical samples and its application to the study of the epidemiology of *Leishmania tropica* in Pakistan. Journal of Clinical Microbiology 1998;36:2877–81.

[100] Hamilton PB, Adams ER, Malele II, Gibson WC. A novel, high-throughput technique for species identification reveals a new species of tsetse-transmitted trypanosome related to the Trypanosoma brucei subgenus, Trypanozoon. Infection, Genetics and Evolution 2008;8:26–33.

[101] Tomas-Perez M, Fisa R, Riera C. The Use of Fluorescent Fragment Length Analysis (PCR-FFL) in the Direct Diagnosis and Identification of Cutaneous *Leishmania* Species. The American Journal of Tropical Medicine and Hygiene 2013;88:586–91.

[102] Da Silva LA, de Sousa CDS, da Graça GC, Porrozzi R, Cupolillo E. Sequence analysis and PCR-RFLP profiling of the hsp70 gene as a valuable tool for identifying *Leishmania* species associated with human leishmaniasis in Brazil.Infection, Genetics and Evolution: Journal of Molecular Epidemiology and Evolutionary Genetics in Infectious Diseases 2010;10:77–83.

[103] Lessa MM, Lessa HA, Castro TWN, Oliveira A, Scherifer A, Machado P, et al. Mucosal leishmaniasis: epidemiological and clinical aspects. Brazilian Journal of Otorhinolaryngology 2007;73:843–7.

[104] Arevalo J, Ramirez L, Adaui V, Zimic M, Tulliano G, Miranda-Verástegui C, et al. Influence of *Leishmania (Viannia)* species on the response to antimonial treatment in patients with American tegumentary leishmaniasis. The Journal of Infectious Diseases 2007;195:1846–51.

[105] Llanos-Cuentas A, Tulliano G, Araujo-Castillo R, Miranda-Verastegui C, Santamaria-Castrellon G, Ramirez L, et al. Clinical and parasite species risk factors for pentavalent antimonial treatment failure in cutaneous leishmaniasis in Peru.Clinical Infectious Diseases: An Official Publication of the Infectious Diseases Society of America 2008;46:223–31.

[106] Thomaz-Soccol V, Velez ID, Pratlong F, Agudelos S, Lanotte G, Rioux JA. Enzymatic polymorphism and phylogenetic relationships in *Leishmania* Ross, 1903 (Sarcomastigophora: Kinetoplastida): a case study in Colombia. Systematic Parasitolog 2000;46:59–68.

[107] Garcia AL, Parrado R, De Doncker S, Bermudez H, Dujardin J-C. American tegumentary leishmaniasis: direct species identification of *Leishmania* in non-invasive clinical samples. Transactions of the Royal Society of Tropical Medicine and Hygiene 2007;101:368–71.

[108] Montalvo AM, Fraga J, Monzote L, Montano I, De Doncker S, Dujardin JC, et al. Heat-shock protein 70 PCR-RFLP: a universal simple tool for *Leishmania* species discrimination in the New and Old World. Parasitology 2010;137:1159–68.

[109] Montalvo AM, Fraga J, Maes I, Dujardin J-C, Van der Auwera G. Three new sensitive and specific heat-shock protein 70 PCRs for global *Leishmania* species identification. European Journal of Clinical Microbiology & Infectious Diseases2011;31:1453–61.

[110] Bensoussan E, Nasereddin A, Jonas F, Schnur LF, Jaffe CL. Comparison of PCR assays for diagnosis of cutaneous leishmaniasis. Journal of Clinical Microbiology 2006;44:1435–9.

[111] Rocha MN, Margonari C, Presot IM, Soares RP. Evaluation of 4 polymerase chain reaction protocols for cultured *Leishmania* spp. typing. Diagnostic Microbiology and Infectious Disease 2010;68:401–9.

[112] Alexander J, Coombs GH, Mottram JC. *Leishmania mexicana* cysteine proteinase-deficient mutants have attenuated virulence for mice and potentiate a Th1 response. Journal of Immunology (Baltimore, Md.: 1950) 1950 1998;161:6794–801.

[113] Mundodi V, Somanna A, Farrell PJ, Gedamu L. Genomic organization and functional expression of differentially regulated cysteine protease genes of *Leishmania donovani* complex. Gene 2002;282:257–65.

[114] Quispe Tintaya KW, Ying X, Dedet J-P, Rijal S, De Bolle X, Dujardin J-C. Antigen genes for molecular epidemiology of leishmaniasis: polymorphism of cysteine proteinase B and surface metalloprotease glycoprotein 63 in the *Leishmania donovani* complex. The Journal of Infectious Diseases 2004;189:1035–43.

[115] Wortmann G, Hochberg L, Houng H-H, Sweeney C, Zapor M, Aronson N, et al. Rapid identification of *Leishmania* complexes by a real-time PCR assay. The American Journal of Tropical Medicine and Hygiene 2005;73:999–1004.

[116] Castilho TM, Camargo LMA, McMahon-Pratt D, Shaw JJ, Floeter-Winter LM. A real-time polymerase chain reaction assay for the identification and quantification of American *Leishmania* species on the basis of glucose-6-phosphate dehydrogenase. The American Journal of Tropical Medicine and Hygiene 2008;78:122–32.

[117] Weirather JL, Jeronimo SMB, Gautam S, Sundar S, Kang M, Kurtz MA, et al. Serial quantitative PCR assay for detection, species discrimination, and quantification of *Leishmania* spp. in human samples. Journal of Clinical Microbiology 2011;49:3892–904.

[118] Tsukayama P, Núñez JH, De Los Santos M, Soberón V, Lucas CM, Matlashewski G, et al. A FRET-based real-time PCR assay to identify the main causal agents of New World tegumentary leishmaniasis. PLoS Neglected Tropical Diseases 2013;7:e1956.

[119] Rioux JA, Lanotte G, Serres E, Pratlong F, Bastien P, Perieres J. Taxonomy of *Leishmania*. Use of isoenzymes. Suggestions for a new classification. Annales de Parasitologie Humaine et Comparée 1990;65:111–25.

[120] Bañuls A-L, Hide M, Prugnolle F. *Leishmania* and the Leishmaniases: A Parasite Genetic Update and Advances in Taxonomy, Epidemiology and Pathogenicity in Humans. Advances in Parasitology., vol. 64, Elsevier; 2007, p. 1–458.

[121] Hide M, Bañuls AL, Tibayrenc M. Genetic heterogeneity and phylogenetic status of *Leishmania (Leishmania) infantum* zymodeme MON-1: epidemiological implications. Parasitology 2001;123:425–32.

[122] Ochsenreither S, Kuhls K, Schaar M, Presber W, Schönian G. Multilocus microsatellite typing as a new tool for discrimination of *Leishmania infantum* MON-1 strains. Journal of Clinical Microbiology 2006;44:495–503.

[123] Jamjoom MB, Ashford RW, Bates PA, Chance ML, Kemp SJ, Watts PC, et al. *Leishmania donovani* is the only cause of visceral leishmaniasis in East Africa; previous descriptions of *L. infantum* and "*L. archibaldi*" from this region are a consequence of convergent evolution in the isoenzyme data. Parasitology 2004;129:399–409.

[124] Zemanová E, Jirků M, Mauricio IL, Miles MA, Lukes J. Genetic polymorphism within the *Leishmania donovani* complex: correlation with geographic origin. The American Journal of Tropical Medicine and Hygiene 2004;70:613–7.

[125] Lukes J, Mauricio IL, Schönian G, Dujardin J-C, Soteriadou K, Dedet J-P, et al. Evolutionary and geographical history of the *Leishmania donovani* complex with a revision of current taxonomy. Proceedings of the National Academy of Sciences of the United States of America 2007;104:9375–80.

[126] Schwenkenbecher JM, Wirth T, Schnur LF, Jaffe CL, Schallig H, Al-Jawabreh A, et al. Microsatellite analysis reveals genetic structure of *Leishmania tropica*. International Journal for Parasitology 2006;36:237–46.

[127] Alam MZ, Haralambous C, Kuhls K, Gouzelou E, Sgouras D, Soteriadou K, et al. The paraphyletic composition of *Leishmania donovani* zymodeme MON-37 revealed by multilocus microsatellite typing. Microbes and Infection / Institut Pasteur 2009;11:707–15.

[128] Williams JG, Kubelik AR, Livak KJ, Rafalski JA, Tingey SV. DNA polymorphisms amplified by arbitrary primers are useful as genetic markers.Nucleic Acids Research 1990;18:6531–5.

[129] Welsh J, McClelland M. Fingerprinting genomes using PCR with arbitrary primers.Nucleic Acids Research 1990;18:7213–8.

[130] Baptista C, Schubach AO, Madeira MF, Leal CA, Pires MQ, Oliveira FS, et al. *Leishmania (Viannia) braziliensis* genotypes identified in lesions of patients with atypical or typical manifestations of tegumentary leishmaniasis: Evaluation by two molecular markers. Experimental Parasitology 2009;121:317–22.

[131] Gomes RF, Macedo AM, Pena SD, Melo MN. *Leishmania (Viannia) braziliensis*: genetic relationships between strains isolated from different areas of Brazil as revealed by DNA fingerprinting and RAPD. Experimental Parasitology 1995;80:681–7.

[132] Mahmoudzadeh-Niknam H, Ajdary S, Riazi-Rad F, Mirzadegan E, Rezaeian A, Khaze V, et al. Molecular epidemiology of cutaneous leishmaniasis and heterogenei-

ty of *Leishmania major* strains in Iran: Molecular epidemiology of cutaneous leishmaniasis. Tropical Medicine & International Health 2012;17:1335–44.

[133] Hamad SH, Khalil EAG, Musa AM, Ibrahim ME, Younis BM, Elfaki MEE, et al. *Leishmania donovani*: genetic diversity of isolates from Sudan characterized by PCR-based RAPD. Experimental Parasitology 2010;125:389–93.

[134] Mauricio IL, Howard MK, Stothard JR, Miles MA. Genomic diversity in the *Leishmania donovani* complex. Parasitology 1999;119 (Pt 3):237–46.

[135] Segatto M, Ribeiro LS, Costa DL, Costa CHN, Oliveira MR de, Carvalho SFG, et al. Genetic diversity of *Leishmania infantum* field populations from Brazil. Memórias Do Instituto Oswaldo Cruz 2012;107:39–47.

[136] Martinez E, Alonso V, Quispe A, Thomas MC, Alonso R, Piero JE, et al. RAPD method useful for distinguishing *Leishmania* species: design of specific primers for *L. braziliensis*. Parasitology 2003;127:513–7.

[137] Ikram G, Dellagi K, Ismaïl RB. Random amplified polymorphic DNA technique for identification and differentiation of old world *Leishmania* species. The American Journal of Tropical Medicine and Hygiene 2002;66:152–6.

[138] Khanra S, Bandopadhyay SK, Chakraborty P, Datta S, Mondal D, Chatterjee M, et al. Characterization of the recent clinical isolates of Indian Kala-azar patients by RAPD-PCR method. Journal of Parasitic Diseases: Official Organ of the Indian Society for Parasitology 2011;35:116–22.

[139] Smith DF, Searle S, Ready PD, Gramiccia M, Ben-Ismail R. A kinetoplast DNA probe diagnostic for *Leishmania major*: sequence homologies between regions of *Leishmania* minicircles. Molecular and Biochemical Parasitology 1989;37:213–23.

[140] Gramiccia M, Smith DF, Angelici MC, Ready PD, Gradoni L. A kinetoplast DNA probe diagnostic for *Leishmania infantum*. Parasitology 1992;105 (Pt 1):29–34.

[141] Laskay T, Kiessling R, Rinke deWit TF, Wirth DF. Generation of species-specific DNA probes for *Leishmania aethiopica*. Molecular and Biochemical Parasitology 1991;44:279–86.

[142] Rodríguez N, Guzman B, Rodas A, Takiff H, Bloom BR, Convit J. Diagnosis of cutaneous leishmaniasis and species discrimination of parasites by PCR and hybridization. Journal of Clinical Microbiology 1994;32:2246–52.

[143] Brenière SF, Telleria J, Bosseno MF, Buitrago R, Bastrenta B, Cuny G, et al. Polymerase chain reaction-based identification of New World *Leishmania* species complexes by specific kDNA probes. Acta Tropica 1999;73:283–93.

[144] Howard MK, Kelly JM, Lane RP, Miles MA. A sensitive repetitive DNA probe that is specific to the *Leishmania donovani* complex and its use as an epidemiological and diagnostic reagent. Molecular and Biochemical Parasitology 1991;44:63–72.

[145] Van Eys GJ, Guizani I, Ligthart GS, Dellagi K. A nuclear DNA probe for the identification of strains within the *Leishmania donovani* complex. Experimental Parasitology 1991;72:459–63.

[146] Van Eys GJ, Schoone GJ, Ligthart GS, Alvar J, Evans DA, Terpstra WJ. Identification of "Old World" *Leishmania* by DNA recombinant probes. Molecular and Biochemical Parasitology 1989;34:53–62.

[147] Grisard EC, Steindel M, Shaw JJ, Ishikawa EA, Carvalho-Pinto CJ, Eger-Mangrich I, et al. Characterization of *Leishmania* sp. strains isolated from autochthonous cases of human cutaneous leishmaniasis in Santa Catarina State, southern Brazil. Acta Tropica 2000;74:89–93.

[148] Rodriguez N, De Lima H, Rodriguez A, Brewster S, Barker DC. Genomic DNA repeat from *Leishmania (Viannia) braziliensis* (Venezuelan strain) containing simple repeats and microsatellites. Parasitology 1997;115 (Pt 4):349–58.

[149] Rodriguez N, Rodriguez A, Cardona M, Barrios MA, McCann SH, Barker DC. *Leishmania (Viannia) guyanensis*: a new minicircle class exclusive to this specie isolated from a DNA cosmid library useful for taxonomic purposes. Experimental Parasitology 2000;94:143–9.

[150] Schönian G, Mauricio I, Gramiccia M, Cañavate C, Boelaert M, Dujardin J-C. Leishmaniases in the Mediterranean in the era of molecular epidemiology. Trends in Parasitology 2008;24:135–42.

[151] Mauricio IL, Yeo M, Baghaei M, Doto D, Pratlong F, Zemanova E, et al. Towards multilocus sequence typing of the *Leishmania donovani* complex: resolving genotypes and haplotypes for five polymorphic metabolic enzymes (ASAT, GPI, NH1, NH2, PGD).International Journal for Parasitology 2006;36:757–69.

[152] Zemanová E, Jirků M, Mauricio IL, Horák A, Miles MA, Lukeš J. The *Leishmania donovani* complex: Genotypes of five metabolic enzymes (ICD, ME, MPI, G6PDH, and FH), new targets for multilocus sequence typing.International Journal for Parasitology 2007;37:149–60.

[153] Tsukayama P, Lucas C, Bacon DJ. Typing of four genetic loci discriminates among closely related species of New World *Leishmania*. International Journal for Parasitology 2009;39:355–62.

[154] Zhang C-Y, Lu X-J, Du X-Q, Jian J, Shu L, Ma Y. Phylogenetic and Evolutionary Analysis of Chinese *Leishmania* Isolates Based on Multilocus Sequence Typing. PLoS ONE 2013;8:e63124.

[155] Alam MZ, Kovalenko DA, Kuhls K, Nasyrova RM, Ponomareva VI, Fatullaeva AA, et al. Identification of the agent causing visceral leishmaniasis in Uzbeki and Tajiki foci by analysing parasite DNA extracted from patients' Giemsa-stained tissue preparations. Parasitology 2009;136:981.

[156] Gouzelou E, Haralambous C, Amro A, Mentis A, Pratlong F, Dedet J-P, et al. Multilocus microsatellite typing (MLMT) of strains from Turkey and Cyprus reveals a novel monophyletic *L. donovani* sensu lato group. PLoS Neglected Tropical Diseases 2012;6:e1507.

[157] Jamjoom MB, Ashford RW, Bates PA, Kemp SJ, Noyes HA. Towards a standard battery of microsatellite markers for the analysis of the *Leishmania donovani* complex. Annals of Tropical Medicine and Parasitology 2002;96:265–70.

[158] Kuhls K, Keilonat L, Ochsenreither S, Schaar M, Schweynoch C, Presber W, et al. Multilocus microsatellite typing (MLMT) reveals genetically isolated populations between and within the main endemic regions of visceral leishmaniasis. Microbes and Infection 2007;9:334–43.

[159] Jamjoom MB, Ashford RW, Bates PA, Kemp SJ, Noyes HA. Polymorphic microsatellite repeats are not conserved between *Leishmania donovani* and *Leishmania major*. Molecular Ecology Notes 2002;2:104–6.

[160] Azmi K, Schnur L, Schonian G, Nasereddin A, Pratlong F, El Baidouri F, et al. Genetic, serological and biochemical characterization of *Leishmania tropica* from foci in northern Palestine and discovery of zymodeme MON-307. Parasites & Vectors 2012;5:121.

[161] Oddone R, Schweynoch C, Schönian G, de Sousa C dos S, Cupolillo E, Espinosa D, et al. Development of a multilocus microsatellite typing approach for discriminating strains of *Leishmania (Viannia)* species. Journal of Clinical Microbiology 2009;47:2818–25.

[162] Rioux JA, Lanotte G, Serres E, Pratlong F, Bastien P, Perieres J. Taxonomy of *Leishmania*. Use of isoenzymes. Suggestions for a new classification. Annales de Parasitologie Humaine et Comparée 1990;65:111–25.

[163] Schönian G, Cupolillo E, Mauricio I. Molecular Evolution and Phylogeny of *Leishmania*. In: Ponte-Sucre A, Diaz E, Padrón-Nieves M, editors. Drug Resistance in *Leishmania* Parasites,, Vienna: Springer Vienna; 2013, p. 15–44.

[164] Croan DG, Morrison DA, Ellis JT. Evolution of the genus *Leishmania* revealed by comparison of DNA and RNA polymerase gene sequences. Molecular and Biochemical Parasitology 1997;89:149–59.

[165] Berzunza-Cruz M, Cabrera N, Crippa-Rossi M, Sosa Cabrera T, Pérez-Montfort R, Becker I. Polymorphism analysis of the internal transcribed spacer and small subunit of ribosomal RNA genes of *Leishmania mexicana*. Parasitology Research 2002;88:918–25.

[166] Dávila AM, Momen H. Internal-transcribed-spacer (ITS) sequences used to explore phylogenetic relationships within *Leishmania*. Annals of Tropical Medicine and Parasitology 2000;94:651–4.

[167] Waki K, Dutta S, Ray D, Kolli BK, Akman L, Kawazu S-I, et al. Transmembrane molecules for phylogenetic analyses of pathogenic protists: *Leishmania*-specific informative sites in hydrophilic loops of trans- endoplasmic reticulum N-acetylglucosamine-1-phosphate transferase. Eukaryotic Cell 2007;6:198–210.

[168] Asato Y, Oshiro M, Myint CK, Yamamoto Y, Kato H, Marco JD, et al. Phylogenic analysis of the genus *Leishmania* by cytochrome b gene sequencing. Experimental Parasitology 2009;121:352–61.

[169] Cupolillo E, Medina-Acosta E, Noyes H, Momen H, Grimaldi G Jr. A revised classification for *Leishmania* and *Endotrypanum*. Parasitology Today (Personal Ed.) 2000;16:142–4.

[170] Kuhls K, Alam MZ, Cupolillo E, Ferreira GEM, Mauricio IL, Oddone R, et al. Comparative microsatellite typing of new world *Leishmania infantum* reveals low heterogeneity among populations and its recent old world origin. PLoS Neglected Tropical Diseases 2011;5:e1155.

[171] Maurício IL, Stothard JR, Miles MA. The strange case of *Leishmania chagasi*. Parasitology Today (Personal Ed.) 2000;16:188–9.

[172] Spanakos G, Piperaki E-T, Menounos PG, Tegos N, Flemetakis A, Vakalis NC. Detection and species identification of Old World *Leishmania* in clinical samples using a PCR-based method. Transactions of the Royal Society of Tropical Medicine and Hygiene 2008;102:46–53.

[173] Yurchenko VY, Lukes J, Jirku M, Zeledón R, Maslov DA. Leptomonas costaricensis sp. n. (Kinetoplastea: Trypanosomatidae), a member of the novel phylogenetic group of insect trypanosomatids closely related to the genus *Leishmania.* Parasitology 2006;133:537–46.

[174] Banũls AL, Hide M, Tibayrenc M. Molecular epidemiology and evolutionary genetics of Leischmania parasites.International Journal for Parasitology 1999;29:1137–47.

[175] Grimaldi G Jr, Tesh RB. Leishmaniases of the New World: current concepts and implications for future research. Clinical Microbiology Reviews 1993;6:230–50.

[176] Noyes H, Pratlong F, Chance M, Ellis J, Lanotte G, Dedet JP. A previously unclassified trypanosomatid responsible for human cutaneous lesions in Martinique (French West Indies) is the most divergent member of the genus *Leishmania* sp. Parasitology 2002;124:17–24.

[177] Suankratay C, Suwanpimolkul G, Wilde H, Siriyasatien P. Autochthonous visceral leishmaniasis in a human immunodeficiency virus (HIV)-infected patient: the first in thailand and review of the literature. The American Journal of Tropical Medicine and Hygiene 2010;82:4–8.

[178] Sukmee T, Siripattanapipong S, Mungthin M, Worapong J, Rangsin R, Samung Y, et al. A suspected new species of *Leishmania*, the causative agent of visceral leishmaniasis in a Thai patient.International Journal for Parasitology 2008;38:617–22.

[179] Villinski JT, Klena JD, Abbassy M, Hoel DF, Puplampu N, Mechta S, et al. Evidence for a new species of *Leishmania* associated with a focal disease outbreak in Ghana.Diagnostic Microbiology and Infectious Disease 2008;60:323–7.

[180] Rose K, Curtis J, Baldwin T, Mathis A, Kumar B, Sakthianandeswaren A, et al. Cutaneous leishmaniasis in red kangaroos: isolation and characterisation of the causative organisms.International Journal for Parasitology 2004;34:655–64.

[181] Lobsiger L, Müller N, Schweizer T, Frey CF, Wiederkehr D, Zumkehr B, et al. An autochthonous case of cutaneous bovine leishmaniasis in Switzerland. Veterinary Parasitology 2010;169:408–14.

[182] Müller N, Welle M, Lobsiger L, Stoffel MH, Boghenbor KK, Hilbe M, et al. Occurrence of *Leishmania* sp. in cutaneous lesions of horses in Central Europe. Veterinary Parasitology 2009;166:346–51.

[183] Silveira FT, Ishikawa EAY, De Souza AAA, Lainson R. An outbreak of cutaneous leishmaniasis among soldiers in Belém, Pará State, Brazil, caused by *Leishmania (Viannia) lindenbergi* n. sp. A new leishmanial parasite of man in the Amazon region. Parasite (Paris, France) 2002;9:43–50.

[184] Simpson AGB, Stevens JR, Lukeš J. The evolution and diversity of kinetoplastid flagellates. Trends in Parasitology 2006;22:168–74.

[185] Miles MA, Llewellyn MS, Lewis MD, Yeo M, Baleela R, Fitzpatrick S, et al. The molecular epidemiology and phylogeography of *Trypanosoma cruzi* and parallel research on *Leishmania*: looking back and to the future. Parasitology 2009;136:1509–28.

Chapter 9

Non-Invasive Molecular Diagnosis of Canine Visceral Leishmaniasis Using Conjunctival Swab Samples

Antero Silva Ribeiro de Andrade and
Maria Norma Melo

Additional information is available at the end of the chapter

http://dx.doi.org/10.5772/57304

1. Introduction

Leishmaniasis is a neglected tropical disease caused by protozoan parasites of the genus *Leishmania,* which is a public health problem in tropical and subtropical regions of the World. The parasite is transmitted to mammals by the bite of naturally infected species of female sand fly vectors (Diptera, Psychodidae: Phlebotominae). The geographic distribution of leishmaniasis is limited by distribution of the sand fly vectors. Vectors of the genus *Lutzomyia* are responsible for transmitting the disease in the New World and the genus *Phlebotomus* in the Old World [1].

Leishmaniases comprise a complex of diseases caused by at least 22 species of *Leishmania* which are obligatory intracellular parasites surviving within phagolysosomes of the mononuclear phagocytes of mammal host. These parasites produce a wide spectrum of diseases, depending both on the species that initiating infection and on the immunological status of the host, among other factors. The disease ranges from: simple cutaneous lesion developing at the site of the sand fly bite, with skin ulcers that usually appears on exposed part of the body, such as the face, arms and legs, that could be heal within a few months, leaving scars; mucocutaneous form with lesions that can partially or totally destroy the mucous membranes of the nose, mouth and throat cavities and surrounding tissues and producing extensive disfiguring, being difficult to treat; diffuse cutaneous that is rare, but more serious complication which occurs when the immune system fails to react effectively to infection with multiple non ulcerative nodules and visceral leishmaniasis, also known as kala azar, that is characterized by high fever, substantial weight loss, swelling of the spleen and liver, and anemia. If left untreated, the visceral leishmaniasis can have a fatality rate as high as 100% within two years. The disease presents high morbidity in tegumentary leishmaniasis and high mortality levels in visceral leishmaniasis [2].

Reported from 98 countries, in six continents, the leishmaniases are responsible for the second-highest number of deaths due to parasitic infection globally and are still one of the world's most neglected diseases, affecting largely the poorest of the poor, mainly in developing countries. It is associated with malnutrition, displacement, poor housing, illiteracy, gender discrimination, weakness of the immune system and lack of resources. Approximately 0.2 to 0.4 and 0.7 to 1.2 million of visceral leishmaniasis and tegumentary leishmaniasis cases respectively, occur each year, with 350 million people in worldwide living at risk to be infected, based on World Health Organization data. Leishmaniasis is the third most important vector-borne disease, and the estimated disease burden places it second in mortality and fourth in morbidity among tropical infections [3].

More than 90% cases of visceral leishmaniasis occur in six countries: India, Bangladesh, Sudan, South Sudan, Ethiopia and Brazil [3]. Certainly, these data are underestimated, since not all affected nations have a system of compulsory notification of cases, and even those countries where the leishmaniasis is a reportable disease there are logistical problems that increase the imprecision of the estimations [4].

The distribution of tegumentary leishmaniasis is more extensive, occurring in three epidemiological regions, the Americas, the Mediterranean basin and Western Asia from the Middle East to Central Asia. Ten countries have 70-75% of cases worldwide: Afghanistan, Algeria, Colombia, Brazil, Iran, Syria, Ethiopia, North Sudan, Costa Rica and Peru. Mortality data were extremely sparse and generally represent hospital-based deaths only [3].

Several studies have reported the expansion of leishmaniasis worldwide and occurrence of cases in endemic regions have been recurrent and the global number of cases has increased in recent decades. The main reasons given for such increases are related to environmental changes, agricultural development, migration of non-immune people to endemic areas, and, in part, by improved diagnosis, but are also due to other factors such as inadequate reservoir or vector control. More recently, an increased detection of disease associated with opportunistic HIV infections and visceral leishmaniasis, especially in intravenous drug users in Southwestern Europe and other endemic areas was verified. A recent report by the World Health Organization [4] indicated that people with AIDS have become the largest risk group for human visceral leishmaniasis in Southern Europe, and that their co-infection is expected to present an increasing problem in areas were HIV and human visceral leishmaniasis overlap, especially in Brazil, Africa, and India. In areas endemic for visceral leishmaniasis, many people have asymptomatic infection. A concomitant HIV infection increases the risk of developing active visceral leishmaniasis by between 100 and 2320 times [5]. In Southern Europe, up to 70% of cases of visceral leishmaniasis in adults are associated with HIV infection. Sum up this the urbanization, deforestation, the emergence of antileishmanial drug resistance, economic development itself is also increasing exposure, tourism, wars and in some areas military training in forest or desert [6].

A large number of different *Leishmania* species cause tegumentary disease belonging to both subgenera *Leishmania* and *Viannia* (which are present only in the America). Epidemiological studies have revealed that except *Leishmania tropica,* all of other species that cause tegumentary leishmaniasis are zoonoses that initially affect animals (rodents, sylvatic edentates, marsupials and non-human primates) and eventually humans [7].

Visceral leishmaniasis or kala azar, is almost always fatal if not treated. In the Americas as well in Mediterranean Basin, Middle East, West Africa and Central Asia, visceral leishmaniasis is caused by *Leishmania infantum* (=*L. chagasi*) and is a zoonosis with an animal reservoir and occasional human infections. However, visceral leishmaniasis in India and Africa caused by *Leishmania donovani* has an anthroponotic cycle with inter-human transmission. Despite the ecological differences, the disease is very similar in their clinical manifestations. It is characterized by targeting visceral organs and results in the development of syndromes comprised of irregular fever, substantial weight loss, splenomegaly, hepatomegaly, hypergammaglobulinemia, pancytopenia, anemia and hypoalbuminaemia witch is associated with edema and other features such as malnutrition [8].

Patients treated and cured for visceral leishmaniasis caused by *L. donovani* may subsequent develop Post-kala azar dermal leishmaniasis (PKDL). Post-kala azar dermal leishmaniasis is an unusual dermatosis that develops as a sequel in 5–15% of cured cases of kala azar after months or years of treatment in India [9].

L. infantum maintains a zoonotic cycle mostly involved canine host, and canine visceral leishmaniasis is also a veterinary problem. The recommended control methods for the disease have only been partially effective. The continued endemicity of zoonotic visceral leishmaniasis, its recent appearance in urban areas of Latin America [10] and its increasing importance as an opportunistic infection among persons infected with human immunodeficiency virus, indicate that present control methods for the disease are ineffective and that new control strategies are needed. Prevention of the disease in dogs appears to be the best approach for interrupting the domestic cycle of zoonotic visceral leishmaniasis. Not all *L. infantum* infections lead to overt clinical disease. In Brazil were described ratios of 8-18 incident asymptomatic infections to 1 incident clinical case [11].

Zoonotic visceral leishmaniasis is an important emerging parasitic disease of humans and dogs. The most feasible approach would seem to be a canine vaccine that protects dogs from developing disease and from becoming peridomestic reservoirs of the parasite. There are two vaccines developed in Brazil, but not used for routine immunization against zoonotic visceral leishmaniasis. There is clear evidence that in the zoonotic visceral leishmaniasis the parasites are maintained through the bite of infected female phlebotomine sand flies, and the prevalence of disease has been expanding throughout the world [12].

Many studies suggest that *L. infantum* in urban and peri-urban settings is a phenomenon reported in several countries when zoonotic visceral leishmaniasis is endemic. Dogs are the only confirmed primary reservoir of infection. Meta-analysis studies confirm that infectiousness is higher in symptomatic infection; infectiousness is also higher in European than South

American studies [13]. A high prevalence of infection has been reported from an increasing number of domestic and wild mammals; updated host ranges are provided.

The domestic dog is the most important domestic reservoir in urban and rural areas [14]. The dogs have intense cutaneous parasitism, favoring infection of vectors and play an important role in the epidemiological chain of human visceral leishmaniasis. Therefore, although visceral leishmaniasis remains more prevalent among dogs than humans, the presence of infected dogs may increase the risk for human infection in some situation [15]. There is a close canine relationship with human in both rural and urban areas, and canine cases usually precede human cases.

The strategies of the control of leishmaniasis have varied very little for decades, but in recent years there have been exciting advances in diagnosis, treatment and prevention. These include an immunochromatographic dipstick for diagnosing visceral leishmaniasis; the licensing of miltefosine, the first oral drug for visceral leishmaniasis; and evidence that the incidence of zoonotic visceral leishmaniasis in children can be reduced by providing dogs with deltamethrin collars. In the context of zoonotic visceral leishmaniasis measures of control transmission vary according to local epidemiology [10].

The canine visceral leishmaniasis is clinically alike to human infection, but with dermal lesions normally found in infected-symptomatic dogs. The infection in dogs carries a wide-ranging clinical signs related to high antileishmanial antibody levels and lack of a cell-mediated response. *Leishmania* are intracellular parasites and, under immunodeficiency conditions, they multiply and migrate from lymphoid tissue to other organs, displaying severe clinical and pathological changes which could leads to animal death. Although, infections in endemic areas are high, not all dogs infected develop the disease, in some dogs several clinical signs of disease appear in short time after infection. Part of dog remains infected for a long time, but without clinical signs of disease. There are evidences that the host's genetics could play a major role in susceptibility or resistance [16]. Canine visceral leishmaniasis has a high prevalence of infection, involving as much as 63-80% of the population [17, 18] and is accompanied by a lower rate of apparent clinical disease.

Dogs have also been found to be infected with other *Leishmania* spp., and their role in these infections is probably more than incidental. In the wide geographical range of *L. infantum*, there are many contrasting situations, depending on whether the dogs are domestic, stray or feral and on the animals' place in society. Naturally infected asymptomatic dogs have been demonstrated to be easily infective to sand flies under experimental conditions (xenodiagnosis). Therefore, the role they may play in the cycle should not be underestimated, as more than 50% of all infected dogs are asymptomatic carriers. This is due to the high degree of parasitism on the skin of the infected animal and greater susceptibility to disease in many of them [19]. Thus, occurrence of infection in endemic regions of sand flies is facilitated, and the dog plays a decisive role in keeping the disease cycle transmission under favorable conditions, with high population density vector and dogs, the infection spreads rapidly and extensively in the population of vectors and also in the canine population [20, 21].

http://dx.doi.org/10.5772/57304

In the Mediterranean basin, human cases and canine cases are treated with antileishmanial drugs. In this area the use of individual measures to protect dogs from sand fly bites using insecticides are common practices, but no public health surveillance and control interventions such as applied, for example, in Brazil are in place [22]. Despite years of effort using control measures the number of infected dogs in South-western Europe alone are approximately at 2.5 million [23] and the number of infected dogs in South America also is estimated in millions. In Latin America the strategies of control of visceral leishmaniasis are based in the diagnosis of human and canine visceral leishmaniasis, treatment of human cases, control of infected dogs using immunological test to diagnose *L. infantum* infections and to cull putative infected animals and also vector control by spraying insecticides with residual action. Animal reservoir control through environmental management is expensive and difficult to implement; the efficacy of dog culling is questionable [24].

In the context of visceral leishmaniasis prophylaxis, the rapid and accurate diagnosis of infected dogs is critical for the control. The correct diagnosis is essential for detection of *L. infantum* infection in both symptomatic and asymptomatic dogs. Reliable clinical signs of canine visceral leishmaniasis are not obvious until late in the disease. The precise diagnosis of canine visceral leishmaniasis is complex and must be performed combined to parasitological, immunological and molecular tests [25]. Although, the disease burden persists due to technical, managerial, financial and political constraints [24].

Current diagnosis methods of zoonotic visceral leishmaniasis are based on parasite demonstration in tissue stained smears. *Leishmania* amastigotes can be demonstrated in impression smears made from fine needle aspirates of lymph nodes, spleen or bone marrow, and stained with Giemsa or a quick stain such as Rapid Panotic (Laborclin®). In dogs impression smears can also be made from dermal lesions, such as those found on the tip of the ear, after scraping of the skin. The material is used for culture, cytology or examination of the parasites presence. Although demonstration of even a single amastigote upon microscopic examination of tissue smears is considered sufficient for positive diagnosis of disease, the sensitivity of the tissue examination varies, being splenic aspirate more sensitivity, than bone marrow or the lymph node aspiration. The specificity is high, but the sensitivity, except in the case of spleen aspirate, is low. However, spleen aspiration can be complicated by life threatening hemorrhages in ~0.1% of the cases. The identification of amastigotes requires considered expertise and training and is subject to the ability of the observer [26]. Diagnosis may also be established by the inoculation of hamsters with infected tissues and monitoring their clinical signs. This technique is used mostly in research parasite identification, requires considerable expertise and training and in our own experience is can be laborious and time consuming.

Other several methods are described to diagnosis human and canine visceral leishmaniasis and the most employed are immunodiagnostic tests for antibody detection. Serodiagnosis is particularly useful in zoonotic visceral leishmaniasis, since humans and dogs present hypergammaglobulinemia. Dogs with canine visceral leishmaniasis infection, either symptomatic or asymptomatic, will almost always demonstrate a specific humoral response. The serological test used crude antigen preparations and they are limited in both specificity and assay reproducibility, and there are cross-reactions with other *Leishmania* species and with *Trypano-*

soma cruzi. Weak responses in some dogs and presence of antibodies in some healthy individuals are inherent limitations with antibody based diagnostics according our own observations. The use of crude *Leishmania* antigens is thought to underestimate the prevalence of canine visceral leishmaniasis [27, 28].

In Latin America, mainly in Brazil, the serological test is extensive used as part of control campaigns to remove seropositive animals for euthanasia often not with the agreement of the owners. The Brazilian Ministry of Health, through the Control Program of Visceral Leishmaniasis, has instituted specific measures to control of the disease using immunofluorescent antibody test (IFAT) and enzyme-linked immunosorbent assay (ELISA). To date, however, the actions of this program have had little impact. Control strategy based on the euthanasia of seropositive dogs depended on mass serological surveys usually with blood samples collected generally on filter paper. According reliable diagnostic test is essential for detection of *L. infantum* infection. This complex panorama certainly generates significant changes in the measures of accuracy of the serological tests and this negative outcome has been ascribed to delays in detecting and eliminating infected dogs, the tendency to replace infected dogs by susceptible puppies, the low sensitivity of the available serological methods, the high incidence of infected dogs and the presence of cross reactions in the used IFAT and ELISA methods [29, 30]. Thus, to remove seropositive dogs is insufficient as a measure for eradicating visceral leishmaniasis in dogs. However, the force of transmission of infection among dogs can be reduced by such programs. The results of this intervention study suggest that the elimination of the majority of seropositive dogs may affect the cumulative incidence of seroconversion in dogs temporarily and may also diminish the incidence of human cases of visceral leishmaniasis [31].

IFAT has low specificity, demand highly trained personnel, it is time consuming and expensive, thus is not adaptable to large-scale epidemiological studies (although it is used in Latin America) and the requirement of sophisticated laboratory conditions prohibit its application in the field. ELISA is the most commonly used test for immunodiagnosis of canine visceral leishmaniasis. The antigen used are traditionally derived from promastigotes cultivated *in vitro* and consist of a repertoire of a least 30 somatic antigens and several surface components. It results that most immunodiagnostic methods have been hampered by problems of cross-reactivity of species within the trypanosomatids as well microorganisms phylogenetically distant [32]. According WHO (2010) [5] serology existing tools (IFAT and ELISA) are difficult to decentralize, direct agglutination test (DAT) can be used at the periphery but needs cold chain and shaking during transportation frequently hampers the antigen. Parasitological existing tools (spleen, bone marrow and lymph node aspirates) are either invasive methods and difficult to decentralize (spleen and bone marrow) or of low sensitivity (lymph nodes).

The recombinant antigens rK9, rK26, rK39 used in the ELISA test seemed to be most suited for point-of-care diagnosis of symptomatic cases of dogs but lack sensitivity for asymptomatic ones [32, 29].The K39 test was not able to detect active infection in dogs with low IFAT titers, in the range of 1:40 to 1:320. Other tests such as DAT, agglutination screen test (FAST), that is a DAT modified, rapid tests like the immunochromatographic-dipstick TRALD (Test Rapid *Leishmania donovani*) and other using the recombinant rK9, rK26 and rK39 proteins of *L. infantum* are used in the routine diagnosis in several countries but not in Latin America [33]. The direct agglutination test, in which stained parasites are agglutinated by serum antibodies, is popular in Iran and Africa, but variation between batches and the high cost of commercially

http://dx.doi.org/10.5772/57304

available antigen are limiting factors. The most recent platform for serodiagnosis by immunochromatography technology is the Dual Path Platform (DPP®), which may in the near future replace other immunochromatographic tests [31]. In Brazil, the Dual Path Platform test began to be incorporated to epidemiological routines [34].

Due to the problems presented by serological tests, different molecular methods have been evaluated for leishmaniasis diagnosis and Polymerase Chain Reaction (PCR) is presently the principal method for molecular diagnosis of *Leishmania.* PCR-based methods for detecting *Leishmania* species in clinical samples have been developed which amplify rRNA and miniexon genes, kinetoplast DNA (kDNA) and repeated nuclear DNA sequences. These methods are of variable specificity; some are generic and can detect all *Leishmania* species while other methods identify the infecting *Leishmania* parasite to the species level. These techniques mostly have a high sensitivity although some, such as PCR with a subsequent hybridization increase the sensitivity of the assay [35]. The real-time PCR was recently introduced for detection and typing of *Leishmania* [36, 37, 38] with the advantages of speed and reduced risk of sample contamination, since monitoring of amplification is conducted as the reaction proceeds. Many studies have reported that real-time PCR has greater sensitivity than conventional PCR for canine visceral leishmaniasis diagnosis and is reproducible in diagnostic routines [39]. PCR based assays are being suggested as useful methods to detect subclinical infections and as a possible addition to serological methods to definitively diagnose inconclusive cases that show low antibody titers or cross reactivity [26].The molecular diagnostics using PCR has demonstrated high sensitivity shown by different studies, than other conventional diagnostic techniques for diagnosis of the canine visceral leishmaniasis, on other hand, PCR methods can vary according to the biological sample examined [40]. This technique has several advantages over other detection methods, especially in the field situation. PCR advantages included, the ability to use very small amounts of target material, the fast detection of *Leishmania* in all material that are used for diagnosis, including skin biopsies, touch preparations, aspirates from lymph nodes, bone marrow, spleen, buffy coat and blood spots collected on filter paper and can be used to simultaneous detection and typing of the parasite [26].

PCR based assays can disclose the presence of parasite DNA very early on, even before seroconversion [21]. The detection of *Leishmania* DNA based on PCR represents an alternative for visceral leishmaniasis diagnosis with highly sensitive, specific and versatile methods [10]. PCR are consistently been shown to be better than microscopy or parasite culture, particularly in samples with low parasite loads [6]. As stated above, several types of canine clinical samples have been used for diagnosis with these techniques [41, 42, 43, 44]. The skin is the principal access point for the phlebotomines and hence represents the principal pathway for infection. Different studies have demonstrated high positive indices for PCR using skin samples of dogs with different clinical signs, and it has been suggested that these techniques based on use of ear skin could be the best procedure for diagnosing canine visceral leishmaniasis [44]. The collection of this sample, however, is painful, bloody and invasive, requiring local anesthesia and aseptic manipulation. The parasites show natural tropism towards lymphoid tissues and many studies have shown that these tissues are a good source for *Leishmania* DNA detection. PCR performed using bone marrow has shown high sensitivity [45], but the procedure of bone marrow sampling is very invasive and traumatic. Complete anesthesia of the animal is necessary, which usually results in opposition by dog owners. Lymph node are one of the preferred internal tissues for *L. infantum* multiplication and lymph node aspirates also allow high sensitivities by PCR [45, 46], but again the collection procedure is invasive, offering risk of infection for the animal and demands very well trained personnel. These limitations make these samples unsuitable for large-scale surveys. Blood is considered a less invasive sample type. The evaluation of blood for the diagnosis of canine visceral leishmaniasis by PCR is still contradictory. Some studies provided evidence that this clinical sample showed a good performance by PCR [42, 47, 48, 49]. In contrast, other authors encountered problems with the use of blood related to DNA preparation, high frequency of PCR inhibitors in dog blood, variations of the parasite load in the course of infection and low sensitivity [40, 41, 50].

Besides to provide high sensitivity, the ideal source of biological material for molecular diagnosis of canine visceral leishmaniasis would be a non-invasive, painless and easily obtained sample, which could be more accepted by the dog-owners and obtained outside veterinary centers. The conjunctival swab sample is acquired by a non-invasive procedure that uses a sterile swab for sampling the dog conjunctiva (Figure 1) and fulfills these criteria.

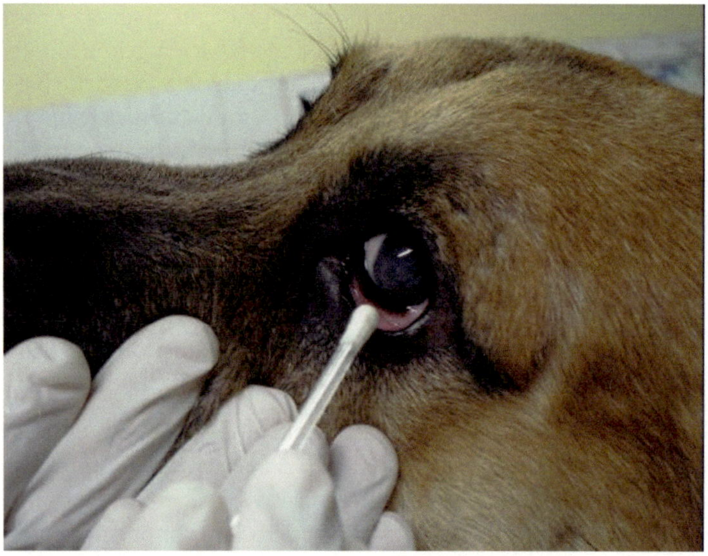

Figure 1. Conjunctival swab sampling method

2. Conjunctival swab

Previous studies had initially pointed that the conjunctiva of infected dogs was a good source of *Leishmania* DNA. Berrahal et al. (1996)[51] investigating asymptomatic carriers was able to identify 15 of 16 dogs (93.8%) by PCR using 5mg of conjunctiva biopsies. In the same study 9 of 14 asymptomatic dogs (64.3%) were positive for skin samples PCR. All these dogs were negative for ELISA and IFAT but immunoblotting detected specific antibodies in 66% of the animals. Solano-Gallego et al. (2001)[17] identified by PCR 32 out 100 dogs (32%) using conjunctiva biopsies while in the same group 17 out of 95 animals (17.8%) had positive bone marrow and 51 out of 100 (51%) presented positive skin. Reithinger et al. (2002)[52] in a study dealing with tissue tropism and parasite dissemination in two domestic dogs was also able to detect by PCR and histology *Leishmania (Viannia)* spp. in conjunctiva biopsies of both animals.

The first work using the conjunctival swab was performed by Strauss-Ayali et al. (2004)[50]. Ninety-eight dogs were examined in this study and divided in four groups. The group A included 24 seropositive symptomatic animals; in the group B were incorporated 65 seronegative dogs; the group C was formed by six male five-month-old beagle dogs that were experimentally infected with *L. infantum*; and the group D included nine seronegative beagle dogs with no clinical signs of leishmaniasis. In the group A, 83% of the conjunctival samples from either the right or the left conjunctivas were positive by ITS1-PCR and 92% of the dogs were found positives when results from both eyes were combined. Skin scrapings obtained from two areas of the back and from skin lesions were positive for 29%, 41% and 46% of the samples, respectively. Sixty five percent of the dogs were found positive if all skin tests were combined. ITS1-PCR from buffy coat and blood were positive for 57% and 17% of the dogs in that order. Spleen and lymph node aspirates were PCR positives for 77% and 67% of the dogs, respectively. Positives cultures were obtained from 61% and 37% of the spleen and lymph node samples and 74% of the dogs were positive considering the sum of results of both cultures. All group B seronegative dogs were found to be negative by ITS1-PCR in both conjunctival samples and buffy coat. In this study a sensitivity of 92% and a specificity of 100% were found for detection of *L. infantum* DNA in naturally symptomatic infected dogs by using conjuntival swab samples. The experimentally infected dogs (group C) were evaluated every two weeks for 90 days. Forty five days after infection 5 (83%) of the 6 dogs had at least one conjunctival sample found to be positive by PCR while the correspondent optical density values for ELISA were still below the cutoff value. After 60 days of infection the number of positive dogs by conjunctival PCR remained the same but all dogs have seroconverted. At 75 and 90 days after infection, at least one conjunctival sample from 100% of the dogs was found to be positive. Conjunctival, spleen and buffy coat samples were PCR negative for group D control animals (seronegative beagle dogs) and spleen cultures were also negative for *L. infantum.* The study demonstrated that sensitivity obtained by the conjunctival swab PCR was superior to that obtained by culture or by PCR using invasively obtained samples. The work also showed that conjunctival PCR was positive in the experimentally infected dogs before the seroconvertion and was superior to serologic testing for early diagnosis.

A study evaluating the conjunctival swab for canine visceral leishmaniasis diagnosis by the kDNA PCR-hybridization method in a Brazilian endemic region of leishmaniasis in Belo Horizonte, Minas Gerais State, was accomplished by Ferreira et al. (2008)[41]. In the kDNA PCR-hibridization method the PCR amplified products (a 120 bp conserved region of kDNA minicircles) are hybridized with minicircle cloned probes labeled with ^{32}P radionuclide. The study also evaluated two procedures of DNA extraction from conjunctival swabs: phenol chloroform and boiling. The efficiency of the two DNA extraction methods was first evaluated, *in vitro,* using cotton swabs seeded with different numbers of *L. infantum* promastigotes. By using the phenol chloroform method of DNA extraction, the kDNA PCR-hybridization procedure was able to detect down to a single parasite per swab, while the limit of detection for the boiling method was 25 parasites. Afterward, two groups of 23 seropositive symptomatic dogs were evaluated. Conjunctival swab samples were obtained from both eyes of each animal. The DNA extraction was performed by the phenol chloroform method in group 1 and by boiling in group 2. Blood was also collected from each animal so that 30μL were spotted onto filter paper and 1.0ml was treated to obtain the buffy coat. The DNA extraction from the buffy coat and filter paper was accomplished by identical procedures in both groups using commercial kits. After hybridization step, the positivities calculated for conjunctival swab combining the results of the right (RC) and left conjunctivas (LC), were 91.3% and 65.2% for groups 1 and 2, respectively. The kDNA PCR-hybridization positivities calculated for the RC and LC separately were 73.9% (17/23) for RC and 91.3% (21/23) for LC in group 1, 52.2% (12/23) for RC and 56.5% (13/23) for LC in group 2. The results obtained for buffy coat and filter paper were 21.7% (5/23) and 30.4% (7/23) in the group 1, 34.8% (8/23) and 43.5% (10/23) in group 2, respectively. All the seronegative control dogs were negative for the kDNA PCR-hybridization assay in conjunctival swab, filter paper and buffy coat. The highest frequency of positivity was obtained by the association between conjunctival swab samples and DNA extraction by phenol chloroform.

Di Muccio et al. (2008)[53] evaluated the conjunctival swab for the early detection of *Leishmania*-Dog contacts in a group of Italian dogs. The following samples were also examined: peripheral blood for IFAT serology, bone marrow and lymph node aspirates for culture, and bone marrow and peripheral blood buffy coat for molecular analysis. Fifty three sets of samples were obtained from 38 dogs. The conjuntival swab (from left and right conjunctivas) PCR was positive for 50 samples (94.3%) while bone marrow plus peripheral blood PCR was positive for 41 samples (77.4%). The IFAT and cultures (bone marrow and lymph node) were positive for 66% and 38.9% of the samples in that order. The PCR sensitivity obtained from conjunctival swab samples proved to be superior to that of systemic samples and much higher than antibody detection. The study highlights that conjunctival swab positives included some asymptomatic animals, as well as drug-treated infected dogs converted to negative at the bone marrow PCR.

The sensitivity of four molecular methods for conjunctival swab samples was compared by Pilatti et al. (2009)[54] in a group of seropositive symptomatic animals. The following methods were used: kDNA PCR-hybridization, kDNA seminested PCR (kDNA snPCR), internal transcribed spacer 1 nested PCR (ITS-1 nPCR) and *Leishmania* nested PCR (LnPCR). All methods had two steps: a first amplification followed by hybridization or by a new amplification (nested or semi-nested).Two methods (kDNA PCR-Hybridization and kDNA snPCR) used primers targeted to the minicircles of kinetoplast DNA (kDNA) and the other two methods to the coding (LnPCR) and intergenic noncoding regions (ITS-1 nPCR) of ribosomal rRNA genes. For all methods DNA samples of 1.0μl were used. The kDNA PCR–Hybridization was positive for 22/23 dogs (95.6%) and for 40/46 samples (86.9%), considering the right and the left conjunctivas. kDNA snPCR was positive for 21/23 dogs (91.3%) and for 40/46 samples (86.9%). The ITS 1 nPCR and LnPCR were both able to detect the parasites in 17/23 dogs (73.9%)

and respectively 29/46 (63%) and 30/46 (65.2%) samples. The positivities of the kDNA based methods were significantly higher. The authors credited this result to the fact that there are ~10, 000 kDNA minicircles per parasite, while the SSU rRNA and ITS-1 targets have less than 200 copies per cell. In this study the conjunctival swab associated with the most sensitive kDNA PCR based assays showed sensitivities above of 90% for symptomatic dogs.

The first study investigating the efficacy of conjunctival swab PCR for visceral leishmaniasis diagnosis in naturally infected asymptomatic dogs was performed by Leite et al. (2010)[40]. Asymptomatic animals may represent a high percentage of infected dogs in areas of endemicity and they serve as reservoir for vector transmission to susceptible animals and humans. Symptomatic dogs usually produce high levels of specific antibodies which can be easily detected, but the sensitivity of antibody detection is generally lower in early or in asymptomatic canine infections. In this report conjunctival swab sensitivity was compared to two less invasive samples potentially useful for massive screening of dogs: blood and skin biopsies. The study was performed with 30 asymptomatic dogs, all presenting serological and parasitological positive tests. The samples were analyzed by two PCR methods: kDNA PCR-hybridization and ITS-1 nPCR. Using conjunctival swab samples the kDNA PCR-hybridization was able to detected parasite DNA in 24/30 dogs (80%) using the right conjunctiva (RC) and 23/30 dogs (76.6%) with the left conjunctiva (LC). The positivity obtained combining RC and LC results was of 90% (27/30 dogs). A total of 17/30 dogs (56.7%) were positive by means of skin biopsies and 4/30 dogs (13.3%) with Blood. The assay of conjunctval swab samples by ITS-1 nPCR revealed that 25/30 dogs (83.3%) were positive when using RC and 20/30 dogs (66.6%) were positive when using LC. The conjunctival swab positivity obtained by ITS-1 nPCR combining RC and LC was of 83.3%. Via the same method 15/30 dogs (50.0%) were positive by skin biopsies and 17/30 dogs (56.7%) with blood. The kDNA PCR-hybridization and ITS-1 nPCR methods showed similar sensitivities for conjunctival swab and skin biopsy samples. On the other hand, for blood samples, the positivity of ITS-1 nPCR was significantly higher than the one obtained by the kDNA PCR-hybridization, indicating that sensitivity of PCR methods can vary according to the biological sample examined. This study demonstrated the conjunctival swab potential to detect *Leishmania* DNA in asymptomatic dogs and that the sensitivities obtained with asymptomatic animals were similar to the ones observed in previous studies for conjunctival swab PCR in symptomatic dogs [41, 50].

A research conducted by Gramiccia et al. (2010)[55], in a public kennel for stray dogs in Santa Maria Capua Vetere (Campania region, Southern Italy), evaluated the diagnostic performance of conjunctival swab associated to a nested PCR assay for both the early and the late detection of *Leishmania* contacts in dogs exposed to risk of transmission. The nested PCR assay was performed using primers addressed to the small subunit rRNA gene. Two groups of animals were used: (A) a cohort of 65 IFAT and conjunctival swab PCR negative dogs exposed to and followed up during a full sand fly season (July-November 2008), and (B) a cohort of 17 IFAT and conjunctival swab PCR negative dogs but positive at the peripheral blood buffy-coat PCR at July 2008. These animals were examined again in September and November 2008, by buffy coat PCR and in May 2009 along with conjunctival swab PCR. None of group A dogs converted to positive by conjunctival swab PCR or IFAT during the transmission season. In relation to group B dogs, all remained IFAT seronegative till the end of the study, except for one animal. The results of buffy coat PCR showed an intermittent tendency with transient or full conversion to negative involving 4 and 11 dogs respectively, till November 2008. Eight two percent of the dogs (14/17) converted to negative on May 2009 by buffy coat PCR. However, the conjunctival swab PCR was negative for all dogs at November 2008, but 71% of the animals (12/17) converted to positive by this technique on May 2009. The positive control group, in which were included 10 asymptomatic dogs positives at high IFAT titres at the initial screening performed in 2008, when examined again in May 2009 presented 80% of the dogs positives by conjunctival swab PCR and 60% positive by buffy coat PCR. The conjunctival PCR was not found effective for the very early detection of infection, but this investigation demonstrated a slowly conversion of conjunctival PCR to positive in a high rate of dogs even in absence of seroconversion. The buffy coat PCR although could represent an early marker of leishmanial infection tends to be transient and prone to negative conversion. The authors considered the conjunctival swab PCR as a non-invasive alternative to current serological and molecular methods to asses *Leishmania* exposure in dogs.

Leite et al. 2011[56] carried out a comparison between the diagnosis by conjunctival swab PCR and serology in a group of 42 police dogs vaccinated against visceral leishmaniasis. The dogs belonged to the Military Police of the State of Minas Gerais (PMMG), Brazil. All dogs were vaccinated against visceral leishmaniasis with Leishmune® vaccine (Fort Dodge, Brazil) according to the manufacturer's protocol. The serologic assays were performed one year after vaccination independently by three laboratories: Laboratories 1 and 2 were private laboratories and Laboratory 3 was the National Reference Laboratory of Brazil. ELISA and IFAT were the serologic tests used. The laboratory 1 analyzed all 42 dogs and found 15 positive animals and 4 were identified as indeterminate. Laboratory 2 confirmed only 3 reactive dogs and 2 were classified as indeterminate. Laboratory 3 confirmed 7 reactive dogs and found 3 indeterminate animals. The consolidated serologic result was considered positive when ELISA and IFAT were simultaneously reagents or ELISA was non reagent and IFAT showed fluorescence at sera dilution of 1:80. The results were considered indeterminate when ELISA was non reagent and IFAT showed fluorescence at sera dilution of 1:40 or ELISA was reagent and IFAT was non reagent. Although the three laboratories used the same official diagnostic kits to perform the serologic assays, a significant difference in the results were verified among them. For this reason only the seven cases confirmed by Lab 3 (the National Reference Laboratory) were considered for euthanasia. The autopsy of the euthanized animals showed organ and tissue morphologic changes related to visceral leishmaniasis, except for one dog. The molecular diagnosis by PCR using the conjunctival swab procedure was performed in all 42 animals and was able to detect *Leishmania* DNA in 17 dogs. Comparing the PCR results with those obtained by serologic assay of Laboratory 1, PCR was positive for 10 reactive and one indeterminate case, but was negative for 5 reactive and 3 indeterminate cases. Conjunctival swab PCR was also positive for 5 non-reactive dogs, all of them asymptomatic. The reactive cases according to Laboratory 1 that were PCR-negative tested negative in the serologic assays of Laboratories 2 and 3, and may represent false positives. The same occurred with the three indeterminate cases from Laboratory 1 that were PCR negatives. For the Laboratories 2 and 3 the PCR was positive for all reactive and indeterminate cases. The PCR assay also confirmed all cases simultaneously reactive in the serologic tests of two laboratories. The study suggested the use of molecular methods as complementary tools for an accurate diagnosis of canine visceral leishmaniasis and pointed that the conjunctival swab procedure could be especially useful as a confirmatory diagnosis for asymptomatic vaccinated dogs that test positive in the serologic assay, since a fraction of these animals might test positive due the vaccination.

A real-time PCR method based on TaqMan which amplifies a 122 bp fragment of the highly conserved kDNA minicircles of *L. infantum* was developed and standardized by Galleti et al. (2011)[57]. In order to evaluate the method, clinical samples of bone marrow, lymph node aspirates, blood and conjunctival swab were collected from 88 dogs for a total of 177 samples. Additional samples of spleen, kidney, lung and liver were also obtained from dead dogs. Twenty seven samples derived from 15 dogs tested positive in the assay. Three of these positive samples corresponded to conjunctival swabs, for which were found a mean number of parasites for PCR reaction of 29.4, 0.35 and 170. The author's opinion was that the conjunctival swab might be suitable for diagnosis of *Leishmania* infection only in case of high parasitic load, but improvements in the sampling and DNA extraction procedures could enhance the sensitivity obtained.

The diagnostic utility of conjunctival swab to detect *Leishmania* infection in a canine population of highly endemic area of leishmaniasis was investigated by Lombardo et al. (2012)[58]. One hundred sixty-three dogs, randomly recruited in various provinces of Sicily, were enrolled. The real-time PCR based on TaqMan (Applied Biosystems) using primers targeting the constant region of the minicircle Kinetoplast DNA, was the molecular assay used. Samples of blood, lymph node, conjunctival and oral swabs were obtained for the molecular assay. From 138 dogs the conjunctival swabs were collected from one eye (Group A) whereas from an additional 25 animals (Group B) both eyes were sampled. Indirect fluorescent antibody test (IFAT), delayed-type hypersensitivity reaction to leishmanin (DTH) and physical examination were also performed. The positivity found for serology and DTH were 27.0% and 73.8%, in that order. The positive PCR percentages for lymph node, conjunctival swab, oral swab and blood were: 24.5%, 22.1%, 8.7% and 5.5%, respectively. The positivity obtained for conjunctival swab in group B, in which both eyes were sampled, increased for 52.0%. The following median parasite load (parasites/ml) was found for each sample: conjunctival swab 10 (range 1-5000), oral swab 7 (range 2-100), lymph node aspirates 16, 500 (range 2-75, 000) and blood 7 (range 2-14). The similar positive PCR percentages obtained for lymph node aspirates and conjunctival swab, based on at least one conjunctival sample, reinforced the use of this non-invasive alternative for the detection of *Leishmania* infected dogs. The study did not show significant association between antibody titers and percentage of positive conjunctival swab PCR, but seropositive and lymph node PCR positives dogs showed a high likelihood to be positive by conjunctival PCR. No association was also found between clinical status and individual molecular results, in especial between the presence of ocular lesions and positive conjunctival PCR. Interestingly, the study demonstrated the presence of *Leishmania* DNA in oral swabs of dogs without any evidence of oral lesions. Therefore oral swab PCR was not a sensitive diagnostic method, the study emphasized that further studies should investigate the importance of this finding for risk of *Leishmania* transmission by licking or bites.

The work of Ferreira et al. (2012)[25] corroborated the conjunctival swab applicability for canine visceral leishmaniasis diagnosis. In this study the kDNA PCR-hybridization and the quantitative real-time PCR were used, respectively, for diagnosis and assessment of parasite load in clinical samples of 80 naturally infected dogs. The dogs were divided in two groups: without clinical manifestations (1) and presenting clinic signs associated with visceral leishmaniasis (2). All animals had positive ELISA and IFAT and/or parasitological positive test. The negative control group included 10 health dogs that tested negative in the serological and parasitological tests. The kDNA PCR-hybridization positive results rates for the clinical samples in the Group 1 were as follow: right conjunctiva, 77.5% (31/40); left conjunctiva, 75.0% (30/40); skin, 45.0% (18/40); bone marrow, 50.0% (20/40) and blood, 27.5% (11/40). By combining the results of both conjunctivas the positivity was 87.5% (35/40). For the group 2 the PCR-hybridization allowed the following results: right conjunctiva, 95% (38/40); left conjunctiva 87.5% (35/40); bone marrow, 77.5% (31/40) and blood 22.5% (9/40). A positivity of 95.0% (38/40) was obtained considering the positive results of both conjunctivas. For qualitative molecular diagnosis the conjunctival swab samples showed the best results for both dogs groups. The quantitative real-time PCR was performed using primers addressed to a fragment of a single-copy-number *L. infantum* DNA polymerase gene. Canine housekeeping β-actin gene was used as endogenous control. The results were defined as the number of parasites per 104 canine cells. For both groups the parasite burdens determinate by the quantitative real time PCR in conjunctival swab and bone marrow were statistically equivalent, by the other side the parasite load in the skin was higher than the other clinical samples. When compared between groups the parasite load from conjunctival swab in group 2 was higher than in group 1. The same relationship was found for bone marrow. However, no differences were observed in skin load between groups. The high parasite burdens detected in skin from both symptomatic and asymptomatic animals emphasized the role of infected dogs, especially the asymptomatic, as reservoir. The article considered the conjunctival swab sampling procedure suitable form molecular diagnosis of canine visceral leishmaniasis and suggested their widespread use.

An interesting study to evaluate the conjunctical swab diagnostic performance in different stages of infection and also for the follow up of dogs undergoing antileishmanial treatment was conducted by Di Muccio et al. (2012)[59]. To achieve the first objective 253 dogs from areas of endemicity from central Italy were submitted to a cross-sectional survey. For the second aim was performed a longitudinal study using 20 sick dogs under treatment. The molecular assay was a nested PCR using primes addressed to the small-subunit rRNA gene. Among the 253 animals the rates of *Leishmania* infection were 21.73% for conjunctival swab PCR, 21.34% for IFAT, 14.22% for popliteal lymph node cytological examination and 8.69% for buffy coat PCR. Seventy two dogs were positive by at least one test and considered positives for canine visceral leishmaniasis. Among these 72 dogs 76.38% were positive for conjunctival swab PCR, 75.0% for IFAT, 50.0% for lymph node cytological examination and 30.55% for buffy coat PCR. The conjunctival swab PCR showed the best performance and presented a high concordance in relation to IFAT ($\kappa = 0.75$). Test correlation with infection and clinical staging were analyzed in 54 IFAT seropositive dogs. Seven dogs were classified as exposed (low IFAT titer plus negative cytology and negative PCR), 38 as infected (low IFAT titer plus positive cytology and/or positive PCR but without clinical signs) and 9 as sick (high IFAT titer plus positive cytology and with at least one clinical sign). The conjunctival swab PCR showed the best positivity in the infected group (84.2%, 32/38 dogs) followed by lymph node cytological examination (77.8%, 7/9 dogs) and buffy coat PCR (42.1%, 16/38). The positivity of conjunctival swab PCR was also high in the symptomatic group (77.8%, 7/9 dogs), the lymph node cytological examination detected 9/9 dogs (100%) and buffy coat PCR 33.3% (3/9 dogs). In the group exposed, none of the three methods was able to detect infection. Eighteen dogs were negative by IFAT and 16 of these dogs were positive by conjunctival swab PCR and 3 by buffy coat PCR. In the longitudinal study using 20 sick dogs, all of them were positive by IFAT and conjunctival swab PCR (100%) at the beginning of the study, whereas 17 tested positive in the lymph node cytological examination (85%) and 9 in the buffy coat PCR (45%). After three months, the therapy protocols promoted a total remission of clinical signs and decrease of antibody titers with reduction in the positivity rates for conjunctival PCR (30%), lymph node cytological examination (10%) and buffy coat PCR (5%). After six months of treatment was verified an increase in the positivity for conjunctival swab PCR (88.89%) and buffy coat PCR (44.44%) and a less marked increase in lymph node cytological examination positivity (22.22%), without reappearance of clinical signs or increase in serological titers. These results demonstrated that conjunctival swab PCR was sensitive for the early detection of relapses and suitable to monitor the evolution of infection after therapy.

Ferreira et al. (2013) [60] compared conjunctival and nasal swabs with other clinical samples in 62 naturally infected dogs (58 of them symptomatic). *L. donovani* complex specific primers addressed to kDNA minicircle conserved region were used. The following frequencies of positive results were obtained: nasal swab, 87% (54/62); conjunctival swab, 76% (47/62); skin biopsy, 81% (50/62); bone marrow biopsy, 90% (56/62). Positivity obtained using nasal swabs was statistically equivalent to those obtained with the other samples, but in this study the conjunctival swab showed a lower frequency of positivity than that calculated for bone marrow samples, probably due to the PCR protocol used. The parasite load was estimated by qPCR, using primers addressed to the parasite DNA polimerase gene and the canine β-actin gene as a housekeeping gene. The parasite load from conjunctival and nasal samples were equivalent, but lower than verified in bone marrow and skin samples. Oral and ear swabs were also evaluated in a smaller group of 28 animals. Positive results were: oral swab, 79% (22/28) and ear swab, 43% (12/28). The results of this study indicated that conjunctival, nasal and oral swabs were effective in detecting *Leishmania* in naturally infected dogs. The authors suggested that a combination of these samples would be useful in large-scale screening of dogs.

3. Conclusions

In the Mediterranean, Southern Europe and South and Central America, with approximately 500, 000 new human visceral leishmaniasis cases reported annually and millions of dogs infected, being dogs considered to be the major reservoirs for the disease, the accurate diagnosis in these animals is extremely important. Diagnosis of canine visceral leishmaniasis is performed mainly by direct parasitological methods that can yield false-negative results, either because of the very low number of *Leishmania* spp. organisms in clinical samples (bone marrow and lymph nodes) or because morphological identification is difficult. In addition, these methods are invasive. Another problem mentioned is that serology is not sufficient as a criterion for eliminating infected dogs. Conventional serological techniques are limited by cross-reactivity with other parasitic diseases, because several technical procedures have not been standardised and due the low sensitivity of the available serological methods in the initial stages of infections.

In dogs PCR-based assay is currently the more sensitive and specific technique for detection of *Leishmania* and it allows using different clinical samples. The conjunctival swab is a non-invasive sample recently reported and up to moment few studies have been performed using this approach. Nevertheless, its high sensitivity and applicability for molecular diagnosis of canine visceral leishmaniasis have been confirmed, independently, by different research groups.

The studies demonstrated that the method allows the identification of infected dogs before the seroconversion and that conjunctival swab sensitivity for molecular diagnosis was superior or equivalent to obtained by invasive samples of either symptomatic or asymptomatic animals. The conjunctival swab was also proved useful to monitor the dogs during drug therapy. The molecular diagnosis using non-invasive samples such conjunctival swab is of great relevance in epidemiological studies when large numbers of dogs are sampled and also for clinical or experimental purposes, that implies repeated samplings. The standardization of this sampling procedure can help to become viable and widespread the molecular diagnosis of canine visceral leishmaniasis. The DNA extraction protocol and the sensitivity of PCR assay used are important variables to be considered in order to obtain the best results. Field studies in wide heterogeneous populations including seronegative and seropositive animals and works that follow up PCR positive seronegative dogs are still lacking and are very important for the method validation.

Molecular tests are yet comparatively expensive in relation to other diagnostic techniques available and require technological expertise, but considering the data presented above, a sensitive, specific and practical test could provide very cost-effective alternatives to currently available diagnostic tests, especially when used in mass-screening surveys.

Author details

Antero Silva Ribeiro de Andrade[1*] and Maria Norma Melo[2]

*Address all correspondence to: antero@cdtn.br

1 National Nuclear Energy Commission, Centre for the Development of Nuclear Technology, Laboratory of Radiobiology, Belo Horizonte, Brazil

2 Federal University of Minas Gerais, Institute of Biological Sciences, Department of Parasitology, Belo Horizonte, Brazil

References

[1] Bates PA. Transmission of *Leishmania* metacycles promastigotes by phlebotomine sand flies. International Journal for Parasitology 2007;37(10) 1097-1106.

[2] WHO, 2012. World Health Organization. Leishmaniasis: Geneva: Special Programme for Research and Training in Tropical Diseases (TDR) 2012; http://www.who.int/tdr/diseases-topics/leishmaniasis/en/index.html/ (accessed 18 September, 2012).

[3] Alvar J, Velez ID, Bern c, Herrero M, Desjeux P. Cano, J, Jannin J, den Boer M, Team WLC. Leishmaniasis Worldwide and Global Estimates of its incidence. Plos One 2012;7(5) e35671.

[4] Control of the Leishmaniasis: report of a meeting of the WHO Expert Committee on the control of Leishmaniasis, Geneva, World Health Organization. 2010.

[5] Bern C, Maguire JH, Alvar J. Complexities of assessing the disease burden attributable to leishmaniasis. Plos Neglected Tropical Disease 2008;2(10):e313.

[6] Reithinger R, Dujardin JC. Molecular Diagnosis of Leishmaniasis: Current Status and Future Applications. Journal Clinical Microbiology 2007;45(1) 21–25.

[7] Lainson R, Shaw JJ, Evolution, classification and geographical distribution. In W Peters, R Killick-Kendrick (eds) The Leishmaniases in Biology and Medicine, Vol. 1, Academic Press, London, 1987. p1-120.

[8] Murray HW, Berman JD, Davies CR, Saravia NG. Advances in leishmaniasis. Lancet 2005; 366(9496)1561-1577.

[9] Vidya NRD, Krishna P, Neena VCSL, Sanjeev B, Roshan KT, Singh D, Niyamat AS, Rakesh B V, Pradeep D. Development of Post–Kala-Azar Dermal Leishmaniasis (PKDL) in Miltefosine-treated visceral leishmaniasis. American Journal Tropical Medicine and Hygiene 2009; 80(3) 336-338.

[10] Gontijo CMF, Melo MN. Visceral Leishmaniasis in Brazil: current status, challenges and prospects. Revista Brasileira de Epidemiologia 2004; 7(3) 338-349.

[11] Costa CH, Stewart JM, Gomes RB, Garcez LM, Ramos PK, Bozza M. Satoskar A, Dissanayake S, Santos RS, Silva MR, Shaw JJ, David JR, Maguire JH. Asymptomatic human carriers of *Leishmania chagasi.* American Journal of Tropical Medicine and Hygiene 2002;66(4) 334-337.

[12] Shaw JJ.The leishmaniasis-survival and expansion in a changing world. A mini-review. Memórias do Instituto Oswaldo Cruz 2007;102(5) 541-547.

[13] *Romero* GAS, Boelaert M. Control of Visceral *Leishmaniasis* in Latin America. A Systematic Review. PLoS Neglected Tropical Disease 2010 4(1) e584.

[14] Gomes AH, Ferreira IM, Lima ML, Cunha EA, Garcia AS, Araújo MF, Pereira-Chioccola VL. PCR identification of *Leishmania* in diagnosis and control of canine Leishmaniasis. Veterinary of Parasitology 2007;144(3-4) 234-241.

[15] Werneck GL, Costa CH, Walker AM, David JR, Wand M, Maguire JH. The urban spread of visceral leishmaniasis: clues from spatial analysis. Epidemiology 2002;13(3)364-367.

[16] Baneth G, Koutinas AF, Solano-Gallego L, Bourdeau P, Ferrer L. Canine leishmaniosis - new concepts and insights on an expanding zoonosis: part one. Trends Parasitology 2008;24(7) 324-330.

[17] Solano-Gallego L, Morell P, Arboix M, Alberola J, Ferrer L. Prevalence of *Leishmania infantum* Infection in Dogs Living in an Area of Canine Leishmaniasis Endemicity Using PCR on Several Tissues and Serology. Journal of Clinical Microbiology 2001;39(2) 560-563.

[18] *Berrahal F*, Mary C, Roze M, Berenger A, Escoffier K, Lamouroux D, Dunan S. Canine leishmaniasis identification of asymptomatic carries by polymerase chain reaction and immunobloting. American Journal Tropical Medicine and Hygiene 1996 55(3) 273-277.

[19] Palatnik- de-Souza Cb, dos Santos WR, França-Silva JC, da Costa RT, Reis AB, Palatinik M, Mayrink W, Genero O. Impact of canine control on the epidemiology of canine and human visceral leishmaniasis in Brazil. American Journal Tropical Medicine and Hygiene 2001;65 (5) 510-517.

[20] Quinnell RJ, Courtenay O, Garcez LM, Kaye PM, Shaw MA, Dye C, Day MJ. IgG subclass responses in a longitudinal study of canine visceral leishmaniasis. Veterinary Immunology and Immunopathology. 2003;91(3-4)161-168.

[21] Oliva G, Scalone A, Manzillo VF, Grammicia M, Pagano A, Di Muccio T, Grandoni L. Incidence and time course of *Leishmania infantum* infections examined by parasitological, serologic, and nested-PCR techniques in a cohort of naïve exposed to three consecutive transmission seasons. Journal of Clinical Microbiology 2006;44(4) 1318–1322.

[22] Dujardin JC, Campino L, Cañavate C, Dedet JP, Gradoni L, Soteriadou K, Mazeris A, Ozbel, Y Boelaert.M. Spread of vector-borne diseases and neglect of Leishmaniasis, Europe. Emerging infectious diseases, 2008;14 (7) 1013-1018.

[23] Moreno J, Alvar L, Moreno J, Alvar J. Canine leishmaniasis: epidemiological risk and the experimental model.Trends in Parasitology 2002;18(9) 399-405.

[24] Costa CHN. How effective is dogs culling in controlling zoonotic visceral leishmaniasis? A critical evaluation of the science, politics and ethics behind this public health policy. Revista da Sociedade Brasileira de Medicina Tropical 2011:44 (2) 0232-242.

[25] Ferreira AS, Leite Rl, Ituassu LT, Almeida GG, Suza D M, Fujiwara T R, Andrade ASR, Melo MN. Canine skin and conjunctival swab samples for the detection and

quantification of *Leishmania infantum* DNA in an endemic urban area in Brazil. Plos Neglected Tropical Disease 2012;6(4) e1596.

[26] Tavares CA, Fernandes AP, Melo MN. Molecular Diagnosis of leishmaniasis Expert Review of Molecular Diagnostics 2003;3(5) 657-667.

[27] Dye C, Vidor E, Dereure J. Serological diagnosis of leishmaniasis: on detecting infection as well as disease. Journal Epidemiology and Infection 1993;110(3) 647-56.

[28] Rosário, EY, Genaro O, França-Silva JC, Da Costa RT. Evaluation of enzyme-linked immunosorbent assay using crude *Leishmania* and recombinant antigens as a diagnostic marker for canine visceral leishmaniasis. Memórias do Instituto Oswaldo Cruz 2005;100(2) 197–203.

[29] Braga MD, Coelho IC, Pompeu MM, Evans TG, MacAullife IT, Teixeira MJ, Lima JW. Control of canine visceral leishmaniasis comparison of results from a rapid elimination program of serum-reactive dogs using an immunoenzyme assay and slower elimination of serum-reactive dogs using filter paper eluation indirect immunofluorescence. Revista da Sociedade Brasileira Medicina Tropical 1998;31(5) 419-424.

[30] Kar K. Serodiagnosis of *Leishmania*. Critical Reviews in Microbiology 1995;21(2) 123-152.

[31] Grimaldi GJ, Teva A, Ferreira AL, dos Santos CB, Pinto IS, de-Azevedo CT, Falqueto A. Evaluation of a novel chromatographic immunoasssay based on canine visceral leishmaniasis. Transactions of the Royal Society Tropical Medicine Hygiene 2012;106(1) 54-59.

[32] Otranto D, Paradies P, Sasanelli M, Spinelli R, Brandonisio O. Rapid immunochromatographic test for serodiagnosis of canine leishmaniasis. Journal Clinical Microbiology 2004;42(6) 2769–2770

[33] Genaro O, Costa RT, França-Silva JC. Reis AB, Vieira EP, Arias JR. Evaluation of an immunocromatographic assay for the diagnosios of dogs experimentally and naturally infected with *Leishmania chagasi* in Brazil. Acta Parasitolologica Turcica 1997;21(1): 93.

[34] Ministério da Saúde. Nota técnica conjunta nº 01/2001 – CGDT/DEVIT/SUS/MS. Esclarecimento sobre a substituição do protocolo diagnóstico da leishmaniose visceral canina (LVC). Brasil: Brasília-DF; 2011.

[35] Degrave W, Fernandes O, Campbell D, Bozza M, Lopes U. Use of molecular probes and PCR for detection and typing of *Leishmania* – a mini-review. Memórias do Instituto Oswaldo Cruz 1994;89(3) 463-469.

[36] Schulz A, Mellenthin K, Schonian G, Fleischer B, Drosten C. Detection, differentiation and quantitation of pathogenic *Leishmania* organisms by fluorescence resonance energy transfer-based real-time PCR assay. Journal of Clinical Microbiology 2003;41(4) 1529–1535.

[37] Mary C, Faraut F, Lascombe L, Dumon H. Quantification of *Leishmania infantum* DNA by a real-time PCR assay with high sensitivity. Journal of Clinical Microbiology 2004;42(11) 5249–5255.

[38] Van der Meide W, Schoone GJ, Faber WR, Zeegelaar JE, de Vries HJ, Ozbel Y, Lai A, Fat RF, Coelho LI, Kassi M, Schallig HD. Quantitative nucleic acid sequence-based assay as a new molecular tool for detection and quantification of *Leishmania* parasites in skin biopsy samples. Journal of Clinical Microbiology 2005;43(11) 5560–5566.

[39] Francino O, Altet L, Sanchez-Robert E, Rodriguez A, Solano-Gallego L, Alberola J, Ferrer L, Sanchez A, Roura X. Advantages of realtime PCR assay for diagnosis and monitoring of canine leishmaniosis. Veterinary Parasitology 2006;137(3-4) 214–221.

[40] Leite R., Ferreira SA, Ituassu LT, Melo MN, de Andrade ASR. PCR Diagnosis of Visceral Leishmaniasis in Asymptomatic Dogs Using Conjunctival Swab Samples. Veterinary Parasitology 2010;170(3-4) 201-206.

[41] Ferreira SA, Ituassu LT, Melo MN, de Andrade ASR. Evaluation of the Conjunctival Swab for Canine Visceral Leishmaniasis Diagnosis by PCR-hibridization in Minas Gerais State, Brazil. Veterinary Parasitology 2008;152(3-4) 257-263.

[42] Maia C, Ramada J, Cristóvão JM, Gonçalves L., Campino L. Diagnosis of canine leishmaniasis: Conventional and molecular techniques using different tissues. The Veterinary Journal 2009:179( )142–144.

[43] Maia, C, Campino, L. Methods for diagnosis of canine leishmaniasis and immune response to infection.The Veterinary Parasitology 2008;158(4) 274-287.

[44] Xavier SC, Andrade HM. Monte SJH. Chiarelli IM, Lima WG, Michalick MSM. Tafuri WL. Comparison of paraffin-embedded skin biopsies from different anatomical regions as sampling methods for detection of *Leishmania* infection in dogs using histological, immunohistochemical and PCR methods. BMC, Veterinary Research 2006;8(2) 17.

[45] Fisa R, Riera C, Gállego M, Manubens J, Portús M, Nested PCR for diagnosis of canine leishmaniosis in peripheral blood, lymph node and bone marrow aspirates. Veterinary Parasitology 2001;99(2) 105-111.

[46] Almeida ABPF, Souza VRF, Gasparetto ND, da Silva GFR, Figueiredo FB, Dutra V, Nakazato L, Madeira MF. Canine visceral leishmaniasis: diagnostic approaches based on polymerase chain reaction employing different biological samples. Diagnostic Microbiology and Infectious Disease 2013;77(3) 321-324

[47] Manna L, Vitale F, Reale S, Caracappa S, Pavone LM, Morte RD, Cringoli G, Staiano N, Gravino AE. Comparison of different tissue sampling for PCR-based diagnosis and follow-up of canine visceral leishmaniosis. Veterinary Parasitology 2004;125(3-4) 251-262.

[48] Lachaud L, Marchergui-Hammami S, Chabbert E, Dereure J, Dedet JP, Bastien P. Comparison of six PCR methods using peripheral blood for detection of canine visceral leishmaniasis. Journal of Clinical Microbiology 2002 ;40(1) 210–215.

[49] Mohammadiha A, Mohebali M, Haghighi A, Mahdian R, Abadi AR, Zarei Z, Yeganeh F, Kazemi B, Taghipour N, Akhoundi B. Comparison of real-time PCR and conventional PCR with two DNA targets for detection *of Leishmania (Leishmania) infantum* infection in human and dog blood samples. Experimental Parasitology 2013;133 (1) 89–94.

[50] Strauss-Ayali D, Jaffe CL, Burshtain O, Gonen L, Baneth G. Polymerase Chain Reaction Using Noninvasively Obtained Samples, for the Detection of *Leishmania infantum* DNA in Dogs. The Journal of Infectious Diseases 2004;189(9) 1729-1733.

[51] Berrahal F, Mary C, Roze M, Berenger A, Escoffier K, Lamouroux D, Dunan S. Canine Leishmaniasis: Identification of Asymptomatic Carriers by Polymerase Chain Reaction and Immunoblotting. American Journal of Tropical Medicine and Hygiene 1966;55(3) 273-277.

[52] Reithiger R, Lambson BE, Barker DC, Counihan H, Espinoza JC, González JS, Davies CR. *Leishmania (Viannia) spp*. Dissemination and Tissue Tropism in Naturally Infected Dogs *(Canis familiaris)*. Transaction of the Royal Society of Tropical Medicine and Hygiene 2002;96(1) 76-78.

[53] Di Muccio T, Fiorentino E, Manzillo F, Cappiello S, Oliva G, Gradoni L, Gramiccia M. The Potential Role of Conjunctival Swab Analysis for the Early Detection of *Leishmania*-Dog Contacts: a Preliminary Study. Parassitologia 2008;50 (suppl.) 1-2.

[54] Pilatti MM, Ferreira SA, Melo MN, de Andrade ASR. Comparison of PCR Methods for Diagnosis of Canine Visceral Leishmaniais in Conjunctival Swab Samples. Research in Veterinary Sciences 2009;87(2) 255-257.

[55] Gramiccia M, Di Muccio T, Fiorentino E, Scalone A. Bongiorno G, Cappiello S, Paparcone R., Manzillo VF, Maroli M, Gradoni L, Oliva G. Longitudinal Study on the Detection of Canine *Leishmania* Infections by Conjunctival Swab Analysis and Correlation with Entomological Parameters. Veterinary Parasitology 2010;171(3-4) 223-228.

[56] Leite RS, Mendes VC, Ferreira A.C, de Andrade ASR. The Use of Conjunctival Swab Samples for PCR Screening for Visceral Leishmaniasis in Vaccinated Dogs. Revista Brasileira de Parasitologia Veterinária 2011;20(1) 36-41.

[57] Galletti E, Bonilauri P, Bardasi L, Fontana MC, Ramini M, Renzi M, Dosa G, Merialdi G. Development of a Minor Groove Binding Probe Based Real-Time PCR for the Diagnosis and Quantification of *Leishmania infantum* in Dog Specimens. Research in Veterinary Sciences 2011;91(2) 243-245.

[58] Lombardo G, Pennisi MG, Lupo T, Migliazzo A, Capri A, Solano-Gallego L. Detection of *Leishmania infantum* DNA by Real-Time PCR in Canine Oral and Conjunctival

Swabs and Comparison with Other Diagnostic Techniques. Veterinary Parasitology 2012;184(1) 10-17.

[59] Di Muccio T, Veronesi F, Antognoni MT, Onofri A, Fioretti DP, Gramiccia M. Diagnostic Value of Conjunctival Swab Associated with Nested PCR for Different Categories of Dogs Naturally Exposes to *Leishmania infantum* Infection. Journal of Clinical Microbiology 2012;50(8) 2651-2659.

[60] Ferreira SA, Almeida GG, Silva SO, Vogas GP, Fujiwara RT, Andrade ASR, Melo MN. Nasal, oral and ear swabs for canine visceral leishmaniasis diagnosis: new practical approaches for detection of *Leishmania infantum* DNA. Plos Neglected Tropical Disease 2013;7(4) e2150.

Chapter 10

Sporotrichoid Cutaneous Leishmaniasis in Central Tunisia: Epidemiological and Clinical Aspects

Moncef Ben Saïd, Fatma Saghrouni,
Yusr Saadi-Ben Aoun, Najet Ghariani, Alia Yaacoub,
Henda Ach, Mohamed Denguezli,
Ikram Guizani and Akila Fathallah-Mili

Additional information is available at the end of the chapter

http://dx.doi.org/10.5772/57413

1. Introduction

Three forms of cutaneous leishmaniasis (CL) are known to occur in Tunisia: the sporadic CL (SCL), the chronic CL (CCL) and the zoonotic CL (ZCL) caused by *Leishmania infantum, L. killicki* and *L. major* respectively [1, 2]. The ZCL is by far the most frequent and the most widely distributed form. It is endemo-epidemic in extended areas of central and southern Tunisia where it constitutes a major public health problem. Rodents of Genus *Psammomys* and *Meriones* are the well-established reservoirs of the disease [1, 2]. One of the characteristics of ZCL is its seasonal occurrence as most cases are diagnosed between October and January [1]. All ages are affected with a median of 20-28 years. Clinically, ZCL usually presents as single or most often multiple ulcerated lesions that involve the face and limbs, and scar in a few months (4 to 8) [3]. However, some patients with ZCL develop sporotrichoid nodules (SN) in the vicinity of the primary lesions [4, 5, 6]. The sporotrichoid condition is characterized by the development of nodules that progress, starting from the primary lesion, along the dermal and subcutaneous lymphatics.

The aim of the present study was to evaluate the frequency of SN in patients from Central Tunisia and to assess the epidemiological and clinical features and the outcome of the disease in the affected patients.

2. Materials and methods

Our study is a retrospective one that includes all CL diagnosed in the laboratory of Parasitology of the Farhat Hached teaching hospital, Sousse, Tunisia, between 1st January 2000 and 31th December 2012. Most of the patients were addressed to the laboratory for suspected CL by the department of Dermatology of the same hospital. Patients' data including age, sex, geographical origin, place of contamination, clinical presentation, treatment and outcome were collected.

The diagnosis of CL was achieved by the demonstration of amastigotes in Giemsa-stained cutaneous smears. Patients with lesions very evocative of CL but found negative on direct examination were further submitted to PCR, known to be more sensitive. Culture on NNN or coagulated rabbit serum (CRS) medium was mainly carried out for the purpose of typing strains either by isoenzymes' electrophoresis or molecular techniques.

3. Results

1. Cutaneous leishmaniasis cases

Over the 13 year study period, 2128 cases of CL were diagnosed in the laboratory, the majority of them by the demonstration of *Leishmania* amastigotes in dermal smears. Ninety five per cent of the affected patients originate from one of the following Central Tunisia Governorates (Districts), known to be endemic or highly endemic for ZCL [1, 2]: Sidi Bouzid, Kairouan, Mahdia and Sousse. The 5% remaining patients originate from Northern or Southern areas or from neighboring countries (Lybia, Algeria). Out of the 2128 cases, 2059 were confirmed (by typing strains) or very likely ZCL cases (according to the geographical origin or place of contamination, seasonal occurrence, large amastigotes on stained smears, outcome, additional cases in families and neighbors). The 96 remaining cases were mostly *L. infantum* SCL, and few *L. killicki* CCL. The age of patients ranged from 1 month to 91 years (median 26.8 years). One thousand two hundred thirty four (1234) patients were females and 894 males (sex ratio F/M: 1.38).

Most of the patients presented with single or more often multiple ulcerated lesions located on the limbs, the face and to a lesser extent on the trunk. According to patients' declarations, the lesions appeared 10 days to > one year prior to first examination.

Patients with a few lesions (< 5) were treated with intralesional meglumine antimoniate (Glucantime®) and/or cryotherapy. Those with more lesions were treated with intramuscular Glucantime® for 14 to 20 days.

In most treated patients, scarring was obtained in 2 to 8 weeks. In a few of them, however, lesions persisted for a longer period and additional cures were delivered.

2. Cases with sporotrichoid nodules:

http://dx.doi.org/10.5772/57413

Out of the 2059 patients with ZCL, 34 (1.7%) developed SN. Fifteen of them were from Mahdia Governorate, 9 from Kairouan Governorate, 6 from Sousse Governorate and 4 from Sidi Bouzid Governorate. It is worth mentioning that Sidi Bouzid region, known to include the most active foci of ZCL in Central Tunisia, was less represented then the 3 remaining Governorates. Inside Governorates, the contamination of all 34 patients took place in areas known to be highly endemic for ZCL.

According to gender, females were more represented then males (23 *vs.* 11) and F/M sex ratio was higher as compared to common ZCL cases (2.1 *vs.* 1.4).

The age of patients with sporotrichoid form ranged from 2.5 years to 81 years. Median (47.8 years) was higher as compared to cases without SN (26.8 years).

In 28 (82.4%) patients, the nodules appeared spontaneously a few days to 3 weeks after the onset of the primary lesions. In 5 (4.7%) patients, the SN developed after intralesional antimonial treatment and in one patient after a 3 day cure of intramuscular Glucantime®.

In the 34 patients, primary ulcers appeared 2 weeks to 5 months prior to the date of diagnosis (median 2.2 months). Their number ranged from 1 to 12 (median: 3.5). They measured 0.5 cm to 6 cm; ninety per cent were between 0.5 cm and 3 cm. They were mainly located on upper limbs: 27.4% on forearms, 26.2% on hands and fingers, 11.9% on arms, 9.5% on wrists and 4.8% on elbows. Lower limbs and other sites (nose, neck, eyelids, cheeks, back) were much less involved. Both sides of the body were equally represented.

The number of SN per patient ranged from 2 to > 10. Most of patients (76.5%) had 2 to 4 nodules; 5 had > 10 nodules.

The size of nodules ranged between 0.5 cm to 3 cm; the majority of them (90.7%) measured 0.5% cm to 1 cm.

Nodules mainly developed on forearms (59.5%) and arms (23.8%). Lower limbs and other sites were much less affected. The left side of the body was slightly more represented than the right one (56.1% *vs.* 43.9%).

In 3 out of the 34 patients, biopsy of nodules was performed. In none of them amastigotes could be demonstrated.

Leishmania strains isolated from 10 out the 34 patients were typed either by enzymes' electrophoresis or by PCR according to Tordini et al. [7]. Nine strains were found to be *L. major* and one *L. killicki*.

Whenever SN were observed in patients initially treated with intralesional infiltrations of antimonials, the treatment was switched to the intramuscular form. Thirty three patients responded well to treatment and SN together with primary lesions scared in 2 to 8 weeks. In the last patient, the primary lesions and the nodules persisted up to 13 months. This patient was suffering of scleroderma and submitted to a long-term corticotherapy. In addition, she developed symptoms of antimonial toxicity while receiving intramuscular Glucantime®.

4. Discussion

The sporotrichoid form (SF) of cutaneous leishmaniasis is defined by the development of palpable (and often visible) painless subcutaneous nodules distributed in a linear fashion along the lymphatics and extending proximally from a cutaneous lesion. In the Old World, sporotrichoid leishmaniasis has mainly been associated with *L. major* ZCL [8, 9, 10, 11]. Its incidence ranges from 6% in Iran [12], to 10% in Saudi Arabia [10] and 11 to 22 % in Sudan [8, 9], whereas it seems to be less frequent in other *L. major* endemic areas like Turkey and Pakistan [13, 14].

In Tunisia, where ZCL is highly endemic, a previous study conducted by Masmoudi et al. [15] showed the SF to be common among patients originating from ZCL endemic areas in Sfax, Sidi Bouzid and Kasserine Governorates, with an incidence of 18%. In our study, which covered a much longer period and a higher number of patients, the incidence was much lower (1.7%). These contrasting results are difficult to explain. One of the factors could be a difference in the pathogenicity of infecting *Leishmania* strains according to the transmission areas. In a study conducted by Gaafar et al. [9] in Sudan and Saudi Arabia, it was shown that the incidence of the SF could be related to the causative *L. major* zymodeme. Yet, all characterized Tunisian *L. major* strains whatever obtained from patients, animal reservoirs or sand flies were found to belong to the single MON 25 zymodeme [2, 16, 17]. Nevertheless, we may consider that this zymodeme includes strains with a variable virulence, unevenly distributed over the transmission foci. An additional explanation may be the degree of immunization of infected populations, those living in emergent foci (like Sfax and Kasserine) being more susceptible to dissemination than those living in more ancient foci. In our series, nearly the 2/3 of patients with the SF came from Mahdia and Sousse Governorates where the ZCL epidemics occurred much later as compared to Kairouan Governorate (where the outbreak first arose) and Sidi Bouzid Governorate, now considered to include the more active foci in the region [1, 2].

The typing of strains obtained from 10 out of our 34 patients showed that most of them (9 strains) were, as expected, *L. major*. Interestingly the last one was *L. killicki*. This finding is not too surprising as the patient came from Ain Jloula, a recent emerging focus of *L. killicki* [2, 16]; and means that *L. killicki* may be a causal agent of SF.

Histopathologic studies show the subcutaneous nodules to consist of a granulomatous reaction with lymphocytes, plasma cells, macrophages and giant cells [9, 15, 18, 19]. They are supposed to represent an immunological reaction against the lymphatic spread of the parasite or its antigens [10, 11]. The factors that trigger lymphatic dissemination are unclear but some data suggest that the host immune status could influence this dissemination [10, 11]. Indeed, Sadeghian et al. [20] showed that the leishmanin skin test (LST) was negative in 72% of SF cases and that none was strongly positive in LST positive patients. They concluded that the SF of CL is at least partially due to a decrease in cellular immunity. However, the role of immunity should be considered with caution because if the immune response is actually involved, it cannot be the sole or the determinant factor as in this situation the age of patients with SF is expected to be lower than that of those with the common ZCL form, the children being much more affected. Yet, this is not the case in our study neither in that of Masmoudi et al. [15]. where the median age of patients with SF was higher as compared to patients with the common form (47.8 years and 26.8 years respectively).

In our study, females were more represented then males (F/M sex ratio = 2.1). A similar finding (F/M sex ratio = 1.7) was reported by Masmoudi et al. [15]; whereas in other previous studies, no significant association of subcutaneous nodules with sex was reported [9].

The time to appearance of nodules is variable. It ranges from a few days to a few weeks or months; nodules may even appear after complete healing of the primary cutaneous lesions [8], with a delay reaching 1 or 2 years in some reported cases [15, 21]. In most of our patients, the nodules appeared in less than one month after the onset of the primary lesions.

Among the factors that trigger the lymphatic dissemination of parasites away from the primary lesions, many reports suggest the intralesional antimonial treatment to play a role [9, 10, 11, 22]. The reason for that is unclear. Nevertheless, this factor appears not to be determinant as only 6 out of our 34 patients (17.6%) had received intralesional Glucantime®; in the remaining 28 patients the nodules appeared spontaneously. The same finding was reported in Masmoudi et al. study [15] where 74% of patients did not receive any Glucantime® infiltrations before the development of nodules.

The number of sporotrichroïd nodules is reported to be variable, but they often are multiple [10, 11, 19, 21]. In our patients the number ranged from 2 to > 10; most of patients had 2 to 4 nodules as shown in figure 1. In the series of Masmoudi et al. [15], this number reached 20 nodules in one patient, with a mean of 7 nodules.

When mentioned, the size of nodules is usually 1 to 2 cm [11, 15, 19]. In our patients, most nodules sized between 0.5 to 1 cm, the largest being 3 cm.

In our 34 patients, nodules mainly developed on forearms and arms; the lower limbs and other sites of the body were much less represented. This finding was expected as the distribution of nodules overall reflects that of primary lesions which mainly involved the upper limbs. This result is very similar to that of Masmoudi et al. [15] where nodules were located on upper limbs in 80% of cases, together with the primary ulcers. Nevertheless, other sites can be affected; indeed, in some of our patients, SN developed on the legs, the cheeks, the eyelids, the nose and the back.

The diagnosis of CL in all of our 34 patients was confirmed by the demonstration of amastigotes in ulcerated primary lesions, while SF was diagnosed on the basis of clinical criteria. In the 3 patients where the biopsy of nodules was performed, no parasites could be shown. According to previous reports, amastigotes may or may not be demonstrable on smears or impressed biopsies nodules [8, 10, 15, 19, 23]. The diagnosis of the SF is usually suspected when nodules develop in the vicinity of a previously confirmed primary CL lesion, and resolve under antimonial treatment. As stated above, the amastigotes may or may not be demonstrated in SN. Similar conditions mainly include sporotrichosis that, to our knowledge, has never been reported in Tunisia. Cutaneous tuberculosis and atypical mycobacteriosis can also be considered but both conditions are unresponsive to antimonials.

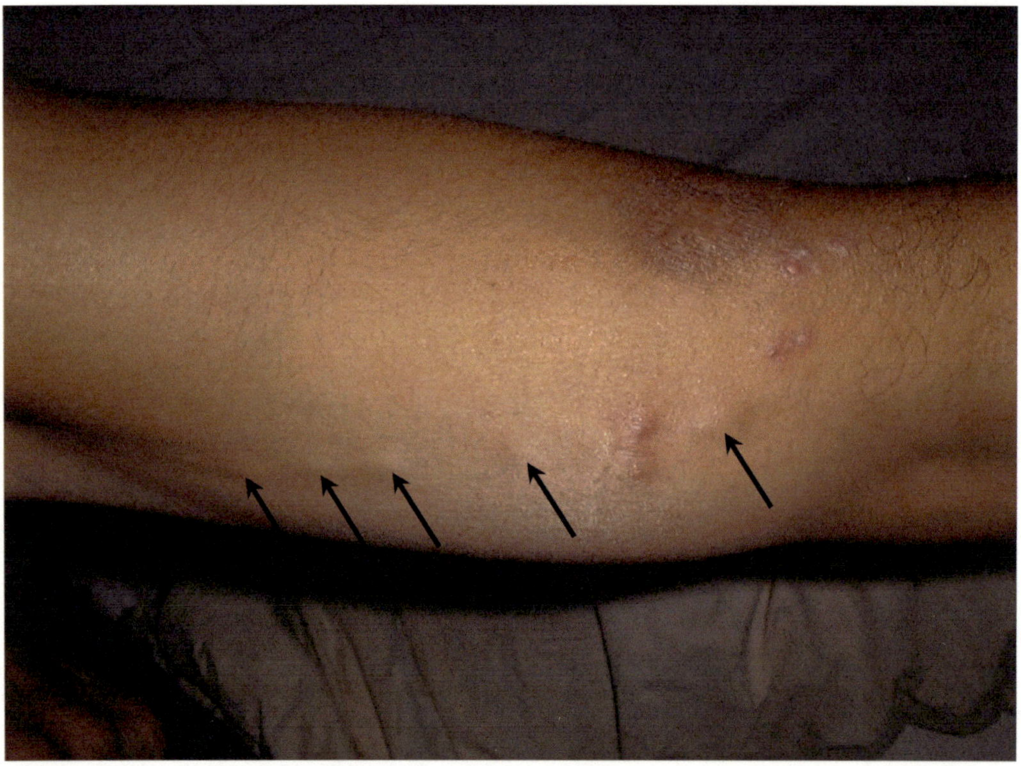

Figure 1. Sporotrichoid nodules (arrows) on the forearm of a patient.

While in localized CL local treatment such as intralesional infiltrations of pentavalent antimonials and /or cryotherapy may be helpful and sufficient, such treatment is of no value in disseminated disease where systemic antimonials must be started [23, 24]. In most reported patients with SF, systemic treatment was successful and outcome favorable [5, 14, 15], even though some patients were reported to be unresponsive to antimonials [11, 19, 22]. Thirty three (97%) of our patients responded well to systemic Glucantime® and SN together with primary lesions scared in 2 to 8 weeks. In the last patient, both primary ulcers and SN persisted up to 13 months. It is worth mentioning that this patient was receiving a long term corticotherapy and developed symptoms of antimonials toxicity which led to the interruption of the Glucantime® cure.

5. Conclusion

The SF of CL appears to be a rather rare event in Central Tunisian SCL foci. In patients affected, outcome is similar to uncomplicated cases.

http://dx.doi.org/10.5772/57413

Author details

Moncef Ben Saïd[1*], Fatma Saghrouni[1], Yusr Saadi-Ben Aoun[2], Najet Ghariani[3], Alia Yaacoub[1], Henda Ach[1], Mohamed Denguezli[3], Ikram Guizani[2] and Akila Fathallah-Mili[1]

*Address all correspondence to: moncef.bensaid@rns.tn

1 Laboratory of Parasitology, Farhat Hached Hospital, Sousse, Tunisia

2 Laboratory of Parasitic Epidemiology and Ecology (LEEP)-LR00SP04, Institut Pasteur, Tunisia

3 Service of Dermatology, Farhat Hached Hospital, Sousse, Tunisia

References

[1] Ben Rachid, M.S., Ben Ismail, R. & Ben Said, M. The ecology of visceral and cutaneous leishmaniasis in Tunisia. In. "Proceedings of the international workshop on leishmaniasis control strategies", 25-29 nov. 1991, Merida, Mexico, IDRC and UPCH eds. (1992), pp. 131-154.

[2] Fathallah, A., Saghrouni, F. Ben Saïd, Z., Saadi-Ben Aoun, Y., Guizani, I. & Ben Saïd, M. Retrospective analysis of leishmaniasis in Central Tunisia : An update on emerging epidemiological trends. In: Current Topics in Tropical Medicine, 2012, Dr. Alfonso Rodriguez Morales (Ed.), ISBN: 978-953-51-0274-8, In Tech, chp.15, pp: 228-252.

[3] Chaffai, M, Ben Rachid, M.S., Ben Ismail, R., Ben Osman, A. & Makni, N. Clinico-epidemiological forms of cutaneous leishmaniasis in Tunisia. Ann Dermatol venereol. (1988), 115: 1255-1260.

[4] Bryceson, A. D. M. Tropical dermatology: Cutaneous leishmaniasis. Br J Dermatol. (1976), 94: 223-226.

[5] Lopez-Escobar, M., Drake-Monfort, M., Salesa-Gutierrez de Rosas, R. & Hermana-Ramirez, S. Sporotrichoid cutaneous leishmaniasis. Actas Dermo Sifiliogr. (2007), 98: 441-445.

[6] Spier, S., Medenica, M., McMillan, S. & Virtue, C. Sporotrichoid leishmaniasis. Arch Dermatol. (1977), 113: 1104-1105.

[7] Tordini, G., Giaccherini, R., Pacenti, L., Miracco, C., Zazzi, M., & Zanelli, G. Cutaneous leishmaniasis: usefulness of PCR on paraffin-embedded skin biopsies as part of routine investigation. Ann Trop Med Parasitol. (2007), 101: 745-749.

[8] El-Safi, S.H., Peters, W., El –Toam,B., El-kadarow, A. & Evans, D. A. Studies on the leishmaniases in the Sudan. 2. Clinical and parasitological studies on cutaneous leishmaniasis. Trans R Soc Trop Med Hyg. (1991), 85: 457-464.

[9] Gaafar, A., Fadl, A., El Kadaro, A.Y., El Hassan, M.M., Kemp, M., Ismail, A.I.A., Morgos, S.A. & El Hassen A.M. Sporotrichoid cutaneous leishmaniasis due to *Leishmania major* of different zymodemes in the Sudan and Saudi Arabia: a comparative study. Trans R Soc Trop Med Hyg. (1994), 88: 552-554.

[10] Kubba, R., El Hassan, A.M., Al-Gindan, Y., Omer, A.H., Kutty, M.K. & Saeed, M.B. Dissemination in cutaneous leishmaniasis. II-Satellite papules and subcutaneous induration. Int J Dermatol. (1988), 27: 702-706.

[11] Morelli, P., Gianelli, E., Calattini, S., Corbellino,M., Antinori, S. & Meroni, L. Itraconazole can be effective in the treatment of sporotrichoid leishmaniasis. J Travel Med. (2004); 11: 328-330.

[12] Talari, S.A., Talaei, R., Shajari, G., Vakili, Z. &Taghaviardakani A. Childhood cutaneous leishmaniasis: report of 117 cases from Iran. Korean J Parasitol. (2006), 44: 355-360.

[13] Gülru Erdogan, F., Gül Çakir, A., Gököz, ö. & Gürler, A. A case of sporotrichoid cutaneous leishmaniasis. Turkderm (2011), 45: 100-103.

[14] Iftikhar, N., Bari, I. & Ejaz, A. Rare variants of cutaneous leishmaniasis: whitlow, paronychia, and sporotrichoid. Int J Dermatol. (2003), 42: 807-809.

[15] Masmoudi, A., Ayadi, N., Khabir, A., Bouzid, L., Bouassida, S., Meziou, T.J., Akrout, F., Zahaf, A., Boudawara, T. & Turki, H. Sporotrichoid cutaneous leishmaniasis in Tunisia: a clinical and histological study. Ann Dermatol Venereol. (2008), 135:63-67.

[16] Aoun, K., Amri, F., Chouihi, E., Haouas, N., Bedoui, K., Ben Khelef, R. & Bouratbine A. Epidemiology of *Leishmania* (*L*) *infantum*, *L. major* and *L. killicki* in Tunisia : results and analysis of the identification of 226 human and canine isolates. Bull Soc Pathol Exot. (2008), 101: 323-328.

[17] Haouas, N., Gorcii, M., Chargui, N., Aoun, K., Bouratbine, A., Messaadi-Akrout, F., Masmoudi, A., Zili, J., Ben Saïd, M., Pratlong, F., Dedet, J.P., Mezhoud, H., Azaiez, R. & Babba, H. Leishmaniasis in central and southern Tunisia: current geographical distribution of zymodemes. Parasite (2007); 14: 239-246.

[18] Kibbi, A.G., Karam, P.G. &Kurban, A.K. Sporotrichoid leishmaniasis in patients from Saudi Arabia: clinical and histological features. J Am Acad Dermatol. (1987), 17: 759-764.

[19] Neva, F.A., Wyler, D. & Nash, T. Cutaneous leishmaniasis – A case with persistent organisms after treatment in presence of normal immune response. Am J Trop Med Hyg. (1979), 28: 467-471.

[20] Sadeghian, G., Ziaei, H., Bidabadi, L.S. & Nilforoushazdeh, M.A. Evaluation of leishmanin skin test reaction in different variants of cutaneous leishmaniasis. Int J Dermatol. (2013), 58: 239.

[21] Ejaz, A., Raza, N. & Iftikhar, N. Recurrent cutaneous leishmaniasis presenting as sporotrichoid abscesses: a rare presentation near Afghanistan border. Dermatology Online Journal (2007), 13: 15.

[22] Cozzani, E., Satta, R., Fausti, V., Cottoni, F. & Parodi A. Cutaneous sporotrichoid leishmaniasis resistant to pentavalent antimonial therapy: complete resolution with itraconazole. Clin Exp Dermatol. (2011), 36: 49-51.

[23] Tobin, E.H. & Jih, W.W. Sporotrichoid lymphocutaneous infections: etiology, diagnosis and therapy. Am Fam Physician. (2001), 63: 326-332.

[24] Killick-Kendrick, R. & Peters, W. Leishmaniasis in Arabia: an annotated bibliography. Am J Trop Med Hyg. (1991), 44, supplement p.31.

Chapter 11

Diagnosis of Leishmaniasis in Children

A K M Mamunur Rashid

Additional information is available at the end of the chapter

http://dx.doi.org/10.5772/58237

1. Introduction

Leishmaniasis, a group of protozoan diseases caused by *leishmania* parasites, is transmitted by the bite of some species of sand fly. This affects various age groups depending on the infecting *leishmania* species, geographical location, and disease reservoir and host immunocompetence. [1] Leishmaniasis is estimated to affect 10-50 million people in endemic tropical and subtropical regions on all continents except Australia and Antarctica. [2] The prevalence is the highest in central and south America, southern Europe, central Africa, and parts of southern and central Asia. The extent and presentation of the disease depends on several factors, including the humoral and cell mediated immune response of the host, the virulence of the infecting species, and the parasite burden. Children are at greater risk than adults in endemic areas. Malnutrition contributes to the development of disease, and incomplete therapy of initial disease is a risk factor for recurrence of leishmaniasis. [1]

Localized cutaneous leishmaniasis (LCL) is caused by *L. major* and *L. tropica* in North Africa, the Middle East, central Asia, and the Indian subcontinent. *L. aethiopica* is a cause of LCL and diffuse cutaneous leishmaniasis (DCL) in Kenya and Ethiopia. Visceral leishmaniasis (VL) in the Old World is caused by *L. donovani* in Kenya, Sudan, India, Pakistan, and China and by *L. infantum* in the Mediterranean basin, Middle East, and Central Asia. *L. infantum* is also a cause of LCL (without visceral disease) in this same geographic distribution. *L. tropica* also has been recognized as an uncommon cause of visceral disease in the Middle East and India. In the new world, *L. mexicana* causes LCL in a region stretching from southern Texas through Central America. *L. amazonensis, L. pifanoi, L. garnbami,* and *L. venezuelensis* cause LCL in South America, the Amazon basin, and northward. Members of the Viannia subgenus *L. braziliensis, L. panamensis, L. guyanensis,* and *L. peruviana* cause LCL from the northern highlands of Argentina northward to Central America. Members of the Viannia subgenus also cause mucosal leishmaniasis (ML) in a similar geographic distribution. VL in the New World is caused by *L. chagasi* (now considered by the same organism as *L. infantum*), which is distributed from

Mexico (rare) through central and south America. Like *L. infantum, L. chagasi* can also cause LCL in the absence of visceral disease. [2]

The emergence of the leishmaniasis in new areas is the result of 1. Movement of a susceptible population in to existing endemic areas, usually because of agricultural or industrial development or timber harvesting; 2. Increase in vector and/or reservoir population as a result of agriculture development projects; 3. Increase in anthroponotic transmission owing to rapid urbanization in some focuses; and 4. Increase in sand fly density resulting from a reduction in vector control programs.

The cutaneous form of the disease is generally mild but may cause cosmetic disfigurement. Mucosal and visceral leishmaniasis is associated with significant morbidity and mortality.

2. Type of Leishmaniasis

Two forms of leishmaniasis; cutaneous and visceral are seen in humans. Some texts also distinguish a mucocutaneous form, while others consider it to be a subset of cutaneous leishmaniasis. The form of the disease and the usual clinical signs vary with the species of leishmania. Some infections remain asymptomatic.

- Cutaneous leishmaniasis (Figure-1)
    - Localized cutaneous leishmaniasis/oriental sore (LCL)
    - Diffuse cutaneous leishmaniasis (DCL)

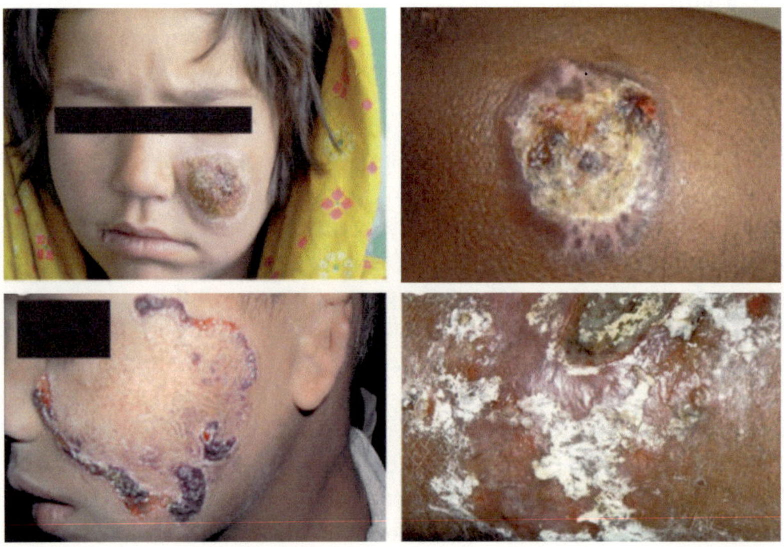

Figure 1. Features of cutaneous leishmaniasis in children

http://dx.doi.org/10.5772/58237

• Mucosal leishmaniasis /Espundia (ML) (Figure-2)

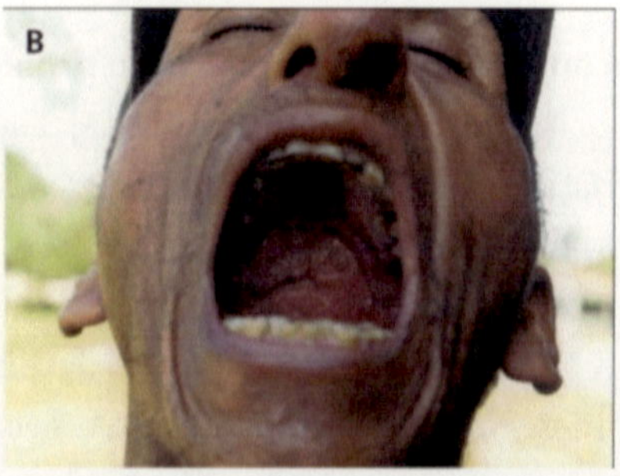

Figure 2. Lesion in palate in Mucosal Leishmaniasis/Espundia (ML)

• Visceral leishmaniasis (Figure-3 & 4)

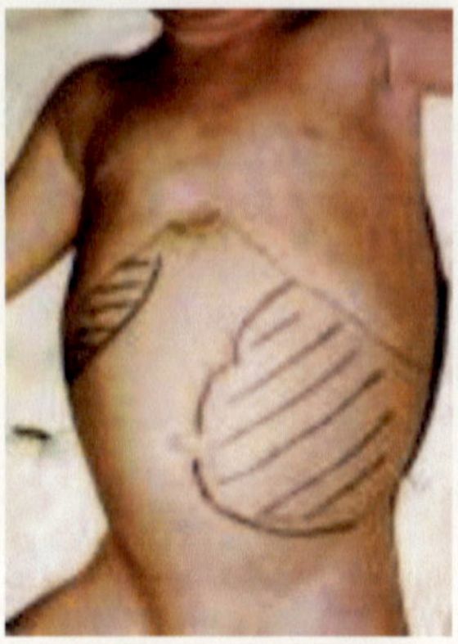

Figure 3. Hepatosplenomegaly in children of VL

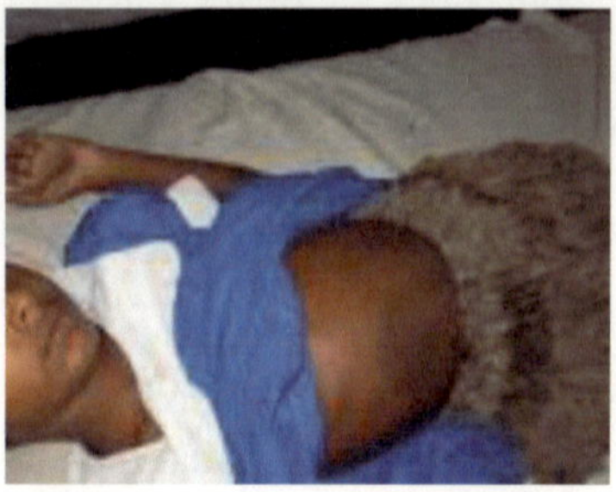

Figure 4. Blackish appearance of skin in children of VL

2.1. Cutaneous leishmaniasis

2.1.1. Localized cutaneous leishmaniasis (LCL)

LCL can affect individuals of any age but children are the primary victims in many endemic regions. Most infections probably remain symptomless. [3] The first sign of an infection is typically a small erythema that develops after a variable prepatent period at the site where an infected sand fly has bitten the host. The erythema develops in to a papule then a nodule that progressively ulcerates over a period of 2 weeks to 6 months to become the lesion that is characteristic of LCL. It typically presents 1 or a few lesions located on exposed skin, such as the face and extremities. Rarely >100 lesions have been recorded. Papule enlarges to 1-3 cm in diameter. The ulcers are usually non-tender, and surrounded by sharp, indurated, erythematous margins. There are no drains, unless a bacterial super infection develops. Lymphatic spread and lymph gland involvement, which may precede lesion development, [4] are common and there is a variable tendency for lesions to self cure within approximately 2-6 months e.g *L. major*, 3-9 months e.g *L. mexicana*, or 6-15 months e.g *L. tropica*, *L. brazilensis*, *L. panamensis* of disease onset. Regional lymphadenopathy and palpable nodules or lymphatic cords, the so-called sporotrichoid appearance is also more common when the patient is infected with organisms of the viannia subgroups [5, 6, 7, 8, 9].

Spontaneous healing usually results in lifelong protection from disease, which may or may not be restricted to the same *Leishmania* species. Resolution of disease results in a lifelong scar, which depending on its size and location may case substantial trauma in affected individuals. [10]

2.1.2. Diffuse Cutaneous Leishmaniasis (DCL)

DCL is a rare form of leishmaniasis found in parts of south and central America, Ethiopia, and Kenya [11] It is caused by organisms of the *L. mexicana* complex in the New World, and *L. aethiopia* in the Old World. DCL manifests as large non-ulcerating macules, papules, nodules, or plaques that often involve large areas of skin and may resemble lepromatous leprosy. The face and extremities are most commonly involved. Dissemination from the initial lesions usually takes place over several years. It is thought that an immunologic defect underlies this severe form of cutaneous leishmaniasis. [2]

The broad clinical spectrum of cutaneous leishmaniasis makes diagnosis of present and past cases difficult. Differential diagnosis is important because diseases of other causes but with a similar clinical spectrum to leishmaniasis are common in leishmaniasis endemic areas.

Diseases that should be considered in the differential diagnosis of cutaneous leishmaniasis include sporotrichosis, blastomycosis, chromomycosis, lobomycosis, cutaneous tuberculosis, atypical mycobacterial infection, leprosy, ecthyma, syphilis, yaws, and neoplasms. [2]

2.2. Mucosal Leishmaniasis/Espundia (ML)

ML is an uncommon but serious manifestation of leishmanial infection resulting from hematogenous metastases to the nasal or oropharyngeal mucosa from a cutaneous infection. [2]

Mucosal leishmaniasis is most commonly associated with *L. braziliensis* thus it is usually limited to South America. Mucosal involvement is the most serious complication in *L. braziliensis* infections and can have disfiguring and life-threatening mucosal leishmaniasis in a varying proportion of patients. In most endemic areas, 1-10% LCL infections result in ML 1-5 years after LCL has healed, [12] but reports do exist for which ML presented at the same time as LCC [13] or for which up to 25 % of LCL infections resulted in ML. [14]

Patients with ML most commonly have nasal mucosal involvement and present with nasal congestion, discharge, and recurrent epistaxis. Oropharyngeal and laryngeal involvement is less common but associated with severe morbidity. Marked soft tissue, cartilage, and even bone destruction occurs late in the course of the disease, and lead to visible deformity of the nose around mouth, nasal septal perforation, and tracheal narrowing with airway obstruction. [2] ML never heals spontaneously, is very difficult to treat with secondary bacterial infections common, and is potentially fatal. [15]

Differential diagnosis of ML includes syphilis, tertiary yaws, histoplasmosis, paracoccidioidomycosis, sarcoidosis, Wegner granulomatosis, midline granuloma.

2.2.1. *Investigation*

Parasitological diagnosis remains the gold standard in cutaneous and mucosal leishmaniasis, because of its high specificity. It includes microscopic examination of Gimsa-stained biopsy smears or aspirates, histopathological examination of fixed lesion biopsies, or culture of biopsy triturates or aspirates. [16] Microscopic examination is probably the most common diagnostic approach used, because more sophisticated methods are expensive and rarely available at primary, secondary, and tertiary health care levels in endemic areas. Culture methods are probably the most informative, allowing species identification and characterization, but require a wealth of technical expertise, and are time consuming and expensive. The sensitivity of these techniques however, tends to be low and can be highly variable, depending on parasite number and dispersion in biopsy samples, technical expertise, and culture media. Molecular parasitological diagnosis for cutaneous leishmaniasis was developed extensively during the past decades and has been recently reviewed. [17] It is essentially done by PCR based methods and is particularly useful in cases with low parasite load such as mucosal leishmaniasis. Reported specificity is 100%, sensitivity is improved by 20-30% in LCL and 55-70% in ML, when compared with conventional parasitological diagnosis. There has been substantial effort in applying molecular diagnostics in the field (e.g successful detection of parasite DNA in blood or tissue smears; development of rapid PCR oligochromatography), its widespread use is still hampered by the requirement of substantial laboratory infrastructure, technical expertise, and cost. [17]

Serological diagnosis is rarely used in cutaneous or mucous leishmaniasis because of variable sensitivity and specificity. [18] The Montenegro skin test is occasionally used in diagnosis of cutaneous disease (eg.in epidemiological surveys), because of its simple use and high sensitivity and specificity; [19] however, it fails to distinguish between past and present infections.

2.3. Visceral Leishmaniasis/ Kala azar (VL)

More than 90% of the world's VL cases are in India, Bangladesh, Nepal, Sudan, and Brazil. The incidence of Kala-azar in India is among the highest in the world. Male: female ratio of the disease is 2:1 in India. [20] VL is found in all age groups. In India and Brazil, an animal reservoir has not been identified. The epidemiological form of the disease was first described in India, and is known as the Indian type of visceral leishmaniasis. In this form of the disease, children between 5 and 15 years of age are affected. L. donovani is the predominant parasite of this form of leishmaniasis in India, while in the new world the disease is predominantly caused by *L. chagasi*. In Mediterranean basin, VL mainly affects children 1 to 4 years of age; it is caused mainly by *L. inanum,* transmitted by phlebotomic sand flies, and dogs are the most important reservoir. The African type of VL is again caused by *L. infantum* affecting older children and young adults and rodents are the reservoir hosts. [21, 22]

After inoculation of the organism in to the skin by the sand fly, the child may have a completely asymptomatic infection or an oligosymptomatic illness that either resolves spontaneously or evolves into active Kala-azar. Children with asymptomatic infection are transiently seropositive but show no clinical evidence of disease. Children who are oligosymptomatic have mild constitutional symptoms (malaise, intermittent diarrhea, poor activity tolerance) and intermittent fever; most will have a mildly enlarged liver. In most of these children the illness will resolve without therapy, but in approximately ¼ it will evolve to active Kala-azar within 2-8 months. Extreme incubation periods of several years have rarely been described. During the first few weeks to months of disease development, the fever is intermittent, there is weakness and loss of energy and the spleen begins to enlarge. The classic clinical pictures of high fever, marked splenomegaly, hepatomegaly and severe cachexia typically develop approximately 6 months after the onset of illness; but a rapid clinical course over 1 month has been noted in up to 20% of patients in some series. At the terminal stages of VL the hepatosplenomegaly is massive, there is gross wasting, the pancytopenia is profound, and jaundice, edema, and ascities may be present. Anaemia may be severe enough to precipitate heart failure. Bleeding episodes, especially epistaxis are frequent. The late stage of illness is often complicated by secondary bacterial infection.

A young age at the time of infection and underlying malnutrition may be a risk factor for the development and more rapid development of active VL. VL has been increasingly recognized as an opportunistic infection associated with HIV infection.

In an African study, clinical symptoms on VL patients include fever 95.8%, weight loss 85.9%, abdominal pain 67.7%, Loss of appetite 56.3%, cough 39.4%, epistaxis 29.6%, joint pain 29.6%, diarrhea 25.4%.. In the same study clinical signs of VL were splenomegaly (93%), pallor (83%), emaciation (76.1%), hepatomegaly (73.2%), lymphadenopathy (50.7%), oedema of lower limbs (14.1%), skin darkness (08.5%), ascitis (08.5%). [23]

Intermittent fever (95%), pallor (77%), refusal to feed or anemia (40%), weight loss (18%), abdominal distension (18%), cough (16%), vomiting (15%) and diarrhea (12%) were the commonest presenting complaints in a study in southern Greece. Massive splenomegaly (99%), hepatomegaly (85%), lymphadenopathy (39%), and echymoses or gingival bleeding (2%) were other common manifestations noted on physical examination. The investigators also reported certain unusual manifestations in the form of tachycardia (80%), cardiac murmur (75%), petechiae or echymoses (30%), and jaundice (20%). Abdominal distension was observed in 80% of their cases. [1]

The most common clinical features are anemia, fever, splenomegaly that presents in > 90% of cases in southern and northwest Iran. Hepatomegaly is less frequent than splenomagaly. Jaundice, edema, and ascitis are reported less frequently. It seems that all of signs and symptoms are compatible with Mediterranean type except for the absence of significant lymphadenopathy. [24]

In a series of seven Kala azar cases in children presented with jaundice, 42% were diagnosed clinically as chronic liver disease, 8% as congenital hemolytic anemia, and 50% as Kala azar. Kala azar may present with various clinical manifestation in children and adult. Jaundice can be considered to be a common manifestation particularly in pediatric Kala azar patients otherwise, it may mislead to another diagnosis if it is taken as rare feature. [25]

2.4. Post-Kala azar Dermal leishmaniasis (PKDL) (Figure 5)

A small percentage of patients previously treated for VL develop diffuse skin lesions, a condition known as post Kala azar dermal leishmaniasis. PKDL occurs in a very high percentage in the 0-9 years age group. [20] These lesions may appear during or shortly after therapy (Africa) or up to several years later (India). [2]

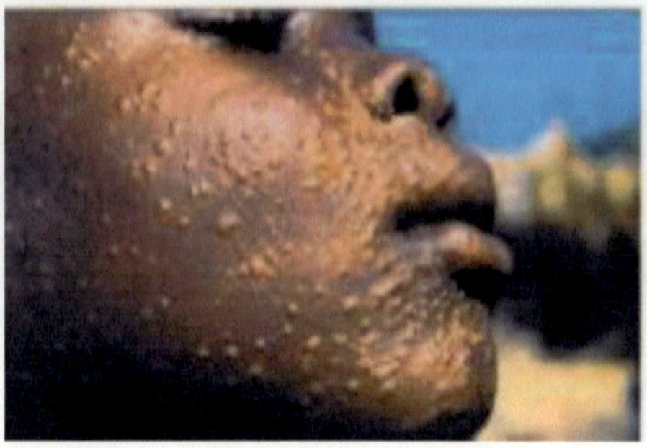

Figure 5. Nodular lesions in children of PKDL

This syndrome is characterized by a maculopapular, macularnodular rash around the mouth, which spreads. It commonly involves the face and torso. They may persist for several months or many years. [2] In India PKDL is seen in 1-3% of successfully treated cases of VL. [1] The clinical features of PKDL have remained almost the same over the years. [20]

The clinical picture of VL may also be consistent with that of malaria, typhoid fever, miliary tuberculosis, scistosomiasis, brucellosis, and leukemia. PKDL should also be differentiated from yaws, syphilis, leprosy, and muco-cutaneous leishmaniasis. [1, 2]

2.4.1. Investigation

Laboratory findings associated with classic Kala azar include anemia (hemoglobulin 5-8 mg/dl), thrombocytopenia, leucopenia (2000-3000 cells/μL), elevated hepatic transaminase levels, and hyper globulinemia (> 5gm/dl) that is mostly immunoglobulin G (IgG). [2]

3. Demonstration (microscopy) and isolation of parasite (culture) (Figure 6)

Direct visualization of amastigotes in clinical specimens is the diagnostic gold standard in regions where tissue aspiration is feasible and microscopy and technical skill are available. [24] Microscopy of bone marrow aspirates is the safest diagnostic approach for paediatric patients, with amastigotes seen in more than 90% of cases by an experienced observer. The higher diagnostic efficacy of the bone marrow examination in children is probably related to the heavier parasitisation encountered in children. Microscopic examination of splenic aspirates offers the highest sensitivity (up to 98%), but is assoiated with the risk of lfe-threatening haemorrhage in cases with profound thrombocytopenia. [1] The results of culture in Novy-McNeal-Nicole (NNN) and RPMI 1640 media have been disappointing in one study. [24]

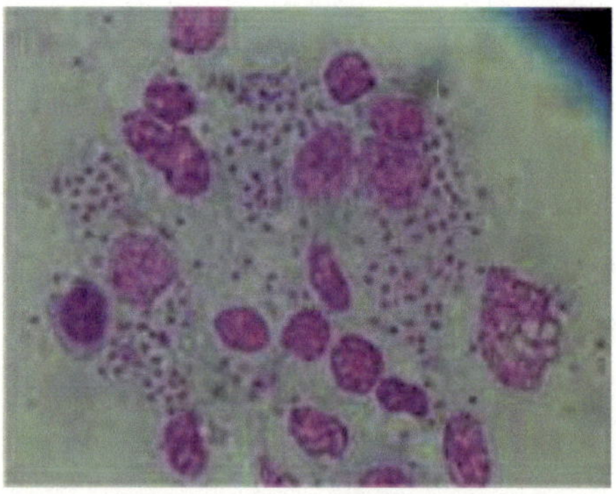

Figure 6. Amastigotes forms of *Leishmania spp* by Giemsa stain

4. Serological methods

Serological methods are highly sensitive and non-invasive. They are comparatively more suited for diagnosing VL in endemic regions. These methods are either based on detection of antibodies (produced against parasite by polyclonal activation of B cells) or antigens. Many conventional methods for antibodies detection for instances, gel diffusion, complement fixation test, indirect haemagglutination test, indirect fluorescent antibody detection test (IFAT), and counter current electrophoresis have been evaluated with varying sensitivities and specificities.

Direct agglutination test (DAT) has been found to be 91-100% sensitive and 72-100% specific in various studies elsewhere in the world. [26]

Detection of anti-K39 by immune-chromatographic strip testing is a rapid and non-invasive method of diagnosing Kala azar. It entails a good sensitivity and specificity. In symptomatic patients, anti-K39 strip-test sensitivity is high (90-100%), while specificity might vary by region. [3]

Two urinary antigens of 72-75 and 123 kDa have been reported to be very useful in diagnosis and prognosis of Kala azar with sensitivity of 96% and specificity of 100%. [26]

DNA detection methods: a variety of nucleic acid detection methods targeting both DNA and RNA have been developed. The most suitable target for the DNA based diagnosis is kinetoplast DNA minicircle (K-DNA). The leishmania polymerase chain reaction (PCR) assays using peripheral blood as clinical specimen showed to be a highly efficient non-invasive alternative with sensitivity varying from 80-100%. [27]

The *Leishmania* skin test (LST): LST is a measure of delayed hypersensitivity to leishmanial antigen. The test remains negative through the period of active disease. The change from negative to a positive LST is regarded as a prognostic sign. [28]

Author details

A K M Mamunur Rashid

Department of Paediatrics, Khulna Medical College, Khulna, Bangladesh

References

[1] Kafetzis DA. An overview of paediatric leishmaniasis. JPGM 2003; 49 (1): 31-8.

[2] Peter CM. Leishmaniasis. In: Kliegman RM, Jenson HB, Behrman RE, Stanton BF, editors. Nelson Textbook of Pediatrics. 18th edn. Philadelphia: WB Saunders; 2008.

[3] Murray HW, Berman JD, Davies CR, Saravia NG. Advances in leishmaniasis. Lancet 2005; 366: 1561-77.

[4] Barral A, Guerreiro J, Bomfim G, Correia D, Barral-Netto M, Carvalho FM. Lymphadenopathy as the first sign of human cutaneous infection by leishmania braziliensis. A J Trop Med Hyg 1995; 53: 256-59.

[5] Nassiri-Kashani M, Firooz A, Kharmesipour A et al. a randomized double-blind placebo-controlled clinical trial of itraconazole in the treatment of cutaneous leishmaniasis. J Eur Acad Dermatol Venereol 2005; 19; 80-3.

[6] Soto J, Arana BA, Toledo J. et al, Miltefosine for New World cutaneous leishmaniasis. Clin Infect Dis 2004; 38: 1266-72.

[7] Dowlati Y. Cutaneous leishmaniasis clinical aspect. Clin Dermatol 1996; 14 : 425-31.

[8] Navin TR, Arana BA, Arana FE, Berman JD, Chajon JF. Placebo-controlled clinical trial of sodium stibogluconate (Pentostam) versus ketoconazole for treating cutaneous leishmaniasis in Guatamala. J infect Dis 1992; 165: 528-34.

[9] Soto JM, Toledo JT, Gutierrez P, et al. Treatment of cutaneous leishmaniasis with a tropical antileishmanial drug (WR279396): phase 2 pilot study. Am J Trop Med Hyg 2002; 66: 147-51.

[10] Yanik M, Gurel MS, Simsek Z, Kati M. The psychological impact of cutaneous leishmaniasis. Clin Exp Dermatol 2004; 29: 464-67.

[11] Peters W, Killick-Kendrick R. eds. The leishmaniases in biology and medicine. Clinical aspects and control. Vol 2. London: Academic Press, 1987.

[12] Davies CR, Reithinger R, Campbell-Lendrum D, Feliciangeli D, Borges R, Rodrigues N. The epidemiology and control of leishmaniasis in Andean countries. Cad Saude Publica 2000; 16: 925-50.

[13] Boaventura Vs, Café V, Costa J, et al. concomitant early mucosal and cutaneous leishmaniasis in Brazil. Am J Tro Med Hyg 2006; 75: 267-69.

[14] Dimier-David I, David C, Munoz M, et al. Epidemiological, clinical and biological features mucocutaneous leishmaniasis in Bolivia after a 221 patient sample. Bull Sac Pathol Exot 1993; 86: 106-11.

[15] Marsden PD. Mucosal leishmaniasis ("espundia" Escomel. 1911) Trans R Soc Trop Med Hyg 1986; 80: 859-76.

[16] Escobar MA, Martinez F, Scott Smith D, Palma GI. American cutaneous and mucocutaneous leishmaniasis (tegumentary): a diagnostic challenge. Trop Doct 1992; 22: 69-78.

[17] Reithinger R, Jean-Claude D, Louzir H, Pirmez C, Alexander B, Brooker S. Cutaneous leishmaniasis. Lancet 2007; vol 7 september: 581-96.

[18] Kar K. serodiagnosis of leishmaniasis. Crit Rev Microbiol 1995; 21: 123-53.

http://dx.doi.org/10.5772/58237

[19] Weigle KA, de Davalos M, Heredia P, Molineros R, Saravia NG, D Alessandro A. Diagnosis of cutaneous and mucocutaneous leishmaniasis in Colombia: a comparison of several methods. Am J Trop Med Hyg 1987; 36: 489-96.

[20] Bora D. Epidemiology of visceral leishmaniasis in India. The National Medical Journal of India 1999; vol. 12(2): 62-8.

[21] Herwaldt BL. Leishmaniasis. Lancet 1999; 354: 1191-9.

[22] Murray W. Leishmaniasis. In: Feigin RD, Cherry JD, editors. Textbook of pediatric infectious disease. 4th edn. Philadelphia: WB Saunders; 1998.

[23] Abdelsalam M. Nail, Abdelmageed M. Imam. Visceral leishmaniasis: Clinical and demographic features in an African population. Pak J Med Sci 2013; 29(2): 485-89.

[24] Abdolvahab Alborzi, Pouladfar GR, Aelami MH. Visceral leishmaniasis; literature review and Iranian experience. Iranian Journal of Clinical Infectious Disease 2007; 2(2); 99-108.

[25] AKMM Rashid, Ashrafuzzaman MD, Mamun AA, Mahboob AA. Jaundice in pediatric visceral leishmaniasis (Kala-azar) patients. Asian Pac J Trop Med 2009; 2(2): 27-9.

[26] Attar ZJ, Chance ML, el-Safi S, et al. Latex agglutination test for the detection of urinary antigens in visceral leishmaniasis. Acta Trop. 2001;78: 6-11.

[27] Singh RK, Pandey HP, Sundar S. Visceral leishmaniasis (kala-azar): challenges ahead. Indian J Med Res 2006; 123:331-44.

[28] Wilsona ME, Jeronimob SMB, Pearson RD. Immunopathogenesis of infection with the visceralizing leishmania species. Microb pathol 2005; 38: 147-60.

Chapter 12

New Advances in the Diagnosis of Canine Visceral Leishmaniasis

Patrícia Sampaio Tavares Veras,
Deborah Bittencourt Mothé Fraga,
Manuela da Silva Solcà and
Carlos Eduardo Sampaio Guedes

Additional information is available at the end of the chapter

http://dx.doi.org/10.5772/57573

1. Introduction

Visceral leishmaniasis (VL) is a serious public health problem of great medical and veterinary importance. This disease is endemic in Brazil and in many other countries of Latin America, Asia, Africa and Europe (1). According to recent review (2), approximately 0.2 to 0.4 million cases of VL occur each year and although worldwide distributed, higher prevalence of the disease is concentrated in six countries, including India, Bangladesh, Sudan, South Sudan, Ethiopia and Brazil, that undertake for more than 90% of the cases. The clinical importance of VL resides in the severity of the disease that results in death of unrecognized cases and even for individuals with treatment access, death occurs in 10 to 20% of the cases [2-8].

Most of the VL cases are caused by the *Leishmania* species from *Leishmania donovani* complex. Parasites from the *Leishmania* genus are diphasic and are transmitted as promastigote form to vertebrate hosts through the bites of female sand flies [9-12]. The genetic similarities between Old World and New World strains, respectively, of *L. infantum* and *L. infantum* (syn. *chagasi*) from different regions in Latin America, indicate these parasites belong to the same origin [11, 12].

The notion that dogs are the main urban domestic reservoir for this *Leishmania* in certain part of the globe is supported by the facts including: i) cases of canine visceral leishmaniasis (CVL) have been reported in 50 of the 88 countries where VL is endemic [13], ii) canine cases precede the onset of human cases [14], iii) high rates of prevalence in dogs, and iv) frequency of parasites is high in dog skin [15-18].

Control strategies include performing accurate and early diagnosis of CVL to identify infected animals [19, 20]. CVL diagnosis is a difficult task since clinical signs of the disease in dogs can be confused with other diseases [19]. In endemic areas, a large percentage of infected animals are asymptomatic or present low number of discrete signs. The role these animals play in parasite transmission is still largely unknown. Several diagnostic strategies have been implemented based on parasitological, serological or molecular methods in association with clinical and epidemiological parameters [21]. Parasite culturing has been considered as gold standard for disease diagnosis [22, 23]. Although offering a high specificity since allows parasite identification, it offers very low sensitivity, besides it is laborious, time-consuming and largely dependent on the expertise of the observer [24, 25].

Serological tests are the most common diagnostic method employed for CVL diagnosis [3]. Several serological methods have been implemented for diagnosis of CVL, including direct agglutination assay (DAT), enzyme linked immunoassay (ELISA) and indirect immunofluorescent antibody test (IFI) [26]. However, most of these classical serological tests present important limitations for CVL diagnosis, including high consumption of time, and lack of sensitivity and specificity, mainly when animals present low antibody titers. This causes underestimation of disease, reflecting in failures in control measures, as well as the maintenance of infected untreated dogs in endemic areas [27, 28]. New methods based on immunochromatography have been implemented for serodiagnosis of CVL and have shown excellent results [29]. These techniques offer several advantages since they are rapid tests easily performed even in field areas, and more specific since they use recombinant DNA technology that additionally facilitates reproducibility and large-scale production. These advantages result in better identification of infected dogs. However, the efficacy of immunochromatographic techniques for CVL diagnosis needs to be improved [30]. In Brazil, a rapid test based in dual path platform (TR DPP®LVC - Biomanguinhos) had been recently implemented as screening test for CVL. This technique seems to be adequate to disease diagnosis in public health system. However, the TR DPP®LVC has shown an excellent performance identifying 98% of symptomatic dogs, it showed less efficacy for diagnosis of asymptomatic dogs (47%) [31]. Since there is evidence that asymptomatic dogs can participate in natural transmission cycle of VL, new strategies should be implemented in order to improve CVL diagnosis [16, 32-34]. For serological diagnosis one strategy can be the development of rapid tests based on impregnation of multi-antigen that would offer more sensitivity, as well specificity.

Finally, it would be important to include more specific confirmatory tests for control strategies that can be advantageous to diagnose inconclusive cases. There is evidence that molecular diagnosis of *Leishmania* spp. provides high levels of sensitivity and specificity when compared to other diagnostic methods [7, 17]. The use of quantitative methods in molecular level allows not only a more accurate detection but also monitoring tissue parasite load in dogs following anti-leishmanial treatment [35-37].

2. Importance of CVL diagnosis

Since the discovery of canine visceral leishmaniasis (CVL) in Tunisia by Nicolle & Comte (1908), several reports have shown that dog and man share a common etiologic agent. The notion that dog is the main reservoir of visceral leishmaniasis (VL) in urban centers [38] is supported by several evidences including the high cutaneous parasitism observed in dogs infected by *Leishmania* [15-18], the high rates of prevalence observed among dogs in endemic areas, and the observation that the appearance of canine cases precedes the emergence of human cases [14]. Some studies conducted in endemic regions, where VL occurs in a zoonotic cycle, point to a prevalence of approximately 20% of VL-positive dogs, as described in China [39], Greece [40], and Mexico [41]. In other endemic areas, rates of *Leishmania* infection detected in dogs range between 60 and 80% [4, 42-44]. However, in spite of the high prevalence of *Leishmania* infection, not all dogs exhibit signs of clinical disease and sick dogs may display clinical signs of variable intensity [4, 42, 45]. Differences in clinical manifestations among dogs as the number of clinical signs and the time to onset of the disease may vary depending on the individual immune response of the infected dog. Three forms of progression of infection by *L. infantum* have been described: about 46% of infected dogs acquire the infection and develop the disease immediately, another 44% of dogs develop the disease later and 10% of them never develop CVL [46-48]. Similar to that which occurs in humans, characteristics such as genetic factors, age and nutritional status may influence the progression of VL in dogs [13, 49, 50].

Some studies have shown a correlation between the presence of clinical signs in infected animals and transmissibility of the parasite to the vector and, consequently, a correlation with the occurrence of human cases [16, 32, 51]. In accordance with these studies, Travi et al. (2001) and Verçosa et al. (2008) showed that asymptomatic dogs did not transmit the parasite to the vector [38, 51]. There is not a consensus about this idea, since there is a wide variation in the rates of infectivity (70 to 90%) between asymptomatic and symptomatic dogs. Studies show that, regardless of the clinical presentation, any dog has the ability to transmit *Leishmania* to the vector, even though the symptomatic animals are more likely to disseminate the disease [16, 32, 52, 53], being more capable of transmitting the parasite to the vector and, consequently, to another dog or a human [33, 34, 54, 55]. Based on studies showing that the dog can transmit the disease regardless of its clinical form, in some countries such as Brazil, dog culling is recommended as a control strategy. This control measure is not well accepted, having its effectiveness questioned and demanding studies to increase the diagnostic methods performance. Additionally, identification of new antigens will allow not only improvement of diagnosis, but also differentiation of dogs that transmit, from those that do not transmit the parasite in an endemic area.

3. Visceral leishmaniasis diagnosis in dogs

The diagnosis of VL in the dog must consider the association between clinical, laboratory and epidemiological data. As discussed above, clinical diagnosis is problematic and difficult for veterinarians to perform due to the great variability of clinical signs that *Leishmania*-infected dogs may present, as long as to its similarity with clinical profiles of other diseases. In clinical practice, identification of characteristic manifestations should be confirmed by ascertaining the infection using laboratory techniques [56] that vary in accuracy [57, 58].

There are several laboratorial diagnosis methods for leishmaniasis: i) parasitological methods (detection of the parasite), ii) serological methods (detection of anti-*Leishmania* antibodies), iii) molecular methods (amplification of parasite DNA) and iv) assay of cell-mediated immunity. This last method not being widely applied to routine diagnosis and will not be discussed in the present report. It should be noted that, although there is a wide variety of diagnostic techniques for CVL, none of them offer 100% of sensitivity or specificity [35, 59].

In spite of serological techniques such as enzyme-linked immunosorbent assay (ELISA) and indirect immunofluorescence assay (IFAT) being the most widely used methods for the diagnosis of CVL [60] parasitological methods, such as direct examination of slides and isolation from tissue cultures, allow the parasite to be detected and can be used as confirmatory diagnostic methods for CVL [61]. In recent decades, molecular techniques such as polymerase chain reaction (PCR) have been introduced for the diagnosis of CVL, exhibiting high sensitivity and specificity [21]. These techniques detect the genetic material of the parasite, which can be used as confirmatory methods in cases of recently infected or asymptomatic animals, which tend not to be diagnosed serologically, and in most cases, do not show seroconversion, having a low parasite load [4, 60]. In a study conducted in Belo Horizonte-MG, a VL-endemic area in Brazil, among 1,443 dogs evaluated, 15.3% of them were seropositive, while 84.7% showed negative serology. Interestingly, among serologically negative dogs, 24.4% showed up as positive using the molecular diagnostic technique, and most of these (97.6%) would not be diagnosed, since they consist of asymptomatic dogs with negative serology [19].

3.1. Clinical diagnosis

Dogs from endemic areas considered resistant remain clinically normal and asymptomatic without exhibiting clinical signs. There is evidence that the parasites in these animals are effectively eliminated at the infection site [62, 63]. However, in susceptible animals, a large number of parasites are detected in infected tissues. In these animals, the presence of the parasite may occur in multiple organs, accompanied by a granulomatous inflammatory reaction and production of immune-mediated phenomena, probably responsible for the appearance of various types of clinical signs [64].

Initial clinical signs of CVL include: hypertrophy of the lymph nodes, changes in skin appendages such as onychogryphosis, swelling of the footpad, localized alopecia, skin ulcers and nasal and periocular dermatitis. Alopecia and non-pruritic exfoliative dermatitis can spread to other parts of the animal's body. Weight loss may also be present, as well as cachexia, anorexia and conjunctivitis. Internal organs such as spleen, liver, kidney and lymph nodes may also be affected, when kidney injuries are present may lead to the dogs death [13, 65]. Fever, apathy, diarrhea, epistaxis, intestinal bleeding, hepatosplenomegaly, hyperkeratosis, keratoconjunctivitis are also found in affected animals [66-68]. Some clinical signs are more frequent than others; skin lesions are the most frequent manifestations affecting approximately 50 to 90% of symptomatic dogs [4, 67, 69, 70], including non-pruritic exfoliative dermatitis, with or without alopecia, which can be generalized or localized to the muzzle, ears and limbs [67, 71, 72]. Other very common signs are weight loss, observed in 25 to 80% of CVL cases,

http://dx.doi.org/10.5772/57573

including onychogryphosis in 30 to 75%, and ocular abnormalities in 16 to 24% [28]. The most common clinical signs of VL in dogs are depicted in Figure 1.

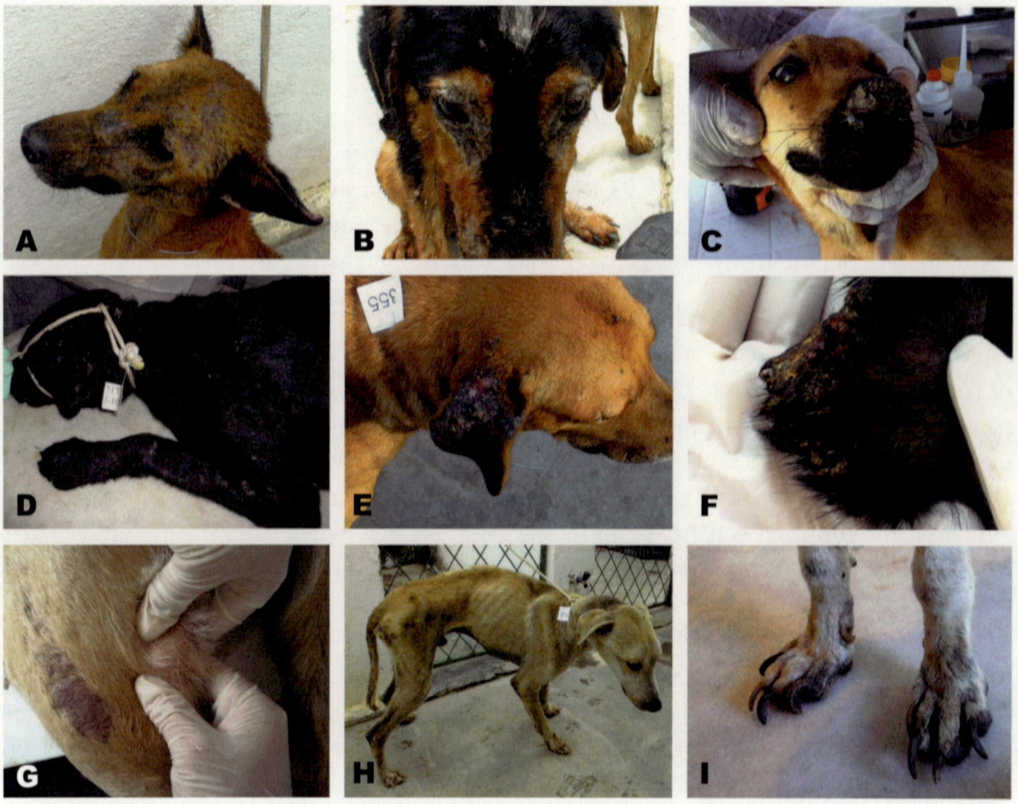

Figure 1. Major clinical signs associated with CVL. A: alopecia on the muzzle, B: periocular dermatitis with keratoconjunctivitis and hyperkeratosis; C: hyperkeratosis of the nasal mucosa; D: generalized non-pruritic exfoliative dermatitis; E: ulcerated lesion in the ear; F: crust with vascular injury on the tip of the ear; G: lymphadenomegaly of the popliteal lymph node; H: cachexia; I: onychogryphosis. Photos of animals infected by *L. infantum* belong to archives from Laboratory of Pathology and Biointervention(LPBI - CPqGM).

In dogs with CVL, clinical-pathological changes may occur such as intestinal lesions, renal and hepatic abnormalities [73]. The main biochemical laboratory findings from CVL are hyperglobulinemia, mainly due to increased production of antibodies, and hypoalbuminemia, attributed to chronic inflammation, as long as renal and hepatic failure [66]. The result of these changes is a reduction in the albumin/globulin ratio and hyperproteinemia [28]. Additionally, severe CVL is associated with changes in hematological parameters such as severe anemia and leukopenia, associated with lymphopenia, eosinopenia and monocytopenia [66, 74, 75].

Immune-mediated thrombocytopenia also occurs accounting for episodes of bleeding such as epistaxis, hematuria and hemorrhagic diarrhea [76].

Finally, nonspecific signs of illness that are mistaken for other diseases such as babesiosis, ehrlichiosis and canine trypanosomiasis also contribute to make CVL clinical diagnosis imprecise and difficult to perform [13].

3.2. Parasitological diagnosis

The detection by optical microscopy of the parasite by direct observation of stained smears from spleen aspirate, lymph node and bone marrow tissues has high specificity, allowing confirmation of CVL diagnosis [3, 53, 61, 77]. However, the sensitivity of this method is less than 30%, since the direct parasite identification may be limited, especially in mildly and asymptomatic dogs that have low parasitic load, producing false negative results [3, 53, 61, 77].

Another method that can identify the parasite in tissues is the culturing of tissue fragments or aspirates, preferably in a biphasic medium [78], composed by Novy-MacNeal-Nicolle (NNN), or Tobie modified medium or United States Army Medical Research Units (USAMRU) as solid phase medium and, most often, Schneider as liquid phase medium. This parasitological diagnostic method offers high specificity allowing isolation and characterization of parasites, as well as determination of which species and/or variants are circulating in endemic areas [79]. However, the culturing consists of an indirect test, because when the parasites are isolated from various tissues, they are present in amastigote form and during cultivation they transform into the promastigote form. This process may be impaired as a result of parasite death due to a failure of temperature-control during transport of the tissue sample, or contamination during collection or cultivation [13]. Additionally, a culturing is time consuming and may take up to 4 weeks of observation for definitive diagnosis [13, 79]. Furthermore, specific media for promastigote isolation are not easily obtained, being a technique restricted to specialized laboratories [70, 80], in which the outcome also depends on the experience of the observer [24, 25]. Although culturing offers greater sensitivity compared to direct viewing of amastigotes in tissue [35], it still remains at very low levels.

In summary, parasitological techniques have high specificity but low sensitivity, especially for the detection of dogs, recently infected, asymptomatic or those presenting low parasite load. In addition, the need for skilled personnel and the long delays to obtain the results prevent parasitological techniques to be used in epidemiological surveys [4, 23, 61, 81-84].

3.3. Serological diagnosis

Serological tests are based on the presence of specific humoral immune responses against the pathogen or purified fraction or recombinant proteins of the pathogen. These tests allow detection of immunoglobulin (IgG) levels, thus becoming an essential tool for the diagnosis of CVL. These methods are simple to carry out and therefore they are frequently used to determine the prevalence of leishmaniasis in epidemiological studies [85].

A wide variety of serological methods are available for CVL diagnosis, presenting variations in sensitivity and specificity. The performance of these diagnostic techniques varies depending on the type of antigen used and the detection of anti-*Leishmania* antibody system.

The most commonly employed serological tests for the diagnosis of CVL, including ELISA, indirect immunofluorescence test (IFAT), and direct agglutination test (DAT), uses parasite or crude extract of *Leishmania,* as the antigen source. More recently, serological methods based on ELISA or rapid tests have been developed using a purified fraction of the parasite or a specific purified recombinant protein, such as rK39 or a chimeric protein as rK28 (rK9 + rK26 + rK39).

Despite the practicality and simplicity of serological tests, they do not have 100% sensitivity because some dogs, especially those that are resistant or in the early stages of the disease, have negative results. Thus, the results of such tests should be evaluated carefully, always associating test results with epidemiological history, clinical state of the animal, and the result of a more specific diagnostic test [86]. In addition, since titers of anti-*Leishmania* antibodies remain detectable for long periods, serological tests are not a good alternative for assessing healing or monitoring dogs after treatment [71].

• IFAT

IFAT is a test in which anti-immunoglobulin antibodies labeled with fluorochromes react with parasites immobilized in a slide. IFAT is a laborious technique that presents difficulties for both standardization and interpretation of the results Therefore, detection of antigen-antibody reaction by fluorescence microscopy depends on the observer experience, compromising reproducibility of this test in different laboratories. Thus, it is not considered a simple and practical technique for evaluating a large number of canine sera [57]. In spite of these limitations, it is still being used as a diagnostic method for mass screening of infected dogs [87]. This method varies in its performance, with sensitivity ranging from 68 to 100% and specificity of 60 to 90% [5, 88-90].

In a study evaluating IFAT for the diagnosis of CVL, the efficacy of the test was evaluated using 254 sera from infected and uninfected dogs and sera from animals with other parasitic diseases. The authors observed low sensitivity (72%) and specificity (52%), as well as cross-reactions when sera from dogs infected with other pathologies, such as *Trypanosoma cruzi, Leishmania braziliensis,* and *Ehrlichia canis* were tested. In this study, the reproducibility of the results among different laboratories yielded a moderate rate of 0.74 [5]. A similar result was obtained by Lira et al. (2006) that using IFAT, found a low sensitivity and specificity of 68% and 87.5%, respectively [88]. By contrast, it was shown by Alves and colleagues that the IFI-CVL kit, IFAT produced by Biomanguinhos (Brazil), provides high sensitivity (100%), detecting all dogs with CVL, although presenting a low specificity of 70%, levels similar to those observed in studies described above. This low level of specificity was due to false positive results from sera of dogs infected with *Trypanosoma caninum* (48.7%) and healthy dogs (10.3%) [90]. Thus, the Brazilian Ministry of Health withdrew the IFI-CVL kit from the CVL control program, due to data in literature that support IFAT has both low sensitivity, which led to maintenance of false-negative dogs in the endemic areas, and low specificity, which promoted the culling of false-positive dogs [65, 91, 92].

- DAT

The direct agglutination test (DAT) is an alternative method for the diagnosis of VL, first described in 1975 and adapted for the diagnosis of human and canine infection in the late 1980s [93, 94]. DAT is a method that uses whole stained promastigotes as antigen, either in suspension or freeze-dried [35]. The advantage of this test lies in its low cost when compared with other tests [93]. However, this test is not desirable for screening large numbers of samples, since it is a laborious procedure, due to the production process for crude *Leishmania* antigen, as well as the need to perform serial dilutions of serum [95, 96]. Regarding the accuracy of DAT, there is some controversy in the literature, the sensitivity appears relatively variable between 88 and 93% and specificity of 70 to 100% [5, 59, 96, 97]. It is likely that these variations are related to how the cutoff is defined, since cutoffs using smaller dilutions reduce sensitivity but raise the specificity, while those using higher dilutions increase sensitivity and reduce specificity [98].

Changes to the DAT protocol have been proposed by Gómez-Ochoa *et al.* (2003) in order to decrease the cost of the procedure and the preparation time of the antigen, while maintaining the same sensitivity and specificity of conventional DAT. One of the proposed changes for DAT protocol is the fast agglutination-screening test (FAST), which combines a higher concentration of parasites with a smaller test volume. FAST requires a single serum dilution and the results can be read in 3 hours [95, 96]. However, in spite of the sensitivity of this technique being greater than that of conventional DAT, which varies from 93 to 98%, the specificity values were similar to those from the conventional DAT, between 78-89% [95, 96].

- ELISA

For various reasons, ELISA tests based on whole parasites or crude lysate of parasite antigens for the diagnosis of CVL do not provide satisfactory results, as follows: i) it is a laborious technique, which leads to a delay in the delivery of results and, consequently, the implementation of treatment or the removal of infected dogs from endemic areas [68, 99]; ii) leads to the appearance of cross-reactions with sera from individuals infected with other *Leishmania* species or even with a variety of other pathogens such as *Toxoplasma gondii, Ehrlichia canis* [23, 24, 29, 100-103],and parasites of the Trypanosomatidae family such as *Trypanosoma cruzi* [5, 29] or *Trypanosoma caninum* [90] iii) there are reports of low reproducibility between batches of ELISA based on whole parasites or crude antigens, since different isolates of *Leishmania* sp. were used and depending on the culturing batch, distinct antigenic compositions can be detected [104].

A study using 234 domesticated dogs in an endemic area for CVL assessed the efficacy of ELISA, IFAT and DAT for the diagnosis of CVL. In this study, dogs were also parasitologically evaluated for identification of *Leishmania* amastigotes in both skin samples and bone marrow aspirates. The sensitivity of IFAT was 72% and ELISA was 95%. When the tests were evaluated against sera from dogs infected with other pathogens, *T. cruzi, E. canis* and *L. braziliensis,* the specificity of these tests shown to be very low 52% for IFAT and 64% for ELISA [5].

Using sera from dogs with CVL, a comparison of an ELISA test using crude soluble antigen of *L. infantum* (SLA) and another ELISA test based on ribosomal protein of *L. infantum* (LRP) was made. The sensitivity of the two tests was similar when evaluated against sera from symptomatic animals (100%), but the ELISA based on LRP showed also higher sensitivity, reaching 100% in the detection of asymptomatic dogs, when compared with ELISA using SLA (19%). Additionally, the LRP-based ELISA showed high specificity (98%), with no cross-reactivity with sera from dogs with other diseases [102].

Thus, the search for tests with higher sensitivity and specificity for dogs with a variety of conditions became necessary for control of CVL, which would lead to a reduction of errors in actions taken for treatment or control. In countries that adopt culling of seropositive dogs as a control measure, low sensitivity of diagnostic tests can lead to the maintenance of dogs that transmit disease and lack of specificity can result in unnecessary culling of healthy dogs. The identification of new proteins of *Leishmania sp.* in order to compose diagnostic tests for CVL can improve both sensitivity and specificity of diagnostic techniques and allow infected dogs to be differentiated from the uninfected ones [5, 29, 87, 105, 106].

Another way to overcome the obstacles of ELISA based on whole parasites or crude parasite antigen was the development of ELISA tests based on parasite fractions such as that using the parasite surface molecule, fucose-mannose ligand antigen (FML). The FML-based ELISA showed a high sensitivity, which was similar in detecting either oligosymptomatic (90%) or symptomatic (90%) dogs. Regarding specificity, ELISA using crude parasite antigen for the diagnosis of oligosymptomatic dogs was superior, achieving 100% in comparison to FML-based ELISA that was 93.3%. However, for symptomatic dogs the specificity of the FML-based ELISA showed similar results of 96.7% compared to that obtained by ELISA based on crude parasite antigen (93.3%) [101].

Other ELISA assays based on recombinant antigens such as rA2 from *L. donovani*, rK26 or rK39 from *L. infantum* have been developed. When compared to an ELISA test based on crude antigen, taking IFAT as the gold standard, and tested against sera from symptomatic dogs, sensitivities was higher for ELISA based on rK26 or rK39 from *L. infantum*, respectively, of 94% and 100% in comparison to 88% for ELISA based on crude antigen and 70% for ELISA based on rA2 from *L. donovani*. However, ELISA based on rA2 showed the highest specificity value of 96% in comparison to those from ELISA based on crude parasite antigen or parasite recombinant antigens rK26, rK39, that showed values of, respectively, 87%, 90%, and 85% [29]. Although good enough for diagnosis of symptomatic dogs, the use of ELISA tests based on recombinant antigens for the diagnosis of asymptomatic dogs seems to be disadvantageous. ELISA based on rA2 gave the lowest sensitivity of 30%, followed by rK26 and rK39 that sensitivity yielded greater, but still stayed low with value of 66% for both tests, in comparison to the sensitivity of 88% for ELISA based on crude parasite antigen. By contrast, another in a multicenter study conducted in 5 regions of Italy using IFAT as gold standard, ELISA based on the recombinant antigen rK39 gave higher levels of sensitivity and specificity of 97.1% and

98.8%, respectively [107]. It is possible that the differences found in relation to the performance of the ELISA containing these proteins may be related to the study design, characterization of serum samples and the experimental protocols of the ELISA assays.

Interestingly, the association of the recombinant proteins enhanced test performance both for detection of symptomatic and asymptomatic infected dogs. Indeed, using IFAT as the gold standard, ELISA based on the mix of rK9, rK26 and rK39 from *L. donovani* showed sensitivity of 95-100% and specificity of 100% against a panel of serum from parasitologically positive dogs, using parasitologically and serologically negative dogs as controls [108]. Furthermore, ELISA containing a chimeric protein rK28, containing reactive epitopes of the three recombinant proteins described above (rK9, rK26 and rK29), shown to present high levels of sensitivity and specificity of 99% and 96%, respectively when tested against a panel of serum from dogs parasitologically positive or serologically positive using IFA, and sera from parasitologically negative dogs as controls [87]. In this study, the authors didn't evaluate rK28-based ELISA against sera from asymptomatic dogs.

The combination of these findings reinforces the notion that the use of multiple antigens in diagnostic tests enhances test performance and the need to search for new antigens that may compose a diagnostic test able to better diagnose asymptomatic dogs.

New recombinant proteins are being evaluated. Faria *et al.* (2011) performed predictions on B-cell epitopes, identifying 360 peptides that were synthesized onto nitrocellulose membranes [105]. The 10 most reactive were evaluated in an ELISA platform. The sensitivity and specificity of the ELISA based on these peptides varied from 70.96% to 88.7% and 55% to 95.0%, respectively, a better result than that obtained with EIE-CVL kit, which gave a sensitivity of 13.8% and specificity of 100%.

Another study evaluated the performance of the ELISA based on another recombinant antigens of *L. infantum*, rLci1A and rLci2B, against a panel of canine sera (n = 256). ELISA based on rLci1A gave sensitivity of 96% and specificity of 92% for rLci1A and sensitivity of 100% and specificity of 95% for rLci2B. The recombinant antigens showed no cross-reactivity with sera from dogs infected with *Trypanosoma caninum, Babesia canis* and *Ehrlichia canis.* Cross-reaction against sera from dogs infected with *Leishmania braziliensis* was observed for rLci1A-based ELISA (11.7%) and for rLci2B-based ELISA (2.9%) [109].

In summary, most studies using ELISA suggest that in comparison to tests based on crude antigen, those based on recombinant antigens improves accuracy, increasing sensitivity and specificity for the diagnosis of symptomatic dogs. Although improved, test accuracy is still low for the detection of asymptomatic animals.

- Rapid tests

Recently, rapid immunodiagnostic tests have begun to be employed as routine laboratory tests for detection of diseases such as leishmaniasis. The recombinant antigens of the parasite are impregnated onto nitrocellulose membranes and serum samples are applied in the rapid test platform. Antigens impregnated in nitrocellulose membranes are recognized by specific immunoglobulin present in the serum of infected individuals. This reaction is revealed by the interaction of protein A coupled to colloidal gold particles, with the Fc portion of the immunoglobulins associated with the recombinant antigens. The use of immunochromatographic assays as diagnostic methods has the main advantages of being rapid, completed in around 15 minutes, easy to carry out and can dispense with the need for equipment to read the results [110]. Furthermore, these tests are easily stored, and test supplies and samples do not need to be maintained at low temperatures and can it even be performed at the place of collection. These tests are already widely used to detect HIV [111] and H1N1 [112] infection. For the diagnosis of CVL and human VL, among the tested and commercially available recombinant proteins, the most widely used for composing immunochromatographic tests is the recombinant protein rK39. This protein contains repetitive sequences of 39 amino acids from a protein related to kinesin of kinetoplast from *L. infantum*, and has been widely used in ELISA platform as described above [30, 31, 91, 96, 97, 110, 113-119].The efficacy of rK39-based rapid lateral flow test was compared with the IFAT against sera of parasitologically positive dogs from Italy. Both tests offered similar sensitivities of 97% for the lateral flow test in the dipstick format and 99% for the DAT, as well as the maximum specificity of 100% in both tests [120]. Similar results were obtained in other study which detected sensitivity of 97% and specificity of 100% using the rK39 dipstick for diagnosis of CVL, indicating that the rK39 dipstick is promising for both large-scale screening in endemic areas and for veterinary clinical practice [121]. However, other studies also conducted in endemic areas for CVL showed that the dipstick based on the recombinant protein rK39 offered inferior performance to that of the studies described above, with sensitivity values of 61-75% and specificity of 72-84.9% [122, 123]. These differences in performance between these studies using dipsticks tests based on rK39 may be related to the use of sera from dogs with different conditions and therefore with varying concentrations of specific immunoglobulins [29-31, 118, 122]. Effectively, another study employing the rapid test based on the recombinant protein rK39 dipstick offered a sensitivity of 96.7% for sera from symptomatic dogs, compared to a sensitivity of 52.9% when evaluating sera from asymptomatic dogs [119]. Similarly, another study found that using sera from asymptomatic dogs that the sensitivity of the dipstick based on rK39 was 75% compared to sensitivities of 88% and 84% for sera from oligosymptomatic and polisymptomatic dogs, respectively [118]. In the same study, an ELISA based on crude parasite antigens yielded a sensitivity of 94% tested using sera from asymptomatic and oligosymptomatic and 95% using sera of polisymptomatic dogs.

Recently, a meta-analysis was performed in order to broadly assess the performance of rapid tests using rK39 as the antigen in the diagnosis of CVL. The combined analysis of 16 studies using rapid tests based on rK39 offered a sensitivity of 86.7% (95% CI: 76.9–92.8%) for the detection of clinical disease and 59.3% (95% CI: 37.9–77.6%) for identification of *Leishmania* infection with a specificity of 98.7% (95% CI: 89.5–99.9%). In summary, this study supports the idea that the rapid test based on rK39 is useful to confirm the disease in dogs with clinical suspicion. However, given its low sensitivity for the diagnosis of asymptomatic dogs, its use is not recommended for large-scale epidemiological studies or VL control programs [30].

First author and year of publication	Serology		Sample			Results	
	Technique	Antigen	(n) Infected dogs confirmed by other techniques	(n) Non-infected dogs	(n) Dogs infected with others pathologies	Sensitivity (%)	Specificity (%)
Harith *et al.*, 1989	DAT	*L. infantum* promastigotes	44	6	176	98.9	100
Barbosa-de-Deus *et al.*, 2002	ELISA	LMS	188	1582	55	98.0	95.0
Scalone *et al.*, 2002	ELISA	K39	209	81	62	97.1	98.8
Schallig *et al.*, 2002	DAT	*L. donovani* promastigotes	79	67	24	88.6	96.7
	FAST	*L. donovani* promastigotes	79	67	24	93.6	89.0
Rosati *et al.*, 2003	ELISA	K26	202	20	0	100	100
	ELISA	K9	202	20	0	95	95
	ELISA	K39	202	20	0	95	95
Mohebali, *et al.*, 2004	Dipstick	rK39	268*	0	0	70.9	84.9
Boarino *et al.*, 2005	ELISA	K9-K39-K26 chimera	232	362	0	95.8	99.1
Mettler *et al.*, 2005	Rapid test	rK39	47	50	26	A: 52.9 S: 96.7	94
	IFAT	*L. infantum* promastigotes	47	50	26	A: 29.4 S: 90.0	100
Lira *et al.*, 2006	EIE® - LVC	*L. major* lysate	25	16	11	72.0	87.5
	IFI® - LVC	*L. major* like promastigotes	25	16	11	68.0	87.5
Ferreira *et al.*, 2007	EIE® - LVC	*L. major* lysate	234*	20	20	96.0	100
	IFI® - LVC	*L. major* like promastigotes	234*	20	20	72.0	100
	DAT	*L. donovani* promastigotes	234*	20	20	93.0	100
Ferroglio *et al.*, 2007	SNAP® CLATK CTA		59	124	0	91.1	99.0
Porrozzi *et al.*, 2007	ELISA	rK26	100	25	14	A: 66.0 S: 94.0	90.0

First author and year of publication	Serology: Technique	Serology: Antigen	Sample: (n) Infected dogs confirmed by other techniques	Sample: (n) Non-infected dogs	Sample: (n) Dogs infected with others pathologies	Results: Sensitivity (%)	Results: Specificity (%)
	ELISA	rK39	100	25	14	A: 66.0 S: 100	85.0
	ELISA	rA2	100	25	14	A: 88.0 S: 70.0	96.0
	ELISA	CTA	100	25	14	A: 30.0 S: 88.0	87.0
Cândido *et al.*, 2008	ELISA	CTA	60	30	0	O: 86.7 P: 90.0	O: 100 P: 93.3
	ELISA	FML	60	30	0	O: 90.0 P: 86.7	O: 93.3 P: 96.7
Lemos *et al.*, 2008	RDTs	rK39	76	33	0	83	100
	ELISA	*L. chagasi* lysate	76	33	0	95	100
Babakhan *et al.*, 2009	FAST	*L. infantum* promastigotes	73	74	0	98.6	78.7
Coelho *et al.*, 2009	ELISA	LRP	111	47	14	100	98.2
	ELISA	CTA	111	47	14	96.0	100
Troncarelli *et al.*, 2009	IFAT	*L. major* like promastigotes	51	0	0	83.0	92.5
Figueiredo *et al.*, 2010	EIE® - LVC	*L. major* lysate	305*	0	0	100	96.6
	IFI® - LVC	*L. major* like promastigotes	305*	0	0	22.2	97.0
de Lima *et al.*, 2010	ELISA	CTA	52	52	0	91.5	94.7
	RDTs	rK39	52	52	0	100	91.2
Marcondes *et al.*, 2011	SNAP® CLATK	CTA	283	86	31	94.7	90.6
Alves *et al.*, 2012	EIE® - LVC	*L. major* lysate	39	39	39	100	68.0
	ELISA	*L. chagasi* lysate	39	39	39	100	93.6
	IFI® - LVC	*L. major* like promastigotes	39	39	39	100	70.5
	IFAT	*L. chagasi* lysate	39	39	39	100	61.5

First author and year of publication	Serology		Sample			Results	
	Technique	Antigen	(n) Infected dogs confirmed by other techniques	(n) Non-infected dogs	(n) Dogs infected with others pathologies	Sensitivity (%)	Specificity (%)
	DPP® - LVC	rK28	39	39	39	100	97.5
Grimaldi *et al.*, 2012	DPP® - LVC	rK28	120	59	11	A: 47.0 S: 98.0	96.0
Souza *et al.*, 2012	ELISA	rLci1A	138	119	86	96.0	92.0
	ELISA	rLci2B	138	119	86	100	95.0
Barral-Veloso *et al.*, 2013	ELISA	*L. infantum* promastigotes fixed with β-mercaptoethanol	31	37	45	93.5	97.6
	ELISA	*L. infantum* promastigotes fixed with trypsin	31	37	45	87.1	100
Quinnell *et al.*, 2013	RDTs	rK39	322	59	0	46.0	98.7

* Dogs from an endemic area for CVL without confirmed diagnosis.

A: asymptomatic dogs; S: dogs with clinical signs related to CVL; O: oligosymptomatic dogs (presenting one to three clinical signs of CVL); P: polysymptomatic dogs (presenting more than three clinical signs of CVL).

RDTs = Kalazar Detect - Canine Rapid Test

LMS = *L. major* like promastigotes lysate

CTA = Crude Total Antigen - antigenic fractions of *L. infantum* promastigotes form

FML = Fucose-Mannose Ligand antigen - glycoprotein complex isolated from the surface of *L. donovani*

LRP = *Leishmania* species ribosomal proteins

Table 1. Sensitivity and specificity of some serological techniques by type of antigen, and evaluated population

Efforts have been made to improve the efficacy of rapid tests by developing more sensitive and specific method that could be used in mass screening for the diagnosis of CVL. An alternative proposal is to use a mixture of recombinant proteins or chimeric proteins. The protein rK28 chimeric for the relevant epitopes of three antigens, rK9, rK26 and rK39 [87, 108] that showed promising efficient results in an ELISA based test [124], was recently used to compose a new rapid test in DPP format. This format consists of a double track platform that offers greater sensitivity and specificity [125]. In addition, this rapid test has advantages over previously used serological methods due to greater precision, simplified interpretation of the

http://dx.doi.org/10.5772/57573

data, minimal use of sample volumes, and compatibility with different types of body fluids such as blood, serum, saliva, plasma and urine. In contrast to these advantages, recently Grimaldi et al (2012) showed that rK28-based DPP despite its high sensitivity (98%) and specificity (96%) towards sera from symptomatic dogs, showed low sensitivity of only 47% towards sera from dogs with no signs [31]. With regard to sera from dogs with other diseases, the observed specificity was 96%, with false-positive reactions mainly for some sera of dogs infected with *L. braziliensis*. Thus, *L. infantum* may not be detected in serological investigations of asymptomatic infected dogs, leading for perpetuation of the parasite cycle and, consequently, hampering the efficacy of the disease control measures. This limitation is reason for concern because several studies indicate that asymptomatic dogs are involved in transmission of infection to the vector, although this occurs less frequently than with symptomatic dogs [16, 32-34]. Therefore, it is necessary to implement more effective serodiagnostic tests so that there is broader detection of animals infected with *L. infantum* by public health services, contributing to more efficient control of CVL.

3.4. PCR

In recent decades, due to advances in molecular biology techniques and reduced implementation costs, the polymerase chain reaction (PCR) began to be used in VL diagnosis [23, 126]. Its use has demonstrated superior results to those obtained by ELISA, IFA and culture in detecting animals infected with *Leishmania* sp., exhibiting high sensitivity and specificity [23, 126].

PCR is a technique based on the principle of complementary bases pairing of the DNA molecule, allowing amplification and detection of a particular region of the target genome using a pair of specific oligonucleotide primers. The reaction can produce tens of billions of DNA fragments from a single molecule, and has high sensitivity small quantities of samples to be used. This type of PCR, hereafter referred as "conventional PCR" (cPCR) needs electrophoresis in agarose or polyacrylamide gels along with dyes such as ethidium bromide, SYBR Green or silver nitrate to view the amplified product. This approach is usually qualitative, with analysis of the presence or absence of bands, or semi-quantitative, when densitometry of bands is used in comparison with known standards. Since it uses qualitative or semi-quantitative analysis, it is imprecise and generates false negatives with some frequency.

A variant of cPCR called "quantitative real-time PCR" (qPCR) became popular in the 2000s. It uses a quantitative approach that allows real-time monitoring of the amplification of the target PCR fragment using fluorophores that bind to double stranded DNA or linked to probes. The most commonly used method is SYBR Green: fluorophore binds to double stranded DNA molecules produced during amplification of the target fragment, leading to the emission of fluorescence during the PCR. This method has the disadvantage of not being able to directly discriminate the amplification of nonspecific DNA fragments, which is usually solved by analyzing the dissociation curve. In contrast, the TaqMan method uses a probe containing between 13 and 30 nucleotides, specifically for the target sequence and combined with a fluorophore and a fluorescence inhibitor. During polymerization of the target fragment, DNA polymerase degrades the probe and fluorescence is emitted. The use of this technique enables an increase in the specificity of this method.

Various PCR-based protocols have been developed for the detection of parasite's DNA and CVL diagnosis. However, the methods used may vary with respect to several parameters, such as fluorophores, probes, target regions and tissue used for detection of target DNA (Table 2), making it difficult to do a comparative analysis between the different protocols. It is known that the sensitivity and specificity of PCR for detection of *Leishmania* sp. depends on many factors such as the physico-chemical conditions of the reaction, the concentration and nature of the sample DNA, the probes, and oligonucleotide primers selected for the target region [44, 127, 128]. The protocols standardization based on changes in previous parameters is the key step to increased sensitivity, specificity and reproducibility of the tests.

The PCR protocol sensitivity is also affected by the type of tissue used in the detection of *Leishmania* sp. DNA. A wide variety of clinical samples can be used such as blood, lymph node, bone marrow, conjunctiva, skin and spleen. The sensitivity tends to vary, since the parasitic load is not equally distributed in all tissues [4, 7, 129-133]. However, studies have shown that PCR can detect the presence of *Leishmania* DNA in a similar way, even in different tissues as demonstrated by Manna et al. (2004) in a study using 56 dogs naturally infected with *L. infantum*, which evaluated samples from lymph nodes, skin and blood by cPCR obtaining positivity values of 99%, 95% and 94% respectively [133]. Similarly, Ferreira *et al.* (2013), using qPCR, obtained positivity values on the order of 90% for blood samples, 97% for skin biopsy, 98% for conjunctival swab samples and 100% for bone marrow samples [134]. Other studies showed better results for sensitivity to certain tissue, such as Maya et al. (2009) that evaluated dogs with different clinical profiles and demonstrated that the use of cPCR for parasite DNA detection on lymph node aspirate would be ideal for the early CVL diagnosis in symptomatic animals [132], a finding later corroborated by Lombardo et al. (2012) and Belinchon-Lorenzo (2013) [135, 136]. However, in the absence of lymphadenopathy, other studies showed that bone marrow aspirates offered better sensitivity, since it has a higher parasite load in relation to lymph nodes [132, 137]. Studies indicate bone marrow as the tissue in which PCR has greater sensitivity; as reported by Andrade et al. (2002), where bone marrow aspirate gave a sensitivity of 100% [138]. However Ferreira et al (2008) obtained positivity values of only 50% for bone marrow aspirates from asymptomatic and 77% from symptomatic dogs using cPCR followed by hybridization, using cloned kDNA-probes from mini circles of *L. infantum* [139].

The selection of target region in the parasite genome is important because the variation in the number of copies, depending on the region, influences the sensitivity for detecting the parasite's DNA and for quantification of parasite load. The highly conserved and repetitive regions are the most commonly employed, such as the gene for subunit ribosomal RNA (rRNA) or minicircle kinetoplast DNA (kDNA) [21, 23, 127, 140, 141], that has 40-200 copies per cell, while the kDNA minicircles have about 10,000 copies distributed among 10 different classes of sequences. Using this as a target region confers high sensitivity to PCR [142]. For quantification of the parasitic load is recommended to normalize the amount of parasite gene amplification in relation to a constitutive gene derived from the host genome in order to correct distortions caused by errors in the DNA used in the PCR reaction [127].

	qPCR technique		qPCR internal control			Sample		Results	
First author and year of publication	Method and target	Detection limit	Inhib.[a]	Norm.[b]	Control gene employed	(n)	Tissue evaluated	Study design*	Sensitivity**
Ferreira et al. 2012	Syber α pol DNA	NI	Yes	Yes	ß - canine actin	(80) Infected dogs	Conjunctival swab, blood, bone marrow and skin	Comparative[1,2]	Skin > Bone marrow > Conjunctival swab > Blood
Solcà *et al.* 2014[#]	TaqMan kDNA	0.01 parasites/ reaction	Yes	Yes	18S eukaryotic rRNA	(51) Dogs	Bone marrow, conjunctival swab, lymph node, skin and spleen	Comparative[1,2]	Spleen > Blood > Lymph node > Skin > Bone marrow > Conjunctival swab
Belinchón-Lorenzo et al. 2013	TaqMan kDNA	0.0079 parasites/ reaction	Yes	Yes	18S eukaryotic rRNA	(28) Dogs	Blood, hair and lymph node	Comparative[2]	Lymph node > Hair = Blood
Ferreira et al. 2013	Syber α pol DNA	NI	Yes	Yes	ß - canine actin	(62) CVL positive dogs	Conjunctival, nasal and ear swab, blood, Bone marrow and skin	Comparative[1,2]	Skin = Nasal swab and bone marrow > Conjunctival swab > Oral swab > Ear swab
Geisweid et al. 2013	Syber kDNA	NI	Yes	No	Canine NCX1	(74) CVL suspected dogs	Conjunctival swab, blood, bone marrow and lymph node	Comparative[2]	Bone marrow > Conjunctival Swab
Reis *et al.* 2013	Syber α pol DNA	NI	Yes	No	G3PDH	(60) Seropositive dogs	Skin and spleen	Comparative[1,2]	Spleen > Skin
Pennisi *et al.* 2005	NI kDNA	NI	No	No	---	(6) Treated dogs	Blood, lymph node and skin	Not comparative	---
Francino *et al.* 2006	TaqMan kDNA	0.001 parasites/ reaction	Yes	No	18S eukaryotic rRNA	(15) Dogs with clinical signs suggestive of CVL	Blood and bone marrow	Comparative[1,2]	Bone marrow > Blood
Rodriguez-Cortez *et al.* 2007	TaqMan kDNA	0.001 parasites/ reaction	Yes	Yes	18S eukaryotic rRNA	(6) Experimentally infected dogs	Blood, bone marrow, liver, lymph node, skin and spleen	Not comparative	---
Solano-Gallego *et al.* 2007	Syber kDNA	7 parasites/ml	Yes	No	Canine GAPDH	(10) Symptomatic	Blood, bone marrow and urine	Comparative[2]	Bone marrow > Blood

	qPCR technique		qPCR internal control			Sample		Results	
First author and year of publication	Method and target	Detection limit	Inhib.[a]	Norm.[b]	Control gene employed	(n)	Tissue evaluated	Study design*	Sensitivity**
						dogs naturally infected			> Urine
Manna *et al.* 2008	TaqMan kDNA	0.001 parasites/ml	Yes	Yes	ß - actin	(18) Naturally infected treated dogs	Blood, lymph node and skin	Comparative[2]	Lymph node > Skin > Blood
Manna *et al.* 2009	TaqMan kDNA	NI	Yes	Yes	ß - actin	(56) Dogs	Blood and lymph node	Not comparative	---
Quaresma *et al.* 2009	Syber kDNA	0.1pg DNA/ml	Yes	Yes	ß -canine globin	(35) Dogs	Blood and bone marrow	Comparative[2]	Blood = Bone marrow
Maia *et al.* 2010	TaqMan kDNA	1 parasite / reaction	Yes	No	ß - canine actin	(12) Experimentally infected dogs	Blood, bone marrow, buffy coat, liver, lymph node, skin and spleen	Comparative[1, 2]	Spleen / Buffy coat / Liver / Lymph node / Bone marrow / Skin > Blood
Galletti *et al.* 2011	TaqMan kDNA	0.03 parasite/ reaction	No	No	---	(88) Dogs	Conjunctival swab, Lymph node, bone marrow and blood	Comparative[1]	---
Lombardo *et al.* 2011	TaqMan kDNA	NI	No	No	---	(138) Dogs	Blood, conjunctival and oral swabs and lymph node	Comparative[1]	---
Naranjo *et al.* 2011	TaqMan kDNA	NI	Yes	No	18S eukaryotic rRNA	(22) Sick dogs	Main lacrimal gland, tarsal gland and nictitating membrane gland	Comparative[1]	---

* Study design: Comparative[1]: aim to compare different diagnostic techniques results; Comparative[2]: aim to compare different canine tissue sensitivity; ** Sensitivity: evaluation of *Leishmania* sp. detection in the different canine tissues; NI: Not informed; [#] submitted; [a]: qPCR inhibition control; [b]: qPCR normalization control.

Table 2. List of papers using the qPCR technique for *Leishmania* sp. detection in different canine tissues, comparing the different methodologies and the use of internal control of the reaction

In a cytological study, Reis *et al.* (2006) showed that the spleen is a major organ where parasite density is high throughout the course of CVL in both symptomatic and asymptomatic dogs [74]. Saldarriaga et al. (2006) demonstrated in a study using dogs submitted to intradermal experimental infection with promastigotes of *Leishmania* sp. ninety-six hours after inoculation, parasites were found in the lymph nodes and spleen of infected animals [148]. Another study revealed varying degrees of splenomegaly in most dogs infected with *Leishmania* sp. [132]. Reis et al. (2013) found 100% of positivity in spleen samples of 37 infected animals [149]. These findings make the spleen the best choice for the CVL diagnosis employing molecular techniques [150]. Nevertheless, obtaining spleen samples, even if tolerated by the animal, can incur a risk of hemorrhage and internal lesions [150]. However, in a study performed by Barrouin-Melo et al. (2006) in which 257 splenic punctures were performed, only two animals had the intestinal loop aspirated and one animal experienced bleeding at the puncture site [151]. These risks can be minimized by organ visualization using ultrasound devices, which allow a guided and safe collection of tissue sample [152]. In a recent study performed by the present authors, 1,200 dogs were punctured with the aid of ultrasound machine without any incident (unpublished data).

Splenic collection, bone marrow and lymph node aspirates are considered invasive procedures [153] in addition to having an elevated cost compared to blood collection. Thus, it can be recommended to use samples obtained less invasively, such as blood and conjunctival swabs [136, 154, 155]. These samples are quick and easy to obtain, and it is low-cost compared to more invasive procedures, in addition to their higher acceptance by animal owners [132, 154, 155].

Some studies have shown that detection of parasites in the peripheral blood is less sensitive compared to other tissue samples such as spleen, bone marrow, lymph nodes and skin and tends to have variable parasitic load in accordance with the stage of infection [129, 141, 156]. However, depending on the technique and the target, blood can be used for detection of *Leishmania* sp. infection even when there is a low parasitic load [142, 157]. Maia *et al.* (2009) showed that the use of peripheral blood samples, extracted from soaked filter paper, from 29 infected dogs showed 93.1% positivity in cPCR of kDNA, suggesting that this tissue can be used as a complement for serological diagnosis [132]. However, despite blood has the advantage of being less invasive than spleen, bone marrow and lymph node punctures, this tissue contains hemoglobin that may acts as inhibitor to the PCR reaction, which are usually neutralized by the addition of albumin, and also present a high variability in parasite detection, due to the fluctuation of parasitemia according to the stage of infection.

According to Solano-Gallego *et al.* (2001) in comparison to other tissues, skin has the greatest sensitivity [4]. In a study involving 80 naturally infected dogs, Ferreira et al. (2012) showed that skin is the tissue with the higher parasitic load, showing no significant difference between symptomatic and asymptomatic animals [139]. Reis *et al* (2013) used skin samples from 37 animals and by means of qPCR obtained a sensitivity of 97.3% in identifying infected dogs. Nevertheless, other noninvasive samples are being tested for molecular diagnosis of CVL, such as conjunctival swabs [149]. Using this type of sample with cPCR, Ayali-Strauss et al (2004) were able to detect 92% of the symptomatic animals evaluated in the study, using spleen or lymph node aspirates, they detected 86%whereas using peripheral blood or white blood cells they detected, respectively, only 17% and 57% of the infected dogs [158]. Leite et al (2010) also succeeded in detecting the parasite DNA from conjunctival swabs of asymptomatic animals by the technique of cPCR followed by kDNA-probe hybridization [159]. Lombardo (2012) using qPCR technique with conjunctival swabs obtained similar results to those obtained with more invasive samples such as lymph node aspirates [136]. Ferreira *et al.* (2012) used cPCR followed by kDNA-probe hybridization of blood samples, skin, marrow and conjunctival swabs. The use of swabs gave the best results for detection of infection in both symptomatic and asymptomatic dogs, showing to be a suitable sample for the molecular diagnosis of CVL. Furthermore, Di Muccio et al (2012) argue that the use of nested PCR from conjunctival swabs shown to be the least invasive procedure with the best performance for the diagnosis of CVL in asymptomatic animals [156].

Among other less invasive sample types investigated, Solano-Gallego et al (2007) evaluated urine samples with qPCR technique, but the results described showed positivity only in dogs with severe renal injury [160]. Naranjo et al. (2012) identified the presence of *Leishmania* sp. DNA in lacrimal glands of infected dogs using qPCR, with positive correlation between positivity and the presence of ocular lesions [161]. Recently, Belinchon-Lorenzo (2013), using qPCR, demonstrated the presence of *Leishmania* kDNA in the hair and keratinocytes of infected animals. According to the authors, the use of the non-invasive hair sample for the diagnosis of CVL would be advantageous because it is easy to collect, handle, transport, and store [135]. However, further studies should be conducted to determine the sensitivity of this method.

Laboratory – Country	**Tests Price**			
	Serology	**cPCR**	**qPCR**	**qPCR and Citology**
Elleviti – Torino, Italy	26.80*	---	63.00*	---
Scanelis - Toulouse, France	---	---	60.30*	---
Laboratoire d'Anatomie Pathologique Vétérinaire du Sud-Ouest – Toulouse, France	---	---	---	127.30*
Laboratório Veterinário INNO – Braga, Portugal	20.60*	54.40*	---	---
Instituto Nacional de Investigação Agrária e Veterinária, I.P. – Lisbõa, Portugal	28.00*	41.20*	---	---
Centro de Investigación y Análisis Biológicos – Madrid, Spain	13.60*	60.30*	73.70*	---
Texas Veterinary Medical Diagnostic Laboratory – San Antonio TX, USA	19.20	---	---	---
Cornell University - Ithaca NY, USA	22.50	60.00	---	---
Hermes Pardini - Belo Horizonte MG, Brazil	17.20*	60.20*	---	---
Análisis Biológicos– Chapecó SC, Brazil	9.40*	42.15*	72.25*	--
Laborlife - Rio de Janeiro RJ, Brazil	30.10*	77.40*	---	---

*Prices in Euros (€) and Brazilian Real (R$) converted in US dollars (U$), quotation of November 14th of 2013. €1 = aprox. U$ 1.34 - €1 = aprox.R$ 0.43

Table 3. Cost of the main diagnostic test for CVL in different laboratories consulted in the second semester of 2013 in U$

http://dx.doi.org/10.5772/57573

Despite the high sensitivity and specificity, the use of molecular methods for the CVL diagnosis presents some limitations to its use in epidemiological surveys: i) it has higher costs than other techniques (Table 3) used in the CVL diagnosis, including reagent and equipment costs; ii) it presents relative complexity in its implementation, requiring personnel with training in the execution of PCR reactions. However, this method has advantages in terms of sensitivity and specificity when compared to other diagnostic techniques, which justify its use in confirming cases screened by serology [24, 132]. Particularly due to the possibility of quantifying target DNA, qPCR may be used to monitor the parasitic load of the animal during the experimental infection, or during and after treatment in countries where it is permitted [35-37, 162]. Compared with cPCR, qPCR enables a reduction in the probability of false positives resulting from amplification artifacts and greater speed in obtaining results, once electrophoresis is no longer performed [163].

4. Conclusion

In summary, detailed clinical evaluation complemented with highly sensitive test allows proper identification of infected dogs in an endemic area. Evidence shows that the use of a rapid serological test associated with a molecular diagnostic test with high specificity, such as qPCR, is required for identification of all infected dogs, both asymptomatic and symptomatic. On the other hand, for sick dogs a correct diagnosis is necessary either to perform dog culling in countries where this measure is used as a control strategy of VL or to define treatment. In this case, a detailed clinical evaluation should be associated with biochemistry and hematological tests to identify signs of renal and hepatic failure, in conjunction with a serological test to confirm animal clinical condition.

Author details

Patrícia Sampaio Tavares Veras[1,2*], Deborah Bittencourt Mothé Fraga[1,2,3], Manuela da Silva Solcà[1,3] and Carlos Eduardo Sampaio Guedes[1]

*Address all correspondence to: pveras@bahia.fiocruz.br

1 Laboratório de Patologia e Biointervenção, Centro de Pesquisa Gonçalo Moniz–FIOCRUZ, Salvador, Bahia, Brazil

2 Instituto Nacional de Ciência e Tecnologia em Doenças Tropicais (INCT - DT), Salvador, Bahia, Brazil

3 Escola de Medicina Veterinária e Zootecnia, Universidade Federal da Bahia, Salvador, Bahia, Brazil

References

[1] Desjeux P. Leishmaniasis. Nat Rev Microbiol. 2004;2(9):692.

[2] Alvar J, Velez ID, Bern C, Herrero M, Desjeux P, Cano J, et al. Leishmaniasis worldwide and global estimates of its incidence. PLoS One. 2012;7(5):e35671.

[3] Gomes YM, Paiva Cavalcanti M, Lira RA, Abath FG, Alves LC. Diagnosis of canine visceral leishmaniasis: biotechnological advances. Vet J. 2008;175(1):45-52.

[4] Solano-Gallego L, Morell P, Arboix M, Alberola J, Ferrer L. Prevalence of *Leishmania infantum* infection in dogs living in an area of canine leishmaniasis endemicity using PCR on several tissues and serology. J Clin Microbiol. 2001;39(2):560-3.

[5] Ferreira Ede C, de Lana M, Carneiro M, Reis AB, Paes DV, da Silva ES, et al. Comparison of serological assays for the diagnosis of canine visceral leishmaniasis in animals presenting different clinical manifestations. Vet Parasitol. 2007;146(3-4):235-41.

[6] Troncarelli MZ, Camargo JB, Machado JG, Lucheis SB, Langoni H. *Leishmania* spp. and/or *Trypanosoma cruzi* diagnosis in dogs from endemic and nonendemic areas for canine visceral leishmaniasis. Vet Parasitol. 2009;164(2-4):118-23.

[7] Solca Mda S, Guedes CE, Nascimento EG, Oliveira GG, dos Santos WL, Fraga DB, et al. Qualitative and quantitative polymerase chain reaction (PCR) for detection of Leishmania in spleen samples from naturally infected dogs. Vet Parasitol. 2012;184(2-4):133-40.

[8] Mary C, Faraut F, Lascombe L, Dumon H. Quantification of *Leishmania infantum* DNA by a real-time PCR assay with high sensitivity. J Clin Microbiol. 2004;42(11): 5249-55.

[9] Lainson R, Shaw JJ. Epidemiology and ecology of leishmaniasis in Latin-America. Nature. 1978;273(5664):595-600.

[10] Killick-Kendrick R. The biology and control of phlebotomine sand flies. Clin Dermatol. 1999;17(3):279-89.

[11] Kuhls K, Alam MZ, Cupolillo E, Ferreira GE, Mauricio IL, Oddone R, et al. Comparative microsatellite typing of new world *Leishmania infantum* reveals low heterogeneity among populations and its recent old world origin. PLoS Negl Trop Dis. 2011;5(6):e1155.

[12] Mauricio IL, Stothard JR, Miles MA. The strange case of Leishmania chagasi. Parasitol Today. 2000;16(5):188-9.

[13] Alvar J, Canavate C, Molina R, Moreno J, Nieto J. Canine leishmaniasis. Adv Parasitol. 2004;57:1-88.

[14] Bevilacqua PD, Paixao HH, Modena CM, Castro MCPS. Urbanization of visceral leishmaniose in Belo Horizonte, Brazil. Arq Bras Med Vet Zoot. 2001;53:1-8.

[15] Deane LM, Deane MP. Leishmaniose visceral urbana (no cão e no homem) em Sobral, Ceará. O Hospital 1955;47:113-28.

[16] Molina R, Amela C, Nieto J, San-Andres M, Gonzalez F, Castillo JA, et al. Infectivity of dogs naturally infected with *Leishmania infantum* to colonized *Phlebotomus perniciosus*. Trans R Soc Trop Med Hyg. 1994;88(4):491-3.

[17] Gramiccia M, Gradoni L. The current status of zoonotic leishmaniases and approaches to disease control. Int J Parasitol. 2005;35(11-12):1169-80.

[18] Dye C. The logic of visceral leishmaniasis control. Am J Trop Med Hyg. 1996;55(2): 125-30.

[19] Coura-Vital W, Marques MJ, Veloso VM, Roatt BM, Aguiar-Soares RD, Reis LE, et al. Prevalence and factors associated with *Leishmania infantum* infection of dogs from an urban area of Brazil as identified by molecular methods. PLoS Negl Trop Dis. 2011;5(8):e1291.

[20] Podaliri Vulpiani M, Iannetti L, Paganico D, Iannino F, Ferri N. Methods of Control of the *Leishmania infantum* Dog Reservoir: State of the Art. Vet Med Int. 2011;2011:215964.

[21] Miro G, Cardoso L, Pennisi MG, Oliva G, Baneth G. Canine leishmaniosis--new concepts and insights on an expanding zoonosis: part two. Trends Parasitol. 2008;24(8): 371-7.

[22] Carvalho D, S.; OTMF, D.; BC, Z. MR. An enzyme-linked immunosorbent assay (ELISA) for the detection of IgM antibodies against Leishmania chagasi in dogs. Pesq Vet Bras 2009;29:120-4.

[23] Sundar S, Rai M. Laboratory diagnosis of visceral leishmaniasis. Clinical and diagnostic laboratory immunology. 2002;9(5):951-8.

[24] Moreira MA, Luvizotto MC, Garcia JF, Corbett CE, Laurenti MD. Comparison of parasitological, immunological and molecular methods for the diagnosis of leishmaniasis in dogs with different clinical signs. Vet Parasitol. 2007;145(3-4):245-52.

[25] Ndao M. Diagnosis of parasitic diseases: old and new approaches. Interdiscip Perspect Infect Dis. 2009;2009:278246.

[26] Morales-Yuste M, Morillas-Marquez F, Diaz-Saez V, Baron-Lopez S, Acedo-Sanchez C, Martin-Sanchez J. Epidemiological implications of the use of various methods for the diagnosis of canine leishmaniasis in dogs with different characteristics and in differing prevalence scenarios. Parasitol Res. 2012;111(1):155-64.

[27] de Paula AA, da Silva AV, Fernandes O, Jansen AM. The use of immunoblot analysis in the diagnosis of canine visceral leishmaniasis in an endemic area of Rio de Janeiro. J Parasitol. 2003;89(4):832-6.

[28] Almeida MA, Jesus EE, Sousa-Atta ML, Alves LC, Berne ME, Atta AM. Clinical and serological aspects of visceral leishmaniasis in northeast Brazilian dogs naturally infected with Leishmania chagasi. Vet Parasitol. 2005;127(3-4):227-32.

[29] Porrozzi R, Santos da Costa MV, Teva A, Falqueto A, Ferreira AL, dos Santos CD, et al. Comparative evaluation of enzyme-linked immunosorbent assays based on crude and recombinant leishmanial antigens for serodiagnosis of symptomatic and asymptomatic *Leishmania infantum* visceral infections in dogs. Clin Vaccine Immunol. 2007;14(5):544-8.

[30] Quinnell RJ, Carson C, Reithinger R, Garcez LM, Courtenay O. Evaluation of rK39 rapid diagnostic tests for canine visceral leishmaniasis: longitudinal study and meta-analysis. PLoS Negl Trop Dis. 2013;7(1):e1992.

[31] Grimaldi G, Jr., Teva A, Santos CB, Ferreira AL, Falqueto A. The effect of removing potentially infectious dogs on the numbers of canine *Leishmania infantum* infections in an endemic area with high transmission rates. Am J Trop Med Hyg. 2012;86(6): 966-71.

[32] Courtenay O, Quinnell RJ, Garcez LM, Shaw JJ, Dye C. Infectiousness in a cohort of brazilian dogs: why culling fails to control visceral leishmaniasis in areas of high transmission. J Infect Dis. 2002;186(9):1314-20.

[33] Michalsky EM, Rocha MF, da Rocha Lima AC, Franca-Silva JC, Pires MQ, Oliveira FS, et al. Infectivity of seropositive dogs, showing different clinical forms of leishmaniasis, to Lutzomyia longipalpis phlebotomine sand flies. Vet Parasitol. 2007;147(1-2): 67-76.

[34] Soares MR, de Mendonca IL, do Bonfim JM, Rodrigues JA, Werneck GL, Costa CH. Canine visceral leishmaniasis in Teresina, Brazil: Relationship between clinical features and infectivity for sand flies. Acta Trop. 2011;117(1):6-9.

[35] Maia C, Campino L. Methods for diagnosis of canine leishmaniasis and immune response to infection. Vet Parasitol. 2008;158(4):274-87.

[36] Pennisi MG, Reale S, Giudice SL, Masucci M, Caracappa S, Vitale M, et al. Real-time PCR in dogs treated for leishmaniasis with allopurinol. Veterinary research communications. 2005;29 Suppl 2:301-3.

[37] Martinez V, Quilez J, Sanchez A, Roura X, Francino O, Altet L. Canine leishmaniasis: the key points for qPCR result interpretation. Parasit Vectors. 2011;4:57.

[38] Travi BL, Tabares CJ, Cadena H, Ferro C, Osorio Y. Canine visceral leishmaniasis in Colombia: relationship between clinical and parasitologic status and infectivity for sand flies. Am J Trop Med Hyg. 2001;64(3-4):119-24.

[39] Shang LM, Peng WP, Jin HT, Xu D, Zhong NN, Wang WL, et al. The prevalence of canine *Leishmania infantum* infection in Sichuan Province, southwestern China detected by real time PCR. Parasit Vectors. 2011;4(1):173.

[40] Athanasiou LV, Kontos VI, Saridomichelakis MN, Rallis TS, Diakou A. A cross-sectional sero-epidemiological study of canine leishmaniasis in Greek mainland. Acta Trop. 2012;122(3):291-5.

[41] Pastor-Santiago JA, Chavez-Lopez S, Guzman-Bracho C, Flisser A, Olivo-Diaz A. American visceral leishmaniasis in Chiapas, Mexico. Am J Trop Med Hyg. 2012;86(1): 108-14.

[42] Berrahal F, Mary C, Roze M, Berenger A, Escoffier K, Lamouroux D, et al. Canine leishmaniasis: identification of asymptomatic carriers by polymerase chain reaction and immunoblotting. Am J Trop Med Hyg. 1996;55(3):273-7.

[43] Quinnell RJ, Courtenay O, Davidson S, Garcez L, Lambson B, Ramos P, et al. Detection of *Leishmania infantum* by PCR, serology and cellular immune response in a cohort study of Brazilian dogs. Parasitology. 2001;122(Pt 3):253-61.

[44] Lachaud L, Chabbert E, Dubessay P, Dereure J, Lamothe J, Dedet JP, et al. Value of two PCR methods for the diagnosis of canine visceral leishmaniasis and the detection of asymptomatic carriers. Parasitology. 2002;125(Pt 3):197-207.

[45] Leontides LS, Saridomichelakis MN, Billinis C, Kontos V, Koutinas AF, Galatos AD, et al. A cross-sectional study of *Leishmania* spp. infection in clinically healthy dogs with polymerase chain reaction and serology in Greece. Vet Parasitol. 2002;109(1-2): 19-27.

[46] Lanotte G, Rioux JA, Perieres J, Vollhardt Y. [Ecology of leishmaniasis in the south of France. 10. Developmental stages and clinical characterization of canine leishmaniasis in relation to epidemiology. (author's transl]. Ann Parasitol Hum Comp. 1979;54(3):277-95.

[47] Pozio E, Gradoni L, Bettini S, Gramiccia M. Leishmaniasis in Tuscany (Italy) V. Further isolation of Leishmania from Rattus rattus in the Province of Grosseto. Ann Trop Med Parasitol. 1981;75(4):393-5.

[48] Moreno J, Alvar J. Canine leishmaniasis: epidemiological risk and the experimental model. Trends Parasitol. 2002;18(9):399-405.

[49] Moreno J, Nieto J, Chamizo C, Gonzalez F, Blanco F, Barker DC, et al. The immune response and PBMC subsets in canine visceral leishmaniasis before, and after, chemotherapy. Vet Immunol Immunopathol. 1999;71(3-4):181-95.

[50] Quinnell RJ, Courtenay O, Garcez LM, Kaye PM, Shaw MA, Dye C, et al. IgG subclass responses in a longitudinal study of canine visceral leishmaniasis. Vet Immunol Immunopathol. 2003;91(3-4):161-8.

[51] Vercosa BL, Lemos CM, Mendonca IL, Silva SM, de Carvalho SM, Goto H, et al. Transmission potential, skin inflammatory response, and parasitism of symptomatic and asymptomatic dogs with visceral leishmaniasis. BMC Vet Res. 2008;4:45.

[52] Guarga JL, Lucientes J, Peribanez MA, Molina R, Gracia MJ, Castillo JA. Experimental infection of *Phlebotomus perniciosus* and determination of the natural infection rates of *Leishmania infantum* in dogs. Acta Trop. 2000;77(2):203-7.

[53] Miles MA, Vexenat JA, Furtado Campos JH, Fonseca de Castro JA. Canine leishmaniasis in Latin América: control strategies for visceral leishmaniasis. Canine Leishmaniasis: an update. 1999;Hoechst Roussel Vet.:46-53.

[54] Moshfe A, Mohebali M, Edrissian G, Zarei Z, Akhoundi B, Kazemi B, et al. Canine visceral leishmaniasis: asymptomatic infected dogs as a source of L. *infantum* infection. Acta Trop. 2009;112(2):101-5.

[55] Banuls AL, Hide M, Prugnolle F. Leishmania and the leishmaniases: a parasite genetic update and advances in taxonomy, epidemiology and pathogenicity in humans. Adv Parasitol. 2007;64:1-109.

[56] Grimaldi G, Jr., Tesh RB. Leishmaniases of the New World: current concepts and implications for future research. Clin Microbiol Rev. 1993;6(3):230-50.

[57] Gontijo CM, Melo MN. Visceral Leishmaniasis in Brazil: current status, challenges and prospects. . Rev Bras Epidemiol 2004;7(3):338-49.

[58] Ferrer L. International canine Leishmaniasis forum. Proceedings. 1999:6-10.

[59] Srivastava P, Dayama A, Mehrotra S, Sundar S. Diagnosis of visceral leishmaniasis. Trans R Soc Trop Med Hyg. 2011;105(1):1-6.

[60] Alves WA, Bevilacqua PD. Quality of diagnosis of canine visceral leishmaniasis in epidemiological surveys: an epidemic in Belo Horizonte, Minas Gerais, Brazil, 1993 – 1997. Cad Saúde Pública. 2004;20(1):259-65.

[61] Barrouin-Melo SM, Larangeira DF, Trigo J, Aguiar PH, dos-Santos WL, Pontes-de-Carvalho L. Comparison between splenic and lymph node aspirations as sampling methods for the parasitological detection of Leishmania chagasi infection in dogs. Mem Inst Oswaldo Cruz. 2004;99(2):195-7.

[62] Cabral M, O'Grady J, Alexander J. Demonstration of Leishmania specific cell mediated and humoral immunity in asymptomatic dogs. Parasite Immunol. 1992;14(5): 531-9.

[63] Solano-Gallego L, Llull J, Ramos G, Riera C, Arboix M, Alberola J, et al. The Ibizian hound presents a predominantly cellular immune response against natural Leishmania infection. Vet Parasitol. 2000;90(1-2):37-45.

[64] Saridomichelakis MN. Advances in the pathogenesis of canine leishmaniosis: epidemiologic and diagnostic implications. Vet Dermatol. 2009;20(5-6):471-89.

[65] Benderitter T, Casanova P, Nashkidachvili L, Quilici M. Glomerulonephritis in dogs with canine leishmaniasis. Ann Trop Med Parasitol. 1988;82(4):335-41.

[66] Ciaramella P, Oliva G, Luna RD, Gradoni L, Ambrosio R, Cortese L, et al. A retrospective clinical study of canine leishmaniasis in 150 dogs naturally infected by *Leishmania infantum*. Vet Rec. 1997;141(21):539-43.

[67] Koutinas AF, Polizopoulou ZS, Saridomichelakis MN, Argyriadis D, Fytianou A, Plevraki KG. Clinical considerations on canine visceral leishmaniasis in Greece: a retrospective study of 158 cases (1989-1996). J Am Anim Hosp Assoc. 1999;35(5):376-83.

[68] Mendonça L, Alves LC, Faustino MAG, Vasconcelos JR. Clinical aspects of visceral Leishmania in naturally infected dogs in the of Teresina, Piauí. Revista Brasileira Parasitologia Veterinaria. 1998 8(1):23-5.

[69] Shaw SE, Langton DA, Hillman TJ. Canine leishmaniosis in the United Kingdom: a zoonotic disease waiting for a vector? Vet Parasitol. 2009;163(4):281-5.

[70] Solano-Gallego L, Miro G, Koutinas A, Cardoso L, Pennisi MG, Ferrer L, et al. LeishVet guidelines for the practical management of canine leishmaniosis. Parasit Vectors. 2011;4:86.

[71] Ferrer L, Aisa MJ, Roura X, Portus M. Serological diagnosis and treatment of canine leishmaniasis. Vet Rec. 1995;136(20):514-6.

[72] Ordeix L, Solano-Gallego L, Fondevila D, Ferrer L, Fondati A. Papular dermatitis due to *Leishmania* spp. infection in dogs with parasite-specific cellular immune responses. Vet Dermatol. 2005;16(3):187-91.

[73] Baneth G, Koutinas AF, Solano-Gallego L, Bourdeau P, Ferrer L. Canine leishmaniosis - new concepts and insights on an expanding zoonosis: part one. Trends Parasitol. 2008;24(7):324-30.

[74] Reis AB, Teixeira-Carvalho A, Giunchetti RC, Guerra LL, Carvalho MG, Mayrink W, et al. Phenotypic features of circulating leucocytes as immunological markers for clinical status and bone marrow parasite density in dogs naturally infected by Leishmania chagasi. Clin Exp Immunol. 2006;146(2):303-11.

[75] Tropia de Abreu R, Carvalho M, Carneiro CM, Giunchetti RC, Teixeira-Carvalho A, Martins-Filho OA, et al. Influence of clinical status and parasite load on erythropoiesis and leucopoiesis in dogs naturally infected with *Leishmania (Leishmania) chagasi*. PLoS One. 2011;6(5):e18873.

[76] Cortese L, Sica M, Piantedosi D, Ruggiero G, Pero ME, Terrazzano G, et al. Secondary immune-mediated thrombocytopenia in dogs naturally infected by *Leishmania infantum*. Vet Rec. 2009;164(25):778-82.

[77] Reis AB, Teixeira-Carvalho A, Vale AM, Marques MJ, Giunchetti RC, Mayrink W, et al. Isotype patterns of immunoglobulins: hallmarks for clinical status and tissue para-

site density in Brazilian dogs naturally infected by *Leishmania (Leishmania) chagasi*. Vet Immunol Immunopathol. 2006;112(3-4):102-16.

[78] Palma G, Gutierrez Y. Laboratory diagnosis of Leishmania. Clin Lab Med. 1991;11(4): 909-22.

[79] de Almeida ME, Steurer FJ, Koru O, Herwaldt BL, Pieniazek NJ, da Silva AJ. Identification of *Leishmania* spp. by molecular amplification and DNA sequencing analysis of a fragment of rRNA internal transcribed spacer 2. J Clin Microbiol. 2011;49(9): 3143-9.

[80] Paltrinieri S, Ravicini S, Rossi G, Roura X. Serum concentrations of the derivatives of reactive oxygen metabolites (d-ROMs) in dogs with leishmaniosis. Vet J. 2010;186(3): 393-5.

[81] Fraga DB, Solca MS, Silva VM, Borja LS, Nascimento EG, Oliveira GG, et al. Temporal distribution of positive results of tests for detecting Leishmania infection in stray dogs of an endemic area of visceral leishmaniasis in the Brazilian tropics: a 13 years survey and association with human disease. Vet Parasitol. 2012;190(3-4):591-4.

[82] da Silva RN, Amorim AC, Brandao RM, de Andrade HM, Yokoo M, Ribeiro ML, et al. Real-time PCR in clinical practice: a powerful tool for evaluating Leishmania chagasi loads in naturally infected dogs. Ann Trop Med Parasitol. 2010;104(2):137-43.

[83] Pinelli E, Killick-Kendrick R, Wagenaar J, Bernadina W, del Real G, Ruitenberg J. Cellular and humoral immune responses in dogs experimentally and naturally infected with *Leishmania infantum*. Infect Immun. 1994;62(1):229-35.

[84] Dos-Santos WL, Jesus EE, Paranhos-Silva M, Pereira AM, Santos JC, Baleeiro CO, et al. Associations among immunological, parasitological and clinical parameters in canine visceral leishmaniasis: Emaciation, spleen parasitism, specific antibodies and leishmanin skin test reaction. Vet Immunol Immunopathol. 2008;123(3-4):251-9.

[85] Ferrer L. Clinical aspects of canine leishmaniasis. International Canine Leishmaniasis forum, Barcelona. 1999:6-10.

[86] da Silva ES, van der Meide WF, Schoone GJ, Gontijo CM, Schallig HD, Brazil RP. Diagnosis of canine leishmaniasis in the endemic area of Belo Horizonte, Minas Gerais, Brazil by parasite, antibody and DNA detection assays. Vet Res Commun. 2006;30(6): 637-43.

[87] Boarino A, Scalone A, Gradoni L, Ferroglio E, Vitale F, Zanatta R, et al. Development of recombinant chimeric antigen expressing immunodominant B epitopes of *Leishmania infantum* for serodiagnosis of visceral leishmaniasis. Clin Diagn Lab Immunol. 2005;12(5):647-53.

[88] Lira RA, Cavalcanti MP, Nakazawa M, Ferreira AG, Silva ED, Abath FG, et al. Canine visceral leishmaniosis: a comparative analysis of the EIE-leishmaniose-visceral-

canina-Bio-Manguinhos and the IFI-leishmaniose-visceral-canina-Bio-Manguinhos kits. Vet Parasitol. 2006;137(1-2):11-6.

[89] Ferroglio E, Centaro E, Mignone W, Trisciuoglio A. Evaluation of an ELISA rapid device for the serological diagnosis of *Leishmania infantum* infection in dog as compared with immunofluorescence assay and Western blot. Vet Parasitol. 2007;144(1-2):162-6.

[90] Alves AS, Mouta-Confort E, Figueiredo FB, Oliveira RV, Schubach AO, Madeira MF. Evaluation of serological cross-reactivity between canine visceral leishmaniasis and natural infection by *Trypanosoma caninum*. Res Vet Sci. 2012;93(3):1329-33.

[91] Reithinger R, Davies CR. Canine leishmaniasis: novel strategies for control. Trends Parasitol. 2002;18(7):289-90.

[92] Figueiredo MM, Moura EP, Costa MM, Ribeiro VM, Michalick MS, Tafuri WL, et al. Histopathological and parasitological investigations of ear healthy skin of dogs naturally and experimentally infected with *Leishmania (Leishmania) chagasi*. Histol Histopathol. 2010;25(7):877-87.

[93] el Harith A, Slappendel RJ, Reiter I, van Knapen F, de Korte P, Huigen E, et al. Application of a direct agglutination test for detection of specific anti-Leishmania antibodies in the canine reservoir. J Clin Microbiol. 1989;27(10):2252-7.

[94] el Safi SH, Evans DA. A comparison of the direct agglutination test and enzyme-linked immunosorbent assay in the sero-diagnosis of leishmaniasis in the Sudan. Trans R Soc Trop Med Hyg. 1989;83(3):334-7.

[95] Babakhan L, Mohebali M, Akhoundi B, Edrissian GH, Keshavarz H. Rapid detection of *Leishmania infantum* infection in dogs: a comparative study using fast agglutination screening test (FAST) and direct agglutination test (DAT) in Iran. Parasitol Res. 2009;105(3):717-20.

[96] Schallig HD, Canto-Cavalheiro M, da Silva ES. Evaluation of the direct agglutination test and the rK39 dipstick test for the sero-diagnosis of visceral leishmaniasis. Mem Inst Oswaldo Cruz. 2002;97(7):1015-8.

[97] Sundar S, Maurya R, Singh RK, Bharti K, Chakravarty J, Parekh A, et al. Rapid, noninvasive diagnosis of visceral leishmaniasis in India: comparison of two immunochromatographic strip tests for detection of anti-K39 antibody. J Clin Microbiol. 2006;44(1):251-3.

[98] Mohammadiha A, Haghighi A, Mohebali M, Mahdian R, Abadi AR, Zarei Z, et al. Canine visceral leishmaniasis: a comparative study of real-time PCR, conventional PCR, and direct agglutination on sera for the detection of *Leishmania infantum* infection. Vet Parasitol. 2013;192(1-3):83-90.

[99] Moreira ED, Jr., Mendes de Souza VM, Sreenivasan M, Nascimento EG, Pontes de Carvalho L. Assessment of an optimized dog-culling program in the dynamics of canine Leishmania transmission. Vet Parasitol. 2004;122(4):245-52.

[100] Kar K. Serodiagnosis of leishmaniasis. Crit Rev Microbiol. 1995;21(2):123-52.

[101] Candido TC, Perri SH, Gerzoschkwitz Tde O, Luvizotto MC, de Lima VM. Comparative evaluation of enzyme-linked immunosorbent assay based on crude and purified antigen in the diagnosis of canine visceral leishmaniasis in symptomatic and oligosymptomatic dogs. Vet Parasitol. 2008;157(3-4):175-81.

[102] Coelho EA, Ramirez L, Costa MA, Coelho VT, Martins VT, Chavez-Fumagalli MA, et al. Specific serodiagnosis of canine visceral leishmaniasis using Leishmania species ribosomal protein extracts. Clin Vaccine Immunol. 2009;16(12):1774-80.

[103] Silva DA, Madeira MF, Teixeira AC, de Souza CM, Figueiredo FB. Laboratory tests performed on Leishmania seroreactive dogs euthanized by the leishmaniasis control program. Vet Parasitol. 2011;179(1-3):257-61.

[104] Nolan TJ, Herman R. Effects of long-term in vitro cultivation on Leishmania donovani promastigotes. J Protozool. 1985;32(1):70-5.

[105] Faria AR, Costa MM, Giusta MS, Grimaldi G, Jr., Penido ML, Gazzinelli RT, et al. High-throughput analysis of synthetic peptides for the immunodiagnosis of canine visceral leishmaniasis. PLoS Negl Trop Dis. 2011;5(9):e1310.

[106] Oliveira GG, Magalhaes FB, Teixeira MC, Pereira AM, Pinheiro CG, Santos LR, et al. Characterization of novel *Leishmania infantum* recombinant proteins encoded by genes from five families with distinct capacities for serodiagnosis of canine and human visceral leishmaniasis. Am J Trop Med Hyg. 2011;85(6):1025-34.

[107] Scalone A, De Luna R, Oliva G, Baldi L, Satta G, Vesco G, et al. Evaluation of the Leishmania recombinant K39 antigen as a diagnostic marker for canine leishmaniasis and validation of a standardized enzyme-linked immunosorbent assay. Vet Parasitol. 2002;104(4):275-85.

[108] Rosati S, Ortoffi M, Profiti M, Mannelli A, Mignone W, Bollo E, et al. Prokaryotic expression and antigenic characterization of three recombinant Leishmania antigens for serological diagnosis of canine leishmaniasis. Clin Diagn Lab Immunol. 2003;10(6): 1153-6.

[109] de Souza CM, Silva ED, Ano Bom AP, Bastos RC, Nascimento HJ, da Silva Junior JG. Evaluation of an ELISA for canine leishmaniasis immunodiagnostic using recombinant proteins. Parasite Immunol. 2012;34(1):1-7.

[110] de Lima VM, Fattori KR, Michelin Ade F, da Silveira Neto L, Vasconcelos Rde O. Comparison between ELISA using total antigen and immunochromatography with antigen rK39 in the diagnosis of canine visceral leishmaniasis. Vet Parasitol. 2010;173(3-4):330-3.

[111] Vuylsteke B, Semde G, Sika L, Crucitti T, Ettiegne Traore V, Buve A, et al. HIV and STI prevalence among female sex workers in Cote d'Ivoire: why targeted prevention programs should be continued and strengthened. PLoS One. 2012;7(3):e32627.

[112] Wu W, Huang L, Mendez S. A live *Leishmania major* vaccine containing CpG motifs induces the de novo generation of Th17 cells in C57BL/6 mice. Eur J Immunol. 2010;40(9):2517-27.

[113] Badaro R, Benson D, Eulalio MC, Freire M, Cunha S, Netto EM, et al. rK39: a cloned antigen of Leishmania chagasi that predicts active visceral leishmaniasis. J Infect Dis. 1996;173(3):758-61.

[114] Burns JM, Jr., Shreffler WG, Benson DR, Ghalib HW, Badaro R, Reed SG. Molecular characterization of a kinesin-related antigen of Leishmania chagasi that detects specific antibody in African and American visceral leishmaniasis. Proc Natl Acad Sci U S A. 1993;90(2):775-9.

[115] de Carvalho LP, Soto M, Jeronimo S, Dondji B, Bacellar O, Luz V, et al. Characterization of the immune response to *Leishmania infantum* recombinant antigens. Microbes Infect. 2003;5(1):7-12.

[116] Ferroglio E, Zanet S, Mignone W, Poggi M, Trisciuoglio A, Bianciardi P. Evaluation of a rapid device for serological diagnosis of *Leishmania infantum* infection in dogs as an alternative to immunofluorescence assay and Western blotting. Clin Vaccine Immunol. 2013;20(5):657-9.

[117] Kumar D, Khanal B, Tiwary P, Mudavath SL, Tiwary NK, Singh R, et al. Comparative evaluation of blood and serum samples in rapid immunochromatographic tests for visceral leishmaniasis. J Clin Microbiol. 2013;51(12):3955-9.

[118] Lemos EM, Laurenti MD, Moreira MA, Reis AB, Giunchetti RC, Raychaudhuri S, et al. Canine visceral leishmaniasis: performance of a rapid diagnostic test (Kalazar Detect) in dogs with and without signs of the disease. Acta Trop. 2008;107(2):205-7.

[119] Mettler M, Grimm F, Capelli G, Camp H, Deplazes P. Evaluation of enzyme-linked immunosorbent assays, an immunofluorescent-antibody test, and two rapid tests (immunochromatographic-dipstick and gel tests) for serological diagnosis of symptomatic and asymptomatic Leishmania infections in dogs. J Clin Microbiol. 2005;43(11):5515-9.

[120] Otranto D, Paradies P, Sasanelli M, Spinelli R, Brandonisio O. Rapid immunochromatographic test for serodiagnosis of canine leishmaniasis. J Clin Microbiol. 2004;42(6):2769-70.

[121] Otranto D, Paradies P, Sasanelli M, Leone N, de Caprariis D, Chirico J, et al. Recombinant K39 dipstick immunochromatographic test: a new tool for the serodiagnosis of canine leishmaniasis. J Vet Diagn Invest. 2005;17(1):32-7.

[122] Mohebali M, Khamesipour A, Mobedi I, Zarei Z, Hashemi-Fesharki R. Double-blind randomized efficacy field trial of alum precipitated autoclaved *Leishmania major* vaccine mixed with BCG against canine visceral leishmaniasis in Meshkin-Shahr district, I.R. Iran. Vaccine. 2004;22(29-30):4097-100.

[123] Reithinger R, Quinnell RJ, Alexander B, Davies CR. Rapid detection of *Leishmania infantum* infection in dogs: comparative study using an immunochromatographic dipstick test, enzyme-linked immunosorbent assay, and PCR. J Clin Microbiol. 2002;40(7):2352-6.

[124] Costa MM, Penido M, dos Santos MS, Doro D, de Freitas E, Michalick MS, et al. Improved canine and human visceral leishmaniasis immunodiagnosis using combinations of synthetic peptides in enzyme-linked immunosorbent assay. PLoS Negl Trop Dis. 2012;6(5):e1622.

[125] Pattabhi S, Whittle J, Mohamath R, El-Safi S, Moulton GG, Guderian JA, et al. Design, development and evaluation of rK28-based point-of-care tests for improving rapid diagnosis of visceral leishmaniasis. PLoS Negl Trop Dis. 2010;4(9).

[126] de Paiva Cavalcanti M, Felinto de Brito ME, de Souza WV, de Miranda Gomes Y, Abath FG. The development of a real-time PCR assay for the quantification of *Leishmania infantum* DNA in canine blood. Vet J. 2009;182(2):356-8.

[127] Bastien P, Procop GW, Reischl U. Quantitative real-time PCR is not more sensitive than "conventional" PCR. J Clin Microbiol. 2008;46(6):1897-900.

[128] Lachaud L, Chabbert E, Dubessay P, Reynes J, Lamothe J, Bastien P. Comparison of various sample preparation methods for PCR diagnosis of visceral leishmaniasis using peripheral blood. J Clin Microbiol. 2001;39(2):613-7.

[129] Fisa R, Riera C, Gallego M, Manubens J, Portus M. Nested PCR for diagnosis of canine leishmaniosis in peripheral blood, lymph node and bone marrow aspirates. Vet Parasitol. 2001;99(2):105-11.

[130] Francino O, Altet L, Sanchez-Robert E, Rodriguez A, Solano-Gallego L, Alberola J, et al. Advantages of real-time PCR assay for diagnosis and monitoring of canine leishmaniosis. Vet Parasitol. 2006;137(3-4):214-21.

[131] Galletti E, Bonilauri P, Bardasi L, Fontana MC, Ramini M, Renzi M, et al. Development of a minor groove binding probe based real-time PCR for the diagnosis and quantification of *Leishmania infantum* in dog specimens. Res Vet Sci. 2011;91(2):243-5.

[132] Maia C, Ramada J, Cristovao JM, Goncalves L, Campino L. Diagnosis of canine leishmaniasis: conventional and molecular techniques using different tissues. Vet J. 2009;179(1):142-4.

[133] Manna L, Vitale F, Reale S, Caracappa S, Pavone LM, Morte RD, et al. Comparison of different tissue sampling for PCR-based diagnosis and follow-up of canine visceral leishmaniosis. Vet Parasitol. 2004;125(3-4):251-62.

[134] Ferreira Sde A, Almeida GG, Silva Sde O, Vogas GP, Fujiwara RT, de Andrade AS, et al. Nasal, oral and ear swabs for canine visceral leishmaniasis diagnosis: new practical approaches for detection of *Leishmania infantum* DNA. PLoS Negl Trop Dis. 2013;7(4):e2150.

[135] Belinchon-Lorenzo S, Iniesta V, Parejo JC, Fernandez-Cotrina J, Munoz-Madrid R, Soto M, et al. Detection of *Leishmania infantum* kinetoplast minicircle DNA by Real Time PCR in hair of dogs with leishmaniosis. Vet Parasitol. 2013;192(1-3):43-50.

[136] Lombardo G, Pennisi MG, Lupo T, Migliazzo A, Capri A, Solano-Gallego L. Detection of *Leishmania infantum* DNA by real-time PCR in canine oral and conjunctival swabs and comparison with other diagnostic techniques. Vet Parasitol. 2012;184(1): 10-7.

[137] Quaresma PF, Murta SM, Ferreira Ede C, da Rocha-Lima AC, Xavier AA, Gontijo CM. Molecular diagnosis of canine visceral leishmaniasis: identification of Leishmania species by PCR-RFLP and quantification of parasite DNA by real-time PCR. Acta Trop. 2009;111(3):289-94.

[138] Andrade HM, de Toledo Vde P, Marques MJ, Franca Silva JC, Tafuri WL, Mayrink W, et al. *Leishmania (Leishmania) chagasi* is not vertically transmitted in dogs. Vet Parasitol. 2002;103(1-2):71-81.

[139] Ferreira Sde A, Ituassu LT, de Melo MN, de Andrade AS. Evaluation of the conjunctival swab for canine visceral leishmaniasis diagnosis by PCR-hybridization in Minas Gerais State, Brazil. Vet Parasitol. 2008;152(3-4):257-63.

[140] Antinori S, Calattini S, Longhi E, Bestetti G, Piolini R, Magni C, et al. Clinical use of polymerase chain reaction performed on peripheral blood and bone marrow samples for the diagnosis and monitoring of visceral leishmaniasis in HIV-infected and HIV-uninfected patients: a single-center, 8-year experience in Italy and review of the literature. Clin Infect Dis. 2007;44(12):1602-10.

[141] Reale S, Maxia L, Vitale F, Glorioso NS, Caracappa S, Vesco G. Detection of *Leishmania infantum* in dogs by PCR with lymph node aspirates and blood. J Clin Microbiol. 1999;37(9):2931-5.

[142] Lachaud L, Marchergui-Hammami S, Chabbert E, Dereure J, Dedet JP, Bastien P. Comparison of six PCR methods using peripheral blood for detection of canine visceral leishmaniasis. J Clin Microbiol. 2002;40(1):210-5.

[143] Rodriguez-Cortes A, Ojeda A, Lopez-Fuertes L, Timon M, Altet L, Solano-Gallego L, et al. A long term experimental study of canine visceral leishmaniasis. International journal for parasitology. 2007;37(6):683-93.

[144] Manna L, Gravino AE, Picillo E, Decaro N, Buonavoglia C. *Leishmania* DNA quantification by real-time PCR in naturally infected dogs treated with miltefosine. Ann NY Acad Sci. 2008;1149:358-60.

[145] Manna L, Reale S, Vitale F, Gravino AE. Evidence for a relationship between *Leishmania* load and clinical manifestations. Res Vet Sci. 2009;87(1):76-8.

[146] Maia C, Nunes M, Cristovao J, Campino L. Experimental canine leishmaniasis: clinical, parasitological and serological follow-up. Acta Trop. 2010;116(3):193-9.

[147] Naranjo C, Fondevila D, Altet L, Francino O, Rios J, Roura X, et al. Evaluation of the presence of *Leishmania* spp. by real-time PCR in the lacrimal glands of dogs with leishmaniosis. Vet J. 2011.

[148] Saldarriaga OA, Travi BL, Park W, Perez LE, Melby PC. Immunogenicity of a multicomponent DNA vaccine against visceral leishmaniasis in dogs. Vaccine. 2006;24(11): 1928-40.

[149] Reis LE, Coura-Vital W, Roatt BM, Bouillet LE, Ker HG, Fortes de Brito RC, et al. Molecular diagnosis of canine visceral leishmaniasis: a comparative study of three methods using skin and spleen from dogs with natural *Leishmania infantum* infection. Vet Parasitol. 2013;197(3-4):498-503.

[150] Leveille R, Partington BP, Biller DS, Miyabayashi T. Complications after ultrasound-guided biopsy of abdominal structures in dogs and cats: 246 cases (1984-1991). Journal of the American Veterinary Medical Association. 1993;203(3):413-5.

[151] Barrouin-Melo SM, Larangeira DF, de Andrade Filho FA, Trigo J, Juliao FS, Franke CR, et al. Can spleen aspirations be safely used for the parasitological diagnosis of canine visceral leishmaniosis? A study on assymptomatic and polysymptomatic animals. Vet J. 2006;171(2):331-9.

[152] Watson AT, Penninck D, Knoll JS, Keating JH, Sutherland-Smith J. Safety and correlation of test results of combined ultrasound-guided fine-needle aspiration and needle core biopsy of the canine spleen. Veterinary radiology & ultrasound : the official journal of the American College of Veterinary Radiology and the International Veterinary Radiology Association. 2011;52(3):317-22.

[153] Carvalho D, Oliveira TMFS, Baldani CD, Machado RZ. An enzyme-linked immunosorbent assay (ELISA) for the detection of IgM antibodies against Leishmania chagasi in dogs. Pesq Vet Bras 2009;29:120-4.

[154] Aoun O, Mary C, Roqueplo C, Marie JL, Terrier O, Levieuge A, et al. Canine leishmaniasis in south-east of France: screening of *Leishmania infantum* antibodies (western blotting, ELISA) and parasitaemia levels by PCR quantification. Vet Parasitol. 2009;166(1-2):27-31.

[155] de Almeida Ferreira S, Leite RS, Ituassu LT, Almeida GG, Souza DM, Fujiwara RT, et al. Canine skin and conjunctival swab samples for the detection and quantification of *Leishmania infantum* DNA in an endemic urban area in Brazil. PLoS Negl Trop Dis. 2012;6(4):e1596.

[156] Di Muccio T, Veronesi F, Antognoni MT, Onofri A, Piergili Fioretti D, Gramiccia M. Diagnostic value of conjunctival swab sampling associated with nested PCR for different categories of dogs naturally exposed to *Leishmania infantum* infection. J Clin Microbiol. 2012;50(8):2651-9.

[157] Nasereddin A, Ereqat S, Azmi K, Baneth G, Jaffe CL, Abdeen Z. Serological survey with PCR validation for canine visceral leishmaniasis in northern Palestine. J Parasitol. 2006;92(1):178-83.

[158] Strauss-Ayali D, Jaffe CL, Burshtain O, Gonen L, Baneth G. Polymerase chain reaction using noninvasively obtained samples, for the detection of *Leishmania infantum* DNA in dogs. J Infect Dis. 2004;189(9):1729-33.

[159] Leite RS, Ferreira Sde A, Ituassu LT, de Melo MN, de Andrade AS. PCR diagnosis of visceral leishmaniasis in asymptomatic dogs using conjunctival swab samples. Vet Parasitol. 2010;170(3-4):201-6.

[160] Solano-Gallego L, Rodriguez-Cortes A, Trotta M, Zampieron C, Razia L, Furlanello T, et al. Detection of *Leishmania infantum* DNA by fret-based real-time PCR in urine from dogs with natural clinical leishmaniosis. Vet Parasitol. 2007;147(3-4):315-9.

[161] Naranjo C, Fondevila D, Altet L, Francino O, Rios J, Roura X, et al. Evaluation of the presence of *Leishmania* spp. by real-time PCR in the lacrimal glands of dogs with leishmaniosis. Vet J. 2012;193(1):168-73.

[162] Manna L, Reale S, Picillo E, Vitale F, Gravino AE. Urine sampling for real-time polymerase chain reaction based diagnosis of canine leishmaniasis. J Vet Diagn Invest. 2008;20(1):64-7.

[163] Rolao N, Cortes S, Rodrigues OR, Campino L. Quantification of *Leishmania infantum* parasites in tissue biopsies by real-time polymerase chain reaction and polymerase chain reaction-enzyme-linked immunosorbent assay. J Parasitol. 2004;90(5):1150-4.

Section 3

Prevention and Treatment of Leishmaniasis

Chapter 13

Can Attenuated *Leishmania* Induce Equally Effective Protection as Virulent Strains in Visceral Leishmaniasis?

Joana Cunha, Eugenia Carrillo, Javier Moreno and
Anabela Cordeiro-da-Silva

Additional information is available at the end of the chapter

http://dx.doi.org/10.5772/57214

1. Introduction

The principle of antimicrobial vaccines is to increase immunity against a specific infectious agent so when the individual is challenged by that agent the appropriate immune response is mounted rapidly and efficiently. Vaccines for infectious agents have historically developed from whole live or dead microorganisms to more defined native or recombinant pure fractions, following antigen-coding DNA and the latest approaches of antigen-pulsed dendritic cells. Although bacterial and viral infections have a quite long list of effective vaccines, parasitic infections – from worms to protozoa – have been a hard challenge for researchers to be able to develop proper vaccines. Currently, the most advanced anti-parasitic vaccine is the RTS,S/AS01 for malaria with a protection that covers 30-40% [1]. Despite several attempts during seven decades of research with some promising approaches, so far there is no vaccine available for human leishmaniasis and the options available for veterinary use have zone-restricted market authorization, being inaccessible to many endemic countries.

Traditionally, live vaccines incorporate attenuated strains that after entering the host cause a non-pathological short-lived infection, being rapidly controlled by the innate and adaptive immune systems. In few words, the microorganism is taken up and processed by antigen presenting cells (APCs) that efficiently expose the microbial antigens *via* MHC class I or MHC class II molecules, activating the cognate T cell receptors (TCRs) on the surface of $CD8^+$ or $CD4^+$ T cells, respectively. From here, the effector cellular and humoral machinery develop a specific response aiming to eliminate the aggressor. When a sterile cure (*i.e.* complete elimination of the microorganisms) is achieved, a contraction in all the effectors takes place, though specific central memory T cells and antibodies endure [2], being ready to initiate a stronger response upon a second encounter with a similar microorganism. However, the abidance time of memory is highly dependent on the strength of the primary response. Studies using mice models have shown that small numbers of parasites restricted to the inoculation site, without causing clinical manifestations, are essential for protection from a virulent challenge [3], indicating that antigen persistence is of major importance in a vaccination protocol for leishmaniasis. In fact, this is the concept behind the leishmanization strategy applied in humans.

In this chapter we address some general aspects of the epidemiology of human and canine leishmaniasis to introduce the needs for a vaccine and the desirable immune response to be generated upon vaccination. We present the animal models most commonly used in leishmaniasis vaccine research, the road so far travelled by the scientific community attempting to discover the vaccine for leishmaniasis and its current status. Finally, we show our experimental study in BALB/c mice about the influence of a primary infection of *Leishmania infantum* on the outcome of a *de novo* infection with a homologous or heterologous strain with distinct infectivity and immunomodulation.

1.1. Human leishmaniasis

Leishmaniasis is endemic in 98 countries and 3 territories ranging the Mediterranean Basin, the Middle East, the Indian sub-continent, and the tropical regions from America and Africa [4]. The last WHO report on the epidemiology of leishmaniasis estimates that every year 0.7 to 1.2 million new cases of cutaneous leishmaniasis (CL) are mounted and 0.2 to 0.4 million people develop visceral leishmaniasis (VL) which, in turn, is responsible for 20000 to 40000 deaths [4]. Nevertheless, in endemic countries most of the *L. infantum*- or *L. donovani*- infected people are asymptomatic carriers or self-healers [5, 6].

The relation of leishmaniasis with poverty catalogues it as a neglected tropical disease. In fact, 72 of the endemic countries are developing nations with a burden of 90% of the VL, CL and mucocutaneous leishmaniasis (MCL) [7]. In these regions, the majority of the population lives in rural areas, where higher densities of sand flies are found, and is malnourished, a condition that leads to immunosuppression. In addition, HIV concomitant infection is frequent, contributing to a severe state of immunodeficiency [8]. The close geographical overlap of *Leishmania* and HIV promote the concomitant infection of both pathogens. In fact, HIV infection increases in 100-2320 times the risk of developing VL in the endemic regions. HIV/*Leishmania* coinfections correspond to 2-9% of all the VL cases in endemic countries [9]. Furthermore, leishmaniasis is nowadays an important issue in developed countries due to coinfection cases with HIV where *Leishmania* arises as an opportunistic infectious agent, the third of the parasitic infections after *Toxoplasma gondii* and *Cryptosporidium* spp. [10]. Indeed, 90% of the reported HIV/*Leishmania* cases are from Southern European countries, namely Spain, Portugal, Italy and France [8]. The routine use of highly active antiretroviral therapy (HAART) by the end of 1990's produced a clear decrease of HIV/*Leishmania* coinfection cases in southern Europe, but it is now a growing concern in those major *foci* of leishmaniasis in developing countries like Ethiopia, where the incidence of HIV is still high [9]. In addition, following the climatic changes that currently allow the presence of the vector in higher latitudes and the constant circulation of people and animals crossing frontiers and oceans, nowadays leishmaniasis cannot anymore be considered restricted to the endemic countries but is otherwise spread in the world.

The progression of a *Leishmania* infection to clinical disease comprises multifactorial phenomena, including the tropism of the species and strains, the genetic background of the host and the efficiency of the immune response developed against the parasite [11]. Studies using mice models have helped the scientific community to better understand the host-parasite relationship in leishmaniasis. Interleukin (IL) -12 is considered a key cytokine in the early development of the effective immune response due to its requirement for the activation of natural killer cells and T lymphocytes [12]. Activation of these cells leads to the secretion of interferon-γ (IFNγ), another commander cytokine.

Both in mice as in humans, macrophages are classically activated by IFNγ. This leads to the transcription of inducible nitric oxide synthase (iNOS) and phagocyte NADPH oxidase (phox) that produce nitric oxide (NO) and reactive oxygen species, respectively, specimens generally considered indispensable for macrophage-direct killing of *Leishmania* [13]. Macrophages activated by IL-12-driven IFNγ secretion by Th1 lymphocytes – named M1 macrophages – also produce TNFα, IL-1β and IL-6, pro-inflammatory cytokines that favor the protective response against *Leishmania* infection. These macrophages are, then, both effectors and inducers of the Th1 polarized immune response [14]. Nevertheless, the strong Th1 pro-inflammatory response must be balanced with the secretion of IL-10 and transforming growth factor-β (TGFβ) to avoid immunopathology through excessive tissue damage [15].

Effector $CD4^+$ and $CD8^+$ T cells that were activated by the recognition of *Leishmania* antigens on the cognate TCR and expanded to respond to infection will face a massive contraction on their numbers of about 90% after the elimination of the parasite, leaving a subset of experienced cells that constitute the memory pool. Memory cells are long-lived cells that rapidly expand in response to a secondary challenge with the priming antigen [16]. They form a heterogeneous pool with distinct abilities in proliferation, migration and cytokine production, which allow their classification in central memory (TCM) or effector memory T cells (TEM).

Memory cells were demonstrated to have great importance in the control of leishmaniasis, with distinct roles described for TCM and TEM cells. Zaph *et al.* have shown that in mice both TCM and TEM $CD4^+$ cells require parasite presence to be developed, though maintenance of TCM is independent of antigen persistence [2]. This achievement, however, seems highly dependent on the initial overall T cell response, since in some immunization experiments that used low dose of parasites protection was lost after the elimination of the parasites, possibly due to insufficient expansion of the TCM pool [3]. Adoptive transfer of TCM from *L. major*-infected mice to naïve animals conferred protection upon a challenge. When facing the antigen, TCM expanded in the lymph nodes, acquired effector functions, including CD62L downregulation which allowed their migration to the infection site and effective protection [2]. In accordance, analysis of $CD4^+$ memory T cells from patients with CL stimulated *ex-vivo* with soluble *Leishmania* antigen (SLA) revealed the high proliferative ability and IL-2 production of TCM and high percentage of IFNγ-secreting TEM [17].

Nevertheless, concomitant immunity, *i.e.* efficient protection upon a challenge due to the long-term and simultaneous persistence of the pathogen, seems to be a hallmark in leishmaniasis [18].

1.2. Canine leishmaniasis

Dogs are primary reservoir hosts of zoonotic visceral leishmaniasis (ZVL) caused by *Leishmania infantum* and play a key role in the long-term maintenance of the parasite in the endemic areas of Mediterranean countries, the Middle East, Asia and Latin America. Epidemiological surveys estimate that, for example in western Mediterranean countries, seroprevalence ranges from 5 to 37%, varying from region to region depending on ecological aspects. Nevertheless, surveys based on PCR diagnosis demonstrated high infection rates in endemic areas, for example 80% in Marseille, France [19], and 67% in Majorca, Spain [20]. Longitudinal studies in Italy have also shown high incidences (40-92%) during the season of transmission [21]. Importantly, not all infected dogs develop canine leishmaniasis; more than 50% of infected dogs remain asymptomatic after infection, though it has been shown that these asymptomatic carriers are also infective to sandflies [22].

The high prevalence of infected dogs in endemic areas, their common presence in the domestic surroundings where ZVL transmission occurs, and the high infectiousness of both symptomatic and asymptomatic animals makes that *Leishmania*-infected dogs represent not only a serious veterinary but also an important public health problem. Infected dogs have been associated with the emergence of new *foci* of ZVL, like those in the North of Argentina, where the appearance of human cases is preceded by those of canine leishmaniasis [23], and also with the spread of VL observed in large Brazilian cities [24] and the northward spread of the disease reported in Italy [25]. Therefore, the control of parasite-infected dogs is of prime urgency to reduce the number of cases of human VL by decreasing prevalence in dogs [26].

The outcome of *Leishmania* infection in dogs is variable and depends on the persistence and multiplication of the parasite and the immune response of the animal. Not all the infected dogs will develop clinical disease, part of them can control the expansion of the parasite and spontaneously cure the infection; in others, the infection is subclinical for an undefined time (years or even the whole life) during which the animal remains asymptomatic. Few than 50% of infected animals do not have (or have lost) the capacity to control the parasite, in these cases being distributed extensively throughout the organism: spleen, liver, lymph nodes, bone marrow, kidney, skin, etc., (as opposed to what occurs in humans, where the parasite is normally limited to bone marrow, spleen and liver) [26]. In these dogs the disease progresses, the parasite burden and the *Leishmania*-specific antibody levels increase, and after two to four months of incubation the symptoms of canine leishmaniasis appear [27].

The natural history of canine leishmaniasis mostly depends on the efficacy of the dog´s immune response to *L. infantum* infection which determines the development of resistance or susceptibility to the disease. In general, resistance is associated with low levels of specific antibodies and presence of a predominant Th1 cell-mediated response against the parasite, with the production of IFNγ that is able to stimulate, in collaboration with TNFα, the leishmanicidal activity of macrophages mediated by the induction of iNOS. Absence of symptoms is related with high levels of IFNγ expression in the peripheral blood as detected by quantitative real-time PCR [28]. When dogs develop such parasite-specific cell-mediated immunity, they are able to control parasite dissemination and present an overall low tissue parasitism. This status of resistance is reflected in the development of a positive leishmanin skin test or/and an *in vitro* lymphoproliferative response after stimulation of peripheral blood mononuclear cells (PBMCs) with leishmanial antigens. In these animals, it has been observed that *in vitro* stimulation of PBMCs with *L. infantum* SLA induces the expression of IL-2, IFNγ, TNFα, IL-4 and IL-10, confirming the existence of both *Leishmania*-specific Th1 and Th2 clones [29]. Also, quantification of the cytokine expression by real-time PCR allowed to establish that PBMCs from resistant dogs expressed high levels of IFNγ and TNFα after *in vitro* stimulation with purified parasite antigens [30, 31]. Therefore, the evaluation of IFNγ expression level from PBMCs constitutes a good approach to evaluate the *in vitro* immunogenicity of leishmanial molecules to identify vaccine candidates able to induce the protective cellular immune response to canine leishmaniasis [30, 32].

Different attempts have been made to confirm a correlation between the classes and subclasses of immunoglobulins and the type of response against *Leishmania* infection in dogs. Early studies associated the appearance of specific IgG2 antibodies against *Leishmania* with the asymptomatic state of the dogs, and the preponderance of IgG1 with progression of the disease [33]. However, other studies have failed to show this [34, 35]. Recent reports have proposed the analysis of IgG, IgG1 and IgG2 isotypes as immune biomarkers for the assessment of the immunogenicity of vaccines against canine leishmaniasis. Since IgG1 and IgG2 responses are largely T cell dependent, the evaluation of the specific isotypes has been considered an important aspect to evaluate the overall immunity induced by a specific vaccine. It has been seen that IgG2 induced by vaccination with *L. infantum* excreted/secreted proteins (*Li*ESP) had a potent inhibitory effect on the *in vitro* growth of both amastigotes and promastigotes and that the pre-treatment of amastigotes with this serum reduced significantly their *in vitro* infectivity in canine macrophages [36].

It is important to remark that the lack of *Leishmania*-specific cell mediated immunity constitutes a key aspect in the pathogenesis of canine leishmaniasis and also in the recovery of the animal after treatment. It has been confirmed that successful chemotherapy of the animals correlates not only with the disappearance of external signs of leishmaniasis but also with a significant increment in the percentage of $CD4^+$ T cells and the appearance of a parasite-specific proliferative response of PBMCs [37].

2. Vaccine research for leishmaniasis

The ideal vaccine for leishmaniasis should be safe, effective, long lasting, transversal to all infective *Leishmania* species and affordable, to be available to the populations most in need.

2.1. Animal models for vaccine research for leishmaniasis

Much of the knowledge generated from leishmaniasis research come from experimental infections in animal models. Differently from human population and natural infections, the most common models of disease employed in leishmaniasis research are based on infection of inbred mice with cloned lines of parasites. These experimental settings reduce the variety of factors that play a role on the disease manifestation, such as host's genetic background and immune competence, concomitant infections with other microorganisms, autoimmune or inflammatory diseases or drug treatments that may affect the fitness of the immune system, diversity of parasite's strains and species, site of infection and inoculum dose, infecting sand fly's species, etc. However, in comparison to the natural transmission and disease, the same limitations are also the major advantages, as in laboratorial settings researchers control all those variables and are able to focus on their specific target to unravel the molecular and immunological mechanisms behind leishmaniasis.

Many models of leishmaniasis have been tested, although none is able to mimic the exact pathology of cutaneous and, principally, visceral human diseases, or to develop the same immune responses. Despite valuable information has come from animal models, careful generalizations must be done when transposing it to the human disease.

The animal species applied on studies of human CL is almost exclusively the mouse (*Mus musculus*). Inbred strains are experimentally infected by subcutaneous or intradermal route with millions of promastigotes cultivated *in vitro* or axenic or tissue-derived amastigotes. The mice's genetic background has a major impact on the severity of the disease. For instance, when infected with a high dose BALB/c strain develops extensive skin lesions that spread away from the inoculation site leading to death of the animal, while C57BL/6 and CBA/N are able to control the infection and skin ulcers self-heal with time [38].

Considering animal models for VL, golden hamsters (*Mesocricetus auratus*) are among the best mimicking model of the human disease. Despite the artificial route (intracardiac or intravenous) and the high amount of parasites usually inoculated, *L. infantum*- or *L. donovani*-infected hamsters show heterogeneous phenotypes of infection, with animals that are asymptomatic, oligosymptomatic or polysymptomatic, in quite a good correlation with human and also canine epidemiology in endemic areas. Symptomatology comprise weight loss, uncontrollable increase in the splenic, hepatic and bone marrow parasite loads, hepatosplenomegaly, pancytopenia, hypergammaglobulinemia and ultimately death (Carrillo *et al.*, submitted, 2013 and [39]). Due to the lack of specific reagents needed to study the immunological mechanisms associated with *Leishmania* infection, the hamster model has been put apart and neglected over the mice models. Visceral leishmaniasis in mouse do not fully resemble the human nor canine disease, but the availability of numerous strains genetically modified and an endless offer of anti-mouse antibodies make the mouse the most preferred model to understand the host-parasite interactions and the immunological aspects of visceral leishmaniasis. However, in the scope of vaccine development and drug screening, where more than the mechanism behind the most important read-out is efficacy (*i.e.* parasite loads and pathology), golden hamsters are the most appropriate rodent model for the human disease.

The use of dogs (*Canis lupus familiaris*) as model of leishmaniasis is an advantage in the way that dogs are themselves natural hosts. Some breeds, like German Shepard, Boxer and Doberman, seem to be more susceptible to natural *Leishmania* infection [40]. However, the most common breed used in laboratorial studies is the Beagle. In addition, many research studies are done with field animals. They can be artificially infected or put in natural contact with sand flies in

http://dx.doi.org/10.5772/57214

endemic areas to test the efficacy of vaccines or anti-*Leishmania* drugs for veterinary practice or be used in the scope of model for human VL. Despite the existence of some dog-specific tools that would allow the study of the immune response, working with dogs is not as easy as handling mice, due to their size, the unpredictability of the infection rates, the cost of the experiments and the emotional connection that naturally exist between humans and dogs.

Non-human primates are usually confined to pre-clinical trials in humans. Some models based on artificial inoculation of rhesus macaques (*Macaca mulata*) [41], African vervet monkeys (*Chlorocebus* spp.) [42] or langur monkeys (*Presbytis entellus*) [43, 44] have been tested for *Leishmania* vaccines. Due to the close phylogenetic relation with humans and considerably good mimicking of pathology and immune responses generated upon infection (depending on the parasite and animal species), these models are attractive for vaccine research. But the difficulty on the handling, the very expensive costs and the impossibility of exposing the animals to a natural challenge are drawbacks on the use of non-human primates for *Leishmania* vaccine research.

2.2. Leishmanization

Until date, the only successful, long-lasting strategy for human immunization against leishmaniasis is the leishmanization process. It consists on the inoculation of live virulent parasites in a hidden area of the skin of healthy people with the purpose of development of immunity for protection when the individuals are challenged by a natural infection. Leishmanization showed 100% protection when used as prophylaxis for cutaneous leishmaniasis (CL) throughout the ex-Soviet Union, Asia, and the Middle East [45]. Due to risk of complications in healthy people and difficult standardization of the live *L. major* inoculum, this procedure was mostly abandoned. However, this is still a current practice in Uzbekistan [45] and a few years ago it was reported to be applied in the evaluation of the efficacy of new vaccines [46].

A "natural" form of leishmanization may be the reason why in Sri Lanka so many cases of CL by *L. donovani* are reported while VL is rare [47]. McCall *et al.* have recently reproduced this scenario in the BALB/c model, immunizing the mice subcutaneously with a dermotropic *L. donovani* strain from Sri Lanka followed by intravenous challenge with a viscerotropic autochthonous strain, and indeed, partial protection was obtained in the liver of the infected mice [48]. The authors attributed the ability of the cutaneous strain to protect against the challenge with the visceral strain to a probable great similarity between the two *L. donovani* strains; this hypothesis may justify the opposing phenotype observed by others [49]. Also, an epidemiological study in Sudan indicated that only individuals previously negative for leishmanin (Montenegro skin test) developed VL, thus, though without scientific evidences, leishmanin-positive individuals that were possibly formerly infected with *L. major* were protected against the visceral disease [50].

2.3. First generation vaccines

First generation vaccines comprise whole killed parasites and live attenuated parasites. They were primarily developed to overcome one of the major concerns related to leishmanization:

the risk of disease development in immunocompetent persons and the total improperness for immunosuppressed patients for this same reason.

2.3.1. *Killed parasites*

With more or less success, some examples of killed vaccines include *L. braziliensis* crude antigens tested in dogs [51] and trivalent (*L. braziliensis* + *L. guayanensis* + *L. amazonensis*) phenol-killed whole *Leishmania* promastigotes with bacille Calmette-Guérin (BCG) as adjuvant in Ecuadorian children [52]. According to a meta-analysis conducted in 2009 by Noazin *et.al.* to evaluate the efficacy of the clinical trials performed with whole killed parasites in endemic areas since 1970's, with the exception of this latter in Ecuador, none of the other eight clinical trials considered (based on autoclaved *L. major* (ALM) with BCG tested against CL in the Old World and *L. amazonensis* or multivalent preparations inactivated with merthiolate used against CL in the New World) showed significant protection against natural infection [53]. A new option was tested recently: a killed but metabolically active (KBMA) *L. infantum*. This vaccine showed partial protection in spleen and liver of BALB/c mice 2 and 8 weeks after challenge triggering a mixed Th1/Th2 response but the authors claim that improved results could be obtained by adding TLR agonists and Th1 adjuvants [54].

2.3.2. *Live attenuated parasites*

For the live attenuated parasites many are the works reported whether using physical, chemical or genetic manipulation for reducing the virulence of the strains, or even naturally attenuated strains, like the non-pathogenic *L. tarentolae* [55]. Some of the most successful vaccine candidates for VL based on genetically altered live parasites were *L. donovani* biopterin transporter gene knockout (KO) ($BT1^{-/-}$) [56], *L. donovani* replication deficient centrin gene KO ($Cen^{-/-}$) [57], *L. donovani* cytochrome c oxidase complex component p27 gene KO ($Ldp27^{-/-}$) [58], *L. infantum* silent information regulatory 2 single KO ($SIR2^{+/-}$) [59] and *L. tarentolae* expressing *L. donovani* A2 antigen [60]. Despite showing hopeful efficiency in murine models, the promising candidates that were tested in human and canine diseases failed to protect (reviewed in [61]).

2.4. Second generation vaccines

A different approach relies on recombinant proteins, polyproteins, DNA vaccines, liposomal formulations and dendritic cell vaccine delivery systems [45]; these constitute the second generation vaccines.

2.4.1. *Purified or recombinant Leishmania antigens and engineered polyproteins*

The *Leishmania* antigen that has been more extensively studied in the scope of a vaccine is the gp63 glycoprotein that is expressed on the surface of both the amastigotes and the promastigotes forms. The recombinant and the native proteins have been inoculated in several strains of mice as models of CL, generally showing a protective phenotype (see [62] for details). Also, an early study using monkeys revealed a partial protection against CL by *L. major* [63]. This gp63 is one of the few recombinant antigens studied in the scope of VL; Bhowmick *et al.* showed that gp63 encapsulated in cationic liposomes induced more than 80% reduction of the parasite loads in spleen and liver of BALB/c mice infected with *L. donovani* [64]. In this group of recombinant antigens, some others of the most successful candidates against VL were the amastigote-specific protein rA2, rHASPB1 (hydrophilic acylated surface protein B1), KMP-11 (kinetoplastid membrane protein-11) and rORFF (open reading frame fragment). *Li*ESA (*L. infantum* promastigotes' excreted/secreted antigens), FML (fucose-mannose ligand) and GRP78 (glucose-regulated protein 78) are the few purified antigens tested in vaccines for VL and all of them revealed at least certain degree of protection (see the reviews from Evans and Kedzierski [45] and Nagill and Kaur [62] for details and references). For CL, other antigens tested by several groups, though with conflicting results, are rLACK (*Leishmania* homologue of receptor for activated C kinase) [65-67] and PSA-2 (promastigote surface antigen 2) [68, 69].

Concerning the recombinant polyproteins, rLeish-111f (or LEISH-F1, composed of three molecules fused in tandem: the *L. major* homologue of eukaryotic thiol-specific antioxidant (TSA), the *L. major* stress-inducible protein 1 (LmSTI1) and the *L. braziliensis* elongation and initiation factor (LeIF)) and its non His-tag form rLeish-110f are undoubtedly the best studied and the most promising candidates for a vaccine against leishmaniasis. After having proved to protect mice with CL [70] and VL [71], rLeish-111f with MPL-SE adjuvant has also demonstrated to be safe and well tolerated in humans [72] as well as immunogenic in healthy subjects of endemic areas with or without previous contact to *L. donovani* [73]. Clinical trials in dogs have resulted in disparate conclusions about the efficacy of the vaccine in the prophylaxis of ZVL [74, 75], though survival of infected dogs was increased after vaccination and treatment with glucantime [76]. rLeish-110f with MPL-SE was shown to be immunogenic and protective in BALB/c mice after *L. major* and *L. infantum* challenges [77] (see [78] for complete information about the clinical trials run with rLeish-f111 and rLeish-f110).

Another polyprotein named Protein Q, composed of the fusion of four fragments of the acidic ribosomal protein Lip2a, Lip2b, P0 and histone 2A, has shown 90% protection as measured by parasite clearance in vaccinated dogs using BCG as adjuvant [79]. After testing other adjuvants in mice, 99% protection was achieved against *L. infantum* when administering Protein Q with CpG-ODN [80].

2.4.2. *DNA vaccines*

DNA vaccines are able to activate both $CD4^+$ and $CD8^+$ T cells through the engagement of MHC class II and MHC class I, respectively [38]. In addition, co-administration of cytokines and CpG oligonucleotides allows the modulation of the cellular immune response [81]. Besides being relatively easy to prepare and stable, another unique advantage is the appropriate folding of the intracellularly synthetized peptide on its native structure [38].

The first DNA vaccines to be studied were the classical candidates that have been tested as proteins. As single plasmids or in multicomponent DNA vaccines, there are successful examples that have shown to protect from some *Leishmania* species but not others, or were effective in some animal models but not others (see [62] for an extensive description of DNA vaccines). Among the most investigated are gp63 for CL in mice, LACK and KMP-11 for both

CL and VL tested in mice, hamsters and dogs. Some reports have shown the use of the strategy of heterologous prime-boost using LACK DNA followed by administration of rLACK protein with positive results [82-86].

2.4.3. Dendritic cell vaccine and liposomal formulations delivery systems

The unique capacity of DCs in amplifying the innate defense mechanisms and providing the link between these and the acquired immune responses makes them ideal candidates for anti-*Leishmania* vaccines [87]. In the recent years, DCs pulsed with gp63 or gp63-derived peptides [88, 89], histone H1 [90] or a mixture of histones [91] delivered to mice challenged with *L. major* or DCs pulsed with KMP-11(12-31aa) peptide + CpG ODN [92] against *L. infantum* have shown to decrease lesion size and parasite loads through the production of antigen-specific IFNγ.

On another approach, the concept behind the use of liposomes to deliver *Leishmania* antigens is that they can modulate antigen presentation, enhancing antigen-specific T cell proliferation and humoral responses. Conventional liposomes are presented by MHC class II molecules, whereas the presentation *via* MHC class I requires pH-sensitive liposomes [93]. The encapsulation of rgp63 or rLmSTI1 in liposomes has proven to develop a Th1 response that protected BALB/c mice from *L. major* [94, 95] or *L. donovani* infection [64]. A different strategy using polar phospholipids from *Escherichia coli* to encapsulate *L. donovani* SLA protected hamsters from *L. donovani* infection by the production of $CD4^+$ and $CD8^+$ T cell-specific responses [96]. Importantly, the route of administration of the liposomes may have a crucial role on the generation of the protective response. For example, BALB/c mice that were immunized by intravenous or intraperitoneal routes with liposomal *L. donovani* membrane antigens were protected from a *L. donovani* challenge, whereas the intramuscular or subcutaneous immunizations failed to protect [97].

2.5. Adjuvants

Adjuvants are synthetic or natural highly immunogenic components that are combined with the specific immunizing antigen with the purpose of efficiently stimulate the immune cells to mount a strong response against that antigen. Adjuvants are usually categorized in two classes. Immunostimulatory or non-particulate adjuvants are agonists of the pathogen-recognition receptors (PRRs) that localize at the surface or inside intracellular vesicles of innate immune cells [93]. These are activated by the binding of the cognate pathogen associated molecular patterns (PAMPs) (or their agonists) and signal a complex cascade of events that triggers the secretion of cytokines, chemokines and type I interferons [98]. The other class comprise the particulate adjuvants which are mineral-, lipid- or polymer-based delivery systems that, along with being transporters of the *Leishmania* antigen, are themselves immunostimulators due to their size, charge and composition; their properties can even be further improved by the decoration with other PAMP-like adjuvants [93].

In a vaccine for leishmaniasis, it is expected that adjuvants modulate the immune system towards a Th1 response, with high amounts of secreted IL-12 and IFNγ. Indeed, recombinant

IL-12 has been successfully tested in animal models as a potent adjuvant. However, stimulation with IL-12 was unable to induce a strong memory response to the immunizing antigen in BALB/c mice [99]. Nevertheless, when administered as IL-12 DNA it induced long-lasting protection against *L. major* [100].

MPL® is a purified derivative of the monophosphoryl lipid A hydrophobic moiety of *Salmonella minnesota*'s lipopolysaccharide (LPS). As LPS, MPL® is a potent TLR4 activator, though without the pyrogenicity of the parent molecule [101]. To even increase its efficacy, MPL® has been formulated in an oil-in-water stable emulsion in squalene (MPL-SE) which rendered high levels of IFNγ and low amounts of IL-4 and IL-10 [102]. A similar derivative, GLA-SE (glucopyranosyl lipid adjuvant) has been chemically synthetized in order to obtain a pure molecule, free of biological components, but still maintaining the same multifunctional immunomodulatory activity as the naturally-derived MPL® [103]. Currently, MPL-SE and GLA-SE are undergoing clinical trials with the antigen LEISH-F3 for the first vaccine for human VL (see section 2.6.2).

Other TLR agonists are CpG-containing oligonucleotides (CpG ODNs) and imiquimod, which are ligands for the TLR9 and TLR7/8, respectively. CpG ODNs are strong immunostimulators by the upregulation on macrophages and DCs of CD40 and MHC class II costimulatory receptors [104] and the induction of IFNα, IFNβ and IFNγ, IL-12, IL-18 and TNFα secretion by lymphocytes [105]. In the same direction, imiquimod, a synthetic imidazoquinoline, is a Th1 activator. But noteworthy, imiquimod has itself anti-leishmanial activity through the activation of macrophages leading to the secretion of IL-12 and IFNγ [106]. Also, signal transduction directed to NO production was detected on *L. donovani*-infected macrophages treated with imiquimod [107]. Indeed, a recent report showed the effective application of topic imiquimod on the cutaneous lesions of a child infected with *L. infantum* unresponsive to liposomal amphotericin B [108].

Bacillus Calmette-Guérin (BCG), besides being the most widely administered vaccine in the world, it is also commonly used as adjuvant in numerous vaccine candidates for infectious diseases. In anti-*Leishmania* treatment [109] and vaccine research it has been tested in murine [110-112], hamster [113], canine [114, 115] and non-human primate models [42] (just to mention the most recent works). Its mechanism of immunostimulation relies on the activation of TLR2, TLR 4 and TLR9 [116, 117] in addition to its anti-leishmanial properties revealed in early studies [118, 119].

Saponins are natural products from the *Quillaja saponaria* tree chemically modified in order to increase their adjuvant properties [120]. QuilA is the heterogeneous mixture of saponins obtained from the aqueous extract of the *Quillaja* bark. Due to its high toxicity, purification by HPLC and chemical modifications have originated several saponins which display different toxicity and immunogenicity [121]. Saponins are common adjuvants used in vaccines for *Leishmania*. Indeed, the three approved vaccines for ZVL include saponins in their formulation (see section 2.6.1).

Particulate adjuvants have many properties that can be designed to bias the immune system in the desirable way which make them very versatile adjuvants. They serve as carriers for antigens and non-particulate adjuvants, targeting both vaccine components to the same APC and controlling their release. They can be used to increase the stability of antigens, like proteins, peptides or oligonucleotides, to improve the solubility of hydrophobic compounds or to bypass gastric degradation [93].

Aluminum salts are common in human and veterinary vaccines, though they are not proper adjuvants *per se* to be used in vaccines for leishmaniasis because their immunostimulatory properties drive a Th2 response. However, they have been used as carriers for other adjuvants, like IL-12 [122] or BCG [111], in combination with ALM antigen. Lipid-based vesicles (liposomes and niosomes) have been tested to carry ALM antigen with or without BCG in C57BL/6 [123] and BALB/c mice [124]. Similarly, virosomes are spheres formed by a phospholipid bilayer but that also contain viral glycoproteins (hemagglutinin and neuraminidase from influenza virus) which confer structural stability and enhance the adjuvanticity of these particles [93].

Micelles and emulsions likewise fall in this category of particulate adjuvants as, for example, MPL® and GLA formulated in stable emulsions (MPL-SE and GLA-SE). The oil-in-water emulsion formed with squalene (SE) is itself an adjuvant that has been included in the ongoing clinical trials run by IDRI (see section 2.6.2), though immunization with Leish-110f antigen plus SE led to the development of a Th2 response in BALB/c mice [77].

Finally, thought without great expression in *Leishmania* vaccine research, the most complex particulate adjuvants are the immune stimulating complexes. ISCOMATRIX™ are cage-like structures composed of cholesterol, lipids and QuilA bond together by hydrophobic interactions; they allow the inclusion of several antigens forming ISCOMATRIX™ vaccines [102]. Similar structures that include a hydrophobic antigen are called ISCOMs, while hydrophilic antigens must be held in cationic ISCOMs-like structures named PLUSCOMs [93]. The inclusion of QuilA in these systems allows the reduction of its amount and the bonding to cholesterol, therefore leaving no free QuilA to interact with cell membranes, which decrease its toxicity [93].

2.6. Current status of vaccine research

2.6.1. Vaccines for zoonotic visceral leishmaniasis

In canine vaccinology three authorized vaccine options are available.

Leishmune® was the first vaccine licensed for the prevention of ZVL but is authorized only in Brazil. It consists of *L. donovani* purified fucose-mannose ligand (FML antigen) in combination with a saponin adjuvant. Clinical trials have showed that Leishmune® reduces the risk of infection but also prevents disease progression in already infected dogs, though the manufacturer does not recommend the vaccine as immunotherapy. A transmission-blocking activity was also attributed to this vaccine, making it highly appealing for the control of the zoonosis [125]. After 5 years of spread use among veterinary clinics in all the Brazilian territory, the manufacturer reports an efficacy of 97.3% in 8393 vaccinated *Leishmania*-seronegative dogs exposed to the natural challenge [126]. Strong cellular response (determined as *Leishmania*-

specific lymphoproliferation with high levels of IFNγ in the absence of IL-10 and positive Montenegro skin reaction test) and favorable humoral response (with high titers of *Leishmania*-specific IgG2) are behind this protective response in vaccinated animals [126].

Some years later, Leish-Tec® was released, also only in Brazil. The recombinant A2 protein is the antigen that constitutes the vaccine along with saponin adjuvant. Protection was found to be related to high levels of anti-A2 IgG and IgG2, without the presence of IgG1, and high amounts of specific IFNγ with low levels of IL-10 [127]. However, there is no updated information about the efficacy of the vaccine in the field.

Recently, a new vaccine, CaniLeish®, the only authorized in Europe, has entered the market for the prophylaxis of ZVL. The manufacturer claims that vaccinated dogs have a 4-fold reduced risk of developing the disease compared to non-vaccinated animals [128]. The use of *L. infantum* excreted/secreted proteins associated to QA-21 adjuvant (*Li*ESP/QA-21) leads to the increase of IgG2 specific antibodies, stronger *Leishmania*-specific lymphoproliferation with an increased IFNγ-producing T cell population that is able to activate a significant leishmanicidal macrophage ability *in vitro* due to NO production [129].

2.6.2. *Ongoing clinical trials for a vaccine for VL*

On February 2012 the Infectious Disease Research Institute (IDRI) has launched a phase 1 clinical trial for the first vaccine against VL [130]. Thirty six healthy adult American volunteers were recruited to evaluate the safety, tolerability and immunogenicity of the LEISH-F3 recombinant antigen (composed of two fused proteins) with GLA-SE, MPL-SE or SE adjuvants [131]. About one year and a half later, this first clinical trial was completed and the vaccine was shown to be safe and to induce potent immune responses in healthy volunteers [132]. Later, IDRI partnered with the Indian pharmaceutical company Zydus Cadila to develop, register and market the three vaccine candidates to ensure that the possible future vaccine is affordable and accessible by the people that really need it. Also, in July 2013 this partnership has started phase 1 clinical trials in India to evaluate the effectiveness of the vaccine on individuals from endemic regions [132].

3. Experimental data: Highly infective *Leishmania infantum* strain induces strong central and effector memory CD4$^+$ and CD8$^+$ immunity required for partial protection against re-infection

3.1. Aim of the study

It is well accepted that the broad clinical manifestations described in leishmaniasis are associated with the different cytokine milieu developed in response to the infection, which is highly dependent on the parasite itself. Accordingly, a diversity of immune responses have been described for *L. major* substrains [133] and *L. infantum* strains from the MON-1 zymodeme [134]. These immune responses may have a pivotal importance if the host faces a *de novo Leishmania* infection. In fact, data from endemic countries put on evidence the reality of resistance to re-infection in VL. In the one hand, it is evident the predominance of *L. infantum* infections in children compared to adults [6], which may result from acquired resistance to re-infection in adulthood, and, on the other hand, there are the examples of fully recovered patients that showed resistance to re-infection by the same *Leishmania* species [61].

Some studies on re-infection have been performed in mice as model for visceral leishmaniasis. Streit *et al.* described a partial level of protection against *L. chagasi* when mice were first infected with a high-dose inoculum since it was able to stimulate the immune system towards a Th1 response for counteracting a subsequent infection. On the contrary, an infection with a low dose suppressed IFNγ production and elicited high levels of TGFβ. Also, protective immunity was not achieved if an attenuated *dhfr-ts* knockout strain was used instead for immunization [49]. However, Oliveira *et al.* published opposing results as when they infected mice with a low dose of *L. chagasi* a protective immune response was generated, while a high dose contributed to the development of visceral disease [135].

To our knowledge, there is no previous literature about the concomitant immunity developed with live virulent *L. infantum* infection followed by homologous or heterologous re-infection. Since the severity of the infection and the progression of visceral leishmaniasis are strongly determined by the elicited immune response, in this work we analyzed the ability of two *L. infantum* virulent strains, which have presented different infectivity and immunomodulation, in the generation of an effective adaptive immunity in the context of experimental chronic infection and in the induction of a recall response after re-infection in BALB/c mouse model.

3.2. Development of protection needs highly infective *Leishmania*

Many efforts have been made to understand how *Leishmania*-specific immunity is generated and maintained over time. Nowadays, it is of scientific consensus that early activation of the innate immune system is essential for the production of a reliable adaptive response that leans on $CD4^+$ and $CD8^+$ specific cellular immunity.

To understand the strain-specific immunomodulation mechanisms that lead to protection to re-infection we used two strains of *L. infantum*, one dermotropic (HL) and the other viscerotropic (ST), which presented differential onset and progression of VL in mice. As previously shown [136], HL was able to colonize the spleen, liver and bone marrow in higher extent than ST parasites 6 weeks after infection (Figure 1, Infection bars). We hypothesized that these differences in infectivity could lead to distinct levels of protection. Thus, we re-infected the mice with homologous or heterologous strains.

In our model, mice that were previously imprinted with HL strain and then challenged with the same highly infective strain (Figure 1, Re-inf HL bars) were able to sustain the splenic parasite load and to decrease in about 1 logarithm the number of parasites colonizing the liver and bone marrow. On the contrary, HL re-infection after ST imprinting led to a significant increase of about 1000 times in all the target tissues. Concomitant immunity was more pronounced when the animals were infected with the highly infective HL strain and then challenged with ST due to its lower infectivity (Figure 1, Re-inf ST bars). As such, the infections

http://dx.doi.org/10.5772/57214

in the spleen and liver of HL imprinted mice suffered a significant reduction of ~1000-fold in the parasite loads to levels close to the quantification limit, and in the bone marrow parasitic presence was detected but not quantifiable. Accordingly, ST imprinting and consecutive challenge resulted in a ~10-fold increase in the splenic and hepatic parasite burden compared to the primary infection numbers, though no changes were noticed in the parasite load of the bone marrow.

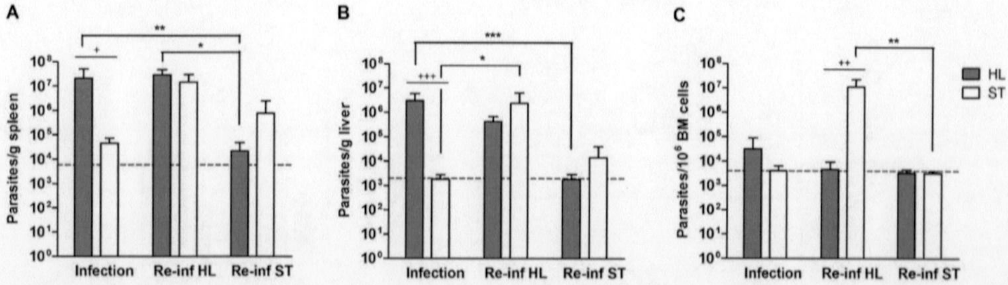

7-8 week-old BALB/c mice were infected by intraperitoneal route with 10^8 HL (grey bars) or ST (white bars) *L. infantum* strains cultivated for 4 days in Novy-MacNeal-Nicolle (NNN) medium at 26 ºC. After 6 weeks of infection mice were anesthetized with isoflurane and sacrificed by cervical dislocation (Infection bars). In the re-infection experiments, animals were infected for 6 weeks with HL or ST strains as before and challenged intraperitoneally with 10^8 promastigotes of the same or the other strain; 6 weeks after challenge they were sacrificed (Re-inf HL and Re-inf ST bars). **(A)** Spleen, **(B)** liver and **(C)** femoral bone marrow were recovered for quantification of the parasite load by real time PCR [136]. Bars represent means ± SD of 5 to 9 animals of one experiment representative of two independent. Statistically significant differences between HL and ST infections were calculated with Mann-Whitney test and are signed with ⁺. Kruskall-Wallis test followed by Dunn's multiple comparison test were used to calculate differences before and after challenge and are depicted with *. Statistical analysis was done in GraphPad Prism 5 (GraphPad Software). Dashed line indicates the limit of detection for quantification for each tissue.

Figure 1. Parasite load after infection and challenge with *L. infantum* strains presenting different infectivities

Based on the data exposed above, in terms of parasitological analysis we established that the onset of pathology (set as hepatosplenomegaly (data not shown; see [136]) and high parasite loads) by an infective *L. infantum* strain confers a degree of protection over a re-infection episode which correlates with the infectivity of both the imprinting and the challenging strains that are inoculated in the host. Similar findings were reported previously, when a high-dose of *L. chagasi* promastigotes was required for the development of protection against re-infection, whereas a low-dose immunization either had no effect or slightly exacerbated disease [49].

3.3. Infectivity may influence downstream adaptive response-triggering events

To understand the immune response behind this protective phenotype, we analyzed the splenic populations and the T cells functionality. We observed that infection with HL produced a significant increase in the total cellularity and major leukocyte populations when compared to naïve animals, which was not noticed when mice were infected with ST strain (Figure 2A-E).

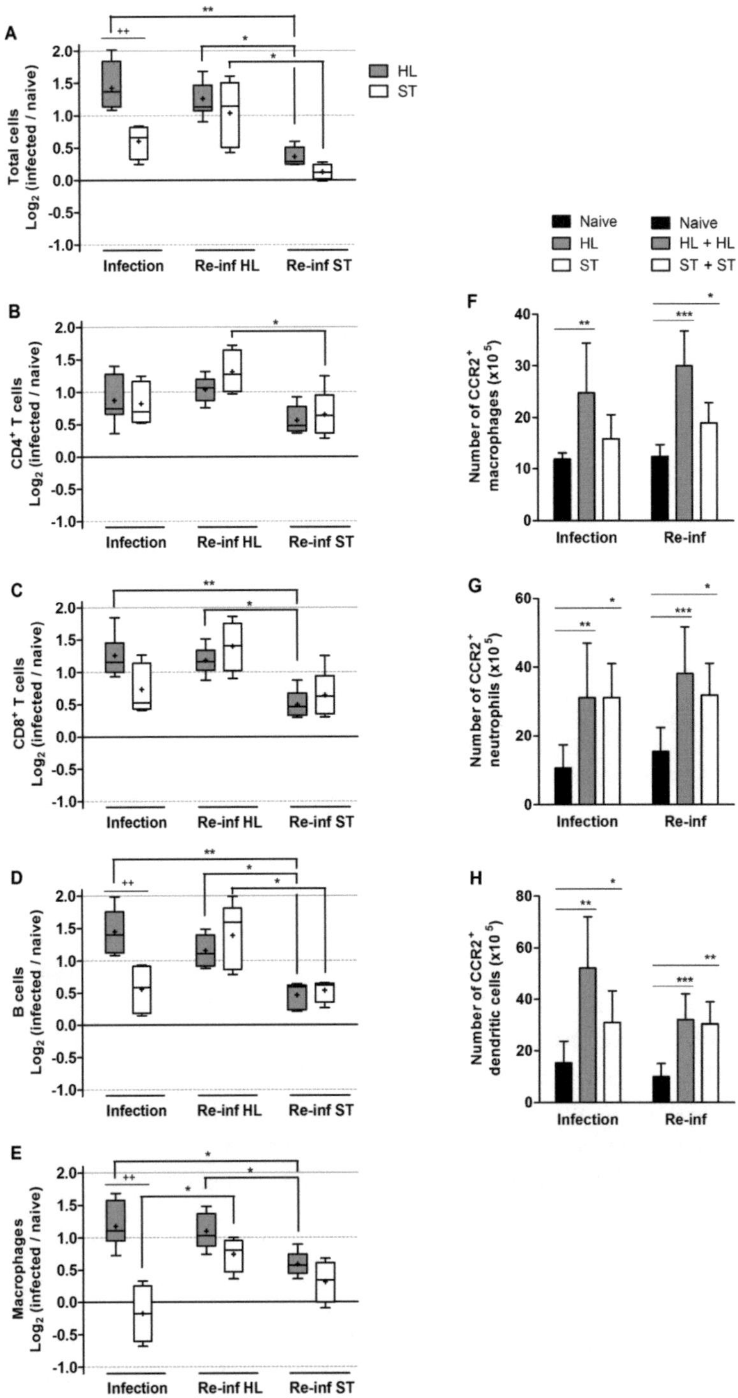

(A-E) After infection and consequent challenge with both HL and ST strains, splenocytes were recovered and surface-stained for identification of major leukocytes populations. **(A)** Total cells were counted and **(B)** CD4+ T cells (CD3+CD4+), **(C)** CD8+ T cells (CD3+CD8+), **(D)** B cells (CD19+) and **(E)** macrophages (CD11b+Ly6C+) were evaluated by

http://dx.doi.org/10.5772/57214

flow cytometry in a FACSCanto (BD Bioscences). Cell numbers from infected mice were normalized with respective values from age-matched naïve mice and results are presented as log_2 of the fold change relative to naïve animals, with dashed and solid lines indicating 2- and 4-fold difference. Boxes and whiskers with 5-95 percentile and mean (showed with +) of 5 to 9 animals of one experiment representative of two independent. Mann-Whitney test was run to calculate statistically significant differences between mice infected with HL or ST and results are depicted with $^+$. Differences before and after challenge are indicated with * for $p<0.05$ or ** for $p<0.01$ and were calculated with Kruskall-Wallis test followed by Dunn's multiple comparison test in GraphPad Prism 5 (GraphPad Software). **(F-H)** Number of **(F)** inflammatory macrophages ($CD11b^+Ly6C^+$ $CCR2^+$), **(G)** inflammatory neutrophils ($CD11b^+Ly6G^+CCR2^+$) and **(H)** activated dendritic cells ($CD11c^+CCR2^+$) in infected mice before (Infection bars) and after homologous challenge (Re-inf bars). Bars represent means ± SD of 5 to 9 animals of one experiment representative of two independent. Statistically significant differences were calculated in GraphPad Prism 5 (GraphPad Software) with Mann-Whitney test between naïve and infected or challenged animals and show * $p<0.05$, ** $p<0.01$ and *** $p<0.001$.

Figure 2. Splenic cellular populations after infection and challenge with highly and low infective *L. infantum* strains

Interestingly, when the animals were subjected to a secondary infection by HL, regardless of the infectivity of the imprinting strain, we detected the same increase in the number of splenocytes, while after challenge with ST there was no change in the cellularity.

Inflammatory macrophages/monocytes and neutrophils, besides its recognition as host cells [137, 138], have been implicated in the remodeling of the spleen during splenomegaly in leishmaniasis [139, 140], as well as in the modulation of the specific $CD4^+$ T cells response in late phases of infection, at least with *L. major* [141]. Infiltration of neutrophils [142], DCs [143] and macrophages [144] in inflamed tissues is tightly regulated by the CC chemokine receptor 2 (CCR2) that also participates in important processes related to anti-*Leishmania* defense [143, 144].

As these are the first cells that need to be committed, we determined the number of inflammatory macrophages, DCs and neutrophils by the expression of CCR2 (Figure 2F-H). Infection and challenge with HL led to the significant increase of these inflammatory cells in the spleen. Similarly, infection with ST also significantly increased the inflammatory DCs and neutrophils, but only with a second wave of parasites the $CCR2^+$ macrophages arisen in numbers significantly higher than in uninfected animals. However, this difference in the number of $CCR2^+$ macrophages relates with the total macrophages present in the spleen, as the relative percentages were similar between HL and ST (data not shown). These $CCR2^+$ macrophages exert an important role in the defense against *Leishmania*, since it has been previously described that optimal parasite killing require the recruitment of $CCR2^+$ macrophages, followed by stimulation with combined monocyte chemotactic protein 1 (MCP-1) and IFNγ [144].

Thus, monocyte and neutrophil activation showed no major differences between HL and ST strains, similarly to the findings of Meddeb-Garnaoui *et al.* that compared the cytokine profile of human monocytes infected with dermotropic and viscerotropic *L. infantum* strains which presented respectively high and low infectivity *in vitro* [145]. In their *in vitro* setup, no differences were found in the ability of those two strains in the modulation of monocyte-secreted cytokines [145], indicating that the infectivity of a *Leishmania* strain not always produces a direct effect on the innate immune response. Nonetheless, *in vivo*, where other factors that influence macrophage function are present, the effect of the infectivity was not evaluated. We hypothesize that despite monocyte and neutrophil activation were similar, HL- and ST-activated cells should present divergent efficiencies when triggering the adaptive immune response, which may be indicative of intrinsic characteristics of the strains in modulating downstream events.

3.4. Highly infective *L. infantum* triggers memory and effector $CD4^+$ and $CD8^+$ T cells

We have studied the generation of $CD4^+$ and $CD8^+$ memory T cells 6 weeks post-infection and upon challenge with the same strain by the surface expression of CD44 and CD62L (Figure 3).

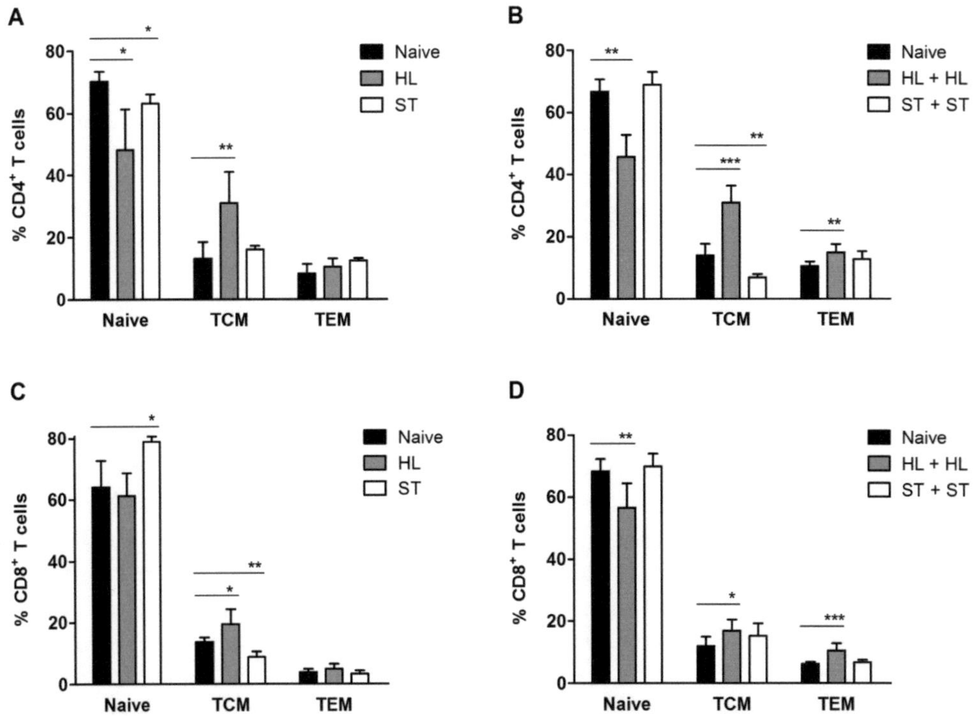

(A, B) $CD4^+$ and (C, D) $CD8^+$ T cells were analyzed by flow cytometry in a FACSCanto (BD Bioscences) according to their surface expression of CD44 and CD62L. Naïve ($CD44^{lo}CD62L^+$), central memory (TCM; $CD44^{hi}CD62L^+$) and effector memory (TEM; $CD44^{hi}CD62L^-$) subpopulations were quantified before **(A, C)** and after **(B, D)** challenge. Bars show means ± SD of 5 to 9 animals of one experiment representative of two independent and statistically significant differences between naïve and infected mice are depicted with * for $p<0.05$, as calculated by two-tailed Mann Whitney test run in GraphPad Prism 5 (GraphPad Software).

Figure 3. T cell memory repertoire of mice subjected to infection and homologous re-infection with HL and ST *L. infantum* strains

HL infection potentiated the expansion of central memory $CD8^+$ (Figure 3C, TCM bars) and especially $CD4^+$ T cells (Figure 3A, TCM bars) that doubled in percentage compared to uninfected mice. These memory populations are probably an important factor in the control of the parasite load in the spleen, as presented before (Figure 1A), when the animals were subjected to re-infection. Memory cells constitute a source of experienced-antigen cells that are able to rapidly respond to face a similar challenge. While TEM cells display protective effector functions, TCM are thought to replenish the TEM pool [146].

In fact, after challenge with HL, both $CD4^+$ (Figure 3B) and $CD8^+$ (Figure 3D) TCM pools remained high and TEM cells also significantly increased compared to naïve mice. Moreover, taking into account that the total numbers of T lymphocytes in the infected animals were significantly increased in relation to naïve mice (Figure 2B and C), the number of memory ($CD44^{hi}$) T cells was even more expressive in the spleens of those HL re-infected animals. On the contrary, ST strain showed no potential in clonal expansion of memory populations or at least in their high number maintenance in order to bring advantage upon re-infection. Neither in the imprinting infection nor after challenge could we detect $CD4^+$ or $CD8^+$ central or effector memory T cells in a percentage higher than that of the naïve animals. The decrease in the $CD8^+$ TCM cells 6 weeks after ST infection (Figure 3C) was considered not to have any biological meaning since, when adjusted to total number of cells, both naïve and infected mice have similar amounts of that subpopulation.

From the data exposed, we justified the partial protection that a primary infection with HL *L. infantum* strain can generate upon an homologous re-infection. This strain has the ability to activate the innate defenders (DCs, macrophages and neutrophils) for mobilization to the spleen where they can drive an effective generation and expansion of memory $CD4^+$ and $CD8^+$ T cell subsets.

3.5. Double producers $CD4^+IFN\gamma^+IL\text{-}10^+$ and $CD8^+IFN\gamma^+TNF\alpha^+$ T cells arise after re-infection

To appreciate the mechanisms underlying the protection observed after re-infection with a highly infective strain, we analyzed the magnitude of the developed T cell response in infected and re-infected mice with HL strain. After infection, we detected high levels of IFNγ-producing $CD4^+$ and $CD8^+$ T cells (Figures 4A and C, respectively). This finding was suspected after having noticed the massive cellular infiltrate of leukocytes in the spleen (Figure 2) and also the existence of approximately 15 % of effector memory lymphocytes (combined $CD4^+$ and $CD8^+$) that classically secrete this cytokine [147]. Upon re-infection (Figures 4B and D), however, a more interesting panel of effector cells has emerged. Along with the same $IFN\gamma^+$ cells, detected in both $CD4^+$ and $CD8^+$ lymphocytes, we identified $IL\text{-}10^+$ in ~1.5 % and $IFN\gamma^+IL\text{-}10^+$ double producers in ~0.75 % of the $CD4^+$ T cells, which represent an increment of ~1.7 and ~3.1, respectively, compared to uninfected animals.

$CD4^+$T-$bet^+IFN\gamma^+IL\text{-}10^+$ cells were recently described by us and others upon infection of BALB/c mice with *L. infantum* [148] or *L. donovani* [149]. This Th1 population is driven by $CD4^+$ T cells activation by the infected DCs and leads to an unprotective phenotype that accentuates the infection. However, a protective role was previously attributed to $CD4^+CD25^-Foxp3^-IFN\gamma^+IL\text{-}10^+$ cells in a vaccination study with *L. donovani* LdCen1$^{-/-}$ [57] and in a non-healing model of CL with *L. major* [150], which were claimed to arise after a strong inflammatory stimulus as a feedback control of Th1 responses to avoid tissue damage.

In $CD8^+$ T cells, conversely, cytokine double producing cells were found for $IFN\gamma^+TNF\alpha^+$, in a representation of ~0.86 %, meaning an increase of ~3.4 fold compared to naïve mice. IFNγ and

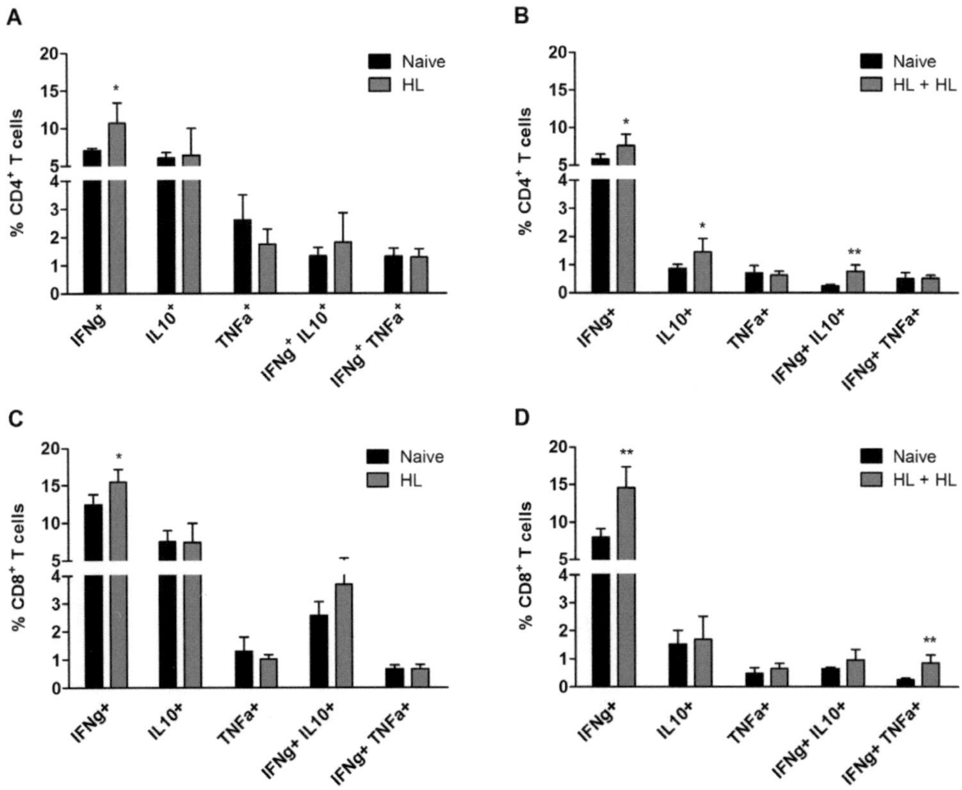

IFNγ, IL-10 and TNFα production was analyzed by flow cytometry in CD4+ **(A, B)** and CD8+ **(C, D)** lymphocytes. Splenocytes were stimulated *ex-vivo* with phorbol 12-myristate 13-acetate (PMA), ionomycin and brefeldin A, stained for surface and intracellular molecules and analyzed in a FACSCanto flow cytometer (BD Bioscences). Cytokine single and double producers in each lymphocyte population are depicted from naïve, infected **(A, C)** or challenged **(B, D)** mice. Bars represent means ± SD of 4 to 9 animals of one experiment with statistically significant differences between naïve and infected mice indicated with * when p<0.05, as calculated by two-tailed Mann Whitney test run in GraphPad Prism 5 (GraphPad Software).

Figure 4. Intracellular cytokines of CD4+ and CD8+ lymphocytes of HL infected and re-infected animals

TNFα concomitant production by Th1 and CD8+ T cells has for long proven to be more efficient in the killing of *L. major* [151, 152] and other unrelated microorganisms (*e.g. Mycobacterium tuberculosis* [153]) than the production of IFNγ or TNFα alone. More recently, IFNγ+TNFα+ high quality CD4+ and CD8+ T cells were described to be generated after several vaccination protocols against *L. major* and correlate with prognosis of protection much better than IFNγ single producers [154]. Moreover, those double producers CD4+ T cells, which can also be IL-2+, were determined to belong to the central memory subset, providing long-term protection [154, 155]. As for CD8+IFNγ+TNFα+ T cells, they were described to have enhanced cytolytic activity compared to IFNγ+ single producer cells in HIV-infected patients [156]. However, in our study, we could not detect any difference in the cytotoxicity mediated by CD8+ T cells from

http://dx.doi.org/10.5772/57214

HL infected and challenged mice compared to that from naïve animals (data not shown), which may indicate that cytolytic activity of those cells was not required in the containment of the parasites in the spleen or, instead, the persistence of the splenic parasite load is due to an incomplete effector function of the $CD8^+$ T cells.

3.6. Conclusions

Taken together, our results show that HL *L. infantum* strain promotes a robust activation of the immune system upon infection initiated by a strong recruitment of leukocytes to the spleen which stimulates the development of an effective adaptive response. This is a mixed response as considered by the detection of single producers $IFN\gamma^+$ and $IL\text{-}10^+$ $CD4^+$ T cells that become more evident when the antigen is re-loaded (*i. e.* re-infection). $CD8^+$ T cells also exert their effector function by the production of IFNγ. After re-infection, double producers $CD8^+IFN\gamma^+TNF\alpha^+$ and $CD4^+IFN\gamma^+IL\text{-}10^+$ T cells arise, probably from the expansion of the central and effector memory subsets, to contain the parasites that colonized the spleen and to efficiently resolve the infection in the liver and bone marrow, controlling tissue damage by IL-10 production. To confirm this hypothesis, adoptive transfer of these memory cells produced after re-infection with our highly infective *L. infantum* strain could be performed to evaluate the protective phenotype of such pools of $CD4^+$ and $CD8^+$ T cells in naïve animals challenged with a subsequent *L. infantum* infection.

Taking the fact that HL is a dermotropic strain that caused CL in a human patient, its tropism is possibly justified by the inflammatory potential of the strain that impedes a silent entry into the host. A protective response may immediately be mounted in the skin, abrogating any chance of the parasite to reach internal organs and visceralize [157]. Concerning the ST strain, an agent of human VL, the initial activation of the innate immune system does not translate into efficient adaptive immunity as no memory cells were detected. With this, a primary infection does not serve as imprinting, since a re-infection with the same strain led to the increase of the parasite load in the spleen and liver.

With this work we contributed to the better understanding of the complex modulation that *Leishmania* parasites do to surmount the protective strategies developed by the host's immune system. Much of the knowledge acquired so far by the scientific community was based on *L. major*-infection models that have a clear Th1/Th2 dichotomy on protection/progression of the disease, and more studies with VL models are needed to clarify the intriguing modulation that viscerotropic *Leishmania* strains provide to take advantage of their host.

4. Final remarks

Leishmaniasis is a tropical neglected disease that urgently needs control measures, as vaccination, since nowadays the global population is at risk. As some vaccines are available for ZVL, the discovery of an effective human vaccine for VL is near. Choosing the right antigen coupled with the appropriate adjuvant for the formulation is crucial to have an effective vaccine, but immunogenicity sometimes countervail safety and complicates the scenario.

Effective immunization requires the presentation of the antigen by proper APCs to mount a strong immune response and develop immunological memory, as well as it entails antigen persistence. As described previously, live vaccines produce more robust immune responses than dead parasites or defined protein or peptides but they represent an important health risk, mainly in immunosuppressed people. Furthermore, the immune response developed against live *Leishmania infantum* strains that display differences in infectivity is also unique and characteristic of each strain, being infectivity related with a stronger induction of an immune response, as showed by our experimental data.

In this chapter, we have updated the main aspects to consider when a vaccination study against *Leishmania* is planned. We aimed to show that vaccination is an effective way, and hopefully a soon reality, to prevent the spread of leishmaniasis, limiting the outcome of the disease and avoiding the parasite transmission. While successful research is close, many efforts are still needed for achieving an efficient human vaccine for leishmaniasis accessible to everyone in need.

5. Abbreviations

ALM autoclaved *Leishmania major*

APCs antigen presenting cells

CL cutaneous leishmaniasis

IL interleukin

MCL mucocutaneous leishmaniasis

MPL purified derivative of the monophosphoryl lipid A

NO nitric oxide

PAMP pathogen-associated molecular pattern

PBMCs peripheral blood mononuclear cells

SE squalene-based oil-in-water stable emulsion

TCM central memory T cell

TCR T cell receptor

TEM effector memory T cell

TLR Toll-like receptor

VL visceral leishmaniasis

ZVL zoonotic visceral leishmaniasis

http://dx.doi.org/10.5772/57214

Acknowledgements

We thank Doctor Maria da Luz Duarte from São Marcos Hospital, Braga, Portugal, for kindly providing us the skin sample infected with HL strain of *L. infantum*. We thank Joana Tavares from the Parasite Disease Group, IBMC, Porto, Portugal, for the isolation of HL strain and preparation of live stocks and Carmen Chicharro from WHO Collaborating Center for Leishmaniasis, National Center of Microbiology, Instituto de Salud Carlos III, Majadahonda, Spain, for analyzing its zymodeme. We thank Ricardo Silvestre and Mariana Resende from the Parasite Disease Group, IBMC, Porto, Portugal, for the help in animal experiments and flow cytometry analysis.

This work was funded by FEDER funds through the Operational Competitiveness Programme – COMPETE and by National Funds through FCT – Fundação para a Ciência e a Tecnologia under the projects FCOMP-01-0124-FEDER-019648 (PTDC/BIA-MIC/118644/2010) and FCOMP-01-0124-FEDER-011058 (PTDC/SAU-FCF/101017/2008) as well as the MICINN's project number PIM2010-ENI00627. The research leading to these results has also received funding from the European Community's Seventh Framework Programme under grant agreement No.603181 (Project MuLeVaClin).

Author details

Joana Cunha[1], Eugenia Carrillo[2], Javier Moreno[2] and Anabela Cordeiro-da-Silva[3*]

*Address all correspondence to: cordeiro@ibmc.up.pt

1 Parasite Disease Group, IBMC – Institute for Molecular and Cellular Biology, Institute for Biomedical Sciences Abel Salazar and Faculty of Medicine, University of Porto, Porto, Portugal

2 WHO Collaborating Center for Leishmaniasis, National Center for Microbiology, Instituto de Salud Carlos III, Majadahonda, Madrid, Spain

3 Parasite Disease Group, IBMC – Institute for Molecular and Cellular Biology and Laboratory of Microbiology, Department of Biological Sciences, Faculty of Pharmacy, University of Porto, Porto, Portugal

References

[1] WHO. Initiative for Vaccine Research (IVR). Parasitic Diseases. Malaria. 2013. Available from: http://www.who.int/vaccine_research/diseases/soa_parasitic/en/index4.html.

[2] Zaph C, Uzonna J, Beverley SM, Scott P. Central Memory T Cells Mediate Long-Term Immunity to *Leishmania major* in the Absence of Persistent Parasites. Nat Med. 2004 Oct;10(10):1104-1110. PubMed PMID: 15448686.

[3] Uzonna JE, Wei G, Yurkowski D, Bretscher P. Immune Elimination of *Leishmania major* in Mice: Implications for Immune Memory, Vaccination, and Reactivation Disease. J Immunol. 2001 Dec 15;167(12):6967-6974. PubMed PMID: 11739516.

[4] Alvar J, Velez ID, Bern C, Herrero M, Desjeux P, Cano J, *et al*. Leishmaniasis Worldwide and Global Estimates of Its Incidence. PLoS One. 2012;7(5):e35671. PubMed PMID: 22693548. Pubmed Central PMCID: 3365071.

[5] Michel G, Pomares C, Ferrua B, Marty P. Importance of Worldwide Asymptomatic Carriers of *Leishmania infantum* (*L. chagasi*) in Human. Acta Trop. 2011 Aug;119(2-3): 69-75. PubMed PMID: 21679680.

[6] Chappuis F, Sundar S, Hailu A, Ghalib H, Rijal S, Peeling RW, *et al*. Visceral Leishmaniasis: What Are the Needs for Diagnosis, Treatment and Control? Nat Rev Microbiol. 2007 Nov;5(11):873-882. PubMed PMID: 17938629.

[7] WHO. World Health Organization Web Page on Leishmaniasis. Burden of the Disease. 2013. Available from: http://www.who.int/leishmaniasis/burden/en/.

[8] WHO. Report of the Fifth Consultative Meeting on *Leishmania*/HIV Co-Infection. Addis Ababa, Ethiopia. 2007.

[9] Alvar J, Aparicio P, Aseffa A, Den Boer M, Canavate C, Dedet JP, *et al*. The Relationship between Leishmaniasis and AIDS: The Second 10 Years. Clin Microbiol Rev. 2008 Apr;21(2):334-359, table of contents. PubMed PMID: 18400800. Pubmed Central PMCID: 2292576.

[10] Ready PD. Leishmaniasis Emergence in Europe. Euro Surveill. 2010 Mar 11;15(10): 19505. PubMed PMID: 20403308.

[11] Rivas L, Moreno J, Canavate C, Alvar J. Virulence and Disease in Leishmaniasis: What Is Relevant for the Patient? Trends Parasitol. 2004 Jul;20(7):297-301. PubMed PMID: 15193556.

[12] Liese J, Schleicher U, Bogdan C. The Innate Immune Response against *Leishmania* Parasites. Immunobiology. 2008;213(3-4):377-387. PubMed PMID: 18406382.

[13] Silvestre R, Santarem N, Tavares J, Silva AM, Cordeiro-da-Silva A. Recognition of *Leishmania* Parasites by Innate Immunity. Immunology Endocrine & Metabolic Agents - Medicinal Chemistry (Formerly Current Medicinal Chemistry - Immunology Endocrine & Metabolic Agents). 2009 //;9(2):106-127.

[14] Tomioka H, Tatano Y, Maw WW, Sano C, Kanehiro Y, Shimizu T. Characteristics of Suppressor Macrophages Induced by Mycobacterial and Protozoal Infections in Relation to Alternatively Activated M2 Macrophages. Clin Dev Immunol. 2012;2012:635451. PubMed PMID: 22666284. Pubmed Central PMCID: 3361169.

[15] Raes G, Beschin A, Ghassabeh GH, De Baetselier P. Alternatively Activated Macrophages in Protozoan Infections. Curr Opin Immunol. 2007 Aug;19(4):454-459. PubMed PMID: 17628461.

[16] Surh CD, Boyman O, Purton JF, Sprent J. Homeostasis of Memory T Cells. Immunol Rev. 2006 Jun;211:154-163. PubMed PMID: 16824125.

[17] Keshavarz Valian H, Nateghi Rostami M, Tasbihi M, Miramin Mohammadi A, Eskandari SE, Sarrafnejad A, *et al*. CCR7$^+$ Central and CCR7$^-$ Effector Memory CD4$^+$ T Cells in Human Cutaneous Leishmaniasis. J Clin Immunol. 2013 Jan;33(1):220-234. PubMed PMID: 22990666.

[18] Belkaid Y, Piccirillo CA, Mendez S, Shevach EM, Sacks DL. CD4$^+$CD25$^+$ Regulatory T Cells Control *Leishmania major* Persistence and Immunity. Nature. 2002 Dec 5;420(6915):502-507. PubMed PMID: 12466842.

[19] Berrahal F, Mary C, Roze M, Berenger A, Escoffier K, Lamouroux D, *et al*. Canine Leishmaniasis: Identification of Asymptomatic Carriers by Polymerase Chain Reaction and Immunoblotting. Am J Trop Med Hyg. 1996 Sep;55(3):273-277. PubMed PMID: 8842114.

[20] Solano-Gallego L, Morell P, Arboix M, Alberola J, Ferrer L. Prevalence of *Leishmania infantum* Infection in Dogs Living in an Area of Canine Leishmaniasis Endemicity Using Pcr on Several Tissues and Serology. J Clin Microbiol. 2001 Feb;39(2):560-563. PubMed PMID: 11158106. Pubmed Central PMCID: 87775.

[21] Oliva G, Scalone A, Foglia Manzillo V, Gramiccia M, Pagano A, Di Muccio T, *et al*. Incidence and Time Course of *Leishmania infantum* Infections Examined by Parasitological, Serologic, and Nested-PCR Techniques in a Cohort of Naive Dogs Exposed to Three Consecutive Transmission Seasons. J Clin Microbiol. 2006 Apr;44(4):1318-1322. PubMed PMID: 16597857. Pubmed Central PMCID: 1448675.

[22] Quinnell RJ, Courtenay O. Transmission, Reservoir Hosts and Control of Zoonotic Visceral Leishmaniasis. Parasitology. 2009 Dec;136(14):1915-1934. PubMed PMID: 19835643.

[23] Cruz I, Acosta L, Gutierrez MN, Nieto J, Canavate C, Deschutter J, *et al*. A Canine Leishmaniasis Pilot Survey in an Emerging *Focus* of Visceral Leishmaniasis: Posadas (Misiones, Argentina). BMC Infect Dis. 2010;10:342. PubMed PMID: 21122107. Pubmed Central PMCID: 3002360.

[24] Maia-Elkhoury AN, Alves WA, Sousa-Gomes ML, Sena JM, Luna EA. Visceral Leishmaniasis in Brazil: Trends and Challenges. Cad Saude Publica. 2008 Dec;24(12): 2941-2947. PubMed PMID: 19082286.

[25] Maroli M, Rossi L, Baldelli R, Capelli G, Ferroglio E, Genchi C, *et al*. The Northward Spread of Leishmaniasis in Italy: Evidence from Retrospective and Ongoing Studies on the Canine Reservoir and Phlebotomine Vectors. Trop Med Int Health. 2008 Feb; 13(2):256-264. PubMed PMID: 18304273.

[26] Alvar J, Canavate C, Molina R, Moreno J, Nieto J. Canine Leishmaniasis. Adv Parasitol. 2004;57:1-88. PubMed PMID: 15504537.

[27] Moreno J, Alvar J. Canine Leishmaniasis: Epidemiological Risk and the Experimental Model. Trends Parasitol. 2002 Sep;18(9):399-405. PubMed PMID: 12377257.

[28] Manna L, Reale S, Viola E, Vitale F, Foglia Manzillo V, Pavone LM, *et al.* Leishmania DNA Load and Cytokine Expression Levels in Asymptomatic Naturally Infected Dogs. Vet Parasitol. 2006 Dec 20;142(3-4):271-280. PubMed PMID: 16920264.

[29] Chamizo C, Moreno J, Alvar J. Semi-Quantitative Analysis of Cytokine Expression in Asymptomatic Canine Leishmaniasis. Vet Immunol Immunopathol. 2005 Jan 10;103(1-2):67-75. PubMed PMID: 15626462.

[30] Carrillo E, Ahmed S, Goldsmith-Pestana K, Nieto J, Osorio Y, Travi B, *et al.* Immunogenicity of the P-8 Amastigote Antigen in the Experimental Model of Canine Visceral Leishmaniasis. Vaccine. 2007 Feb 9;25(8):1534-1543. PubMed PMID: 17178178. Pubmed Central PMCID: 2571115.

[31] Strauss-Ayali D, Baneth G, Shor S, Okano F, Jaffe CL. Interleukin-12 Augments a Th1-Type Immune Response Manifested as Lymphocyte Proliferation and Interferon Gamma Production in *Leishmania infantum*-Infected Dogs. Int J Parasitol. 2005 Jan; 35(1):63-73. PubMed PMID: 15619517.

[32] Carrillo E, Crusat M, Nieto J, Chicharro C, Thomas Mdel C, Martinez E, *et al.* Immunogenicity of HSP-70, KMP-11 and PFR-2 Leishmanial Antigens in the Experimental Model of Canine Visceral Leishmaniasis. Vaccine. 2008 Mar 28;26(15):1902-1911. PubMed PMID: 18321614.

[33] Deplazes P, Smith NC, Arnold P, Lutz H, Eckert J. Specific Igg1 and Igg2 Antibody Responses of Dogs to *Leishmania infantum* and Other Parasites. Parasite Immunol. 1995 Sep;17(9):451-458. PubMed PMID: 8552413.

[34] Solano-Gallego L, Riera C, Roura X, Iniesta L, Gallego M, Valladares JE, *et al.* *Leishmania infantum*-Specific IgG, IgG1 and IgG2 Antibody Responses in Healthy and Ill Dogs from Endemic Areas. Evolution in the Course of Infection and after Treatment. Vet Parasitol. 2001 Apr 19;96(4):265-276. PubMed PMID: 11267753.

[35] Quinnell RJ, Courtenay O, Garcez LM, Kaye PM, Shaw MA, Dye C, *et al.* IgG Subclass Responses in a Longitudinal Study of Canine Visceral Leishmaniasis. Vet Immunol Immunopathol. 2003 Feb 10;91(3-4):161-168. PubMed PMID: 12586479.

[36] Bourdoiseau G, Hugnet C, Goncalves RB, Vezilier F, Petit-Didier E, Papierok G, *et al.* Effective Humoral and Cellular Immunoprotective Responses in Li ESAp-MDP Vaccinated Protected Dogs. Vet Immunol Immunopathol. 2009 Mar 15;128(1-3):71-78. PubMed PMID: 19046774.

[37] Moreno J, Nieto J, Chamizo C, Gonzalez F, Blanco F, Barker DC, *et al.* The Immune Response and PBMC Subsets in Canine Visceral Leishmaniasis before, and after,

Chemotherapy. Vet Immunol Immunopathol. 1999 Nov 30;71(3-4):181-195. PubMed PMID: 10587300.

[38] Handman E. Leishmaniasis: Current Status of Vaccine Development. Clin Microbiol Rev. 2001 Apr;14(2):229-243. PubMed PMID: 11292637. Pubmed Central PMCID: 88972.

[39] Melby PC, Chandrasekar B, Zhao W, Coe JE. The Hamster as a Model of Human Visceral Leishmaniasis: Progressive Disease and Impaired Generation of Nitric Oxide in the Face of a Prominent Th1-Like Cytokine Response. J Immunol. 2001 Feb 1;166(3): 1912-1920. PubMed PMID: 11160239.

[40] Abranches P, Santos-Gomes G, Rachamim N, Campino L, Schnur LF, Jaffe CL. An Experimental Model for Canine Visceral Leishmaniasis. Parasite Immunol. 1991 Sep; 13(5):537-550. PubMed PMID: 1956700.

[41] Porrozzi R, Pereira MS, Teva A, Volpini AC, Pinto MA, Marchevsky RS, *et al. Leishmania infantum*-Induced Primary and Challenge Infections in Rhesus Monkeys (*Macaca mulatta*): A Primate Model for Visceral Leishmaniasis. Trans R Soc Trop Med Hyg. 2006 Oct;100(10):926-937. PubMed PMID: 16455120.

[42] Mutiso JM, Macharia JC, Taracha E, Gicheru MM. *Leishmania donovani* Whole Cell Antigen Delivered with Adjuvants Protects against Visceral Leishmaniasis in Vervet Monkeys (*Chlorocebus aethiops*). J Biomed Res. 2012 Jan;26(1):8-16. PubMed PMID: 23554725. Pubmed Central PMCID: 3596075.

[43] Dube A, Sharma P, Srivastava JK, Misra A, Naik S, Katiyar JC. Vaccination of Langur Monkeys (*Presbytis entellus*) against *Leishmania donovani* with Autoclaved *L. major* Plus BCG. Parasitology. 1998 Mar;116 (Pt 3):219-221. PubMed PMID: 9550214.

[44] Misra A, Dube A, Srivastava B, Sharma P, Srivastava JK, Katiyar JC, *et al*. Successful Vaccination against *Leishmania donovani* Infection in Indian Langur Using Alum-Precipitated Autoclaved *Leishmania major* with BCG. Vaccine. 2001 May 14;19(25-26): 3485-3492. PubMed PMID: 11348715.

[45] Evans KJ, Kedzierski L. Development of Vaccines against Visceral Leishmaniasis. J Trop Med. 2012;2012:892817. PubMed PMID: 21912561. Pubmed Central PMCID: 3170777.

[46] Khamesipour A, Dowlati Y, Asilian A, Hashemi-Fesharki R, Javadi A, Noazin S, *et al*. Leishmanization: Use of an Old Method for Evaluation of Candidate Vaccines against Leishmaniasis. Vaccine. 2005 May 25;23(28):3642-3648. PubMed PMID: 15882524.

[47] Karunaweera ND. *Leishmania donovani* Causing Cutaneous Leishmaniasis in Sri Lanka: A Wolf in Sheep's Clothing? Trends Parasitol. 2009 Oct;25(10):458-463. PubMed PMID: 19734098.

[48] McCall LI, Zhang WW, Ranasinghe S, Matlashewski G. Leishmanization Revisited: Immunization with a Naturally Attenuated Cutaneous *Leishmania donovani* Isolate

from Sri Lanka Protects against Visceral Leishmaniasis. Vaccine. 2013 Feb 27;31(10): 1420-1425. PubMed PMID: 23219435.

[49] Streit JA, Recker TJ, Filho FG, Beverley SM, Wilson ME. Protective Immunity against the Protozoan *Leishmania chagasi* Is Induced by Subclinical Cutaneous Infection with Virulent but Not Avirulent Organisms. J Immunol. 2001 Feb 1;166(3):1921-1929. PubMed PMID: 11160240.

[50] Zijlstra EE, el-Hassan AM, Ismael A, Ghalib HW. Endemic Kala-Azar in Eastern Sudan: A Longitudinal Study on the Incidence of Clinical and Subclinical Infection and Post-Kala-Azar Dermal Leishmaniasis. Am J Trop Med Hyg. 1994 Dec;51(6):826-836. PubMed PMID: 7810819.

[51] Giunchetti RC, Correa-Oliveira R, Martins-Filho OA, Teixeira-Carvalho A, Roatt BM, de Oliveira Aguiar-Soares RD, *et al*. Immunogenicity of a Killed *Leishmania* Vaccine with Saponin Adjuvant in Dogs. Vaccine. 2007 Nov 1;25(44):7674-7686. PubMed PMID: 17913311.

[52] Armijos RX, Weigel MM, Aviles H, Maldonado R, Racines J. Field Trial of a Vaccine against New World Cutaneous Leishmaniasis in an at-Risk Child Population: Safety, Immunogenicity, and Efficacy During the First 12 Months of Follow-Up. J Infect Dis. 1998 May;177(5):1352-1357. PubMed PMID: 9593024.

[53] Noazin S, Khamesipour A, Moulton LH, Tanner M, Nasseri K, Modabber F, *et al*. Efficacy of Killed Whole-Parasite Vaccines in the Prevention of Leishmaniasis: A Meta-Analysis. Vaccine. 2009 Jul 30;27(35):4747-4753. PubMed PMID: 19540273.

[54] Das A, Ali N. Vaccine Prospects of Killed but Metabolically Active *Leishmania* against Visceral Leishmaniasis. Expert Rev Vaccines. 2012 Jul;11(7):783-785. PubMed PMID: 22913255.

[55] Breton M, Tremblay MJ, Ouellette M, Papadopoulou B. Live Nonpathogenic Parasitic Vector as a Candidate Vaccine against Visceral Leishmaniasis. Infect Immun. 2005 Oct;73(10):6372-6382. PubMed PMID: 16177308. Pubmed Central PMCID: 1230936.

[56] Papadopoulou B, Roy G, Breton M, Kundig C, Dumas C, Fillion I, *et al*. Reduced Infectivity of a *Leishmania donovani* Biopterin Transporter Genetic Mutant and Its Use as an Attenuated Strain for Vaccination. Infect Immun. 2002 Jan;70(1):62-68. PubMed PMID: 11748164. Pubmed Central PMCID: 127620.

[57] Selvapandiyan A, Dey R, Nylen S, Duncan R, Sacks D, Nakhasi HL. Intracellular Replication-Deficient *Leishmania donovani* Induces Long Lasting Protective Immunity against Visceral Leishmaniasis. J Immunol. 2009 Aug 1;183(3):1813-1820. PubMed PMID: 19592661.

[58] Dey R, Meneses C, Salotra P, Kamhawi S, Nakhasi HL, Duncan R. Characterization of a *Leishmania* Stage-Specific Mitochondrial Membrane Protein That Enhances the Activity of Cytochrome C Oxidase and Its Role in Virulence. Mol Microbiol. 2010 Jul; 77(2):399-414. PubMed PMID: 20497506. Pubmed Central PMCID: 2909329.

[59] Silvestre R, Cordeiro-Da-Silva A, Santarem N, Vergnes B, Sereno D, Ouaissi A. Sir2-Deficient *Leishmania infantum* Induces a Defined IFN-gamma/IL-10 Pattern That Correlates with Protection. J Immunol. 2007 Sep 1;179(5):3161-3170. PubMed PMID: 17709531.

[60] Mizbani A, Taheri T, Zahedifard F, Taslimi Y, Azizi H, Azadmanesh K, *et al*. Recombinant *Leishmania tarentolae* Expressing the A2 Virulence Gene as a Novel Candidate Vaccine against Visceral Leishmaniasis. Vaccine. 2009 Dec 10;28(1):53-62. PubMed PMID: 19818721.

[61] Selvapandiyan A, Dey R, Gannavaram S, Lakhal-Naouar I, Duncan R, Salotra P, *et al*. Immunity to Visceral Leishmaniasis Using Genetically Defined Live-Attenuated Parasites. J Trop Med. 2012;2012:631460. PubMed PMID: 21912560. Pubmed Central PMCID: 3168768.

[62] Nagill R, Kaur S. Vaccine Candidates for Leishmaniasis: A Review. Int Immunopharmacol. 2011 Oct;11(10):1464-1488. PubMed PMID: 21616175.

[63] Russell DG, Alexander J. Effective Immunization against Cutaneous Leishmaniasis with Defined Membrane Antigens Reconstituted into Liposomes. J Immunol. 1988 Feb 15;140(4):1274-1279. PubMed PMID: 3257774.

[64] Bhowmick S, Ravindran R, Ali N. gp63 in Stable Cationic Liposomes Confers Sustained Vaccine Immunity to Susceptible BALB/c Mice Infected with *Leishmania donovani*. Infect Immun. 2008 Mar;76(3):1003-1015. PubMed PMID: 18195029. Pubmed Central PMCID: 2258822.

[65] Gurunathan S, Prussin C, Sacks DL, Seder RA. Vaccine Requirements for Sustained Cellular Immunity to an Intracellular Parasitic Infection. Nat Med. 1998 Dec;4(12): 1409-1415. PubMed PMID: 9846579.

[66] Coelho EA, Tavares CA, Carvalho FA, Chaves KF, Teixeira KN, Rodrigues RC, *et al*. Immune Responses Induced by the *Leishmania* (*Leishmania*) *donovani* A2 Antigen, but Not by the LACK Antigen, Are Protective against Experimental *Leishmania* (*Leishmania*) *amazonensis* Infection. Infect Immun. 2003 Jul;71(7):3988-3994. PubMed PMID: 12819086. Pubmed Central PMCID: 162020.

[67] Pinto EF, Pinheiro RO, Rayol A, Larraga V, Rossi-Bergmann B. Intranasal Vaccination against Cutaneous Leishmaniasis with a Particulated Leishmanial Antigen or DNA Encoding LACK. Infect Immun. 2004 Aug;72(8):4521-4527. PubMed PMID: 15271911. Pubmed Central PMCID: 470668.

[68] Handman E, Symons FM, Baldwin TM, Curtis JM, Scheerlinck JP. Protective Vaccination with Promastigote Surface Antigen 2 from *Leishmania major* Is Mediated by a Th1 Type of Immune Response. Infect Immun. 1995 Nov;63(11):4261-4267. PubMed PMID: 7591056. Pubmed Central PMCID: 173605.

[69] Sjolander A, Baldwin TM, Curtis JM, Bengtsson KL, Handman E. Vaccination with Recombinant Parasite Surface Antigen 2 from *Leishmania major* Induces a Th1 Type of

Immune Response but Does Not Protect against Infection. Vaccine. 1998 Dec;16(20): 2077-2084. PubMed PMID: 9796067.

[70] Coler RN, Skeiky YA, Bernards K, Greeson K, Carter D, Cornellison CD, *et al.* Immunization with a Polyprotein Vaccine Consisting of the T-Cell Antigens Thiol-Specific Antioxidant, *Leishmania major* Stress-Inducible Protein 1, and *Leishmania* Elongation Initiation Factor Protects against Leishmaniasis. Infect Immun. 2002 Aug;70(8): 4215-4225. PubMed PMID: 12117930. Pubmed Central PMCID: 128156.

[71] Coler RN, Goto Y, Bogatzki L, Raman V, Reed SG. Leish-111f, a Recombinant Polyprotein Vaccine That Protects against Visceral Leishmaniasis by Elicitation of $CD4^+$ T Cells. Infect Immun. 2007 Sep;75(9):4648-4654. PubMed PMID: 17606603. Pubmed Central PMCID: 1951162.

[72] Velez ID, Gilchrist K, Martinez S, Ramirez-Pineda JR, Ashman JA, Alves FP, *et al.* Safety and Immunogenicity of a Defined Vaccine for the Prevention of Cutaneous Leishmaniasis. Vaccine. 2009 Dec 11;28(2):329-337. PubMed PMID: 19879995.

[73] Chakravarty J, Kumar S, Trivedi S, Rai VK, Singh A, Ashman JA, *et al.* A Clinical Trial to Evaluate the Safety and Immunogenicity of the Leish-F1+MPL-SE Vaccine for Use in the Prevention of Visceral Leishmaniasis. Vaccine. 2011 Apr 27;29(19): 3531-3537. PubMed PMID: 21414377.

[74] Trigo J, Abbehusen M, Netto EM, Nakatani M, Pedral-Sampaio G, de Jesus RS, *et al.* Treatment of Canine Visceral Leishmaniasis by the Vaccine Leish-111f+MPL-SE. Vaccine. 2010 Apr 26;28(19):3333-3340. PubMed PMID: 20206667. Pubmed Central PMCID: 2874835.

[75] Gradoni L, Foglia Manzillo V, Pagano A, Piantedosi D, De Luna R, Gramiccia M, *et al.* Failure of a Multi-Subunit Recombinant Leishmanial Vaccine (MML) to Protect Dogs from *Leishmania infantum* Infection and to Prevent Disease Progression in Infected Animals. Vaccine. 2005 Nov 1;23(45):5245-5251. PubMed PMID: 16054272.

[76] Miret J, Nascimento E, Sampaio W, Franca JC, Fujiwara RT, Vale A, *et al.* Evaluation of an Immunochemotherapeutic Protocol Constituted of N-Methyl Meglumine Antimoniate (Glucantime) and the Recombinant Leish-110f + MPL-SE Vaccine to Treat Canine Visceral Leishmaniasis. Vaccine. 2008 Mar 17;26(12):1585-1594. PubMed PMID: 18328956.

[77] Bertholet S, Goto Y, Carter L, Bhatia A, Howard RF, Carter D, *et al.* Optimized Subunit Vaccine Protects against Experimental Leishmaniasis. Vaccine. 2009 Nov 23;27(50):7036-7045. PubMed PMID: 19786136. Pubmed Central PMCID: 2783536.

[78] Duthie MS, Raman VS, Piazza FM, Reed SG. The Development and Clinical Evaluation of Second-Generation Leishmaniasis Vaccines. Vaccine. 2012 Jan 5;30(2):134-141. PubMed PMID: 22085553. Pubmed Central PMCID: 3359766.

[79] Molano I, Alonso MG, Miron C, Redondo E, Requena JM, Soto M, *et al.* A *Leishmania infantum* Multi-Component Antigenic Protein Mixed with Live BCG Confers Protec-

tion to Dogs Experimentally Infected with *L. infantum*. Vet Immunol Immunopathol. 2003 Mar 20;92(1-2):1-13. PubMed PMID: 12628759.

[80] Parody N, Soto M, Requena JM, Alonso C. Adjuvant Guided Polarization of the Immune Humoral Response against a Protective Multicomponent Antigenic Protein (Q) from *Leishmania infantum*. A CPG + Q Mix Protects BALB/c Mice from Infection. Parasite Immunol. 2004 Jun-Jul;26(6-7):283-293. PubMed PMID: 15541032.

[81] Restifo NP, Ying H, Hwang L, Leitner WW. The Promise of Nucleic Acid Vaccines. Gene Ther. 2000 Jan;7(2):89-92. PubMed PMID: 10673713. Pubmed Central PMCID: 2241736.

[82] Dondji B, Perez-Jimenez E, Goldsmith-Pestana K, Esteban M, McMahon-Pratt D. Heterologous Prime-Boost Vaccination with the LACK Antigen Protects against Murine Visceral Leishmaniasis. Infect Immun. 2005 Aug;73(8):5286-5289. PubMed PMID: 16041057. Pubmed Central PMCID: 1201228.

[83] Gomes DC, Pinto EF, de Melo LD, Lima WP, Larraga V, Lopes UG, *et al*. Intranasal Delivery of Naked DNA Encoding the LACK Antigen Leads to Protective Immunity against Visceral Leishmaniasis in Mice. Vaccine. 2007 Mar 8;25(12):2168-2172. PubMed PMID: 17240003.

[84] Ramos I, Alonso A, Marcen JM, Peris A, Castillo JA, Colmenares M, *et al*. Heterologous Prime-Boost Vaccination with a Non-Replicative Vaccinia Recombinant Vector Expressing LACK Confers Protection against Canine Visceral Leishmaniasis with a Predominant Th1-Specific Immune Response. Vaccine. 2008 Jan 17;26(3):333-344. PubMed PMID: 18093705.

[85] Tapia E, Perez-Jimenez E, Lopez-Fuertes L, Gonzalo R, Gherardi MM, Esteban M. The Combination of DNA Vectors Expressing IL-12 + IL-18 Elicits High Protective Immune Response against Cutaneous Leishmaniasis after Priming with DNA-P36/LACK and the Cytokines, Followed by a Booster with a Vaccinia Virus Recombinant Expressing P36/LACK. Microbes Infect. 2003 Feb;5(2):73-84. PubMed PMID: 12650765.

[86] Perez-Jimenez E, Kochan G, Gherardi MM, Esteban M. MVA-LACK as a Safe and Efficient Vector for Vaccination against Leishmaniasis. Microbes Infect. 2006 Mar;8(3):810-822. PubMed PMID: 16504562.

[87] Moll H, Berberich C. Dendritic Cells as Vectors for Vaccination against Infectious Diseases. Int J Med Microbiol. 2001 Nov;291(5):323-329. PubMed PMID: 11727816.

[88] Jardim A, Alexander J, Teh HS, Ou D, Olafson RW. Immunoprotective *Leishmania major* Synthetic T Cell Epitopes. J Exp Med. 1990 Aug 1;172(2):645-648. PubMed PMID: 1695670. Pubmed Central PMCID: 2188333.

[89] Tsagozis P, Karagouni E, Dotsika E. Dendritic Cells Pulsed with Peptides of gp63 Induce Differential Protection against Experimental Cutaneous Leishmaniasis. Int J Immunopathol Pharmacol. 2004 Sep-Dec;17(3):343-352. PubMed PMID: 15461868.

[90] Agallou M, Smirlis D, Soteriadou KP, Karagouni E. Vaccination with *Leishmania* Histone H1-Pulsed Dendritic Cells Confers Protection in Murine Visceral Leishmaniasis. Vaccine. 2012 Jul 20;30(34):5086-5093. PubMed PMID: 22704924.

[91] Carrion J, Nieto A, Soto M, Alonso C. Adoptive Transfer of Dendritic Cells Pulsed with *Leishmania infantum* Nucleosomal Histones Confers Protection against Cutaneous Leishmaniosis in BALB/c Mice. Microbes Infect. 2007 May;9(6):735-743. PubMed PMID: 17400015.

[92] Agallou M, Margaroni M, Karagouni E. Cellular Vaccination with Bone Marrow-Derived Dendritic Cells Pulsed with a Peptide of *Leishmania infantum* KMP-11 and CPG Oligonucleotides Induces Protection in a Murine Model of Visceral Leishmaniasis. Vaccine. 2011 Jul 12;29(31):5053-5064. PubMed PMID: 21569815.

[93] Badiee A, Heravi Shargh V, Khamesipour A, Jaafari MR. Micro/Nanoparticle Adjuvants for Antileishmanial Vaccines: Present and Future Trends. Vaccine. 2013 Jan 21;31(5):735-749. PubMed PMID: 23219436.

[94] Jaafari MR, Ghafarian A, Farrokh-Gisour A, Samiei A, Kheiri MT, Mahboudi F, *et al.* Immune Response and Protection Assay of Recombinant Major Surface Glycoprotein of *Leishmania* (rgp63) Reconstituted with Liposomes in BALB/c Mice. Vaccine. 2006 Jul 17;24(29-30):5708-5717. PubMed PMID: 16740346.

[95] Badiee A, Jaafari MR, Khamesipour A. Leishmania Major: Immune Response in BALB/c Mice Immunized with Stress-Inducible Protein 1 Encapsulated in Liposomes. Exp Parasitol. 2007 Feb;115(2):127-134. PubMed PMID: 16979165.

[96] Bhowmick S, Ali N. Recent Developments in Leishmaniasis Vaccine Delivery Systems. Expert Opin Drug Deliv. 2008 Jul;5(7):789-803. PubMed PMID: 18590463.

[97] Bhowmick S, Mazumdar T, Ali N. Vaccination Route That Induces Transforming Growth Factor Beta Production Fails to Elicit Protective Immunity against *Leishmania donovani* Infection. Infect Immun. 2009 Apr;77(4):1514-1523. PubMed PMID: 19168736. Pubmed Central PMCID: 2663136.

[98] Kawai T, Akira S. The Role of Pattern-Recognition Receptors in Innate Immunity: Update on Toll-Like Receptors. Nat Immunol. 2010 May;11(5):373-384. PubMed PMID: 20404851.

[99] Gurunathan S, Sacks DL, Brown DR, Reiner SL, Charest H, Glaichenhaus N, *et al.* Vaccination with DNA Encoding the Immunodominant LACK Parasite Antigen Confers Protective Immunity to Mice Infected with *Leishmania major*. J Exp Med. 1997 Oct 6;186(7):1137-1147. PubMed PMID: 9314562. Pubmed Central PMCID: 2199076.

[100] Mendez S, Gurunathan S, Kamhawi S, Belkaid Y, Moga MA, Skeiky YA, *et al.* The Potency and Durability of DNA- and Protein-Based Vaccines against *Leishmania major* Evaluated Using Low-Dose, Intradermal Challenge. J Immunol. 2001 Apr 15;166(8): 5122-5128. PubMed PMID: 11290794.

[101] Coler RN, Reed SG. Second-Generation Vaccines against Leishmaniasis. Trends Parasitol. 2005 May;21(5):244-249. PubMed PMID: 15837614.

[102] Raman VS, Duthie MS, Fox CB, Matlashewski G, Reed SG. Adjuvants for *Leishmania* Vaccines: From Models to Clinical Application. Front Immunol. 2012;3:144. PubMed PMID: 22701453. Pubmed Central PMCID: 3371596.

[103] Coler RN, Bertholet S, Moutaftsi M, Guderian JA, Windish HP, Baldwin SL, *et al*. Development and Characterization of Synthetic Glucopyranosyl Lipid Adjuvant System as a Vaccine Adjuvant. PLoS One. 2011;6(1):e16333. PubMed PMID: 21298114. Pubmed Central PMCID: 3027669.

[104] Klinman DM, Kamstrup S, Verthelyi D, Gursel I, Ishii KJ, Takeshita F, *et al*. Activation of the Innate Immune System by CPG Oligodeoxynucleotides: Immunoprotective Activity and Safety. Springer Semin Immunopathol. 2000;22(1-2):173-183. PubMed PMID: 10944812.

[105] Klinman DM, Yi AK, Beaucage SL, Conover J, Krieg AM. CPG Motifs Present in Bacteria DNA Rapidly Induce Lymphocytes to Secrete Interleukin 6, Interleukin 12, and Interferon gamma. Proc Natl Acad Sci U S A. 1996 Apr 2;93(7):2879-2883. PubMed PMID: 8610135. Pubmed Central PMCID: 39727.

[106] Novak N, Yu CF, Bieber T, Allam JP. Toll-Like Receptor 7 Agonists and Skin. Drug News Perspect. 2008 Apr;21(3):158-165. PubMed PMID: 18560614.

[107] Buates S, Matlashewski G. Treatment of Experimental Leishmaniasis with the Immunomodulators Imiquimod and S-28463: Efficacy and Mode of Action. J Infect Dis. 1999 Jun;179(6):1485-1494. PubMed PMID: 10228071.

[108] Hervas JA, Martin-Santiago A, Hervas D, Rojo E, Mena A, Rocamora V, *et al*. Old World *Leishmania infantum* Cutaneous Leishmaniasis Unresponsive to Liposomal Amphotericin B Treated with Topical Imiquimod. Pediatr Infect Dis J. 2012 Jan;31(1): 97-100. PubMed PMID: 21829140.

[109] Garcia Bustos MF, Barrio AB, Parodi Ramoneda CM, Ramos F, Mora MC, Convit J, *et al*. Immunological Correlates of Cure in the First American Cutaneous Leishmaniasis Patient Treated by Immunotherapy in Argentina. A Case Report. Invest Clin. 2011 Dec;52(4):365-375. PubMed PMID: 22523846.

[110] Nahrevanian H, Jafary SP, Nemati S, Farahmand M, Omidinia E. Evaluation of Anti-Leishmanial Effects of Killed *Leishmania* Vaccine with BCG Adjuvant in BALB/c Mice Infected with *Leishmania major* MRHO/IR/75/ER. Folia Parasitol (Praha). 2013 Feb; 60(1):1-6. PubMed PMID: 23539946.

[111] Soudi S, Hosseini AZ, Hashemi SM. Co-Administration of Rectal BCG and Autoclaved *Leishmania major* Induce Protection in Susceptible BALB/c Mice. Parasite Immunol. 2011 Oct;33(10):561-571. PubMed PMID: 21781137.

[112] Nateghi Rostami M, Keshavarz H, Khamesipour A. Immune Response of BALB/c Mice against an Experimental Vaccine of Alum Precipitated Autoclaved *Leishmania*

major (Alum-Alm) Mixed with Bcg or Mycobacterium Vaccae. Trop Biomed. 2010 Apr;27(1):89-102. PubMed PMID: 20562818.

[113] Tripathi P, Gupta SK, Sinha S, Sundar S, Dube A, Naik S. Prophylactic Efficacy of High-Molecular-Weight Antigenic Fractions of a Recent Clinical Isolate of *Leishmania donovani* against Visceral Leishmaniasis. Scand J Immunol. 2008 Nov;68(5):492-501. PubMed PMID: 18803606.

[114] Trotta T, Fasanella A, Scaltrito D, Gradoni L, Mitolo V, Brandonisio O, *et al*. Comparison between Three Adjuvants for a Vaccine against Canine Leishmaniasis: *In Vitro* Evaluation of Macrophage Killing Ability. Comp Immunol Microbiol Infect Dis. 2010 Mar;33(2):175-182. PubMed PMID: 20061026.

[115] Poot J, Janssen LH, van Kasteren-Westerneng TJ, van der Heijden-Liefkens KH, Schijns VE, Heckeroth A. Vaccination of Dogs with Six Different Candidate Leishmaniasis Vaccines Composed of a Chimerical Recombinant Protein Containing Ribosomal and Histone Protein Epitopes in Combination with Different Adjuvants. Vaccine. 2009 Jul 16;27(33):4439-4446. PubMed PMID: 19500553.

[116] Heldwein KA, Liang MD, Andresen TK, Thomas KE, Marty AM, Cuesta N, *et al*. TLR2 and TLR4 Serve Distinct Roles in the Host Immune Response against *Mycobacterium bovis* BCG. J Leukoc Biol. 2003 Aug;74(2):277-286. PubMed PMID: 12885945.

[117] von Meyenn F, Schaefer M, Weighardt H, Bauer S, Kirschning CJ, Wagner H, *et al*. Toll-Like Receptor 9 Contributes to Recognition of *Mycobacterium bovis* Bacillus Calmette-Guerin by Flt3-Ligand Generated Dendritic Cells. Immunobiology. 2006;211(6-8):557-565. PubMed PMID: 16920494.

[118] Smrkovski LL, Larson CL. Effect of Treatment with BCG on the Course of Visceral Leishmaniasis in BALB/c Mice. Infect Immun. 1977 Apr;16(1):249-257. PubMed PMID: 873609. Pubmed Central PMCID: 421515.

[119] Weintraub J, Weinbaum FI. The Effect of BCG on Experimental Cutaneous Leishmaniasis in Mice. J Immunol. 1977 Jun;118(6):2288-2290. PubMed PMID: 864260.

[120] Modified Saponins Isolated from *Quillaja saponaria* - Us 5443829 A. Available from: https://www.google.com/patents/US5443829.

[121] Sun HX, Xie Y, Ye YP. Advances in Saponin-Based Adjuvants. Vaccine. 2009 Mar 13;27(12):1787-1796. PubMed PMID: 19208455.

[122] Kenney RT, Sacks DL, Sypek JP, Vilela L, Gam AA, Evans-Davis K. Protective Immunity Using Recombinant Human IL-12 and Alum as Adjuvants in a Primate Model of Cutaneous Leishmaniasis. J Immunol. 1999 Oct 15;163(8):4481-4488. PubMed PMID: 10510390.

[123] Nakanishi T, Hayashi A, Kunisawa J, Tsutsumi Y, Tanaka K, Yashiro-Ohtani Y, *et al*. Fusogenic Liposomes Efficiently Deliver Exogenous Antigen through the Cytoplasm into the MHC Class I Processing Pathway. Eur J Immunol. 2000 Jun;30(6):1740-1747. PubMed PMID: 10898512.

[124] Pardakhty A, Shakibaie M, Daneshvar H, Khamesipour A, Mohammadi-Khorsand T, Forootanfar H. Preparation and Evaluation of Niosomes Containing Autoclaved *Leishmania major*: A Preliminary Study. J Microencapsul. 2012;29(3):219-224. PubMed PMID: 22150018.

[125] Dantas-Torres F. Leishmune Vaccine: The Newest Tool for Prevention and Control of Canine Visceral Leishmaniosis and Its Potential as a Transmission-Blocking Vaccine. Vet Parasitol. 2006 Oct 10;141(1-2):1-8. PubMed PMID: 16750885.

[126] Dodge F. Leishmune É Ética, É Legal E Protege. 2009. Available from: http://www.leishmune.com.br/leishmaniose/Leishmune/Outros/Diversos/14682_folheto.pdf.

[127] Fernandes AP, Costa MM, Coelho EA, Michalick MS, de Freitas E, Melo MN, *et al*. Protective Immunity against Challenge with *Leishmania* (*Leishmania*) *chagasi* in Beagle Dogs Vaccinated with Recombinant A2 Protein. Vaccine. 2008 Oct 29;26(46): 5888-5895. PubMed PMID: 18786587.

[128] Virbac. Canileish® Veterinary Brochure - Portuguese Edition 2011 [cited 2013]. Available from: http://www.ruminal.com.ar/sites/default/files/vet%20brochure.pdf.

[129] Moreno J, Vouldoukis I, Martin V, McGahie D, Cuisinier AM, Gueguen S. Use of a LiESP/QA-21 Vaccine (Canileish) Stimulates an Appropriate Th1-Dominated Cell-Mediated Immune Response in Dogs. PLoS Negl Trop Dis. 2012;6(6):e1683. PubMed PMID: 22724031. Pubmed Central PMCID: 3378610.

[130] IDRI. First Vaccine against Fatal Visceral Leishmaniasis Enters Clinical Trial 2012. Available from: http://www.idri.org/press-2-22-12.php.

[131] clinicaltrials.gov. A Phase 1 Clinical Trial to Evaluate the Safety, Tolerability, and Immunogenicity of the Vaccine Candidates Leish-F3 + GLA-SE, Leish-F3 + MPL-SE, and Leish-F3 + SE in Healthy Adult Subjects 2013. Available from: http://clinicaltrials.gov/ct2/show/study/NCT01751048.

[132] IDRI. Idri and Zydus Sign Agreement for Development of Idri's Vaccine Candidate for Visceral Leishmaniasis (Kala-Azar) 2013. Available from: http://www.idri.org/press-07-25-13.php.

[133] Tacchini-Cottier F, Weinkopff T, Launois P. Does T Helper Differentiation Correlate with Resistance or Susceptibility to Infection with *L. major*? Some Insights from the Murine Model. Front Immunol. 2012;3:32. PubMed PMID: 22566916. Pubmed Central PMCID: 3342012.

[134] Baptista-Fernandes T, Marques C, Roos Rodrigues O, Santos-Gomes GM. Intra-Specific Variability of Virulence in *Leishmaniai infantum* Zymodeme MON-1 Strains. Comp Immunol Microbiol Infect Dis. 2007 Jan;30(1):41-53. PubMed PMID: 17109961.

[135] Oliveira DM, Costa MA, Chavez-Fumagalli MA, Valadares DG, Duarte MC, Costa LE, *et al*. Evaluation of Parasitological and Immunological Parameters of *Leishmania*

chagasi Infection in BALB/c Mice Using Different Doses and Routes of Inoculation of Parasites. Parasitol Res. 2012 Mar;110(3):1277-1285. PubMed PMID: 21915627.

[136] Cunha J, Carrillo E, Sanchez C, Cruz I, Moreno J, Cordeiro-da-Silva A. Characterization of the Biology and Infectivity of *Leishmania infantum* Viscerotropic and Dermotropic Strains Isolated from HIV^+ and HIV^- Patients in the Murine Model of Visceral Leishmaniasis. Parasites & Vectors. 2013;6:122. PubMed PMID: 23622683. Pubmed Central PMCID: 3649922.

[137] Peters NC, Egen JG, Secundino N, Debrabant A, Kimblin N, Kamhawi S, *et al*. *In Vivo* Imaging Reveals an Essential Role for Neutrophils in Leishmaniasis Transmitted by Sand Flies. Science. 2008 Aug 15;321(5891):970-974. PubMed PMID: 18703742. Pubmed Central PMCID: 2606057.

[138] Thalhofer CJ, Chen Y, Sudan B, Love-Homan L, Wilson ME. Leukocytes Infiltrate the Skin and Draining Lymph Nodes in Response to the Protozoan *Leishmania infantum chagasi*. Infect Immun. 2011 Jan;79(1):108-117. PubMed PMID: 20937764. Pubmed Central PMCID: 3019875.

[139] Yurdakul P, Dalton J, Beattie L, Brown N, Erguven S, Maroof A, *et al*. Compartment-Specific Remodeling of Splenic Micro-Architecture During Experimental Visceral Leishmaniasis. Am J Pathol. 2011 Jul;179(1):23-29. PubMed PMID: 21703391. Pubmed Central PMCID: 3123882.

[140] Smelt SC, Cotterell SE, Engwerda CR, Kaye PM. B Cell-Deficient Mice Are Highly Resistant to *Leishmania donovani* Infection, but Develop Neutrophil-Mediated Tissue Pathology. J Immunol. 2000 Apr 1;164(7):3681-3688. PubMed PMID: 10725726.

[141] Tacchini-Cottier F, Zweifel C, Belkaid Y, Mukankundiye C, Vasei M, Launois P, *et al*. An Immunomodulatory Function for Neutrophils During the Induction of a $CD4^+$ Th2 Response in BALB/c Mice Infected with *Leishmania major*. J Immunol. 2000 Sep 1;165(5):2628-2636. PubMed PMID: 10946291.

[142] Souto FO, Alves-Filho JC, Turato WM, Auxiliadora-Martins M, Basile-Filho A, Cunha FQ. Essential Role of CCR2 in Neutrophil Tissue Infiltration and Multiple Organ Dysfunction in Sepsis. Am J Respir Crit Care Med. 2011 Jan 15;183(2):234-242. PubMed PMID: 20732989.

[143] Sato N, Ahuja SK, Quinones M, Kostecki V, Reddick RL, Melby PC, *et al*. CC Chemokine Receptor (CCR)2 Is Required for Langerhans Cell Migration and Localization of T Helper Cell Type 1 (Th1)-Inducing Dendritic Cells. Absence of CCR2 Shifts the *Leishmania major*-Resistant Phenotype to a Susceptible State Dominated by Th2 Cytokines, B Cell Outgrowth, and Sustained Neutrophilic Inflammation. J Exp Med. 2000 Jul 17;192(2):205-218. PubMed PMID: 10899907. Pubmed Central PMCID: 2193245.

[144] Conrad SM, Strauss-Ayali D, Field AE, Mack M, Mosser DM. *Leishmania*-Derived Murine Monocyte Chemoattractant Protein 1 Enhances the Recruitment of a Restrictive Population of CC Chemokine Receptor 2-Positive Macrophages. Infect Immun. 2007 Feb;75(2):653-665. PubMed PMID: 17088347. Pubmed Central PMCID: 1828528.

[145] Meddeb-Garnaoui A, Zrelli H, Dellagi K. Effects of Tropism and Virulence of *Leishmania* Parasites on Cytokine Production by Infected Human Monocytes. Clin Exp Immunol. 2009 Feb;155(2):199-206. PubMed PMID: 19040614. Pubmed Central PMCID: 2675250.

[146] Liu D, Uzonna JE. The P110 Delta Isoform of Phosphatidylinositol 3-Kinase Controls the Quality of Secondary Anti-*Leishmania* Immunity by Regulating Expansion and Effector Function of Memory T Cell Subsets. J Immunol. 2010 Mar 15;184(6):3098-3105. PubMed PMID: 20154209.

[147] Mueller SN, Gebhardt T, Carbone FR, Heath WR. Memory T Cell Subsets, Migration Patterns, and Tissue Residence. Annu Rev Immunol. 2012 Dec 3. PubMed PMID: 23215646.

[148] Resende M, Moreira D, Augusto J, Cunha J, Neves B, Cruz MT, *et al.* *Leishmania*-Infected MHC Class II^{high} Dendritic Cells Polarize $CD4^{+}$ T Cells toward a Nonprotective T-bet^{+} IFN-$gamma^{+}$ IL-10^{+} Phenotype. J Immunol. 2013 Jul 1;191(1):262-273. PubMed PMID: 23729437.

[149] Owens BM, Beattie L, Moore JW, Brown N, Mann JL, Dalton JE, *et al.* IL-10-Producing Th1 Cells and Disease Progression Are Regulated by Distinct CD11c(+) Cell Populations During Visceral Leishmaniasis. PLoS Pathog. 2012;8(7):e1002827. PubMed PMID: 22911108. Pubmed Central PMCID: 3406093.

[150] Anderson CF, Oukka M, Kuchroo VJ, Sacks D. CD4(+)CD25(-)Foxp3(-) Th1 Cells Are the Source of IL-10-Mediated Immune Suppression in Chronic Cutaneous Leishmaniasis. J Exp Med. 2007 Feb 19;204(2):285-297. PubMed PMID: 17283207. Pubmed Central PMCID: 2118728.

[151] Bogdan C, Moll H, Solbach W, Rollinghoff M. Tumor Necrosis Factor-alpha in Combination with Interferon-gamma, but Not with Interleukin 4 Activates Murine Macrophages for Elimination of *Leishmania major* Amastigotes. Eur J Immunol. 1990 May; 20(5):1131-1135. PubMed PMID: 2113475.

[152] Liew FY, Li Y, Millott S. Tumor Necrosis Factor-alpha Synergizes with IFN-gamma in Mediating Killing of *Leishmania major* through the Induction of Nitric Oxide. J Immunol. 1990 Dec 15;145(12):4306-4310. PubMed PMID: 2175327.

[153] Chan J, Xing Y, Magliozzo RS, Bloom BR. Killing of Virulent *Mycobacterium tuberculosis* by Reactive Nitrogen Intermediates Produced by Activated Murine Macrophages. J Exp Med. 1992 Apr 1;175(4):1111-1122. PubMed PMID: 1552282. Pubmed Central PMCID: 2119182.

[154] Darrah PA, Patel DT, De Luca PM, Lindsay RW, Davey DF, Flynn BJ, *et al.* Multifunctional Th1 Cells Define a Correlate of Vaccine-Mediated Protection against *Leishmania major*. Nat Med. 2007 Jul;13(7):843-850. PubMed PMID: 17558415.

[155] Seder RA, Darrah PA, Roederer M. T-Cell Quality in Memory and Protection: Implications for Vaccine Design. Nat Rev Immunol. 2008 Apr;8(4):247-258. PubMed PMID: 18323851.

[156] Lichterfeld M, Yu XG, Waring MT, Mui SK, Johnston MN, Cohen D, *et al*. HIV-1-Specific Cytotoxicity Is Preferentially Mediated by a Subset of CD8(+) T Cells Producing Both Interferon-gamma and Tumor Necrosis Factor-alpha. Blood. 2004 Jul 15;104(2): 487-494. PubMed PMID: 15059848.

[157] Maia C, Seblova V, Sadlova J, Votypka J, Volf P. Experimental Transmission of *Leishmania infantum* by Two Major Vectors: A Comparison between a Viscerotropic and a Dermotropic Strain. PLoS Negl Trop Dis. 2011 Jun;5(6):e1181. PubMed PMID: 21695108. Pubmed Central PMCID: 3114756.

Chapter 14

Perspectives for Diagnosis and Control of Leishmaniasis Based on Volatile Organic Compounds

Jailson Bittencourt de Andrade,
Jairo Torres Magalhães Junior,
Paulo Roberto Ribeiro Mesquita,
Fábio Santos Oliveira,
Frederico de Medeiros Rodrigues and
Stella Maria Barrouin-Melo

Additional information is available at the end of the chapter

http://dx.doi.org/10.5772/57279

1. Introduction

During the pathogenesis of an infectious disease the cells of an infected host interact actively with its pathogen resulting in the production of different chemical metabolites. In the case of *Leishmania* infection, the pathophysiology of the disease and the final metabolism due to this infection is dependent on the parasite load in different organs, the type of immune response triggered predominantly in the post-infection, nutritional and physiological condition of the animals, among others [1]. In this way variables related to the host and the parasite must be considered together in metabolomics studies.

Metabolomics is the science applied to systematic study of the profile of metabolics, their composition and the dynamics influenced by genetic modifications, physiological stimuli, environmental, nutritional, among other factors. This field of researches shows great potential for the identification of potential biomarkers and metabolic disorders at an early stage.

In the last decade the study of metabolomics has intensified in order to understand the production and excretion of these metabolites, what are the consequences on sick organisms and especially the possibilities and perspectives resulting from this knowledge. Most of the studies aim to develop new ways of diagnosing diseases based on identification of volatile organic compounds (VOC) as indicative of pathological states. Diseases such as diabetes, breast cancer, lung cancer and chronic obstructive lung disease, among others, have been target of metabolomics studies [2-4]. These diseases have in common the chronic condition in its pathogenesis, such as in leishmaniasis, and may develop over a long period without the manifestation of clinical indications but with the production of metabolites as biomarkers of the disease.

Different biological samples may be used for metabolomic studies and they commonly vary according to the pathogenesis of the disease and anatomical region with greatest pathological involvement. In the case of visceral leishmaniasis hair is noteworthy as a biological matrix for analysis of VOC resulting from final metabolism of *Leishmania* infection and due to the ease of sample collection and the nature of the hair follicle, which has the function to secrete and excrete endogenous produced substances [5].

Therefore, the identification of biomarkers in the dogs with visceral leishmaniasis can serve as a painless diagnostic tool with minimal invasivity, which represents a gain in the field of animal welfare and perspectives for disease control.

We emphasize the use of different techniques for the extraction, separation and identification of these VOCs, as well as the use of univariate and multivariate planning in conducting the work. The use chemometric methods allow the analysis of a large number of variables, identifying similarities in complex samples, where several compounds are analyzed simultaneously.

When metabolomics approach is performed on vector-borne diseases, another important aspect is the possibility of the identified VOC act as chemical attractants for vector insects. VOC produced by hosts which are detected by receivers and antennas of the vectors during the search the process of search and location of food are called kairomones [6]. The ability to detect these volatile compounds makes easier specific recognition of the host and increases the radius of food search by the vector. In the case of leishmaniasis VOC produced from final metabolism of *Leishmania* infection when released into the environment can attract phlebotomine so that the insect feeds from the infected animals, thereby ensuring the dissemination of the parasite and maintenance of disease cycle.

The discovery of attractiveness of these compounds may aid studies about the presence and dispersion of phlebotomine providing subsidies for better understanding of the biology of these insects and in the future to substantiate effective programs to control the disease based on the manipulation of chemical communication of phlebotomine.

The present chapter contributes to a better understanding of the relationship parasite-dog-sandfly in visceral leishmaniasis. Here we summarize the importance of studies involving metabolomics, identification of biomarkers for disease diagnosis, the key techniques and methods of extraction and analysis of VOCs, attract sandflies aspects of the VOC and its application in the control of visceral leishmaniasis.

2. Canine visceral Leishmaniasis and fisiopathology of VOC released from hair

Assumed as a neglected disease by World Health Organization [7], visceral *Leishmania*sis (VL) are recorded in about 62 world counties and it mainly affects children, elderly and immunodeficient people [8, 9]. The VL is a parasitic disease with zoonosis character caused in american continent by *Leishmania infantum*, protozoan transmited between hosts by phlebotomine vector of *Lutzomyia longipalpis* specie [10].

The VL is considered a serious public health problem due to its complex epidemiological characteristics, different reservoirs involved, besides fast geographic expansion as well as expensive and arduous control [11].

Domestic dog (*Canis familiaris*) is considered the main reservoir of urban area due to its high susceptibility to pathogen, the strong cutaneous parasitism and the fact that canine cases precedes humans [11-13]. Thus this species is considered protagonist in studies that aim the development of new forms of control and disease prevention.

In the wild, crab-eating fox *(Cerdocyon thous)*, the hoary fox (*Lycalopex vetulus)*, the common opossum (*Didelphis marsupialis)* and the white-eared opossum (*Didelphis albiventris*) are used as natural reservoirs of infection and it is common to find positive animals in areas of human habitations which are related to the wild [9, 14].

The *Lutzomyia longipalpis* (Lutz & Neiva, 1912) is considered the main vector of VL in the American continent and it is widely studied because of its epidemiological importance for the transmission of this disease [15, 16].

L. longipalpis is one diptera of Psychodidae family and Phlebotominae subfamily. These phlebotomine insects measure approximately 2-3 mm, the body is quite hairy, light colored (light brown or straw color) and are easily recognized by their behavior of flying with small jumps and landing with half open wings [11].

The only proven way of transmission so far is through the bite of phlebotomine females that ingest amastigote forms with blood meal when it feeds from an infected mammal [9]. After undergoing processing in the digestive tract they are transmitted to other hosts already in the promastigote form while females feed for the second time [15, 17]. On the spot of inoculation an inflammatory process takes place and promastigostes are then phagocytosed by macrophages, then they become amastigotes and multiply until macrophages break up and they are released to spread to the whole body [17].

The consequences, progression and severity of the disease depend on the immune response expressed by the animal, especially the cytokine production profile [1]. Cytokine production profile varies with environmental factors, nutritional and genetic aspects of the parasite like the species, strain and inoculum size [18].

In the early periods of post-infection there are changes in populations of T lymphocytes and it has been shown that there is a relationship between the pattern of produced cytokines and the manifestation of clinical signs [19]. This association is a result of the greater intensity of parasite load, when there is a lower production of Th1 cytokines (Lymphocyte T helper type I) in various organs such as lymph nodes [20], spleen [21], bone marrow [22] and skin [23].

Animals that produce Th1-type response develops immunity against the parasite cell type, resulting in resistance to infection [19]. In these animals there is a predominance of IFN-$_{\gamma}$, TNF-α and IL-12 release, which among other things promotes the production and activation of macrophages, nitric oxide and cell apoptosis [24].

Resistant dogs are characterized by low parasitic burden in several organs [25], no development of clinical signs [19], normal erythropoietic and leukopoietic activities [22] and low infectability to phlebotomine [26].

On other hand animals that produce Th2-type (Lymphocyte T helper type II) response are characterized by a humoral immune type response and consequent susceptibility to infection [19]. In these animals there is a predominance of IL4, IL10 and TGF-$_{\beta}$ that inhibit the production of IFN-$_{\gamma}$ and IL-2 then the cell type response [22, 27]. The antibodies produced by humoral response are unable to eradicate the infection resulting in high parasitic burden and expression of clinical signs of disease.

Thus in dogs with active VL the strength of parasite load is directly proportional to the intensity of clinical signs and disease severity (Figure 1). The most important clinical signs are ocular lesions, periocular and cutaneous, kidney diseases and their consequences; respiratory, digestive, cardiovascular and musculoskeletal disorders; hypertrophy of lymphoid organs and hematological disorders [28].

The transmission of *Leishmania* by dogs seems to be related to the extent of clinical manifestations of disease so how much more clinical signs present higher the ratio of infectivity, which is possibly related with high parasite load in different organs, especially skin and lymph nodes [29].

Histological skin evaluations of animals which show the presence of perifollicular dermatitis with inflammatory infiltration generally extending by the sebaceous glands [30] and a predominance of macrophages, lymphocytes and polymorphonuclear neutrophils [31].

The hair is considered an appendix of the skin performing various functions in the body among which are included the secretion and excretion of endogenously produced substances by several metabolic processes [32].

The emission and accumulation of chemical compounds by hair are well-studied, in both humans and animals, for several purposes, either as indicative of the internal metabolism of drugs [33]; for investigation in toxicological forensic [34]; for evaluation of chemical contaminants [35]; post-treatment accumulation of drugs [36] ; alcohol and drugs abuse [37]; evaluation of trace elements [38]; or for anti-doping investigations [39].

Hair is an interesting sample for standardization of biomarkers because of its role to excrete endogenous substances [5]. Furthermore, the exam of dogs hair allowed to find *Leishmania* DNA by standard PCR technique, reingorcing its importance for the diagnosis [40].

http://dx.doi.org/10.5772/57279

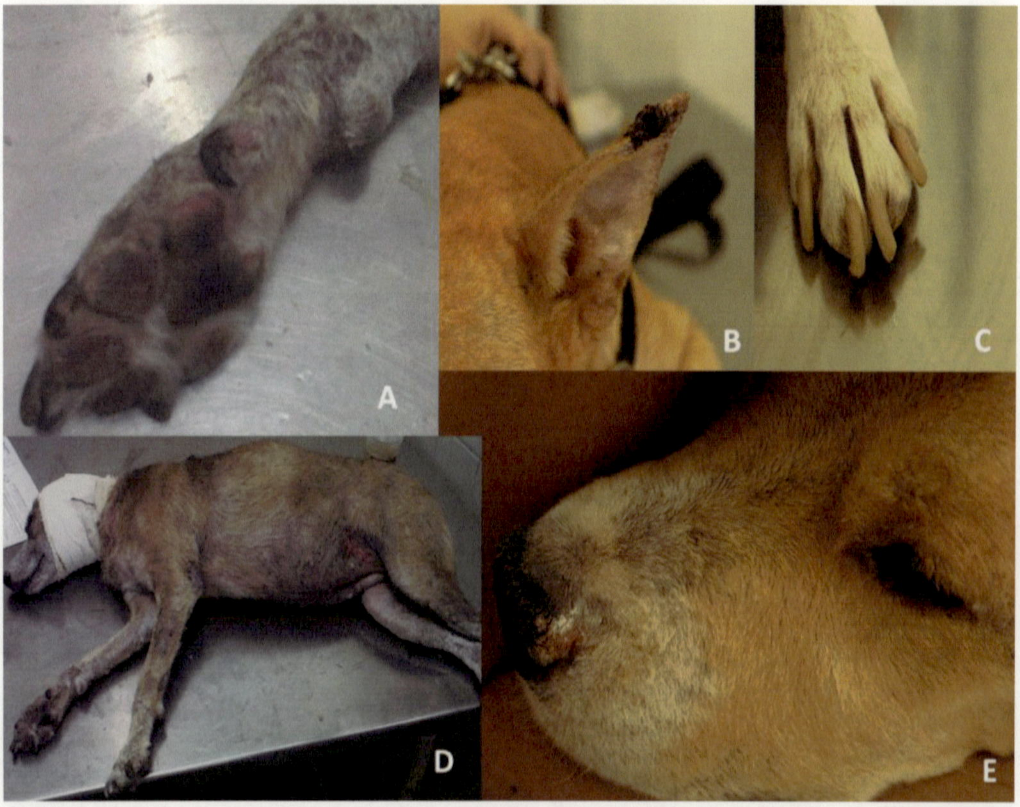

Figure 1. Some clinical signs found in dogs with leishmaniasis: A) Ulcerative erythematous lesions on the plantar surface of the paw; B) Dermatitis tip of ear; C) Onychogryphosis; D) Marked cachexia and generalized exfoliative alopecia; E) Ulcerative nasal mucocutaneous lesions and periocular alopecia.

Following the thought that hair is a biological sample that allows evaluation of internal metabolism of healthy and infected animals, Oliveira et al. [41] demonstrated that volatile organic compounds (VOC) emitted by the dogs clearly differ comparing healthy animals and infected by *Leishmania* sp., previously identified for ELISA and PCR. In this way, VOC profile also varies due to presence and manifestation of clinical signs for dogs infected by *Leishmania* sp. [42].

3. The metabolomics study of its applications

Due to the current compartmentalization model widespread in human medicine and in veterinary gradually been developed a quest for a embracing perspective in life sciences. This trend is a throwback to ancient times where a holistic perspective was predominant [43]. Biological system, which brings together these ideas, is a term that has a recent origin and currently allows different types of research [44]. This attempt to an expanded approach began what the authors call the "omics" age, where genomics, proteomics and metabolomics studies has been carried out (Figure 2) [45].

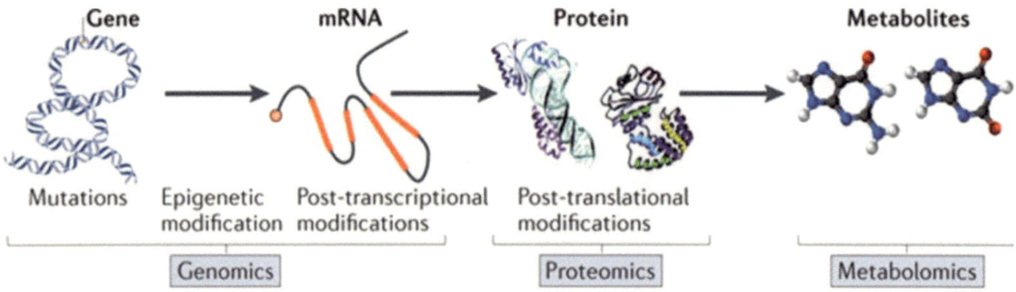

Figure 2. The central dogma of biology and the omic cascade. Adapted of [45].

By definition, genomic characterizes hereditary information of an organism and defines what can happen in a biological system. On other hand, research about proteomics defining the structure and function of the proteins encoded by the genome of an organism is the next logical step for the study of biological systems. Finally, metabolomics systematically analyzes a whole set of chemicals resulting from specific cellular processes, determining the main aspects of the function and regulation of these processes [46].

Metabolomics is also called metabonomics and outlines the study of metabolome [47]. Metabolome in turn is a set of metabolites produced or present in a biological system [47]. Thus, metabolomics can be defined as the study that enables the detection, identification and quantification of the largest number of possible metabolites in biological samples, searching for variations that can be used to discriminate volatile organic compounds between samples [48].

Metabolomics aims to determine a whole set of low molecular weight compounds (less than 1.500 Da) in a given biological sample, getting closer as much as possible of the physiology of the whole system [49]. For samples obtained from healthy subjects and patients, the aim is to identify one or more endogenous metabolites found in clinical samples related to disease [48].

This approach of combining various faces of a biological system allows integrating different details of this complex information network. Thus, this makes possible application of metabolomics in different approaches, such as the study of basic biological models, drug development, human and animal pathophysiological models, toxicology studies, nutritional effects, metabolic consequences from genetic modifications, inborn errors of metabolism and identification of biomarkers of diseases [45, 47, 50, 51].

Currently, analysis involving metabolomics has been successfully performed in several pathogens that infect living beings, such as lineages of uropathogenic *Escherichia coli* [52], Hepatitis B [53], the pathogenic fungi *Aspergillus fumigatus* [54] and protozoan *Plasmodium falciparum*, the major cause of malaria [55]. According Lakshmanan and Daily [50], metabolomics offers a unique and powerful tool to explore the biology of insects vectors and to develop strategies to stop its transmission. It has been shown that in the case of malaria some chemical compounds play a critical role in the development life cycle of *P. falsiparum* within *Anopheles* spp. vector and the interruption of the formation of such metabolites could help to reduce disease transmission [56].

In the case of *Leishmania* sp., most studies involving metabolomics deal mainly with metabolic changes in parasite at cellular level, differences in metabolism pathways of substances, sensitivity and resistance to drugs and other approaches related to the development of the parasite [57-59]. To our knowledge the only work that involves metabolomics with diagnostic purposes was developed in dogs with different clinical profiles for canine visceral leishmaniasis and it was found some of the volatile organic compounds emitted by animals such as potential biomarkers of disease [42].

Metabolomic studies in order to diagnose diseases are quite conducted for other diseases [2, 60]. The idea that chemical components resulting cellular activities can reflect the health status of an individual is old: in China (1500-2000 BC), doctors used ants to detect the presence of glucose in urine of patients with suspected diabetes [43]. The pathophysiological changes observed from metabolomic have a shorter response time in comparison to the development of clinical symptoms for example. This is one of the reasons why metabolomics has been used in an attempt to identify biomarkers for early stage disease, especially those of a chronic nature such as cancer and respiratory diseases, which usually have a later diagnosis [61, 62].

As in metabolomics studies takes into account a systemic approach, theoretically any change in the body, whether physiological or pathological, can influence the results. Thus, to minimize interference unrelated to the objectives of the study it is important that at the experimental design taken into account factors intrinsic and extrinsic to individuals, such as genetic variations, diet, gender, age of individuals, climatic conditions, concomitant infections, among others. Moreover, this multiplicity of effects can be used. For example, metabolomics can be used to identify the impact of nutrients in the diet on the biochemistry of living organisms and their susceptibility / resistance to disease [50].

The metabolites are a wide range of molecular arrangements and that provides a variation in several physical and chemical properties of their components. The degree of diversity is indicated by analysis of organic metabolites with low molecular weight, polar, volatile such as isoprene as nonanol, by analysis of metabolites with higher molecular weight, polar (carbohydrates) and nonpolar (terpenoids and lipid) [63]. To characterize and quantify these compounds is necessary to use specific methodologies and instruments according to the characteristics of each class. Therefore, metabolomics includes several analytical technologies that need to be carefully selected in accordance with the metabolites and metabolic pathway of interest, or the biological question to be answered.

4. Methods for extraction and determination of VOC emitted by hosts

Although in many instances scientists do not collect biological samples that they want to analyze, it must be aware about the history of the samples, to procedures for collecting, type of packaging, added preservatives, stability characteristics and sample processing, in addition to the conditions storage and delivery protocol [48]. These aim to maintain the chemical profile of substances and physico-chemical characteristics, avoiding losses and minimizing contamination risks.

In metabolomic studies involving the diagnosis of dogs infected by *Leishmania* sp. the volatile organic compounds emitted from hair of these animals can be used as biomarkers of infection. Research involving VOC emitted from dog has critical steps such as: i) sampling and sample preparation, ii) choice of the extraction method, and iii) choice of analysis method.

4.1. Sampling and sample storage

The hair has a large amount of VOC, which can be derived from two sources: endogenous and exogenous. Exogenous VOC adhere to hair according to environmental exposure and the longer the residence time at a given location, the greater the extent of adsorption of these compounds. On other hand, endogenous VOC deriving from internal sources and they are products of host metabolism which when emitted through the skin a fraction is adsorbed by hair. Due to this feature, the hair sample is ideal sample both for outdoor exposure evaluation and for identification of biomarkers of metabolism changes.

When sampling hair it should always be removed from the same anatomical region due to possible variations of VOC profile depending on the area in which the host sample was collected (Figure 3). Sterilized gloves, razors and tweezers should be used in order to avoid sample contamination.

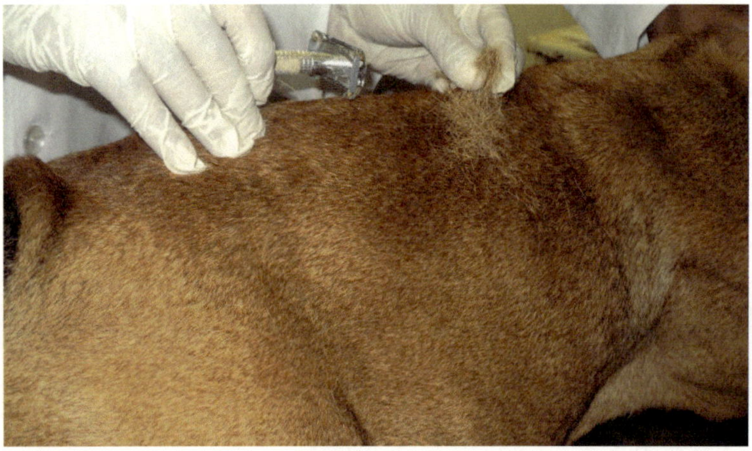

Figure 3. Collect of hair in dorse of dog.

Strategies to reduce exogenous compounds are another important aspect since these compounds can make difficult biomarker identification. For example, dogs can be bathed using mild soap three days before sampling period and the contact of these animals with chemicals must also be avoided.

http://dx.doi.org/10.5772/57279

After collection, the samples should be stored in clean and sterilized plastic bags kept in freezers at -20 º C. As VOC tend to desorb from hair in the course of time, the storage at low temperatures minimizes this process. Anyway, the storage of samples for a long period of time should be avoided.

4.2. Extraction methods

The hair can contain dozens of VOC with different chemical structures and polarities. Therefore, the ideal extraction technique should be suitable for sampling VOC with quite different properties and to prevent sample contamination during the whole procedure.

Currently, the most used techniques for sampling VOC from biological materials are solvent extraction, steam distillation (SD) and with simultaneous extraction (SDE), supercritical fluid extraction (SFE) solid phase extraction and solid phase microextraction (SPME).

Solvent extraction, SD and SDE are conventional and widely used methods for sampling VOC from biological samples. These methods always require a long extraction time, the use of large amounts of organic solvents and the performance of many steps. In addition, many unstable volatiles compounds such as alkenes, esters and some unsaturated volatile organic compounds may be thermally decomposed and degraded during extraction or distillation at high temperatures [64].

However, these procedures still are widely applied for the characterization of fragrances and flavors since they are direct and less complex. Recently, SFE techniques, adsorbent extraction and SPME have attracted much attention from analysts due to its green and innovative features for sampling VOC from biological samples.

4.2.1. Solvent extraction

The solvent extraction is based on the relative solubility of the analyte by an organic solvent. This extraction can be done using a solvent to remove the analytes directly from a solid sample, which typically uses a Soxhlet system.

This extraction technique is perhaps the oldest and has the advantage of being a simple technique with a variety of commercially available pure solvents that provide a wide range of solubility and selectivity. As disadvantages, some of them use large amounts of toxic organic solvents, require a relatively large volume of sample and need ultrapure solvents to avoid sample contamination

The solvent extraction is widely used for sampling of pheromones, because of the lipid nature of many pheromones they are easily dissolved by solvents such as hexane or dichloromethane [65]. When the section of insect that produces pheromone mixture is known, usually a gland may be removed then put in contact with a small volume of solvent for extraction of interesting compounds. However, in this procedure other non-volatile compounds can also be extracted.

4.2.2. Steam distillation and extraction by simultaneous distillation

The SD is the original sampling method of VOC from plants. VOC are extracted from plants using water vapor steam distillation system followed by solvent extraction. The SDE techniques couple steam distillation and solvent extraction in order to simplify experimental procedures, to minimize the use of toxic organic solvents and to reduce the losses that occur during the sample transfer [66, 67].

Due to the high temperature during the procedures using SD and SDE, these techniques are not suitable for sampling for VOC from live animals and they can cause thermal decomposition of some thermo-unstable compounds. However, due to the large extraction capacity and the existence of simple SD and SDE experimental devices, they are still considered useful as sampling methods for thermally stable volatile compounds.

Some improvements have been implemented in these conventional sampling techniques to achieve better extraction efficiency. For example, Hashemi et al. [68] combined hydrodistillation with solvent microextraction (HD-SME) for extraction of VOC from Artemisia (a type of plant) and obtained better results than those obtained with conventional hydrodistillation technique. It was also developed by Ferhat et al. [69] a microwave assisted SDE method (MW-SDE) for the analysis of volatile compounds form aromatic herbs. This new technique greatly improves the extraction time and amount of organic solvent due to the introduction of microwave energy as a heat source during extraction.

4.2.3. Supercritical fluid extraction

SFE is a process of separation and extraction by the use of supercritical fluids as the extraction solvents. Supercritical fluids are considered as a clean solvent, less toxic than organic solvents. Carbon dioxide (CO_2) is a widely used supercritical fluid to which sometimes a co-solvent is added, such as ethanol or methanol. SFE is a good alternative to liquid-liquid extraction and proved to be an effective technique for sample preparation. Giannuzzo et al. [70] used a mixture of supercritical CO_2 with ethanol (15 wt.%) for extraction of flavonoid naringin from citrus paradise, obtaining better results when compared with pure supercritical CO_2.

The advantage of carbon dioxide is that it is easy to remove by simply reducing the pressure, which leaves virtually no trace, also being environmentally friendly [71, 72]. However, the SFE has as main drawback the high cost compared with solvent extraction technique. The carbon dioxide used in SFE has limited power for dissolving polar compounds [73]. The study of new supercritical fluid and the development of small scale SFE instruments are required for application of this technique for the study of VOC from biological samples. The SFE is widely used in the extraction of bioactive compounds from vegetables [74].

4.2.4. Extraction with adsorbents

In the extraction with solid adsorbent a pre-purified inert gas is used as carrier gas that flows continuously through the sample and extracts the VOC. Then, the volatile organic compounds are retained on a solid adsorbent, usually Tenax [75]. Finished the extraction time of VOC, an

http://dx.doi.org/10.5772/57279

organic solvent such as hexane is directed through a tube containing the adsorbent for elution of the compounds. Another possibility is to carry out thermal desorption of VOC retained in the adsorbent tube before analysis.

Different types of adsorbents may be used to obtain a more selective sampling, depending on characteristics of VOC present in the sample. The choice of adsorbents must take into account their specific surface area and ability to retain VOC of interest. If thermal desorption mode is used, it should also be assessed the ability to attain complete and rapid desorption of the analytes, the existence of homogeneous and inert surface to prevent the formation of artifacts and irreversible adsorption during sampling, storage of tubes and desorption; low water affinity to avoid hydrolysis reactions and damage to the stationary phase used for chromatographic analysis, high mechanical and thermal stability [76]. The most used adsorbent materials are sub-classified into activated carbon [77], carbon molecular sieves (Carboxen, Carbosphere e Carbosieve) [78, 79] and porous organic polymers (Tenax, Chromosorb e Porapak) [80, 81].

This technique has great potential for the identification of disease biomarkers. Sporing et al. [82] monitored the release of VOC by a lineage of lung cancer cells using solid adsorbents and analysis by thermal desorption and gas chromatography-mass spectrometry (TD-GC/MS) where several aldehydes and ethers were identified.

4.2.5. Solid-phase microextraction (SPME)

Solid-phase microextraction (SPME) was developed by Arthur e Pawliszyn [83], it has been regarded as one of the most innovative inventions in the field of VOC extraction in the last years. SPME integrates the steps of extraction, concentration and introduction to analysis, reducing sampling time and increasing the sensitivity when compared to other extraction methods.

This is a technique that has been successfully used for the extraction of compounds from environmental samples [84], pharmaceuticals [85], biological [86] and study of fragrances and flavors [87].

Headspace solid-phase microextraction (HS-SPME) is the most widely used form for sampling VOC from different matrices, including biological samples from animals [88-90], vegetables [91-94] e microbes [95, 96].

In recent years, SPME has been applied to the monitoring of compounds in living systems [97]. This application has advantages such as the possibility of sampling compounds without changing the actual condition of the system and to carry out studies about temporal progression of a disease of a subject over time without the need to sacrifice one specimen for each sampling point [98]. For example, Bai et al. [99] used SPME technique in vivo for determination of off-flavor compounds in live fish. Geosmin and 2-methylisoborneol (2-MIB), produced by cyanobacteria and actinomycetes, were quantified in fish muscles which give the flavor of "land" and "clay" to fish.

In the area of Leishmaniasis there is only one work reported in literature about VOC extraction. HS-SPME was used by de Oliveira et al. [41] for extraction of VOC from hair of dog healthy and infected by *Leishmania infantum,* followed by GC-MS analysis which detected about 274 compounds, mostly ketones, aldehydes and hydrocarbons

4.3. Methods of analysis

After extraction VOC from samples it is necessary to identify each component to obtain quantitative and qualitative information about samples. Since the invention and development of gas chromatography technique the analysis of volatile compounds in biological becomes much easier.

GC is an excellent analytical technique for separating compounds which can be volatilized at the temperature applied to the injector device. Therefore, when GC is coupled to a detector it becomes a powerful technique for analysis of VOC in biological samples [100].

Nowadays gas chromatography coupled to flame ionization detector (GC-FID) and GC-MS are the main techniques used for VOC analysis and the GC-MS technique is more powerful due to the great identification ability of mass spectrometry (MS).

In recent years, the development of multi-dimensional CG has significantly improved separation of VOC from complex samples, making easier than before to obtain bio-information related to compounds present in samples [101]. Bean et al. [102] applied comprehensive two-dimensional chromatography coupled to time-of-flight mass spectrometry (GCxGC-TOF-MS) technique to identify the profile of VOC from the metabolism of *Pseudomonas aeruginosa* bacteria. The method enabled better separation and identification of a wider number of compounds compared to the GC-MS technique, enabling the discovery of 28 new VOC characteristic of *P. aeruginosa.*

Another innovative application was proposed by Stadler et al. [103] that used TD × GC-TOF-MS for the identification of VOC released from a pig carcass, which allowed to define of the profile of compounds released during the decomposition of different tissues

5. Biomarkers in diagnostic of disease

Using the techniques of extraction and identification of VOC allows the discovery of biomarkers that are measurable biomolecules that represent the normal physiological state or changes of an individual related with a pathophysiological process or treatment. Generally biomarkers may be (a) proteins that represent the cellular and enzymatic changes or (b) small organic molecules called metabolites. These compounds may help in early detection and monitoring the progress of a disease, and its response to the use of a drug or therapeutic intervention [104].

Currently biomarker discovered using "omics" technologies, such as proteomics and metabolomics wherein sample biochemical profiles, are determined (mainly biofluids) from patients and healthy individuals. Compounds that after an appropriate statistical analysis appear over or under-expressed in samples from patients when compared to healthy controls may be considered as potential biomarkers of disease [105].

It is highlighted that finding metabolites present at significantly different levels in samples from patients does not necessarily make them useful biomarkers. The route for the validation and use of biomarkers requires extensive studies. This validation must address two issues: a) the metabolite whose concentration levels differ significantly between samples of a test population is indicative of a specific pathophysiology? b) there is an abnormal level of this specific metabolite clearly stating a specific pathophysiology when all other symptoms are considered? In addition, biomarkers need to provide adequate levels of sensitivity and specificity (> 80%) for correct detection and classification of disease [106].

The strategy most often used to develop biomarkers involves a discovery phase in a restrict number of samples, followed by validation of biomarker with potential using a larger number of samples from patients before this compound can be adopted as a clinical tool.

The use of chromatographic techniques combined with the power of mass spectrometry allows the identification of dozens of compounds and this when coupled with the large number of samples studied generates an immense amount of data that must be processed, analyzed and interpreted.

The purpose of the data processing is to extract quantitative information from data related to detected metabolites obtained from chromatographic and mass spectrometry. This extracted information can be arranged in an matrix which later be will used in the multivariate analysis[107].

The main multivariate techniques used for biomarker discovery are Principal Component Analysis (PCA), Partial Least-Squares – Discriminant Analysis (PLS-DA) and orthogonal PLS-DA (OPLS-DA) [108]. PCA is commonly implemented as a starting point for the data manipulation to obtain an overview about cluster tendencies and to detect outliers.

PLS-DA is used to deal with specific studies class where a linear relationship between metabolites in the matrix X and category information in the matrix Y is established. This technique can enhance the separation of classes and improve the interpretability of statistical models [109]. In OPLS-DA model partition variance matrix X in predictive and non-predictive classes (orthogonal classes) not only improves the discrimination metabolic profiles but also the transparency of models [110].

Many biomarkers of disease from different samples have been discovered by the application of different techniques for extraction and analysis. Table 1 summarizes some of these biomarkers.

Table 1 shows already discovered biomarkers for various diseases such as Melitus diabetes, myocardial ischemia, galactosemia, breast cancer, ovarian carcinoma, renal cell carcinoma, colorectal carcinoma, etc [4].

Sample	Disease	Technique	Biomarkers	References
Urine	Colorectal carcinoma	UPLC-TOF-MS	Nucleosides, carnitines	Wang et al [111]
Blood serum	Diabetes melitus	LC-MS	Leucine, isoleucine, valine, phenylalanine, tyrosine	Wang et al [112] Langenberg and Savage [113]
Blood serum	Type I diabetes	UPLC and GC-TOF-MS	Lipids and polar metabolites	Oresic et al [114]
Urine	Breast cancer, ovarian carcinoma, cervical carcinoma	HPLC-MS	Hormones, nucleosides	Woo et al. [115]
Blood plasma	Myocardial ischemia	HPLC-MS	Sugars, ribonucleotides, amino acids	Sabatine et al [116]
Dried blood	Galactosemia	LC-MS/MS	Hexose monophosphates	Jensen et al. [117]
Blood serum	Renal cell carcinoma	LC-MS	Phospholipids, phenylalanine and cholesterol metabolites	Liu et al. [118]
Blood plasma and serum	Onchocerciasis	LC-MS	Fatty acids, protein, sterol lipid, etc	Denery et al. [119]
Breath	Lung cancer	GC-TOF-MS	Propane,carbon disulfide, 2-propenal, ethylbenzene and isopropyl alcohol	Rudnicka et al. [120]
Breath	Cysticfibrosis	GC-MS	Carbonyl sulphide, alkanes	Phillips et al. [121]
Breath	Chronic ostructive pulmonary disease	TD-GC-TOF-MS	Hexanal, nonanal, decanal, undecanal, pentadecanal, dodecanal, etc	Basanta et al. [3]
Urine	Lung cancer	GC-MS	2-heptanone, o-toluidine, nitromethane, etc	Matsumura et al. [122]

Table 1. Biomarkers identified for different diseases.

Most of the identified biomarkers are non-volatile, such as proteins, lipids and other high molecular weight compounds. However, several volatile biomarkers have been discovered in recent years.

In this context, the discovery of VOC that may serve as biomarkers of infectious diseases such as leishmaniasis is presented as a promising possibility. The first work in this direction has been reported in the literature by Oliveira et al. [41] which proposed a noninvasive diagnostic method for detection of visceral leishmaniasis in dogs. HS-SPME/GC-MS techniques were developed and applied to identify the VOC emitted from hair of 8 healthy dogs and 16 dogs infected by *Leishmania infantum* and 274 compounds were detected (Figure 4).

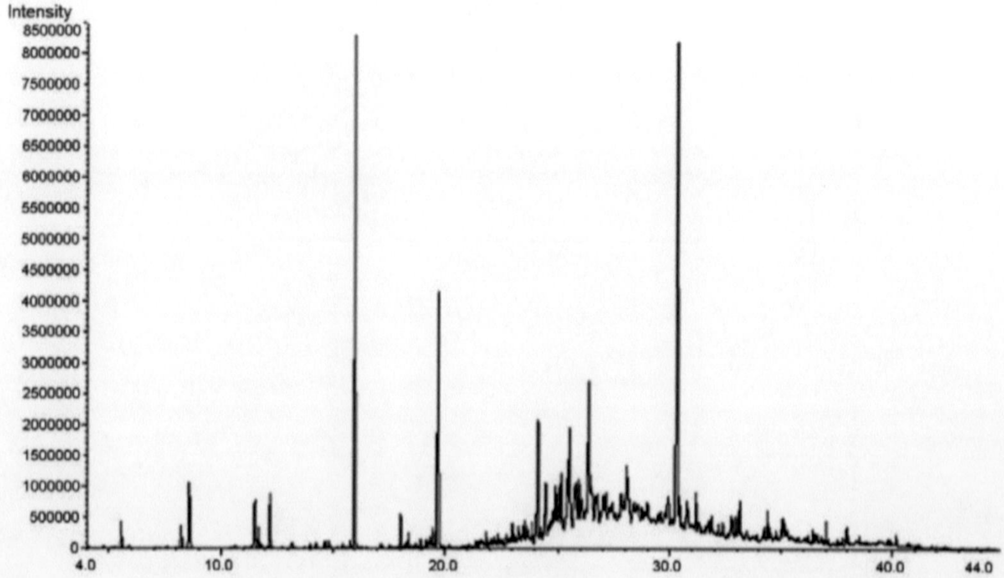

Figure 4. Chromatograms obtained by HS-SPME/GC–MS analysis of canine hair samples, for all VOC [41].

So, multivariate Principal Component Analysis (PCA) and Soft Independent Modeling of Class Analogy (SIMCA) were used to discriminate healthy and infected groups of dogs. Figure 5 shows the PCA scores graph.

The majority of identified VOC belonged to the class of ketones, aldehydes and hydrocarbons, and compounds such as benzaldehyde, 2-hexanone and 2,4-nonadienal showed greater discriminatory power between the two groups, therefore potential this later compounds are candidates for biomarkers of canine visceral leishmaniasis.

Continuing this work, Magalhães-Junior et al [42] investigated that the profile of VOC emitted from infected dogs change according to symptomatology or not of their conditions. For this 36 dogs living in endemic areas for leishmaniasis were studied, which were divided into three groups according to (1) absence of the disease, (2) presence of clinical infection or (3) sub-clinical *Leishmania infantum*. In this study, infection was confirmed for parasitological test by culture and microscopy and PCR.

The authors used HS-SPME/GC-MS techniques for identification of VOC from dogs and after multivariate analysis using PCA and PLS-DA they found that the profile of these compounds emitted differ between the three groups. There still differences among infected dogs showing clinical disease from those with subclinical infection. They were also identified 10 new compounds with potential use as biomarkers of infection. These studies show that the use of VOC as biomarkers of infection by *Leishmania sp*. as a promising approach. However, many studies must still be performed until confirmation of biomarkers capable of being used in clinical practice, including potential application for humans.

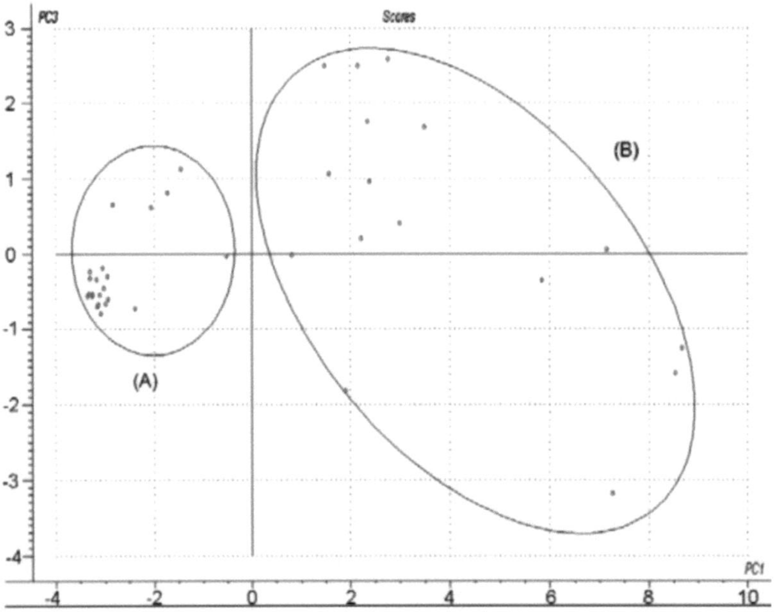

Figure 5. PCA scores graph based on chromatographic peak areas of VOC of the hair of leishmaniasis infected (A) and non-infected dogs (B) [41].

6. Attraction of phlebotomine to volatile organic compounds

It is well known that insects use olfactory and visual stimuli during different stages of its life cycle like for the search for a blood source or suitable place for oviposition [123]. In the case of olfactory stimuli, the orientation of these insects towards the sources of attractive odors depends on the time and space distribution of odorant molecules spread on the environment. The molecules associated with olfactory responses are volatile organic compounds that disperse following the gas laws, forming clouds of odors and are responsible for chemical communication between the vector insect and host [124].

6.1. Chemical ecology of insects

The chemical communication occurs when an individual (transmitter) sends chemicals which are transmitted through a medium (air, water, substrate) and are captured by another individual (receiver). These chemicals are called semiochemicals and can be toxins, nutrients, or the substances responsible for the proper transmission of information, infochemicals [125].

Infochemicals are chemical substances that provide information during the interaction between two individuals, resulting in a behavior or physiological response of the receptor. Communication is considered intraspecific when infochemicals called pheromones are secreted by an individual and released to the environment, resulting on a specific behavior reaction of another individual of the same specie [6].

The substances involved in the case of interspecific communication are called allelochemicals and are classified based on harm and benefits to the organisms. The kairomone is a type of allelochemicals which evokes an adaptive response that is unfavorable to the transmitter, but favorable to the receiver [6]. Typical example of kairomone are the volatile organic compounds produced by hosts and are detected by receivers and antennae of insects during the search process and location of food source [126]. The ability to detect these volatile compounds makes easier the specific recognition of the host and increases the range foraging by the vector [127].

Several animals produce a huge number of volatile compounds derived from their own skin, breathing, urine and feces. The detectability of these substances by receivers depends upon the amount that are produced and dispersed over the environment, distance between the insect and the host; wind speed, turbulence and specificity of these molecules to receptor cell of insects which are primarily present in the antennas of insects [128].

The importance of some chemical compounds to the guidance of hematophagous insects has been demonstrated. Carbon dioxide is a by-product of cellular respiration that is released in large amounts by potential hosts and it is a wildly studied semiochemical such as its attractive effect has already been reported for *Aedes aegipty* [129], *Culex quinquefasciatus* [130], *Lutzomyia* sandflies [131] and some species of tsetse fly (*Glossina* spp.) [132]. Another extensively studied compound is 1-octen-3ol which was initially identified from volatile compound of expiration of bovine animals and its attractive effect was evaluated in several species of hematophagous insects [123], including sandflies [124]. Lactic acid is the main component of human sweat and effect was evaluated, being considered attractive when used together with CO_2 [133].

These chemical compounds are produced in large scale by several species of animals, therefore they can be regarded as universal kairomones. They attract insects that have opportunistic feeding habits, since they indicate the presence of live vertebrate at a nonspecifically way [134]. Additionally, these orientation behaviours are complicated and potentially plastic, may be modulated by environmental factors [135].

6.2. Chemical ecology of phlebotomines

Among the studies performed to identify VOC involved in chemical communication of phlebotomines most of them use *L. longipalpis* as target species, which is why there are few knowledge about other species of phlebotomines.

In the late 80s the sex pheromone of *L. longipalpis* was discovered and since then many studies have been carried out. The pheromone is produced in glandular tissue located in the abdomen of males [136, 137] and is primarily composed of terpenes, a class of natural products that contains in their structure three or four isoprene units with five carbon atoms. More recent works have shown that there are differences in the chemical composition of the sexual pheromone according to the geographical location of *L. longipalpis* the male that produces it, suggesting that this variation is a result of reproductive isolation [138]. This result supports the hypothesis that the *L. longipalpis* is formed by a complex of cryptic species with different morphological and behavioral characteristics [139, 140].

Despite the proven efficacy of sexual pheromone for attraction of *L. longipalpis* by both laboratory [141] as well as field studies [142], this variation in chemical composition restricts the practical use of pheromone at different locations, increasing the importance of the study of kairomones for chemical ecology of phlebotomines. Furthermore, Bray e Hamilton [143] when conducting behavioral studies in the laboratory, they found that the attractiveness of females of *L. longipalpis* nearly doubled when the odor of hosts was added to sex pheromone.

Even so, there are few studies in the literature that evaluate the attractiveness of the phlebotomine to host odors. For example, Hamilton and Ramsoondar [144] found that females and males of *L. longipalpis* were attracted by emitted volatile organic compounds from human skin and there was a difference in attractiveness among the volunteers.

Likewise Rebollar-Tellez *et al.* [145] found different levels of attractiveness to human volunteers, suggesting that this variation may be due to different VOCs emitted by humans. It was also observed that females of *L. longipalpis* preferred to bite human's ear over other parts of the body, considering the number of bites over the exposed area. It has been shown that insects were attracted by odors extracted from human ear, showing that this preference is related to the VOC emitted this region of body [145]. Also in this work, females of *L. longipalpis* coming from the city of Jacobina (Bahia, Brazil) were more anthropophilic than insects from other geographical locations (Marajó, Pará, Brazil and Curiágua, Venezuela). This difference in response of female of *L. longipalpis* from different sites was also found by Rebollar-Tellez *et al.* [146] suggesting that there is a local adaptation of the complex of *L. longipalpis* species to particular hosts or to a specific set of odors and this behavior is inborn and genetically controlled.

For other host species it had been shown that sixteen chemical compounds from anal and caudal glands of European foxes (*Vulpes vulpes*) perform electrophysiological and behavioral action on *L. longipalpis* [147], suggesting that there is a complexity of components that can act on chemical communication between hosts and phlebotomines.

It has been observed that in the case of canine VL phlebotomines are more attracted to feed from infected dogs than from healthy dogs and this preference is probably related to the different odors emitted by infected animals [128]. As demonstred by Oliveira *et al.* [41], in fact volatile organic compounds emitted by the dog clearly differ between animals infected by *Leishmania sp.* and healthy ones, previously identified for ELISA and PCR. O'Shea *et al.* [148] when studying the attractiveness of *L. longipalpis* to hamsters it was observed that the vector is more attracted by individuals infected by *Leishmania infantum* in comparison with healthy ones. After analyzing the volatile organic compounds emitted by rodents using gas chromatography O'Shea *et al.* [148] described the presence of 10 chromatographic peaks of substances in infected animals which were not detected in those healthy.

6.3. Main techniques used for chemical ecology of phlebotomines

The insects have a well developed sense of smell which odors are mainly picked up by the antennae for the detection and discrimination of chemical compounds present in the environment. This signal reception in most insects is performed by sensilla, small hairs that are located in the antennae, and is processed as follows: when the molecules responsible for the emission of odors reach the antennae sensilla they cross through the cuticle pores until they attain sensillum lymph where they bind to odors ligand protein and they are carried to receiving neuron, generating a cation flow through the membrane of the axon which is then converted to electrical stimulation [149]. This electrical stimulation can be measured by a technique known as electroantennography, wherein the insect antenna is used as a detector of chemical substances. In this technique the amplitude of the voltage produced by the stimulus increases proportionally with concentration of the substance until saturation threshold is reached.

The electroantennography is a sensitive and specific technique since the insect antenna is much more sensitive than equipments usually used for the detection of chemical substances, therefore it is able to detect minimum amounts of a particular substance.

To identify which VOC present in particular extract exhibit biological activity on *L. longipalpis* gas chromatography coupled to an electroantennographic detector (GC-EAD) can be used, which is an instrument capable of separating the organic compounds present in the sample and measuring electrical signals emitted by antennae of insects used as biological detectors (Figure 6).

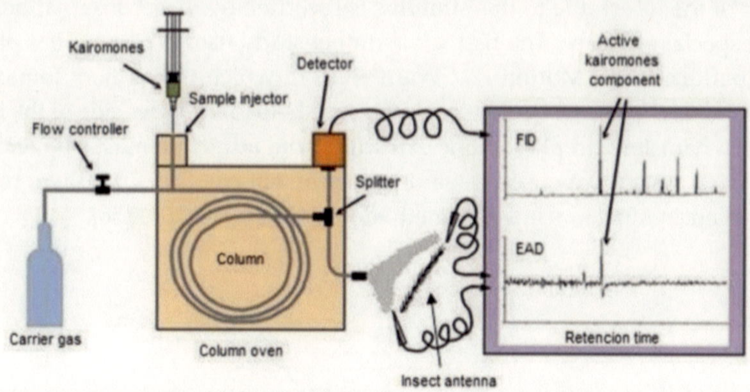

Figure 6. Gas chromatograph coupled with flame ionization detector and electroantennogram recorder, adapted of [150].

Thus, by inserting the sample into the GC injector it is vaporized and the compounds are transported by a carrier gas traveling across the chromatographic column where separation of substances is performed. When leaving the chromatographic column the flow is splitted into two and one part goes to the detector that identifies the chemical compound and the other part goes to the electroantennographic detector. In this way, the first detector provides a chromatogram containing all compounds detected while the second detector produces an electroantennogram exhibiting only the compounds that are biologically active to that insect (Figure 6).

This technique has been used successfully in several studies involving chemical ecology of insects, especially to search for compounds which are used for agricultural pest management [151, 152]. In research involving phlebotomines this procedure has also been used [147, 153], but it is underexplored and still needs further study due to the great potential for discoveries [154]. The electroantennography serves to specify which compound the insect actually reacts [155]. However, to specify the biological role of this compound laboratory bioassays and field tests must be carried out.

The laboratory bioassays are conducted in closed systems attempting to obtain data about the behavior of insects when they are induced to respond to a chemical stimulus. Bioassay in the detector is a living organism or part of your sensory system. In bioassay the detector is a living being or part of its sensory system. For the realization of bioassays can be used olfactometers, wind tunnels, testing arena, among others. It is important to highlight that the design and size of these apparatus vary greatly depending on the size and biological characteristics of each insect.

There are several advantages of performing bioassay under laboratory conditions compared to field tests: (I) control of environmental conditions, (II) control of the physiological conditions of the organism, (III) elimination of external stimuli, (IV) better interpretation of complex responses.

The bioassay most widely used for phlebotomines is the wind tunnel. In this methodology the flight of insects is allowed while they follow a track of chemical compounds established by an air current which is released on the opposite side where the insects are arranged (Figure 7). The behavior of the insect due to this stimulus is recorded by direct observation or by video cameras and special software. The first wind tunnel study using *L. longipalpis* phlebotomine species was performed by Morton and Ward [136] in which the authors found that virgin females aged 3-6 days came faster and in greater numbers to the other side of the tunnel when they were used hamster and pheromone extracted from attractive males as compared to the control. For these tests it was used a wind tunnel of 240 cm, but since then, relatively few studies have been conducted using this methodology [147, 148, 153, 156].

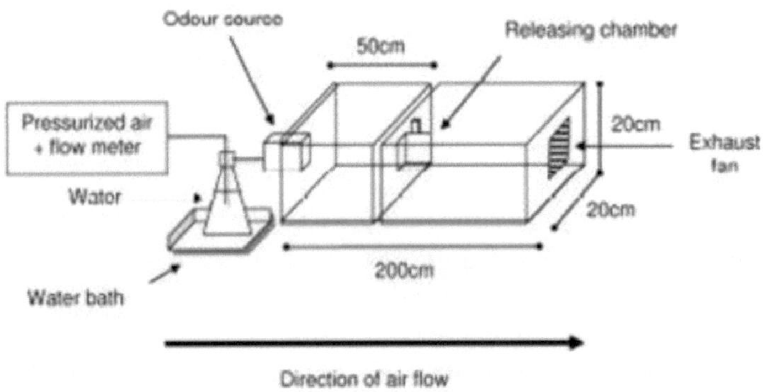

Figure 7. Schematic drawing of wind tunnel [156]

Despite several advantages, bioassays have significant drawbacks: (I) organisms up under laboratory conditions may have different behaviors compared with wild organisms, (II) environment standardization in the laboratory is scarcely repeated at field conditions. Thus, field tests are considered as essential for the validation of a semiochemical and they are the final phase for determining the attraction of phlebotomines to a compound or mixture of compounds. In these studies chemical compounds are placed as bait in traps and their own attractiveness is tested in a proven endemic area for the particular studied insect [124].

6.4. Application of chemical ecology for vector control

Despite recurrent attempts to control and prevent visceral *Leishmania*sis, it is booming worldwide, particularly in Brazil [7, 8].

The situation becomes more alarming when it evaluates the current trend towards urbanization of the disease [10], associated with increasing environmental degradation that favors its spread [157], as well as exposure of susceptible populations and the ineffectiveness of current measures to combat disease [158].

Currently, vector control is based only on the use of environmentally-destructive chemical insecticides [159], however this measure is highly debatable due the risks of environmental contamination and development of resistant insects [160]. Thus, the vector control based on chemical manipulation of vectors is gaining prominence.

In this direction, the identification of semiochemical that can be used as bait in traps to capture phlebotomine can provide a significant improvement for disease control. Light traps are commonly used to monitor populations of phlebotomines and are important for several reasons: (I) enable early identification of the presence of disease vectors in areas previously considered as non-transmission, making it easier to decision making authorities, (II) allow the knowledge about distribution of the vector in a given region as well as monitoring the spread of vector in these locations, (III) and finally, they allow a better understanding of the relationship between parasite, phlebotomine and environment, thus maximizing the attempts to control the disease.

The trap advocated for capture of phlebotomines is the CDC light [11] and these traps have some operational limitations such as the high cost, little specific and contestable accuracy for areas with low phlebotomines occurrence [161]. The use of chemical compounds along with traps aims to make them more specific and efficient, which has also been demonstrated in studies of phlebotomine [124, 162, 163], as well as other insect vectors of diseases [164, 165].

Another option arising from the identification of semiochemicals attractive to phlebotomine is their use integrated with insecticides. The use of semiochemicals with insecticides to control sand fly populations would be an example of integrated vector control. Similar techniques are used to control agricultural pests [152, 166]. Configures as an ecological approach for the control of insect vectors of disease and it is a rational and integrated use of various techniques available and necessary to a unified program.

The use of semiochemicals in integrated vector management reduces the amount of insecticide used, reducing accidents and environmental risks to public health, as well as decreasing risks of development of resistance in insects. The use of semiochemicals has other advantages, such as focus control on single specie, since most compounds is specie-specific, nontoxic, need to be used in small amounts and are biodegradable

In the case of phlebotomines control, Bray *et al.* [167] used sex pheromone of *L. longipalpis* as attractive on walls treated with insecticides and sticky traps, obtaining satisfactory results. However more studies are needed to increase the efficiency of the system, including the use of host odors to maximize the attraction of insects.

7. Conclusion

In this chapter we discuss the possibility of studying visceral leishmaniasis from a metabolomics approach aiming to identify VOC from dogs that can be used as biomarkers of early infection. Studies such as these can contribute for the development of a new diagnostic method which is painless, of minimal invasiveness and able to detect infection even before the animals manifest clinical signs.

In general the results from biological samples such as hair demonstrated high dispersion. This variation is expected, since the matrix is not uniform and several factors intrinsic to samples can influence the analysis. Randomized controlled studies that consider gender, race and age as potential confounding variables are needed to minimize the diversity of competing effects and to highlight subtle differences of expression of odor molecules between several clinical profiles, immunological and parasitological of dogs.

In general the results from biological samples such as by, demonstrated a marked degree of dispersion. This variation is expected, since the matrix is not uniform, and several intrinsic factors can influence the samples in the analysis. To minimize the multiplicity of competing effects and better highlight the differences more subtle expression of odor molecules between different clinical profiles, immunological and parasitological dogs are needed randomized controlled studies that consider gender, race and age as potential confounding variables.

Author details

Jailson Bittencourt de Andrade[1], Jairo Torres Magalhães Junior[2],
Paulo Roberto Ribeiro Mesquita[1,3], Fábio Santos Oliveira[4],
Frederico de Medeiros Rodrigues[3] and Stella Maria Barrouin-Melo[2]

1 Instituto de Química, Universidade Federal da Bahia, Campus Universitário de Ondina, Salvador, Brasil

2 Laboratório de Infectologia Veterinária, Hospital de Medicina Veterinária, Universidade Federal da Bahia (UFBA), CEP Salvador, Bahia, Brasil

3 Empresa Baiana de Desenvolvimento Agrícola S.A. (EBDA), Ondina, Salvador, Brasil

4 Centro de Ciências da Saúde, Universidade Federal do Recôncavo da Bahia, Cajueiro, Santo Antônio de Jesus, Brasil

References

[1] Barral-Netto M, Barral A, Brownell CE, Skeiky Y, Ellingsworth LR, Twardzik DR, et al. Transforming growth factor-beta in leishmanial infection: a parasite escape mechanism. Science. 1992;257(5069):545-8.

[2] Phillips M, Cataneo RN, Saunders C, Hope P, Schmitt P, Wai J. Volatile biomarkers in the breath of women with breast cancer. Journal of Breath Research. 2010;4(2): 026003.

[3] Basanta M, Ibrahim B, Dockry R, Douce D, Morris M, Singh D, et al. Exhaled volatile organic compounds for phenotyping chronic obstructive pulmonary disease: a cross-sectional study. Respiratory research. 2012;13(1):72.

[4] Kartsova L, Obedkova E. Chromatographic and electrophoretic profiles of biologically active compounds for the diagnosis of various diseases. Journal of Analytical Chemistry. 2013;68(4):291-9.

[5] Harkey M. Anatomy and physiology of hair. Forensic science international. 1993;63(1):9-18.

[6] Vilela ED-L, T. Introdução aos semioquímicos e terminologia. In: HOLOS, editor. Feromônios de insetos: Biologia, química e emprego no manejo de pragas. Ribeirão Preto2001. p. 9-12.

[7] Organization WH. Leishmaniasis: worldwide epidemiological and drug access update. In: WHO, editor. Geneva, Switzerland2011.

[8] Alvar J, Vélez ID, Bern C, Herrero M, Desjeux P, Cano J, et al. Leishmaniasis worldwide and global estimates of its incidence. PloS one. 2012;7(5):e35671.

[9] Quinnell RJ, Courtenay O. Transmission, reservoir hosts and control of zoonotic visceral leishmaniasis. Parasitology. 2009;136(14):1915-34.

[10] Lainson R, Rangel EF. Lutzomyia longipalpis and the eco-epidemiology of American visceral leishmaniasis, with particular reference to Brazil: a review. Memorias do Instituto Oswaldo Cruz. 2005;100(8):811-27. Epub 2006/01/31.

[11] Brasil. Manual de Vigilância e Controle da Leishmaniose Visceral. In: Saúde Md, editor. Brasília: Editora do Ministério da Saúde; 2006. p. 120.

[12] Monteiro EM, da Silva JC, da Costa RT, Costa DC, Barata RA, de Paula EV, et al. [Visceral leishmaniasis: a study on phlebotomine sand flies and canine infection in Montes Claros, State of Minas Gerais]. Revista da Sociedade Brasileira de Medicina Tropical. 2005;38(2):147-52. Epub 2005/04/12. Leishmaniose visceral: estudo de flebotomineos e infeccao canina em Montes Claros, Minas Gerais.

[13] Silva AV, Paula AA, Cabrera MA, Carreira JC. [Leishmaniasis in domestic dogs: epidemiological aspects]. Cadernos de saude publica / Ministerio da Saude, Fundacao

Oswaldo Cruz, Escola Nacional de Saude Publica. 2005;21(1):324-8. Epub 2005/02/05. Leishmaniose em caes domesticos: aspectos epidemiologicos.

[14] Sherlock IA. Ecological interactions of visceral leishmaniasis in the state of Bahia, Brazil. Memorias do Instituto Oswaldo Cruz. 1996;91(6):671-83. Epub 1996/11/01.

[15] Soares RP, Turco SJ. Lutzomyia longipalpis (Diptera: Psychodidae: Phlebotominae): a review. Anais da Academia Brasileira de Ciencias. 2003;75(3):301-30. Epub 2003/08/30.

[16] Rangel EF, Vilela ML. Lutzomyia longipalpis (Diptera, Psychodidae, Phlebotominae) and urbanization of visceral leishmaniasis in Brazil. Cadernos de saude publica / Ministerio da Saude, Fundacao Oswaldo Cruz, Escola Nacional de Saude Publica. 2008;24(12):2948-52. Epub 2008/12/17.

[17] Gontijo CMF, Melo MN. Visceral Leishmaniasis in Brazil: current status, challenges and prospects. Revista Brasileira de Epidemiologia. 2004;7(3):338-49.

[18] Grimaldi G, Tesh R. Leishmaniases of the New World: current concepts and implications for future research. Clinical microbiology reviews. 1993;6(3):230-50.

[19] Pinelli E, Killick-Kendrick R, Wagenaar J, Bernadina W, Del Real G, Ruitenberg J. Cellular and humoral immune responses in dogs experimentally and naturally infected with Leishmania infantum. Infection and immunity. 1994;62(1):229-35.

[20] Alves CF, de Amorim IF, Moura EP, Ribeiro RR, Alves CF, Michalick MS, et al. Expression of IFN-γ, TNF-α, IL-10 and TGF-β in lymph nodes associates with parasite load and clinical form of disease in dogs naturally infected with< i> Leishmania</i>(< i> Leishmania</i>)< i> chagasi</i>. Veterinary immunology and immunopathology. 2009;128(4):349-58.

[21] Kenney RT, Sacks DL, Gam AA, Murray HW, Sundar S. Splenic cytokine responses in Indian kala-azar before and after treatment. Journal of Infectious Diseases. 1998;177(3):815-9.

[22] de Abreu RT, das Graças Carvalho M, Carneiro CM, Giunchetti RC, Teixeira-Carvalho A, Martins-Filho OA, et al. Influence of Clinical Status and Parasite Load on Erythropoiesis and Leucopoiesis in Dogs Naturally Infected with Leishmania (Leishmania) chagasi. PloS one. 2011;6(5):e18873.

[23] Souza DM, Oliveira RCd, Sá RG, Giunchetti RC, Carvalho ATd, Martins Filho OA, et al. Cytokine and transcription factor profiles in the skin of dogs naturally infected by Leishmania (Leishmania) chagasi presenting distinct cutaneous parasite density and clinical status. 2011.

[24] Carrillo E, Moreno J. Cytokine profiles in canine visceral leishmaniasis. Veterinary immunology and immunopathology. 2009;128(1):67-70.

[25] Manna L, Reale S, Vitale F, Gravino AE. Evidence for a relationship between< i> Leishmania</i> load and clinical manifestations. Research in veterinary science. 2009;87(1):76-8.

[26] Travi BL, Tabares CJ, Cadena H, Ferro C, Osorio Y. Canine visceral leishmaniasis in Colombia: relationship between clinical and parasitologic status and infectivity for sand flies. The American journal of tropical medicine and hygiene. 2001;64(3-4): 119-24. Epub 2001/07/10.

[27] Sato N, Ahuja SK, Quinones M, Kostecki V, Reddick RL, Melby PC, et al. Cc Chemokine Receptor (Ccr) 2 Is Required for Langerhans Cell Migration and Localization of T Helper Cell Type 1 (Th1)-Inducing Dendritic Cells Absence of Ccr2 Shifts the Leishmania major–Resistant Phenotype to a Susceptible State Dominated by Th2 Cytokines, B Cell Outgrowth, and Sustained Neutrophilic Inflammation. The Journal of experimental medicine. 2000;192(2):205-18.

[28] Barrouin-Melo SM, Larangeira DF, de Andrade Filho FA, Trigo J, Juliao FS, Franke CR, et al. Can spleen aspirations be safely used for the parasitological diagnosis of canine visceral leishmaniosis? A study on assymptomatic and polysymptomatic animals. Vet J. 2006;171(2):331-9. Epub 2006/02/24.

[29] Michalsky ÉM, Rocha MF, da Rocha Lima ACVM, França-Silva JC, Pires MQ, Oliveira FS, et al. Infectivity of seropositive dogs, showing different clinical forms of leishmaniasis, to Lutzomyia longipalpis phlebotomine sand flies. Veterinary parasitology. 2007;147(1–2):67-76.

[30] Solano-Gallego L, Fernandez-Bellon H, Morell P, Fondevila D, Alberola J, Ramis A, et al. Histological and Immunohistochemical Study of Clinically Normal Skin of< i> Leishmania infantum</i>-infected Dogs. Journal of comparative pathology. 2004;130(1):7-12.

[31] Verçosa B, Lemos C, Mendonça I, Silva S, De Carvalho S, Goto H, et al. Transmission potential, skin inflammatory response, and parasitism of symptomatic and asymptomatic dogs with visceral leishmaniasis. BMC veterinary research. 2008;4(1):45.

[32] Stenn K, Paus R. Controls of hair follicle cycling. Physiological reviews. 2001;81(1): 449-94.

[33] Gratacos-Cubarsi M, Castellari M, Valero A, Garcia-Regueiro J. Hair analysis for veterinary drug monitoring in livestock production. Journal of Chromatography B. 2006;834(1):14-25.

[34] Vincenti M, Salomone A, Gerace E, Pirro V. Application of mass spectrometry to hair analysis for forensic toxicological investigations. Mass spectrometry reviews. 2012.

[35] Agusa T, Kunito T, Iwata H, Monirith I, Chamnan C, Tana TS, et al. Mercury in hair and blood from residents of Phnom Penh (Cambodia) and possible effect on serum hormone levels. Chemosphere. 2007;68(3):590-6.

[36] Dorea J, Costa J, Holzbecher J, Ryan D, Marsden P. Antimony accumulation in hair during treatment of leishmaniasis. Clinical chemistry. 1987;33(11):2081-2.

[37] Kintz P, Villain M, Cirimele V. Hair analysis for drug detection. Therapeutic drug monitoring. 2006;28(3):442-6.

[38] Pasa S, Kargin F, Bildik A, Seyrek K, Ozbel Y, Ozensoy S. Serum and hair levels of zinc and other elements in dogs with visceral leishmaniasis. Biological trace element research. 2003;94(2):141-7.

[39] Anielski P. Hair analysis of anabolic steroids in connection with doping control—results from horse samples. Journal of Mass Spectrometry. 2008;43(7):1001-8.

[40] Belinchón-Lorenzo S, Iniesta V, Parejo JC, Fernández-Cotrina J, Muñoz-Madrid R, Soto M, et al. Detection of< i> Leishmania infantum</i> kinetoplast minicircle DNA by Real Time PCR in hair of dogs with leishmaniosis. Veterinary parasitology. 2012.

[41] Oliveira LS, Rodrigues Fde M, Oliveira FS, Mesquita PR, Leal DC, Alcantara AC, et al. Headspace solid phase microextraction/gas chromatography-mass spectrometry combined to chemometric analysis for volatile organic compounds determination in canine hair: a new tool to detect dog contamination by visceral leishmaniasis. Journal of chromatography B, Analytical technologies in the biomedical and life sciences. 2008;875(2):392-8. Epub 2008/10/24.

[42] Magalhães-Junior JTM, P. R. R. ; Rodrigues, F. M. ; Oliveira, W. F. S. ; Franke, C.R.; Andrade, J.B.; Barrouin-Melo, S. M. Identification of biomarkers in the hair of dogs: new diagnostic possibilities in the study and control of visceral leishmaniasis. 2013.

[43] van der Greef J, Smilde AK. Symbiosis of chemometrics and metabolomics: past, present, and future. Journal of Chemometrics. 2005;19(5-7):376-86.

[44] Wilson IDN, J. K. Metabonomics and Global Systems Biology. In: Griffith WJ, editor. Metabolomics, metabonomics, and metabolite profiling: Royal Society of Chemistry; 2008. p. 295-314.

[45] Patti GJ, Yanes O, Siuzdak G. Innovation: Metabolomics: the apogee of the omics trilogy. Nature reviews Molecular cell biology. 2012;13(4):263-9.

[46] Fontana JM, Alexander E, Salvatore M. Translational research in infectious disease: current paradigms and challenges ahead. Translational Research. 2012;159(6):430-53.

[47] Smolinska A, Blanchet L, Buydens L, Wijmenga SS. NMR and pattern recognition methods in metabolomics: from data acquisition to biomarker discovery: a review. Analytica chimica acta. 2012;750:82-97.

[48] Issaq HJ, Van QN, Waybright TJ, Muschik GM, Veenstra TD. Analytical and statistical approaches to metabolomics research. Journal of separation science. 2009;32(13): 2183-99.

[49] Ramautar R, Somsen GW, de Jong GJ. CE-MS for metabolomics: Developments and applications in the period 2010–2012. Electrophoresis. 2013;34(1):86-98.

[50] Lakshmanan V, Rhee KY, Daily JP. Metabolomics and malaria biology. Molecular and biochemical parasitology. 2011;175(2):104-11.

[51] Kell DB. Systems biology, metabolic modelling and metabolomics in drug discovery and development. Drug discovery today. 2006;11(23):1085-92.

[52] Henderson JP, Crowley JR, Pinkner JS, Walker JN, Tsukayama P, Stamm WE, et al. Quantitative metabolomics reveals an epigenetic blueprint for iron acquisition in uropathogenic Escherichia coli. PLoS pathogens. 2009;5(2):e1000305.

[53] Rodgers MA, Villareal VA, Schaefer EA, Peng LF, Corey KE, Chung RT, et al. Lipid metabolite profiling identifies desmosterol metabolism as a new antiviral target for hepatitis C virus. Journal of the American Chemical Society. 2012;134(16):6896-9.

[54] Willger SD, Grahl N, Cramer Jr RA. Aspergillus fumigatus metabolism: clues to mechanisms of in vivo fungal growth and virulence. Medical Mycology. 2009;47(S1):S72-S9.

[55] Olszewski KL, Morrisey JM, Wilinski D, Burns JM, Vaidya AB, Rabinowitz JD, et al. Host-Parasite Interactions Revealed by< i> Plasmodium falciparum</i> Metabolomics. Cell host & microbe. 2009;5(2):191-9.

[56] Arai M, Billker O, Morris HR, Panico M, Delcroix M, Dixon D, et al. Both mosquito-derived xanthurenic acid and a host blood-derived factor regulate gametogenesis of< i> Plasmodium</i> in the midgut of the mosquito. Molecular and biochemical parasitology. 2001;116(1):17-24.

[57] Saunders E, MacRae J, Naderer T, Ng M, McConville M, Likić V. LeishCyc: A Guide to Building a Metabolic Pathway Database and Visualization of Metabolomic Data. In: Navid A, editor. Microbial Systems Biology: Humana Press; 2012. p. 505-29.

[58] Silva AM, Cordeiro-da-Silva A, Coombs GH. Metabolic variation during development in culture of Leishmania donovani promastigotes. PLoS neglected tropical diseases. 2011;5(12):e1451.

[59] Berg M, Vanaerschot M, Jankevics A, Cuypers B, Maes I, Mukherjee S, et al. Metabolic adaptations of Leishmania donovani in relation to differentiation, drug resistance, and drug pressure. Molecular Microbiology. 2013:n/a-n/a.

[60] Phillips M, Cataneo RN, Condos R, Ring Erickson GA, Greenberg J, La Bombardi V, et al. Volatile biomarkers of pulmonary tuberculosis in the breath. Tuberculosis. 2007;87(1):44-52.

[61] Van Berkel J, Dallinga J, Möller G, Godschalk R, Moonen E, Wouters E, et al. A profile of volatile organic compounds in breath discriminates COPD patients from controls. Respiratory medicine. 2010;104(4):557-63.

[62] Zhang A, Sun H, Xu H, Qiu S, Wang X. Cell Metabolomics. Omics: a journal of integrative biology. 2013.

[63] Dunn WB, Ellis DI. Metabolomics: current analytical platforms and methodologies. TrAC Trends in Analytical Chemistry. 2005;24(4):285-94.

[64] Zhang Z, Li G. A review of advances and new developments in the analysis of biological volatile organic compounds. Microchemical Journal. 2010;95(2):127-39.

[65] Kimbaris AC, Siatis NG, Daferera DJ, Tarantilis PA, Pappas CS, Polissiou MG. Comparison of distillation and ultrasound-assisted extraction methods for the isolation of sensitive aroma compounds from garlic (< i> Allium sativum</i>). Ultrasonics sonochemistry. 2006;13(1):54-60.

[66] Chaintreau A. Simultaneous distillation–extraction: from birth to maturity—review. Flavour and fragrance journal. 2001;16(2):136-48.

[67] Pollien P, Chaintreau A. Simultaneous distillation-extraction: Theoretical model and development of a preparative unit. Analytical chemistry. 1997;69(16):3285-92.

[68] Hashemi P, Abolghasemi MM, Fakhari A, Ebrahimi SN, Ahmadi S. Hydrodistillation–solvent microextraction and GC–MS identification of volatile components of Artemisia aucheri. Chromatographia. 2007;66(3-4):283-6.

[69] Ferhat M, Tigrine-Kordjani N, Chemat S, Meklati B, Chemat F. Rapid extraction of volatile compounds using a new simultaneous microwave distillation: solvent extraction device. Chromatographia. 2007;65(3-4):217-22.

[70] Giannuzzo AN, Boggetti HJ, Nazareno MA, Mishima HT. Supercritical fluid extraction of naringin from the peel of Citrus paradisi. Phytochemical Analysis. 2003;14(4):221-3.

[71] Stashenko EE, Jaramillo BE, Martínez JR. Analysis of volatile secondary metabolites from Colombian< i> Xylopia aromatica</i>(Lamarck) by different extraction and headspace methods and gas chromatography. Journal of Chromatography A. 2004;1025(1):105-13.

[72] Stashenko EE, Puertas MA, Combariza MY. Volatile secondary metabolites from< i> Spilanthes americana</i> obtained by simultaneous steam distillation-solvent extraction and supercritical fluid extraction. Journal of Chromatography A. 1996;752(1):223-32.

[73] Crespo MP, Yusty ML. Comparison of supercritical fluid extraction and Soxhlet extraction for the determination of aliphatic hydrocarbons in seaweed samples. Ecotoxicology and Environmental Safety. 2006;64(3):400-5.

[74] Azmir J, Zaidul ISM, Rahman MM, Sharif KM, Mohamed A, Sahena F, et al. Techniques for extraction of bioactive compounds from plant materials: A review. Journal of Food Engineering. 2013;117(4):426-36.

[75] MacLeod G, Ames JM. Comparative assessment of the artefact background on thermal desorption of Tenax GC and Tenax TA. Journal of Chromatography A. 1986;355:393-8.

[76] Dettmer K, Engewald W. Adsorbent materials commonly used in air analysis for adsorptive enrichment and thermal desorption of volatile organic compounds. Analytical and bioanalytical chemistry. 2002;373(6):490-500.

[77] Senf L, Frank H. Thermal-desorption of organic pollutants enriched on activated carbon.5. Desorption behavior and temperature profile. Journal of Chromatography. 1990;520:131-5.

[78] Leboda R, Łodyga A, Gierak A. Carbon adsorbents as materials for chromatography I. Gas chromatography. Materials Chemistry and Physics. 1997;51(3):216-32.

[79] Brown RH. What is the best sorbent for pumped sampling thermal desorption of volatile organic compounds? Experience with the EC sorbents project. Analyst. 1996;121(9):1171-5.

[80] Camel V, Caude M. Trace enrichment methods for the determination of organic pollutants in ambient air. Journal of Chromatography A. 1995;710(1):3-19.

[81] Dettmer K, Felix U, Engewald W, Mohnke M. Application of a unique selective PLOT capillary column for the analysis of oxygenated compounds in ambient air. Chromatographia. 2000;51:S221-S7.

[82] Sponring A, Filipiak W, Ager C, Schubert J, Miekisch W, Amann A, et al. Analysis of volatile organic compounds (VOCs) in the headspace of NCI-H1666 lung cancer cells. Cancer Biomarkers. 2010;7(3):153-61.

[83] Arthur CL, Pawliszyn J. Solid phase microextraction with thermal desorption using fused silica optical fibers. Analytical chemistry. 1990;62(19):2145-8.

[84] Penalver A, Pocurull E, Borrull F, Marcé R. Trends in solid-phase microextraction for determining organic pollutants in environmental samples. TrAC Trends in Analytical Chemistry. 1999;18(8):557-68.

[85] Ulrich S. Solid-phase microextraction in biomedical analysis. Journal of Chromatography A. 2000;902(1):167-94.

[86] Mills GA, Walker V. Headspace solid-phase microextraction procedures for gas chromatographic analysis of biological fluids and materials. Journal of Chromatography A. 2000;902(1):267-87.

[87] Augusto F, Leite e Lopes A, Zini CA. Sampling and sample preparation for analysis of aromas and fragrances. TrAC Trends in Analytical Chemistry. 2003;22(3):160-9.

[88] Grote C, Pawliszyn J. Solid-phase microextraction for the analysis of human breath. Analytical chemistry. 1997;69(4):587-96.

[89] Hyšpler Rr, Crhová Š, Gasparič J, Zadák Z, Čížková M, Balasová V. Determination of isoprene in human expired breath using solid-phase microextraction and gas chromatography–mass spectrometry. Journal of Chromatography B: Biomedical Sciences and Applications. 2000;739(1):183-90.

[90] Wu D, Wang Z, Wang H, Zhang L, Wang X. Analysis of odors in human palm by GC/MS with headspace solid phase microextraction. Modern Scientific Instruments. 2003;4:52-4.

[91] Wang Y, Zhao M. Analysis of volatile constituents of Thymus Amurensis Klokov by gas chromatography-mass spectrometry with solid-phase microextraction. Chinese Journal of Analytical Chemistry. 2004;32(2):272-.

[92] Jirovetz L, Buchbauer G, Ngassoum MB, Geissler M. Aroma compound analysis of< i> Piper nigrum</i> and< i> Piper guineense</i> essential oils from Cameroon using solid-phase microextraction–gas chromatography, solid-phase microextraction–gas chromatography–mass spectrometry and olfactometry. Journal of Chromatography A. 2002;976(1):265-75.

[93] Sánchez-Palomo E, Diaz-Maroto MC, Pérez-Coello MS. Rapid determination of volatile compounds in grapes by HS-SPME coupled with GC–MS. Talanta. 2005;66(5): 1152-7.

[94] Augusto F, Valente ALP, dos Santos Tada E, Rivellino SR. Screening of Brazilian fruit aromas using solid-phase microextraction–gas chromatography–mass spectrometry. Journal of Chromatography A. 2000;873(1):117-27.

[95] Crespo R, Pedrini N, Juárez M, Dal Bello G. Volatile organic compounds released by the entomopathogenic fungus< i> Beauveria bassiana</i>. Microbiological research. 2008;163(2):148-51.

[96] Hachem C, Fazio P, Rao J, Bartlett K, Chaubey YP. Identification and transport investigation of microbial volatile organic compounds in full-scale stud cavities. Building and Environment. 2009;44(8):1691-8.

[97] Souza Silva EA, Risticevic S, Pawliszyn J. Recent trends in SPME concerning sorbent materials, configurations and< i> in vivo</i> applications. TrAC Trends in Analytical Chemistry. 2012.

[98] Ouyang G, Vuckovic D, Pawliszyn J. Nondestructive sampling of living systems using in vivo solid-phase microextraction. Chemical Reviews. 2011;111(4):2784-814.

[99] Bai Z, Pilote A, Sarker PK, Vandenberg G, Pawliszyn J. In Vivo Solid-Phase Microextraction with in Vitro Calibration: Determination of Off-Flavor Components in Live Fish. Analytical chemistry. 2013;85(4):2328-32.

[100] Etiévant PX, Callement G, Langlois D, Issanchou S, Coquibus N. Odor intensity evaluation in gas chromatography-olfactometry by finger span method. Journal of agricultural and food chemistry. 1999;47(4):1673-80.

[101] Sanchez JM, Sacks RD. GC analysis of human breath with a series-coupled column ensemble and a multibed sorption trap. Analytical chemistry. 2003;75(10):2231-6.

[102] Bean HD, Dimandja J-MD, Hill JE. Bacterial volatile discovery using solid phase microextraction and comprehensive two-dimensional gas chromatography–time-of-flight mass spectrometry. Journal of Chromatography B. 2012;901:41-6.

[103] Stadler S, Stefanuto P-H, Brokl M, Forbes SL, Focant J-Fo. Characterization of Volatile Organic Compounds from Human Analogue Decomposition Using Thermal Desorption Coupled to Comprehensive Two-Dimensional Gas Chromatography–Time-of-Flight Mass Spectrometry. Analytical chemistry. 2012;85(2):998-1005.

[104] Dieterle F, Marrer E. New technologies around biomarkers and their interplay with drug development. Analytical and bioanalytical chemistry. 2008;390(1):141-54.

[105] Denoroy L, Zimmer L, Renaud B, Parrot S. Ultra high performance liquid chromatography as a tool for the discovery and the analysis of biomarkers of diseases: A review. Journal of Chromatography B. 2013;927(0):37-53.

[106] Koulman A, Lane GA, Harrison SJ, Volmer DA. From differentiating metabolites to biomarkers. Analytical and bioanalytical chemistry. 2009;394(3):663-70.

[107] Katajamaa M, Orešič M. Data processing for mass spectrometry-based metabolomics. Journal of Chromatography A. 2007;1158(1–2):318-28.

[108] Trygg J, Holmes E, Lundstedt T. Chemometrics in metabonomics. Journal of proteome research. 2007;6(2):469-79.

[109] LU G, WANG J, ZHAO X, KONG H, XU G. Study on gender difference based on metabolites in urine by ultra high performance liquid chromatography/time of flight mass spectrometry. Chinese Journal of Chromatography. 2006;24(2):109-13.

[110] Stella C, Beckwith-Hall B, Cloarec O, Holmes E, Lindon JC, Powell J, et al. Susceptibility of human metabolic phenotypes to dietary modulation. Journal of proteome research. 2006;5(10):2780-8.

[111] Wang W, Feng B, Li X, Yin P, Gao P, Zhao X, et al. Urinary metabolic profiling of colorectal carcinoma based on online affinity solid phase extraction-high performance liquid chromatography and ultra performance liquid chromatography-mass spectrometry. Molecular BioSystems. 2010;6(10):1947-55.

[112] Wang TJ, Larson MG, Vasan RS, Cheng S, Rhee EP, McCabe E, et al. Metabolite profiles and the risk of developing diabetes. Nature medicine. 2011;17(4):448-53.

[113] Langenberg C, Savage DB. An amino acid profile to predict diabetes? Nature medicine. 2011;17(4):418.

[114] Orešič M, Simell S, Sysi-Aho M, Näntö-Salonen K, Seppänen-Laakso T, Parikka V, et al. Dysregulation of lipid and amino acid metabolism precedes islet autoimmunity in

children who later progress to type 1 diabetes. The Journal of experimental medicine. 2008;205(13):2975-84.

[115] Woo HM, Kim KM, Choi MH, Jung BH, Lee J, Kong G, et al. Mass spectrometry based metabolomic approaches in urinary biomarker study of women's cancers. Clinica Chimica Acta. 2009;400(1):63-9.

[116] Sabatine MS, Liu E, Morrow DA, Heller E, McCarroll R, Wiegand R, et al. Metabolomic identification of novel biomarkers of myocardial ischemia. Circulation. 2005;112(25):3868-75.

[117] Jensen UG, Brandt NJ, Christensen E, Skovby F, Nørgaard-Pedersen B, Simonsen H. Neonatal screening for galactosemia by quantitative analysis of hexose monophosphates using tandem mass spectrometry: a retrospective study. Clinical chemistry. 2001;47(8):1364-72.

[118] Liu G, Snapp HM, Ji QC, Arnold ME. Strategy of accelerated method development for high-throughput bioanalytical assays using ultra high-performance liquid chromatography coupled with mass spectrometry. Analytical chemistry. 2009;81(22): 9225-32.

[119] Denery JR, Nunes AA, Hixon MS, Dickerson TJ, Janda KD. Metabolomics-based discovery of diagnostic biomarkers for onchocerciasis. PLoS neglected tropical diseases. 2010;4(10):e834.

[120] Rudnicka J, Kowalkowski T, Ligor T, Buszewski B. Determination of volatile organic compounds as biomarkers of lung cancer by SPME–GC–TOF/MS and chemometrics. Journal of Chromatography B. 2011;879(30):3360-6.

[121] Phillips M, Boehmer JP, Cataneo RN, Cheema T, Eisen HJ, Fallon JT, et al. Prediction of heart transplant rejection with a breath test for markers of oxidative stress. The American journal of cardiology. 2004;94(12):1593-4.

[122] Matsumura K, Opiekun M, Oka H, Vachani A, Albelda SM, Yamazaki K, et al. Urinary volatile compounds as biomarkers for lung cancer: a proof of principle study using odor signatures in mouse models of lung cancer. PloS one. 2010;5(1):e8819.

[123] Logan JG, Birkett MA. Semiochemicals for biting fly control: their identification and exploitation. Pest Management Science. 2007;63(7):647-57.

[124] Andrade AJ, Andrade MR, Dias ES, Pinto MC, Eiras AE. Are light traps baited with kairomones effective in the capture of Lutzomyia longipalpis and Lutzomyia intermedia? An evaluation of synthetic human odor as an attractant for phlebotomine sand flies (Diptera: Psychodidae: Phlebotominae). Memorias do Instituto Oswaldo Cruz. 2008;103(4):337-43. Epub 2008/07/29.

[125] Dicke M, Sabelis MW. Infochemical terminology: based on cost-benefit analysis rather than origin of compounds? Functional Ecology. 1988:131-9.

[126] Kelly DW, Mustafa Z, Dye C. Differential application of lambda-cyhalothrin to control the sandfly Lutzomyia longipalpis. Medical and veterinary entomology. 1997;11(1):13-24. Epub 1997/01/01.

[127] Corrêa A, Sant'Ana J. Ecologia química de insetos. Produtos naturais no controle de insetos São Carlos: Editora UFSCar. 2007:150.

[128] Knols BGJ, Meijerink J. Odors influence mosquito behavior. Science and Medicine. 1997;4:56-63.

[129] Eiras AE, Jepson PC. Host location by Aedes aegypti (Diptera: Culicidae): a wind tunnel study of chemical cues. Bulletin of entomological research. 1991;81(02):151-60.

[130] Mboera L, Takken W, Sambu E. The response of Culex quinquefasciatus (Diptera: Culicidae) to traps baited with carbon dioxide, 1-octen-3-ol, acetone, butyric acid and human foot odour in Tanzania. Bulletin of entomological research. 2000;90(02):155-9.

[131] Pinto MC, Campbell-Lendrum DH, Lozovei AL, Teodoro U, Davies CR. Phlebotomine sandfly responses to carbon dioxide and human odour in the field. Medical and veterinary entomology. 2001;15(2):132-9. Epub 2001/07/04.

[132] Torr S. Dose responses of tsetse flies (Glossina) to carbon dioxide, acetone and octenol in the field. Physiological Entomology. 1990;15(1):93-103.

[133] Kline D, Takken W, Wood J, Carlson D. Field studies on the potential of butanone, carbon dioxide, honey extract, l-octen-3-ol, L-lactic acid and phenols as attractants for mosquitoes*. Medical and veterinary entomology. 1990;4(4):383-91.

[134] Bray DP, Ward RD, Hamilton JG. 9. The chemical ecology of sandflies. Olfaction in vector-host interactions. The Netherlands: Wageningen Academic Publishers; 2010. p. 203.

[135] Grant AJ, O'Connell R. The detection of carbon dioxide and its role in the orientation to hosts by haematophagous insects. Olfaction in vector-host interactions. The Netherlands: Wageningen Academic Publishers; 2010. p. 91-113.

[136] Morton IE, Ward RD. Laboratory response of female Lutzomyia longipalpis sandflies to a host and male pheromone source over distance. Medical and veterinary entomology. 1989;3(3):219-23. Epub 1989/07/01.

[137] Hamilton JGC, Hooper AM, Ibbotson HC, Kurosawa S, Mori K, Muto S-E, et al. 9-methylgermacrene-B is confirmed as the sex pheromone of the sandfly Lutzomyia longipalpis from lapinha, Brazil, and the absolute stereochemistry defined as S. Chemical communications. 1999(23):2335-6.

[138] Hamilton J, Maingon R, Alexander B, Ward R, Brazil R. Analysis of the sex pheromone extract of individual male Lutzomyia longipalpis sandflies from six regions in Brazil. Medical and veterinary entomology. 2005;19(4):480-8.

[139] Rebollar-Tellez E, Hamilton J, Ward R. Biting site selection on a human volunteer by members of the Lutzomyia longipalpis complex. Southwestern Entomologist. 2002;27(1):97-104.

[140] Uribe S. The status of the Lutzomyia longipalpis species complex and possible implications for Leishmania transmission. Memorias do Instituto Oswaldo Cruz. 1999;94(6):729-34.

[141] Jones TM, Hamilton JGC. A role for pheromones in mate choice in a lekking sandfly. Animal behaviour. 1998;56(4):891-8. Epub 1998/12/16.

[142] Bray DP, Alves GB, Dorval ME, Brazil RP, Hamilton JG. Synthetic sex pheromone attracts the leishmaniasis vector Lutzomyia longipalpis to experimental chicken sheds treated with insecticide. Parasites & vectors. 2010;3:16. Epub 2010/03/13.

[143] Bray D, Hamilton JGC. Host odor synergizes attraction of virgin female Lutzomyia longipalpis (Diptera: Psychodidae). Journal of medical entomology. 2007;44(5): 779-87.

[144] Hamilton J, Ramsoondar T. Attraction of Lutzomyia longipalpis to human skin odours. Medical and veterinary entomology. 1994;8(4):375-80.

[145] Rebollar-Tellez E, Hamilton J, Ward R. Response of female Lutzomyia longipalpis to host odour kairomones from human skin. Physiological Entomology. 1999;24(3): 220-6.

[146] Rebollar-Téllez E, Hamilton J, Ward R. Genetic inherence of the response to human kairomones by two allopatric members of the Lutzomyia longipalpis complex. Physiological Entomology. 2006;31(1):94-7.

[147] Dougherty MJ, Guerin PM, Ward RD, Hamilton JGC. Behavioural and electrophysiological responses of the phlebotomine sandfly Lutzomyia longipalpis (Diptera: Psychodidae) when exposed to canid host odour kairomones. Physiological Entomology. 1999;24(3):251-62.

[148] O'Shea B, Rebollar-Tellez E, Ward RD, Hamilton JG, el Naiem D, Polwart A. Enhanced sandfly attraction to Leishmania-infected hosts. Transactions of the Royal Society of Tropical Medicine and Hygiene. 2002;96(2):117-8. Epub 2002/06/12.

[149] Keil TA. Morphology and development of the peripheral olfactory organs. In: Hansson BS, editor. Insect olfaction. Germany, Berlin: Springer; 1999.

[150] Bradbury JW, Vehrencamp SL. Principles of animal communication 2011.

[151] Park KC, Ochieng SA, Zhu J, Baker TC. Odor Discrimination using Insect Electroantennogram Responses from an Insect Antennal Array. Chemical Senses. 2002;27(4): 343-52.

[152] Witzgall P, Kirsch P, Cork A. Sex pheromones and their impact on pest management. Journal of chemical ecology. 2010;36(1):80-100.

[153] Spiegel CN, Jeanbourquin P, Guerin PM, Hooper AM, Claude S, Tabacchi R, et al. (1S,3S,7R)-3-methyl-alpha-himachalene from the male sandfly Lutzomyia longipalpis (Diptera: Psychodidae) induces neurophysiological responses and attracts both males and females. Journal of insect physiology. 2005;51(12):1366-75. Epub 2005/10/18.

[154] Sant'ana AL, Eiras AE, Cavalcante RR. Electroantennographic responses of the Lutzomyia (Lutzomyia) longipalpis (Lutz & Neiva) (Diptera: Psychodidae) to 1-octen-3-ol. Neotropical entomology. 2002;31:13-7.

[155] Trimble R, Marshall D. Quantitative method for pheromone delivery in studies of sensory adaptation of moth antennae. Physiological Entomology. 2007;32(4):388-93.

[156] Pinto MC, Bray DP, Eiras AE, Carvalheira HP, Puertas CP. Attraction of the cutaneous leishmaniasis vector Nyssomyia neivai (Diptera: Psychodidae) to host odour components in a wind tunnel. Parasites & vectors. 2012;5(1):210.

[157] Dias-Lima AG, Guedes ML, Sherlock IA. Horizontal stratification of the sand fly fauna (Diptera: Psychodidae) in a transitional vegetation between caatinga and tropical rain forest, state of Bahia, Brazil. Memorias do Instituto Oswaldo Cruz. 2003;98(6): 733-7. Epub 2003/11/05.

[158] Werneck GL. Forum: geographic spread and urbanization of visceral leishmaniasis in Brazil. Introduction. Cadernos de saude publica / Ministerio da Saude, Fundacao Oswaldo Cruz, Escola Nacional de Saude Publica. 2008;24(12):2937-40. Epub 2008/12/17.

[159] Alexander B, Maroli M. Control of phlebotomine sandflies. Medical and veterinary entomology. 2003;17(1):1-18.

[160] Amóra SS, Bevilaqua CM, Feijó F, Alves ND, Maciel MdV. Control of phlebotomine (Diptera: Psychodidae) leishmaniasis vectors. Neotropical entomology. 2009;38(3): 303-10.

[161] Andrade AJd. Ecologia química de flebotomíneos (Diptera : Psychodidae: Phlebotominae): desenvlvimento de uma armadilha e análise dos hidrocarbonetos cuticulares das espécies. Belo Horizonte, Minas Gerais: Universidade Federal de Minas Gerais; 2010.

[162] Kasili S, Kutima H, Mwandawiro C, Ngumbi PM, Anjili CO. Comparative attractiveness of CO(2)-baited CDC light traps and animal baits to Phlebotomus duboscqi sandflies. Journal of vector borne diseases. 2009;46(3):191-6. Epub 2009/09/03.

[163] Morton IE, Ward RD. Response of female sandflies (Lutzomyia longipalpis) to pheromone-baited sticky traps in the laboratory. Annals of tropical medicine and parasitology. 1990;84(1):49-51. Epub 1990/02/01.

[164] Tchouassi DP, Sang R, Sole CL, Bastos AD, Mithoefer K, Torto B. Sheep skin odor improves trap captures of mosquito vectors of Rift Valley fever. PLoS neglected tropical diseases. 2012;6(11):e1879.

[165] Verhulst NO, Mukabana WR, Takken W, Smallegange RC. Human skin microbiota and their volatiles as odour baits for the malaria mosquito Anopheles gambiae ss. Entomologia Experimentalis et Applicata. 2011;139(2):170-9.

[166] Shani A. Chemical communication agents (pheromones) in integrated pest management. Drug development research. 2000;50(3-4):400-5.

[167] Bray DP, Alves GB, Dorval ME, Brazil RP, Hamilton J. Research Synthetic sex pheromone attracts the leishmaniasis vector Lutzomyia longipalpis to experimental chicken sheds treated with insecticide. 2010.

Chapter 15

Leishmaniasis: Possible New Strategies for Treatment

Alane Beatriz Vermelho, Claudiu T. Supuran,
Verônica Cardoso, Dayanne Menezes,
Jefferson Rocha de Andrade Silva,
Jose Luiz Pinto Ferreira,
Ana Claudia Fernandes Amaral and
Igor A. Rodrigues

Additional information is available at the end of the chapter

http://dx.doi.org/10.5772/57388

1. Introduction

1.1. Leishmaniasis

Leishmaniasis is a vector-born disease caused by protozoan parasites in the genus *Leishmania*. Leishmaniasis is a potentially lethal, neglected disease that mostly affects economically disadvantaged individuals in many developing countries. Human infection occurs through the bite of infected female phlebotomine sand flies followed by injection of promastigote forms into the skin, which penetrate the macrophages and/or other types of mononuclear phagocytic cells. The promastigotes then transform into amastigotes (tissue stage of the parasite) in these cells and replicate, resulting in the bursting of the host cell and infection of other mononuclear phagocytic cells. Sand flies become infected by ingesting amastigote-infected cells during blood meals. These evolutionary forms transform into promastigotes in the gut of the insect and migrate to the proboscis, infecting other people through the bite (Scheme 1).

Depending on the *Leishmania* species involved and the host immune response, infection can lead to tegumentary or visceral manifestations of the disease. The tegumentary form of leishmaniasis (TL) includes cutaneous (CL), mucocutaneous (MCL), and diffuse (DL) clinical manifestations. All tegumentary forms have a major impact on patient life, because the skin lesions can lead to disfigurement and social stigmatization [2, 3]. Visceral leishmaniasis (VL), or Kala-azar, affects organs and internal tissues such as spleen, liver, bone marrow, and lymph

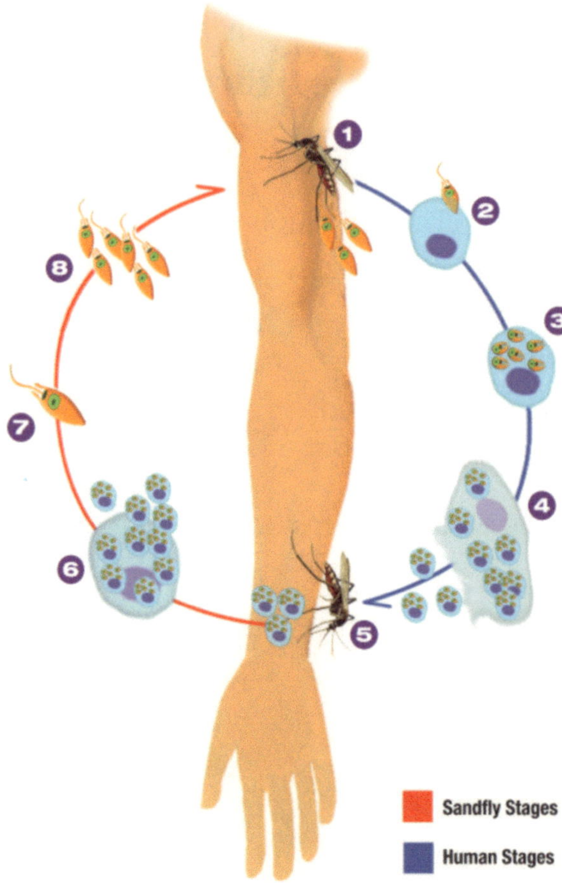

Scheme 1. Leishmaniasis life cycle. 1- sand flies inject promastigotes during blood meals ;2-promastigote infects macrophages and other types of mononuclear phagocytic cells;3-promastigotes transform into amastigotes; 4-amastigotes multiply. 5- sand flies become infected by ingesting macrophages infected with amastigotes during blood meals; 6- parasitized cells ; 7- in sand flies, amastigotes transform into promastigotes, in the gut; 8- promastigotes divide and migrate to proboscis based on CDC, 2013 [1].

nodes. With the progression of VL, splenomegaly and hepatomegaly lead to a distended abdomen and pain. Eventually, VL may lead to death caused by secondary infections, severe anemia, or organ failure [4]. Both TL and VL are endemic diseases in several countries. In fact, the number of cases of leishmaniasis may be underestimated because only 40 of the 88 countries where the disease frequently occurs report cases on a regular basis [5, 6].

The World Health Organization (WHO) estimates that 1.6 million new leishmaniasis cases occur annually, of which 500,000 correspond to VL (90% of them occurring in Bangladesh, Brazil, Ethiopia, India, Nepal, and Sudan) and 1.1 million to CL (90% of them occurring in Afghanistan, Algeria, Brazil, Iran, Peru, Saudi Arabia, Sudan, and Syria) [7]. Leishmaniasis currently affects an estimated 12 million people and approximately 350 million people live at risk of infection [1], whereas an estimated half a million people die annually of VL. In addition, immunosuppressive conditions such as AIDS contribute to the emergence of severe clinical forms of the disease. To date, the greatest prevalence of *Leishmania*-HIV co-infection has been reported in the Mediterranean basin [8, 9]. In some east African regions, up to 40% of patients with VL are co-infected with HIV, which further complicates treatment [10].

2. Current drugs

Currently, most antileishmanial drugs can be considered orphan drugs. In fact, leishmaniasis, Chagas disease, are examples of tropical neglected diseases (TND) as they receive little attention from governments and the pharmaceutical industry. For instance, by the 2000s, global investment in new anti-parasitic drugs was only about 0.1% of global investment in research [11, 12]. Additionally, the lack of human vaccines for leishmaniasis makes chemotherapy the primary method used to control the disease. Despite the existence of several chemotherapics to treat human leishmaniasis, many of them are new formulations of ancient drugs [13]. The chemotherapeutic agents currently used in the treatment of VL and TL such as stibogluconate of sodium (Pentostam®), *N*-methylglucantime (Glucantime®), pentamidine (Pentacarinato®), and amphotericin B (Fungizone®) do not possess activity when orally administered and require parenteral administration for long periods [14]. In addition, those chemotherapeutic agents are very expensive and cause severe side effects due to their high toxicity [15].

Taken together, all these factors contribute to poor patient adherence or abandonment of treatment. In turn, treatment failure has a great impact on the spread of the disease and the emergence of drug-resistant strains. However, the introduction of new chemotherapeutic agents, including liposomal amphotericin B (AmBisome®), paramomycin, and miltefosin has certainly improved the current scenario for the treatment of leishmaniasis. AmBisome® has become the first-choice drug for treating VL in several countries. For instance, this treatment is currently used in Bihar, India, because pentavalent antimonials have become less effective against parasites [16, 17]. However, none of these drugs are free of severe side effects and the development of new strategies and/or alternative therapeutic agents remain crucial.

The incorporation of amphotericin B into lipid formulations has brought new perspectives to the treatment of leishmaniasis, resulting in the incorporation of several other drugs to different lipid formulations, including meglumine antimoniate [18], furazolidone [19], paromomycin sulfate [20] and miltefosin [21]. Conventional chemotherapeutics usually have difficulty reaching target tissues in therapeutic concentrations and are also associated with toxic effects on healthy organs and tissues. Thus, drug delivery approaches should improve the efficacy, specificity, tolerability, and therapeutic index of antiparasitic agents [12]. However, despite advances in the efficacy of existing drugs, the toxic potential of these substances must be considered. Thus, the search for new strategies and/or alternative therapeutic agents is crucial.

3. Natural products and drug delivery systems against leishmaniasis: state-of-the-art

The use of tools and materials at the nanoscale enabled the creation of nanoparticulate formulations such as liposomes, microemulsions, and microcapsules of great interest to the pharmaceutical industry. Drug delivery systems using liposomes are the ones most studied because of their high biocompatibility, ease of preparation, and chemical versatility [22]. Basically, liposomes are microscopic vesicles composed of one or more concentric lipid bilayers separated by aqueous media. Liposomes can encapsulate hydrophilic and lipophilic substances; the former stay in the aqueous compartment, whereas the latter are inserted into the membrane. Because liposomes are biodegradable, biocompatible, and non-immunogenic, they are highly versatile for research, therapeutic, and analytical applications [23]. These vesicles are primarily consisted of phospholipids (either synthetic or natural), sterols, and antioxidants [24]. Lipids with a cylindrical shape such as phosphatidylcholine, phosphatidylserine, phosphatidylglycerol, and sphingomyelin, which tend to form a stable bilayer in aqueous solution, are commonly used in liposomal formulations. Phosphatidylcholine is the most employed lipid in liposomal formulation studies due to its great stability against pH or salt concentration variations in the medium [25]. The pharmacokinetic properties of liposomes can be simply modified by changing the chemical composition of the bilayer components. Moreover, peptides, polysaccharides, or affinity ligands such as antibodies can be incorporated into liposomes [12].

Phospholipid-based liposomes are usually used to change the pharmacokinetics profile of several drugs, either natural or synthetic ones. Natural products such as crude extracts, fractions, or isolated phytocompounds have been incorporated into different colloidal carriers, including liposomes, with promising results. As expected in the incorporation of synthetic drugs, lipid formulations enhance the solubility and bioavailability of extracts and bioactive compounds derived from plants. Additional benefits of phytoformulations include: (i) protection from toxicity; (ii) enhanced pharmacological activity; (iii) enhanced stability; (iv) increased retention time; and (v) protection from physical and chemical degradation [26,22]. The ability of colloidal carriers to improve tissue macrophages distribution may have an impact on *Leishmania* infection. The tendency of nanoformulations, especially liposomes, to be captured by the mononuclear phagocyte system may be an additional advantage in the treatment of leishmaniasis. In fact, intraperitoneal and intravenous administration of liposomes proved to be a good biodistribution system for drugs in the treatment of VL, because it increased drug accumulation in macrophage-rich tissues such as liver and spleen, thus reducing the toxicity level to other tissues and organs [27].

Since ancient times, products from plant, mineral, and animal sources have been used in traditional medicine to fight many human diseases. In fact, for centuries traditional medicine has been the only health care system available for the prevention and treatment of several diseases in different cultures. Currently, the practice of traditional medicine still has a great impact on the health of people who have no access to modern health care practices. In fact, an estimated 80% of people living in developing countries rely almost completely on traditional medicinal practices to meet their primary medication needs [28-30]. Thus, the use of natural products as medicines has attracted the interest of research laboratories around the world

http://dx.doi.org/10.5772/57388

seeking new bioactive molecules. Among the most studied natural products, plants are a valuable source of compounds with antileishmanial activity. Active compounds derived from plant extracts have been described by several laboratories worldwide [31-34]. The antileishmanial activity of several crude extracts and fractions derived from plants has been attributed to compounds belonging to diverse chemical groups, including phenolic compounds (e.g., chalcones, flavonols, aurones, lignans, coumarins, quinines, tannins), terpenoids (monoterpenes, sesquiterpenes, diterpenoids, triterpenes), and alkaloids (indole alkaloids, isoquinoline alkaloids, quinoline alkaloids) [35-37]. In fact, phytoscience may be an important tool in the search for novel antileishmanial agents with fewer side effects and lower potential costs. Secondary metabolites isolated from plant extracts or essential oils can be used in several different ways for the development of drugs. Nanoformulation-based delivery systems are a promising approach to developing novel antileishmanial agents.

Species	Family	Geographical origin (country)	Part used	References
Aesculus hippocastanum	Hipocastanaceae	not cited	Seeds	[40]
Andrographis paniculata	Acanthaceae	(India)	Leaves	[41, 42]
Bacopa monniera	Scrophulariaceae (Plantaginaceae)	(India)	Leaves	[43, 44]
Camptotheca acuminata	Cornaceae	(China)	bark, stem	[45]
Curcuma longa	Zingiberaceae	(India)	rhizome	[46]
Fagopyrum esculentum	Polygonaceae	(India)	not cited	[39, 47]
Mimusops elangii	Sapotaceae	(India)	Seeds	[48]
Peganum harmala	Nitrariaceae	(India)	Seeds	[49, 50]
Piper aduncum	Piperaceae	(Brazil)	inflorescence	[51]
Piper nigrum	Piperaceae	(India)	Seeds	[52, 53]
Swertia chirata	Gentianaceae	Himalayan region (India)	aerial part	[54, 55]
Taxus baccata	Taxaceae	Peloponnese region (Greece)	needles, branches	[56]
Terminalia bellerica	Combretaceae	—	stem bark	[57]
Zanthoxylum chiloperone	Rutaceae	Cordillera (Paraguay)	stem bark	[58, 59]

Table 1. Natural sources of active substances used in nanoformulations against *Leishmania*.

Table 1 lists the natural sources used in nanoformulations to improve the bioavailability of antileishmanial drugs, thus increasing their expected therapeutic efficacy. However, the botanical species used for isolation of the active constituent have not been described in some formulations such as those containing asiaticoside and acaciaside [38], whereas others have a plant origin but were purchased commercially [39]. It should be noted that the most studied species listed in Table 1 are native to developing countries, where the popular use of medicinal plants is widespread.

4. Phytocompound nanoformulations and antileishmanial activity

In the last decades, advances in nanoscience have enabled the development of nano-range materials approved for therapeutic use or in clinical development stage. In fact, many encapsulation matrices have been approved by the Food and Drug Administration (FDA) for use in humans, i.e., a wide range of naturally or chemically modified cyclodextrins that are extensively used in medicine and food fields [60, 61]. Similarly, vesicular systems such as liposomes, niosomes, nanoparticles, and microspheres are very useful and have many advantages in delivering drugs of natural origin, representing a promising approach for the treatment of several diseases, including leishmaniasis. Nanoformulations prepared with compounds from medicinal plants and their antileishmanial activity are summarized in Table 2. Liposomes, niosomes, and nanoparticles are the main formulations investigated.

Saponins (liposomes) and alkaloids (nanoparticles) are among the main plant constituents used to prepare nanoformulations. Liposomes are mainly formed by a mixture of phosphatidyl choline (PC), cholesterol (Chol), and phosphatidic acid (PA), usually in a 7:4:1 molar ratio [55, 38], whereas nanoparticle formulations have polylactide (PLA) as their main ingredient, providing greater stability, biocompatibility, and an efficient delivery system compared to liposomal structures [50, 57]. The antileishmanial properties of each nanoformulation are briefly cited below.

Flavonoids are among the most common phenolic compounds found in the human diet and a variety of members of this family has been described as bioactive agents. Significant antiprotozoal activity of flavonoids has been reported against *Trypanosoma* and *Leishmania* species. Quercetin (Fig. 1) is a widely studied food-derived flavonoid with several biological effects, including antioxidant, antihypertensive, anti-inflammatory, and antiprotozoal activities. Quercetin inhibits parasite arginase activity [62,63] and induces the production of superoxide anion, hydrogen peroxide, and other reactive oxygen species (ROS) by infected cells. Thus, ROS generation induced by quercetin could be crucial for maximal antiparasitic activity, because ROS are naturally generated by macrophages as a mechanism to kill intracellular parasites such as *Leishmania* [64, 65]. In fact, liposomal, niosomal, microspherulated, and nanocapsulated quercetin formulations have been tested to evaluate the best drug delivery system. In hamster models of *L. donovani* infection, all quercetin vesicular formulations reduced the parasite load compared to the free form of the drug. Nanocapsulated quercetin is more effective than non-capsulated quercetin in the control of leishmaniasis (87% reduction in spleen parasite burden) and its pronounced activity may be related to vesicular composition and size. Moreover, drug efficacy may be inversely correlated to the size of vesicular forms [39].

http://dx.doi.org/10.5772/57388

Similarly, the incorporation of terpenoids into nanoparticle carriers has also shown promising results. The search for active molecules to treat leishmaniasis is very laborious, because most molecules have low solubility. The incorporation of andrographolide (Fig. 2), a diterpenoid extracted from the herbaceous species *Andrographis paniculata* (Acanthaceae), with different poly (d,l-lactide-co-glycolide) (PLGA) nanoformulations enhanced the antileishmanial activity of andrographolide against axenic and intracellular amastigote forms of *L. donovani*. Among the formulations tested, the 175 nm andrographolide-loaded nanoparticles exhibited the best antileishmanial activity (IC_{50} = 36 and 28μM for axenic and intracellular amastigotes, respectively) [66]. *Andrographis paniculata* can be considered an interesting source of antileishmanial agents. While 14-deoxy-11-oxoandrographolide (Fig. 2), an andrographolide-derived diterpenoid, reduced spleen parasite load in hamster models of *L. donovani* infection in 39%, liposomal, niosomal, and microspherulated formulations of this substance suppressed spleen parasite load by 78, 91, and 59%, respectively. In addition, the toxicity of 14-deoxy-11-oxoandrographolide to hepatic tissue also decreased after incorporation of 14-deoxy-11-oxoandrographolide into colloidal carriers, as demonstrated by the normal levels of serum alkaline phosphatase (ALP) and serum glutamate pyruvate transaminase (SGPT) in the blood [67]. Interestingly, particle size also proved to be an important factor for drug delivery efficacy. In fact, nanoparticles in a size range below 200 nm have been associated with increased phagocytosis by *Leishmania*-infected macrophages [68].

Formulations	**Active ingredients**	**Administration Route**	**Target and Parasite reduction**	**% Entrapment efficiency**	**References**
Liposomes Niosomes	Amarogentin	SC	*L. donovani* (LP 69% and NS 90%)	33 24	[55]
Mannose-coated Liposomes Liposomes	Piperine	SC	*L. donovani* (ML 90%; LP 77%)	22	[52]
Nanoparticles	2′,6′-dihydroxy-4′-methoxychalcone	IP	*L. amazonensis* (53%)	92	[51]
Liposomes	camptothecin	IP	*L. donovani* (55%)	2.7	[45]
Liposomes Niosomes Micropspheres Nanoparticles	Quercetin	SC	*L. donovani* (LP 51%; NS 68%; MS 44%; NP 87%)	40 50 09 -	[39]
Liposomes Niosomes Nanoparticles Microspheres	bacopasaponin C	SC	*L. donovani* (LP 81%; NS 86%; NP 79%; MS 91%)	30 30 30 50	[44]
Liposomes Niosomes Micropspheres	14-deoxi-11-oxoandrographolide	SC	*L. donovani* (LP 78%; NS 91%; MS 59%)	10 1 10	[42]
Liposomes	Harmine	SC	*L. donovani*	65	[50]

Formulations	Active ingredients	Administration Route	Target and Parasite reduction	% Entrapment efficiency	References
Niosomes Nanoparticles			(LP 60%; NI 70%; NP 80%)	60 20	
Lipid nanospheres	Piperine	IV	*L. donovani* (52-90%)	100	[53]
Liposomes	asiaticoside	nr	*L. donovani* (LP 62%)	Nd	[38]
Liposomes	acaciaside	nr	*L. donovani* (LP 92%)	Nd	
Microemulsion Nanoparticles	bassic acid	SC	*L. donovani* (ME 62%; NP 78%)	100 50	[48]
Nanogels Nanoparticles	arjunglucoside I	SC	*L. donovani* (NG 79%; NP75%)	80 60	[57]
Nanoparticles	andrographolide	*in vitro* assay	*L. donovani* Axenic amastigotes (IC_{50} = 36 ± 4 μM/mL) Amastigotes in macrophage (IC_{50} = 28 ± 2 μM/mL)	80	[66]
Nanoparticles	β-aescin	*in vitro* assay	*L. infantum* Amastigotes (IC_{50} = 1.04 ± 0.23ug/ml)	2.8 – 31.9	[40]
Gold nanoparticles	quercetin	*in vitro* assay	*L. donovani* Axenic amastigotes (IC_{50} = 15 ± 3 μM/ml) Amastigotes in macrophage (IC_{50} 10 ± 2 μM/ml)	77	[69]

LP: liposomes; NS: niosomes; ML: manose-coated liposomes; NP: nanoparticles; MS: microspheres; ME: microemulsions; NG: nanogels.

SC: subcutaneous; IP: intraperitoneal; IV: intravenous.

nr: not reported; nd: not determined.

Table 2. Phytocompound nanoformulations and antileishmanial activity.

Triterpenoidic or steroidal saponins directly reduce cell viability via membrane disruption. The mode of action of saponins is related to its aglycone portion, which binds to membrane sterols, leading to the formation of transmembrane pores and loss of intracellular content. This feature of saponins demonstrates the toxic potential of these molecules, hampering their use as antileishmanial agents. Conversely, polymeric nanoparticles composed of PLGA were successfully used to improve the efficacy of β-aescin (Fig. 2), the main saponin isolated from the seeds of horse-chestnut *Aesculus hippocastanumi* (Sapindaceae), lowering its cytotoxic effect for mammalian cells [40]. Bacopasaponin-C (Fig. 2) was firstly reported as an antileishmanial

http://dx.doi.org/10.5772/57388

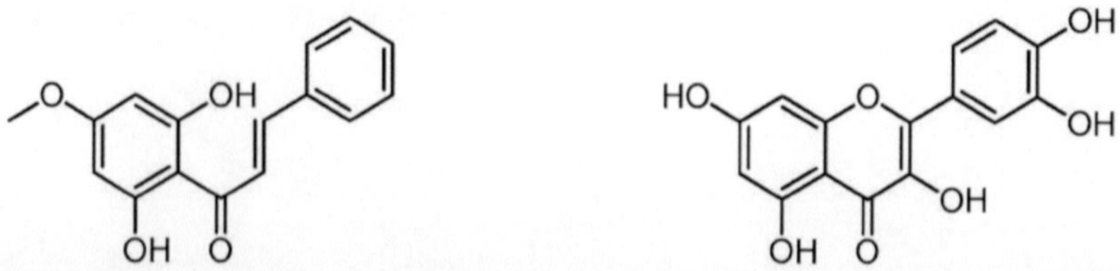

2′,6′-dihidroxy-4′-methoxychalcone **Quercetin**

Figure 1. Structure of phenolic compounds loaded in nanoformulations.

agent in 2002, but its mechanism of action remains unclear. This glycoside extracted from *Bacopa monnieri* (Plantaginaceae) has glucose and rhamnose residues attached to the triterpenoid aglycone moiety. The glucose residue may be responsible for targeting bacopasaponin-C to glucose receptors on the cellular surface. Incorporation of bacopasaponin-C into various delivery carriers (niosomes, microspheres, nanoparticles, and liposomes) improved its antileishmanial activity. After six-day treatment with subcutaneous injections of liposomal, niosomal, microencapsulated, or nanocapsulated formulations of bacopasaponin-C, hamster models of *L. donovani* infection showed a significant reduction in spleen parasite burden (81, 86, 79, and 91%, respectively) compared to free drug-treated animals (40%). At the same dose (1.7 mg/kg), the smallest vesicles had the best efficacy, as follows: nanocapsules > niosomes > liposomes > microspheres [44]. Another glycoside with remarkable activity against *Leishmania* parasites has been isolated from the indigenous plant *Swertia chirata* (Gentianaceae): amarogentin (Fig. 2) is a secoiridoid glycoside with the capacity to inhibit DNA-topoisomerase I, an essential enzyme related to *Leishmania* viability. Liposomal and niosomal formulations of amarogentin (2.5 mg/kg) reduced spleen parasite load by 69 and 90%, respectively, whereas free drug at equivalent dose reduced parasite load by 39%. In addition, both SPTG and ALP activity remained close to normal levels when liposomal or niosomal formulations of this iridoid were used in murine models [55].

The amide alkaloid piperine (Fig. 3) extracted from *Piper nigrum* (Piperaceae), an Indian species commonly used in traditional medicine, has been reported as a potent antileishmanial acting against both visceral (*L. donovani*) and tegumentary (*L. amazonensis*) leishmaniasis [70, 71]. *In vivo* tests have shown that piperine entrapped into liposomes and mannose-coated liposomes were effective against murine models of *L. donovani* infection. After 12-day treatment with liposomal and mannose-coated liposomal formulations of this alkaloid (four doses, 6 mg/mL) administered subcutaneously, a reduction in parasite burden of approximately 77 and 90%, respectively was achieved. Free piperine not only was less effective in reducing parasite burden (29%)but also had higher toxicity to liver compared to the colloidal carriers (ALP = 20.5 μmol of *p*-nitrophenol released/min/dL of sera and SGPT = 77.2 μmol of sodium pyruvate/min/L of sera) [52]. Nevertheless, better results can be achieved by using lipid nanospheres of piperine (LN-P). A single dose (5 mg/kg) of the lipid formulation composed of stearylamine (LN-P-SA) reduced parasite burden in liver and spleen of *L. donovani*-infected hamsters by 90% and 85% after 15 days post infection, respectively. Despite the size of the vesicles (about 884.6 nm), the efficacy of LN-P-SA may be related to the preferential uptake of stearylamine-bearing

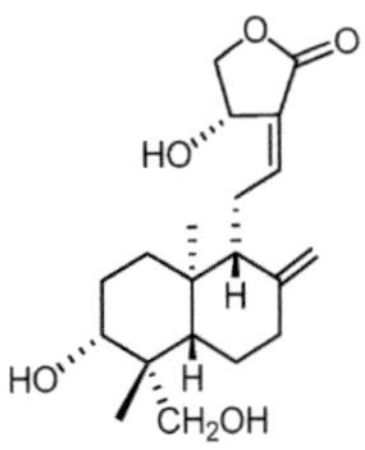

Andrographolide

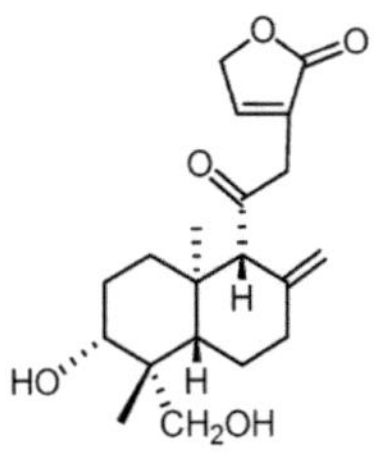

14-deoxy-11-oxoandrographolide

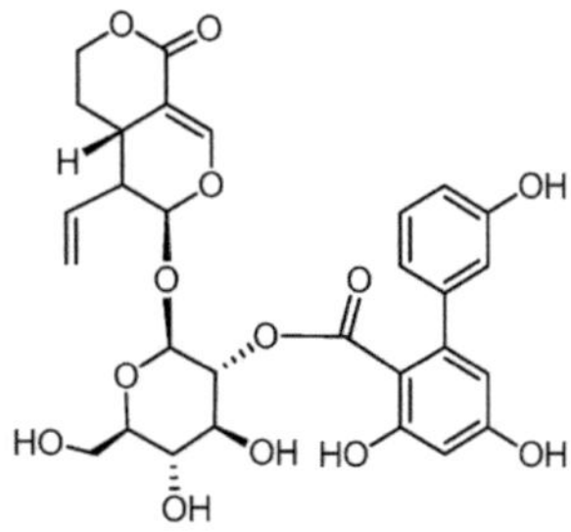

Amarogentin

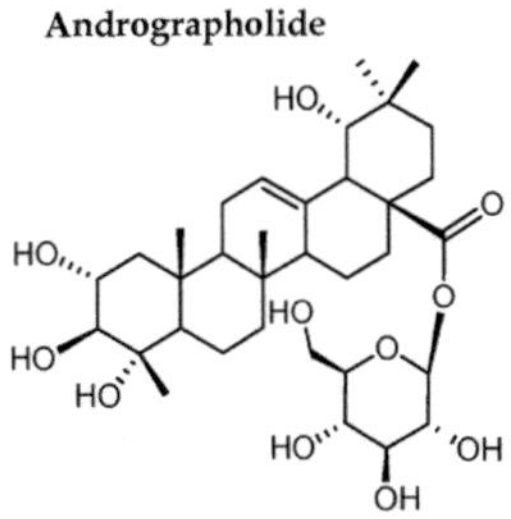

Arjunglucoside I

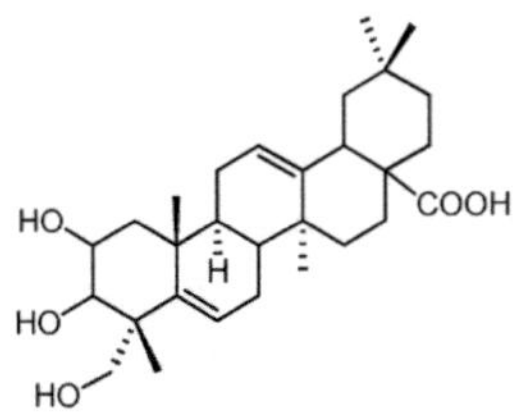

Bassic acid

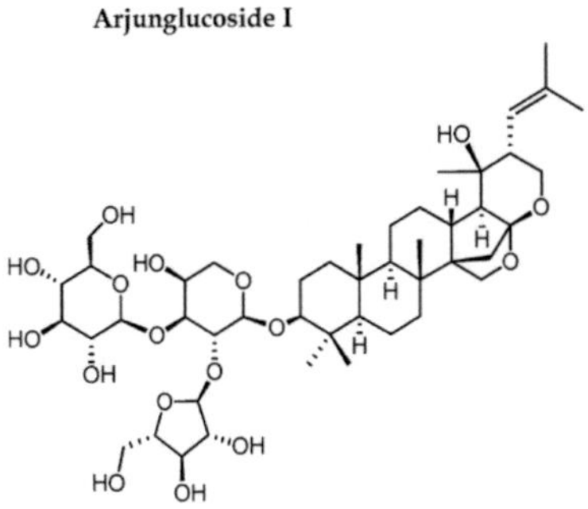

Bacopasaponin-C

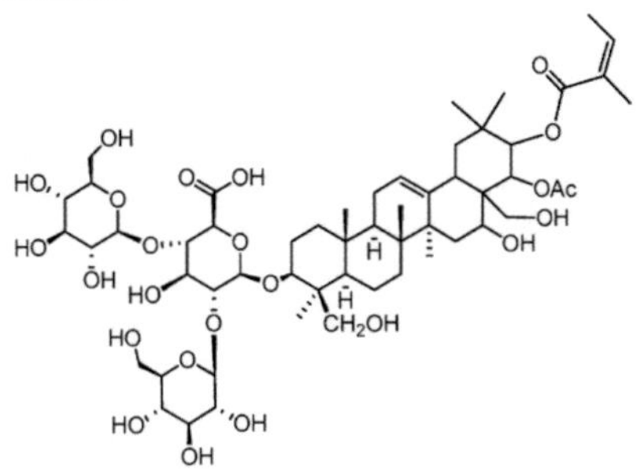

β-aescin

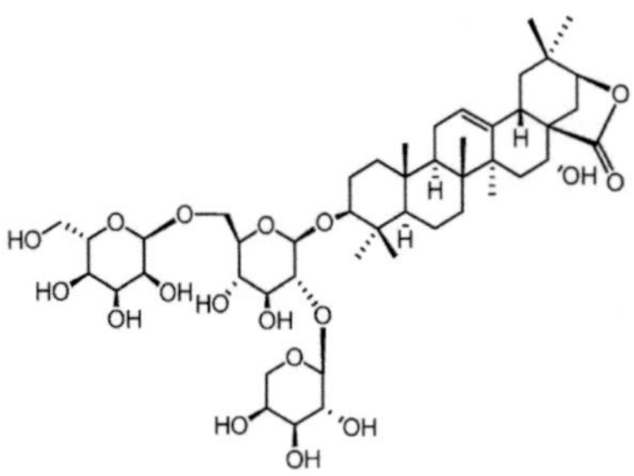

Acaciaside

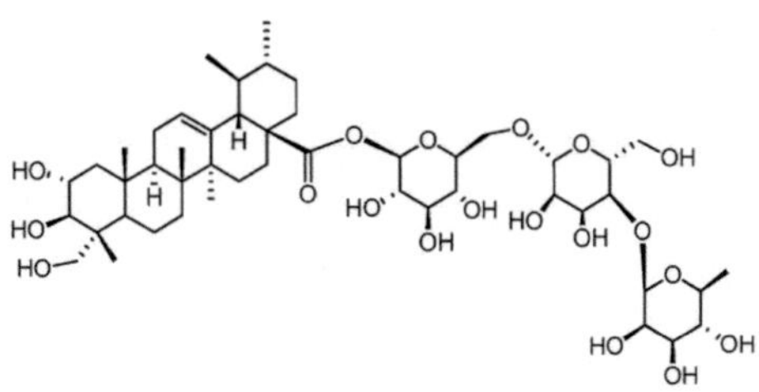

Asiaticoside

Figure 2. Structure of terpenoids loaded in nanoformulations.

positively charged liposomes (+ 24.2 mV) by peritoneal macrophages compared to neutral and negatively charged vesicles [53].

β-carboline alkaloids such as harmane, harmaline, and harmine were initially described as potent psychoactive and hallucinogenic agents. However, a wide range of pharmacological activities have been reported for those compounds, including those against *Leishmania* parasites [72]. Harmine (Fig. 3), isolated from *Peganum harmala* (Nitrariaceae), displays *in vitro* anti-*L. donovani* promastigote activity at 25 μg/mL. Recently, this alkaloid was incorporated into liposomes, niosomes, and nanoparticles at an equivalent dose of 1.5 mg/kg body weight, and after six doses administered subcutaneously to *L. donovani*-infected murine models, all harmine-entrapped vesicular formulations were able to reduce spleen parasite burden, especially nanosomes (a reduction of about 79%). Nevertheless, the mechanism of action of harmine against *Leishmania* remains unclear and may be related to necrotic membrane damage.

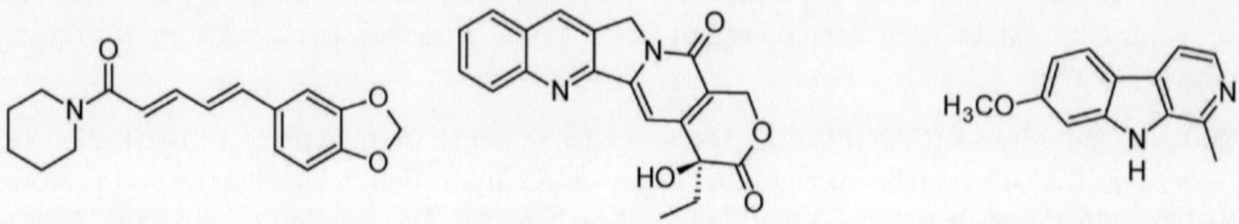

Piperine **Camptothecin** **Harmine**

Figure 3. Structure of alkaloids loaded in nanoformulations.

The search for new compounds with antileishmanial activity in medicinal plants is an interesting strategy, however most studies are still limited to basic research and probably only a few compounds will reach stages of clinical trials and development of new drugs. The combination of phytochemistry and nanoformulations may open up new perspectives in the search for new antileishmanial drugs, because drug delivery systems based on nanoformulations can improve the effectiveness of natural compounds making them more attractive to the development of new therapeutic targets. Due to their structural versatility in terms of size, composition, and ability to incorporate hydrophilic or lipophilic substances, there are many possible applications of nanoparticulate formulations in the treatment and control of leishmaniasis.

5. Parasite targets for new drugs

Parasite resistance, cost, side effects, toxicity, and other therapy issues prompt an urgent need to identify and develop new drugs and alternative targets for leishmaniasis treatment [73, 74, 10]. Metabolic pathways such as glycolytic pathway [75, 76], polyamine biosynthesis [77, 78], glyoxalase pathway [79, 80], uptake and turnover of phospholipids/sphingolipids [81, 82], microtubule biosynthesis [83, 84], and folate metabolism [85] have been targeted.

The development of drugs directed at new targets such as parasite enzymes represents another approach in the search for new antileishmanial drugs. Arginase is a recently described target for the treatment of leishmaniasis. The enzyme is localized in the glycosome, a subcellular organelle found in some trpypanosomatids such as *Leishmania*. Inhibition of the arginase pathway causes inhibits the polyamine biosynthetic pathway, resulting in antileishmanial activity [86].

Other enzyme systems investigated as potential targets for antileishmanial drug action include nitric oxide synthase, DNA topoisomerase, trypanothione redutase, superoxide dismutase enzymes, and hypoxanthine-guanine phosphoribosyltransferase [74]; heme oxygenase-1 [87]; ribose 5-phosphate isomerase B [88]; dihydroorotate dehydrogenase [89]; ornitine decarboxylases [62]; Abl family kinases and phosphoinositide 3-kinase γ [90-93]; and spermidine synthase [94, 95].

A total of 154 peptidases were detected in the *Leishmania major* genome, including serine, cysteine, aspartic, threonine, and metallopeptidases. The cysteine peptidase-specific inhibitor K11777 has shown that these peptidases are necessary for parasite growth [96]. Even though some inhibitors have been developed but failed to kill parasites, peptidases are promising targets [97-99].

Carbonic anhydrases (CAs, EC 4.2.1.1) are a new target that are starting to be studied for *Leishmania*. CAs are metalloenzymes that catalyze CO_2 hydration to bicarbonate and protons, and five CA classes have been identified: α, β, γ, δ, and ζ. The reaction catalyzed by CAs is essential in the regulation of acid-base balance in organisms [100, 101]. A β-carbonic anhydrase was recently cloned and characterized from *Leishmania donovani chagasi*, and enzyme-specific inhibitors were tested against *Leishmania* [102].

The death of the parasite by inhibiting an enzyme or pathway essential for parasite survival and non-essential for the host requires the exploration of differences between these pathways or enzymes [103]. Thus, new *Leishmania* molecules should be studied and the possibility of developing rational and more effective drugs with less harmful side effects for the host investigated. Finally, new *Leishmania* chemotherapeutic targets and new approaches to the development of drugs should be considered [104, 93, 105].

6. Synthetic drugs

No vaccine candidates for leishmaniasis are currently under animal or clinical trials. Thus, new and effectives drugs should be investigated. In the last years, several drugs have been studied to find potential new drugs with desirable characteristics. Leishmaniasis is expanding in developed countries and in North America and Europe, which has alarmed health authorities worldwide [106]. Although leishmaniasis is treatable, it is difficult to control due to the absence of an effective vaccine, the adaptation of the vector and reservoir hosts to human environments, and the emergence of resistant lineages [107]. The first-line chemotherapy drugs available are pentavalent antimonials [108], whereas pentamidine and amphotericin B are second-line therapies, but these are associated with limited effectiveness, a long-term treatment, toxicity,

http://dx.doi.org/10.5772/57388

and significant side effects [109]. Consequently, there is an urgent need to discover new drugs that are effective against leishmaniasis [110].

Some compounds have been studied and regarded as promising new drugs. The stilbene trans-3,4',5-trimethoxy-3'-amino-stilbene (TTAS) showed a LD_{50} of 2.6 lg/mL against *Leishmania infantum* with low toxicity. The action mechanism is the disruption of the mitochondrial membrane potential and the ability to block *Leishmania* parasites during the G2/M phase of cell cycle [111].

N-butyl-1-(4-dimethylamino)phenyl-1,2,3,4-tetrahydro-β-carboline-3-carboxamide has been tested against *Leishmania amazonensis* and ultrastructural alterations, depolarization of the mitochondrial membrane with loss of cell membrane integrity, and increased formation of mitochondrial superoxide anions were detected, indicating that this compound induced mitochondrial dysfunction [111].

Besides the lack of an effective vaccine against leishmaniasis, in some East African regions, up to 40% of patients with visceral leishmaniasis are co-infected with HIV, which complicates the treatment. Peptidase inhibitors, used to treat HIV-infected individuals are a new route that needs more studies. HIV-1 protease inhibitors such as Indinavir, Saquinavir, and others have been tested to treat leishmaniasis and inhibition of parasite growth has been reported at high drugs concentrations [9].

Other synthetic antileishmanial compounds are currently being developed an evaluated for therapeutic use. β-carbolines from various natural and synthetic sources have shown diverse biological activities. A total of 22 compounds were synthesized and tested *in vitro* against *Leishmania donovani*, out of which six compounds (4, 5, 10, 11, 19, and 22) showed more activity than the standard miltefosine (IC_{50} = 12.07 ± 0.82 lM), with compound 4 being the most potent (IC_{50} = 2.16 ± 0.26 lM) [112]. Moreover, a semi-synthetic berberine analogue, 5,6-didehydro-8,8-diethyl-13-oxodihydroberberine chloride showed nanomolar level potency against *in vitro* models of leishmaniasis, malaria, and trypanosomiasis, as well as activity in an *in vivo* visceral leishmaniasis model [113]. Tamoxifen is a synthetic estrogen that has been successfully used to prevent recurrence of breast cancer in women who are estrogen-receptor positive. Miguel *et al.* (2008) [114] reported the leishmanicidal activity of tamoxifen *in vitro* using BALB/c mice infected with *L. amazonensis* and treated with this compound for 15 days.

Diospyrin, a bis-naphthoquinone isolate from the tree *Diospyros montana* and its semi-syntheitic derivatives showed inhibitory activity against *Leishmania* spp. The di-epoxide derivative of diospyrin (D17) was more effective against *L. donovani* promastigotes than diospyrin. The same derivative tested in *L.donovani* BHU1216 selectively inhibited intracellular amastigotes. Computational docking studies demonstrated that D17 could inhibit *L donovani* ornithine decarboxylase but not trypanothione reductase [115].

Therapeutic approaches using drugs that act on structures of vital importance to the parasite but absent or sufficiently different in their hosts have been explored by several research groups. Indotecan and AM13-55, are TopIB poisons with indenoisoquinoline structure. Both compounds were tested against *L infantum* and the results compared with paromomycin, a leishmanicidal drug. The tests were done on a murine BALB/c model of splenocytes infected with *L. infantum*. The results showed that Indotecam reduced more than 80% of the parasite burden of the spleen and liver, indicating that this compound is a potential drug against visceral leishmaniasis [116].

TiO2@Ag nanoparticles (TiAg-Nps) produce reactive oxygen species (ROS), which have an antimicrobial effect, including antileishmanial effects on *Leishmania tropica* and *Leishmania infantum* promastigotes and amastigotes, mainly non-visible light-exposed TiAg-Nps [117]. Twenty-four porphyrin precursors and derivatives were evaluated against *Trypanosoma brucei, L. donovani,* and *Plasmodium* sp. The perforine 4i derivative showed the best activity against *T. brucei* with a MEC value of 6.25 mM, but the compound was not active against intramacrophage amastigotes of *L. donovani* [118].

Another approach used in studies is the combination of drug therapies aimed at finding the most effective and secure one. Pam3Cys (an in-built immunoadjuvant and TLR2 ligand) and miltefosine were combined and the resulting combination was evaluated. All experiments were done in BALB/c mouse. Parasitic inhibition significantly increased in groups treated with combinations of the drugs compared to groups receiving miltefosine and Pam3Cys separately. Moreover, increased production of Th1 cytokines, RNS, ROS, and H_2O_2, as well as increased phagocytosis were observed during the study of immunological alterations [119].

Several aromatic/heterocyclic sulfonamides and 5-mercapto-1,3,4-thiadiazoles were recently investigated against *L. donovani* CAs. The sulfonamides were medium potency-weak inhibitors, but some heterocyclic thiols inhibited the enzyme with KIs in the range of 13.4–52 nM. Microscopic studies revealed cell swelling and structural alterations on the flagellar pocket such as presence of vacuoles. Autophagic vacuoles that cause intracellular damages and parasite death, and accumulation of intracytoplasmic electron-dense granules were also induced by the inhibitors. These result suggest that β-CA from *Leishmania* is a potential new antileishmanial drug target [102].

7. Conclusions

Leishmaniasis is a neglected, potentially lethal infectious disease caused by parasites in the genus *Leishmania* that affects many developing countries. Infection can lead to tegumentary or visceral manifestations of the disease. The tegumentary form of leishmaniasis (TL) includes cutaneous, mucocutaneous, and diffuse clinical manifestations, whereas visceral leishmaniasis (VL), or Kala-azar, affects organs and internal tissues. The treatment of VL is challenging and long. Treated patients need monitoring and hospitalization. Therapeutic problems include toxicity and teratogenicity of the available drugs, and low response in human immunodeficiency virus (HIV)/*Leishmania* co-infections. In addition, drug resistance is increasing. Moreover, leishmaniasis received little attention from governments and the pharmaceutical industry until the last decade. The absence of either prophylactic or preventive vaccine candidates makes it further difficult to control the disease.

The development of new parasite targets and synthetic drugs along with the research on natural products represents a major strategy for the discovery of new compounds against Leishmania sp.

http://dx.doi.org/10.5772/57388

Acknowledgements

This study was supported by grants from Coordenação de Aperfeiçoamento Pessoal de Nível Superior (CAPES), Conselho Nacional de Desenvolvimento Científico e Tecnológico (MCT/CNPq), Fundação Carlos Chagas Filho de Amparo à Pesquisa do Estado do Rio de Janeiro (FAPERJ), and Fundação Oswaldo Cruz (FIOCRUZ). The authors are grateful to Iêda Coleto Miguel de Castro and Silvia Rocha de Souza for technical support.

Author details

Alane Beatriz Vermelho[1*], Claudiu T. Supuran[2,3], Verônica Cardoso[1], Dayanne Menezes[1], Jefferson Rocha de Andrade Silva[4], Jose Luiz Pinto Ferreira[5], Ana Claudia Fernandes Amaral[5] and Igor A. Rodrigues[1,6]

*Address all correspondence to: abvermelho@micro.ufrj.br

1 Biotecnologia – Bioinovar, Instituto de Microbiologia Paulo de Góes, Universidade Federal do Rio de Janeiro, Cidade Universitária, Rio de Janeiro, Brasil

2 Istituto di Biochimica delle Proteine, CNR, Napoli, Italy

3 Università degli Studi di Firenze, NEUROFARBA Dept., Sezione di Scienze Farmaceutiche, Florence, Italy

4 Universidade Federal do Amazonas, Instituto de Ciências Exatas, Departamento de Química, Manaus-AM, Brasil

5 Laboratório de Plantas Medicinais e Derivados, Farmanguinhos, FIOCRUZ, Rio de Janeiro, Brasil

6 Faculdade de Farmácia, Departamento de Produtos Naturais e Alimentos (DPNA), Universidade Federal do Rio de Janeiro, Universitária, Rio de Janeiro, Brasil

References

[1] Centers for Disease Control and Prevention (2013). http://www.cdc.gov/parasites/leishmaniasis/ (accessed 20 august 2013).

[2] David CV., Craft, N. Cutaneous and mucocutaneous leishmaniasis. Dermatology Therapy 2009; 22(6) 491-502.

[3] Toledo JS., Junior PES., Manfrim V., Pinzan CF., Araújo AS., Cruz AK., Emery FS. Synthesis, Cytotoxicity and In Vitro Antileishmanial Activity of Naphthothiazoles. Chemical Biology & Drug Design, 2013; 81(6) 749–756.

[4] Piscopo TV., Mallia AC. Leishmaniasis. Postgraduate Medical Journal 2007; 83(976) 649-657.

[5] Aguilar-Be I., Zardo RS., Souza EP., Borja-Cabrera GP., Rosado-Vallado M., Mut-Martin M., García-Miss MR., Sousa CBP., Dumonteil E. Cross-Protective Efficacy of a Prophylactic *Leishmania donovani* DNA Vaccine against Visceral and Cutaneous Murine Leishmaniasis. Infection and Immunity 2005; 73(2) 812–819.

[6] Croft SL., Sundar S., Fairlamb, AH. Drug Resistance in Leishmaniasis. Clinical Microbiology Reviews 2006; 19(1) 111- 126.

[7] World Health Organization. First WHO report on neglected tropical diseases (2010). http://whqlibdoc.who.int/publications/2010/9789241564090_eng.pdf.

[8] Cruz I., Nieto J., Moreno J., Canavate C., Desjeux P., Alvar J. Leishmania/ HIV co-infections in the second decade. Indian Journal Med. Res. 2006; 123(3) 357–388.

[9] Colomba C., Saporito L., Vitale F., Reale S., Vitale G., Casuccio A., Tolomeo M., Maranto D., Rubino R., Di Carlo P., Titone L.. Cryptic *Leishmania infantum* infection in Italian HIV infected patients. BMC Infectious Diseases 2009; 9(199). http://www.biomedcentral.com/1471-2334/9/199

[10] Griensven J., Diro E., Lopez-Velez R., Boelaert M., Zijlstra LLE., Dujardin JC., Hailu A. HIV-1 protease inhibitors for treatment of visceral leishmaniasis in HIV-co-infected individuals. The Lancet Infectious Diseases 2013; 13(3), 251-259.

[11] Ehrenberg JP., Ault, SK. Neglected diseases of neglected populations: thinking to reshape the determinants of health in Latin America and the Caribbean. BMC Public Health 2005; 5 119. http://www.biomedcentral.com/1471-2458/5/119

[12] Date AA., Joshi MD., Patravale VB. Parasitic diseases: Liposomes and polymeric nanoparticles versus lipid nanoparticles. Advanced drug delivery reviews 2007; 59(6) 505-521.

[13] Croft SI., Yardley V. Chemotherapy of leishmaniasis. Current Pharmaceutical Design 2002; 8(4), 319-342.

[14] Akendengue B., Ngou-Milama E., Laurens A., Hocquemiller R. Recent Advances in the fight against leishmaniasis with natural products. Parasite 1999; 6(1) 3-8.

[15] Chatelain E., Loset JR. Drug discovery and development for neglected diseases: the DNDi model. Drug Design Development and Therapy 2011; 16(5) 175-181.

[16] Griensven J., Diro E. Visceral leishmaniasis. Infectious Disease Clinics of North America 2012; 26(2) 309-322.

[17] Barrett M., Croft S. Management of trypanosomiasis and leishmaniasis. British Medical Bulletin 2012; 104 (1) 175–196. http://www.ncbi.nlm.nih.gov/pmc/articles/PMC3530408/

[18] Borborema SE., Schwendener RA., Osso JA., Andrade HF., Nascimento N. Uptake and antileishmanial activity of meglumine antimoniate-containing liposomes in Leishmania (Leishmania) major-infected macrophages. International Journal of Antimicrobial Agents 2011; 38(4) 341-347.

[19] Tempone AG., Mortara RA., Andrade HF., Reimão JQ. Therapeutic evaluation of free and liposome-loaded furazolidone in experimental visceral leishmaniasis. International Journal of Antimicrobial Agents 2010; 36(2) 159-163.

[20] Jaafari, M. R.; Bavarsad, N.; Bazzaz, B. S.; Samiei, A.; Soroush, D.; Ghorbani, S.; Heravi, M. M. & Khamesipour, A. Effect of topical liposomes containing paromomycin sulfate in the course of *Leishmania major* infection in susceptible BALB/c mice. Antimicrobial Agents and Chemotherapy 2009; 53(6) 2259-2265.

[21] Papagiannaros A., Bories C., Demetzos C., Loiseau PM. Antileishmanial and trypanocidal activities of new miltefosine liposomal formulations. Biomedicine & Pharmacotherapy 2005; 59(10) 545-550.

[22] Chen M., Wang S., Tan M., Wang Y. Applications of nanoparticles in herbal medicine: zedoary turmeric oil and its active compound β-elemene. The American Journal of Chinese Medicine 2011; 39(6) 1093-1102.

[23] Edwards KA., Baeumner AJ. Liposomes in analyses. Talanta 2006; 68 (5), 1432-1441.

[24] Vemuri S., Rhodes C T. Preparation and characterization of liposomes as therapeutic delivery systems: a review. Pharmaceutica Acta Helvetica 1995; 70(2) 95-111.

[25] Batista CM., Carvalho CMB., Magalhães NSS. Lipossomas e suas aplicações terapêuticas: Estado da arte. Brazilian Journal of Pharmaceutical Sciences 2007; 43(2) 167-179.

[26] Ajazuddin SS. Applications of novel drug delivery system for herbal formulations. Fitoterapia 2010; 81(7) 680-689.

[27] Harvier P., Désormeaux A., Gagne N., Tremblay M., Poulin L., Beauchamp D. Bergeron MG. Lymphoid tissues targeting of liposome-encapsulated 2',3'-dideoxyinosine. AIDS 1995; 9(7) 701-707.

[28] Esquenazi D., Wigg MD., Miranda MMFS., Rodrigues HM., Tostes JBF., Rozental S., Silva AJR., Alviano CS. Antimicrobial and antiviral activities of polyphenolics from *Cocos nucifera* Linn. (Palmae) husk fiber extract. Research in Microbiology 2002; 153(10) 647-652.

[29] Kim HS. Do not put too much value on conventional medicines. Journal of Ethnopharmacology 2005; 100(1-2) 37–39.

[30] Firenzuoli F., Gori L. Herbal medicine today: clinical and research issues. Evidence-Based Complementary and Alternative Medicine 2007; 4(1) 37–40. http://www.ncbi.nlm.nih.gov/pmc/articles/PMC2206236/

[31] Braga FG., Bouzada ML., Fabri RL., Matos MO., Moreira FO., Scio E., Coimbra ES. Antileishmanial and antifungal activity of plants used in traditional medicine in Brazil. Journal of Ethnopharmacology 2007; 111(2) 396-402.

[32] Bero J., Hannaert V., Chataigné G., Hérent MF., Quetin-Leclercq J. In vitro antitrypanosomal and antileishmanial activity of plants used in Benin in traditional medicine and bio-guided fractionation of the most active extract. Journal of Ethnopharmacology 2011; 137(2), 998-1002.

[33] Al-Musayeib NM., Mothana RA., Matheeussen A., Cos P., Maes L. In vitro antiplasmodial, antileishmanial and antitrypanosomal activities of selected medicinal plants used in the traditional Arabian Peninsular region. BMC Complementary and Alternative Medicine, 2012; 12(49). http://www.biomedcentral.com/content/pdf/1472-6882-12-49.pdf

[34] González-Coloma A., Reina M., Sáenz C., Lacre, R., Ruiz-Mesia L., Arán VJ., Sanz J., Martínez-Díaz RA. Antileishmanial, antitrypanosomal, and cytotoxic screening of ethnopharmacologically selected Peruvian plants. Parasitology Research 2012; 110(4) 1381-1392.

[35] Salem MM., Werbovetz KA. Natural products from plants as drug candidates and lead compounds against leishmaniasis and trypanosomiasis. Current Medicinal Chemistry 2006; 13(21) 2571-2598.

[36] Rodrigues IA., Amaral ACF., Rosa MSS. Trypanosomatid enzymes as targets for plant-derived compounds: new perspectives for phytotherapeutic approaches. Current Enzyme Inhibition 2011; 7(1) 32-41.

[37] Wink M. Medicinal plants: A source of anti-parasitic secondary metabolites. Molecules 2012; 17(11), 12771-12791. http://www.mdpi.com/1420-3049/17/11/12771

[38] Basu MK. Liposomal Delivery of Antileishmanial Agents. Journal of Applied Research 2005; 5 (1) 221-236.

[39] Sarkar S., Mandal S., Sinha J., Mukhopadhyay S., Das N., Basu, MK. Quercetin: Critical Evaluation as an Antileishmanial Agent In Vivo in Hamsters Using Different Vesicular Delivery Modes. Journal of Drug Targeting 2002; 10(8)573–578.

[40] Van de Ven H., Vermeersch M., Matheeeussen A., Vandervoort J., Weyenberg W., Apers S., Cos P., Maes L., Ludwig A. PLGA Nanoparticles Loaded with the Antileishmanial Saponin β-Aescin: Factor Influence Study and In Vitro Efficaçy Evaluation. International Journal of Pharmaceutics 2011; 420(1) 122-132.

[41] Sinha J., Mukhopadhyay S., Das N., Basu M.K. Targeting of Liposomal Andrographolide to *L. donovani* Infected Macrophages in vivo. Drug Delivery 2000; 7(4) 209-213.

[42] Lala S., Nandy AK., Mahato SB., Basu MK. Delivery in vivo of 14-deoxy-11-oxoandrographolide, an antileishmanial agent, by different drug carriers. Indian Journal of Biochemistry and Biophysics 2003; 40(3) 169-174.

[43] Garai S., Mahato SB., Ohtani K., Yamasaki K. Dammarane-Type Triterpenoid Saponins from *Bacopa monniera*. Phytochemistry 1996; 42(3) 815-820.

[44] Sinha J., Raay B., Das N., Medda S., Garai S., Mahato SB., Basu MK. Bacopasaponin C: critical evaluation of anti-leishmanial properties in various delivery modes. Drug Delivery 2002; 9(1) 55-62.

[45] Proulx ME., Désormeaux A., Marquis JF., Olivier M., Bergeron MG. Treatment of Visceral Leishmaniasis with Sterically Stabilized Liposomes Containing Camptothecin. Antimicrobial Agents and Chemotherapy 2001; 45(9): 2623–2627.

[46] Luz PP., Magalhães LG., Pereira AC., Cunha VR., Rodrigues V., Silva MLA. Curcumin-Loaded into PLGA Nanoparticles : preparation and in vitro schistosomicidal activity. Parasitology Research 2012; 110(2) 593-598.

[47] Basu MK., Lala S. Macrophage Specific Drug Delivery in Experimental Leishmaniasis. Current Molecular Medicine 2004; 4(6) 681-689.

[48] Lala S., Gupta S., Sahu NP., Mandal D., Mondal NB., Moulik SP., Basu MK. Critical Evaluation of the Therapeutic Potential of Bassic Acid Incorporated in Oil-in-Water Microemulsions and Poly-D,L-Lactide Nanoparticles Against Experimental Leishmaniasis. Journal of Drug Targeting 2006; 14(4) 171–179.

[49] Mukhopadhyay S., Banerjee SK., Atal CK., Lin LJ., Cordell, GA. Alkaloids of Corydalis govaniana. Journal of Natural Products 1987; 50(2) 270–273.

[50] Lala S., Pramanick S., Mukhopadhyay S., Bandyopadhyay S., Basu M.K. Harmine Evaluation of its Antileishmanial Properties Invarious Vesicular Delivery Systems. Journal of Drug Targeting 2004; 12(3) 165-175.

[51] Torres-Santos EC., Rodrigues JM., Moreira DL., Kaplan MAC., Rossi-Bergmann B. Improvement of In Vitro and In Vivo Antileishmanial Activities of 2′,6′-Dihydroxy-4′-Methoxychalcone by Entrapment in Poly(D,L-Lactide) Nanoparticles. Antimicrobial Agents and Chemotherapy 1999; 43(7) 1776-1778.

[52] Raay B., Medda S., Mukhopadhyay S., Basu MK. Targeting of piperine intercalated in mannose-coated liposomes in experimental leishmaniasis. Indian Journal of Biochemistry and Biophysics 1999; 36(4) 248-251.

[53] Veerareddy PR., Vobalaboina V., Nahid, A. Formulation and Evaluation of Oil-in-Water Emulsions of Piperine in Visceral Leishmaniasis. Pharmazie 2004; 59(3) 194-197.

[54] Ray S., Majumder K., Chakravarty AK., Mukhopadhyay S., Gil RR., Cordell GA. Amarogentin, a Naturally Occurring Secoiridoid Glycoside and a Newly Recognized Inhibitor of Topoisomerase I from *Leishmania donovani*. Journal of Natural Products 1996; 59(1) 27-29.

[55] Medda S., Mukhopadhyay S., Basu MK. Evaluation of the In Vivo Activity and Toxicity of Amarogentin, an Antileishmanial Agent, in Both Liposomal and Niosomal Forms. Journal of Antimicrobial Chemotherapy 1999; 44(6) 791-794.

[56] Georgopoulou K., Smirlis D., Bisti S., Xingi E., Skaltsounis L., Soteriadou K. In Vitro Activity of 10-Deacetylbaccatin III Against Leishmania donovani Promastigotes and Intracellular Amastigotes. Planta Medica 2007; 73(10) 1081-1088.

[57] Tyagi R., Lala S., Verma AK., Nandy AK., Mahato SB., Maitra A., Basu MK. Targeted Delivery of Arjunglucoside I Using Surface Hydrophilic and Hydrophobic Nanocarriers to Combat Experimental Leishmaniasis. Journal of Drug Targeting 2005; 13(3) 161-171.

[58] Ferreira M.E., Arias ASR., Ortiz ST., Inchausti A., Nakayama H., Thouvenel C., Hocquemiller R., Fournet A. Leishmanicidal Activity of Two Canthin-6-one Alkaloids, Two Major Constituents of Zanthoxylum chiloperone var. angustifolium. Journal of Ethnopharmacology 2002; 80(2-3), 199-202.

[59] Arias JL, Cebrián-Torrejón G., Poupon E., Fournet A. Couvreur P. Biodegradable Polymeric Nanoformulation Based on the Antiprotozoal Canthin-6-one. Journal of Nanoparticle Research 2011; 13(12) 6737-6746. http://link.springer.com/article/10.1007%2Fs11051-011-0580-z#page-1

[60] Hadaruga DI., Hadăruga NG., Bandur GN., Rivis A., Costescu C., Ordodi VL., Ardelean A. Berberis vulgaris extract /β-cyclodextrin nanoparticles synthesis and characterization. Revista de Chimie (Bucharest) 2010; 61(7) 669-675.

[61] Sanna V., Siddiqui IA., Sechi M., Mukhtar H. Nanoformulation of natural products for prevention and therapy of prostate cancer. Cancer Letters 2013; 334(1) 142–151.

[62] Silva AM., Tavares J., Silvestre R., Ouaissi A., Coombs GH., Silva AC. Characterization of Leishmania infantum thiol-dependent reductase 1 and evaluation of its potential to induce immune protection. Parasite Immunology 2012; 34(6) 345-50.

[63] Manjolin LC., Reis MB., Maquiaveli, CC., Santos-Filho OA., Silva, ER. Dietary flavonoids fisetin, luteolin and their derived compounds inhibit arginase, a central enzyme in *Leishmania (Leishmania) amazonensis* infection. Food Chemistry 2013; 141(3) 2253-2262.

[64] Fonseca-Silva, F., Inacio JD., Canto-Cavalheiro MM., Almeida-Amaral EE. Reactive oxygen species production and mitochondrial dysfunction contribute to quercetin in-

duced death in *Leishmania amazonensis*. PLoS One 2011; 6, (2) 14666. http://www.plosone.org/article/info:doi/10.1371/journal.pone.0014666

[65] Fonseca-Silva F., Inacio JD., Canto-Cavalheiro MM., Almeida-Amaral EE. Reactive oxygen species production by quercetin causes the death of *Leishmania amazonensis* intracellular amastigotes. Journal of Natural Products 2013; 76(8) 1505-1508. http://pubs.acs.org/doi/abs/10.1021/np400193m

[66] Roy P., Das S., Bera T., Mondol S., Mukherjee A. Andrographolide nanoparticles in leishmaniasis: characterization and in vitro evaluations. International Journal of Nanomedicine 2010; 5(1) 1113-1121. http://www.ncbi.nlm.nih.gov/pmc/articles/PMC3023240/

[67] Lala S., Nandy AK., Mahato SB., Basu MK. Delivery In Vivo of 14-Deoxy-11-Oxoandrographolide, an Antileishmanial Agent, by Different Drug Carriers. Indian journal of Biochemistry & Biophysics 2003; 40(3) 169-174.

[68] Vasir JK., Reddy MK., Labhasetwar VD. Nanosystems in drug targeting: opportunities and challenges. Current Nanoscience 2005; 1(1) 47–64.

[69] Das S., Roy P., Mondal S., Bera T., Mukherjee, A. One Pot Synthesis of Gold Nanoparticles and Application in Chemotherapy of Wild and Resistant Type Visceral Leishmaniasis. Colloids and Surfaces B: Biointerfaces 2013; 107(1) 27–34.

[70] Kapil A. Piperine: a potent inhibitor of *Leishmania donovani* promastigotes in vitro. Planta Medica 1993; 59(5) 474.

[71] Ferreira C., Soares DC., Barreto-Junior CB., Nascimento MT., Lima LF., Delorenzi JC., Lima M E., Atella GC., Folly E., Carvalho TM., Saraiva EM., Silva LHP. Leishmanicidal effects of piperine, its derivatives, and analogues on *Leishmania amazonensis*. Phytochemistry 2011; 72(17) 2155-2164.

[72] Di Giorgio C., Delmas F., Ollivier E., Elias R., Balansard G., Timon-David P. In vitro activity of the beta-carboline alkaloids harmane, harmine, and harmaline toward parasites of the species *Leishmania infantum*. Experimental Parasitology 2004; 106(3-4), 67-74.

[73] Gil ES., Cunha LC., Paula, J. R., Bezerra JCB., Aguiar FA. Leishmaníase: Arsenal Terapêutico e Alvos Moleculares. Vita et Sanitas 2007; 1(1). http://www.fug.edu.br/revista/artigos/Organizados/Leishmaniase.pdf.

[74] Melos JLR., Echevarria A. Sistemas Enzimáticos de Tripanossomatídeos como Potenciais Alvos. Quimioterápicos. Revista Virtual de Quimíca 2012; 4(4) 374-392.

[75] Genestra M., Guedes SD., Souza WJS., Cysne-Finkelstein L., Bezerra RJS., Monteiro FP., Leon LL. Nitric Oxide Synthase (NOS) Characterization in *Leishmania amazonensis* Axenic Amastigotes, Archives of Medical Research 2006; 37(3) 328-333.

[76] Dias LC., Dessoy MA., Silva JJN., Thiemann OH., Oliva G., Andricopulo AD. Chemotherapy of chagas' disease: state of the art and perspectives for the development of new drugs. Quimica Nova 2009; 32(9) 2444-2457.

[77] Reguera MR., Tekwani BL., Balaña-Fouce R. Poliamine transport in parasites: A potential target for new antiparasistic drug development. Comparative Biochemistry and Physiology. Part C, 2005; 140(2) 151-164. http://europepmc.org/abstract/MED/15907761/reload=0;jsessionid=rJHFy2UYQHdnHPOLt0dI.50

[78] Roberts SC. Genetic manipulation of Leishmania parasites facilitates the exploration of the polyamine biosynthetic pathway as a potential therapeutic target. In: Urbano KV. (ed.) Advances in Genetics Research Hauppauge, NY: Nova Science Publishers; 2013. p 29-54.

[79] Padmanabhan PK., Mukherjee A., Singh S., Chattopadhyaya S., Gowri VS., Myler PJ., Srinivasan N., Madhubala R. Glyoxalase I from *Leishmania donovani*: A potential target for anti-parasite drug. Biochemical and Biophysical Research Communications 2005; 337(4) 1237-1248.

[80] Sousa SM., Gomes RA., Ferreira AE, Ponces FA., Cordeiro C. The glyoxalase pathway: the first hundred years... and beyond. The Biochemical Journal 2013; 453(1) 1-15.

[81] Lepesheva GI., Hargrove TY., Anderson S., Kleshchenko Y., Furtak V., Wawrzak Z., Villalta F., Waterman M. Sterol 14 α-demethylase as a potential target for antitrypanosomal therapy: enzyme inhibition and parasite cell growth. Chemistry and Biology 2007; 14(11) 1283–1293.

[82] Zhang K., Beverle SM. Molecular & Biochemical Parasitology Phospholipid and sphingolipid metabolism in Leishmania Review Article Molecular and Biochemical Parasitology 2010; 170(2) 55-64.

[83] Libusová L., Sulimenko T., Sulimenko V., Hozák P., Dráber P. Gamma- Tubulin in Leishmania: cell cycle-dependent changes in subcellular localization and heterogeneity of its isoforms, Experimental Cell Research 2004; 295(2) 375-386.

[84] Najwa MJA., Abu-Mejdad, Al-Hilfy AAA. Evaluation of therapeutic effects of vicine against *Leishmania donovani*. in vitro. The Journal American Science 2013; 9(5) 115-120. http://www.jofamericanscience.org/journals/am-sci/am0905/016_17646am0905_115_120.pdf

[85] Gangjee A., Jain HD., Kurup S. Recent advances in classical and non-classical antifolates as antitumor and antiopportunistic infection agents: part I. Anticancer Agents in Medicinal Chemistry 2007; 7(5) 524-42.

[86] Takele Y., Abebe T., Weldegebreal T., Hailu A., Hailu W., Hurissa Z., Ali J., Diro E., Sisay, Y., Cloke T., Modolell M., Munder M., Tacchini-Cottier F., Müller, I., Kropf P.

Arginase activity in the blood of patients with visceral leishmaniasis and HIV infection. PLoS Neglected Tropical Diseases 2013; 7 (1) 1-7.

[87] Luz NF., Andrade BB., Feijó, DF., Araújo-Santos T., Carvalho GQ., Andrade D., Abánades DR., Melo EV., Silva AM., Brodskyn CI., Barral-Netto M., Barral A., Mahmoudzadeh-Niknam H., McKerrow JH. *Leishmania tropica*: cysteine proteases are essential for growth and pathogenicity. Experimental Parasitology 2004; 106(3-4) 158-163.

[88] Kaur PK., Dinesh N., Soumya N., Babu NK.; Singh S. Identification and characterization of a novel Ribose 5-phosphate isomerase B from *Leishmania donovani*. Biochemical and Biophysical Research Communications 2012; 421(1) 51-56.

[89] Cordeiro AT., Feliciano, P. R.; Pinheiro, M. P.; Nonato, M. C. (2012). Crystal structure of dihydroorotate dehydrogenase from *Leishmania major*. Biochimie. 8(94) 1739-1748.

[90] Rotella DP. Recent results in protein kinase inhibition for tropical diseases. Bioorganic and Medicinal Chemistry Letters 2012; 22(22) 6788-6793.

[91] Wetze DMl, McMahon-Pratt D., Koleske AJ. The Abl and Arg Kinases Mediate Distinct Modes of Phagocytosis and Are Required for Maximal Leishmania Infection Molecular and Cellular Biolology 2012; 32(15) 3176–3186.

[92] Cummings HE., Barbi J., Reville P., Oghumu S., Zorko N., Sarkar A., Keiser TL., Lu B., Rückle T., Varikuti S., Lezama-Davila C., Wewers MD., Whitacre, C.; Radzioch, D.; Rommel C., Seveau S., Satoskar AR. Critical role for phosphoinositide 3-kinase gamma in parasite invasion and disease progression of cutaneous leishmaniasis. Proceedings of the National Academy Sciences 2012; 109(4) 1251-1256.

[93] Singh N., Kumar M., Singh RK. Leishmaniasis: current status of available drugs and new potential drug targets. Asian Pacific Journal of Tropical Medicine 2012; 5(6) 485-97.

[94] Gilroy C., Olenyik T., Roberts SC., Ullman B. Spermidine synthase is required for virulence of *Leishmania donovani*. Infection and Immunity 2011; 79(7) 2764-2769. http://www.ncbi.nlm.nih.gov/pubmed/21536795

[95] Grover A., Katiyar SP., Singh, SK., Dubey VK., Sundar D. A leishmaniasis study: structure-based screening and molecular dynamics mechanistic analysis for discovering potent inhibitors of spermidine synthase. Biochimica et Biophysica Acta - Proteins and Proteomics 2012; 1824(12) 1476-1483. http://www.sciencedirect.com/science/article/pii/S1570963912001136

[96] Mahmoudzadeh-Niknam H., McKerrow J.H. *Leishmania tropica*: cysteine proteases are essential for growth and pathogenicity. Experimental Parasitology 2004; 106(3-4) 158–163.

[97] Lopez RES. Proteases de Leishmania: novos alvos para o desenvolvimento racional de fármacos. Química Nova 2010; 33(7) 1541-1548.

[98] Swenerton RK., Zhang S., Sajid M., Medzihradszky KF., Craik CS., Kelly BL., McKerrow JH. The oligopeptidase B of Leishmania regulates parasite enolase and immune evasion. The Journal Biology Chemistry 2011; 286(1) 429-40.

[99] Jäger W., Santag S., Weidner-Glunde M., Gellermann E., Kati S., Pietrek M., Viejo-Borbolla A., Schulz TF. The ubiquitin-specific protease USP7 modulates the replication of Kaposi's sarcoma-associated herpesvirus latent episomal DNA. Journal of Virology 2012; 86(12) 6745-6757.

[100] Supuran CT. Carbonic anhydrase inhibition/activation: trip of a scientist around the world in the search of novel chemotypes and drug targets. Current Pharmaceutical Design 2010; 16(29) 3233-3245.

[101] Neri D., Supuran CT. Interfering with pH regulation in tumours as a therapeutic strategy. Nature Reviwens Drug Discovery 2011; 10(10) 767-777. http://www.nature.com/nrd/journal/v10/n10/abs/nrd3554.html

[102] Syrjänen L, Vermelho AB, de Rodrigues IA., Corte-Real S, Salonen T, Pan P, Vullo D, Parkkila S, Capasso C, Supuran CT. Cloning, Characterization, and Inhibition Studies of a β-Carbonic Anhydrase from *Leishmania donovani chagasi*, the Protozoan Parasite Responsible for Leishmaniasis. Journal of Medicinal Chemistry 2013; 56(18) 7372-7381.

[103] Urbina JA. Specific chemotherapy of Chagas disease: relevance, current limitations and new approaches. Acta Tropica 2010; 115(1-2) 55-68.

[104] Schetelma RA., Decuypere S., T'Kindt R., Dujardin JC., Coombs GR., Breitling G. The potential of metabolomics for Leishmania research in the post-genomics era. Parasitology 2010; 137(9) 1291–1302.

[105] Ogungbe VI., Setzer WN. In-silico Leishmania Target Selectivity of Antiparasitic Terpenoids Molecules 2013; 18(7) 7761-7847.

[106] Antinori S., Schifanella L., Corbellino M. Leishmaniasis: new insights from an old and neglected disease. European Journal of Clinical Microbiology and Infectious Diseases 2011; 31(2) 109–118.

[107] Alvar J., Croft S., Olliaro P. Chemotherapy in the treatment and control of leishmaniasis. Advances in Parasitology 2006; 61(1) 223–274. http://www.sciencedirect.com/science/article/pii/S0065308X05610068

[108] Cardenas R., Sandoval CM., Rodrıguez-Morales AJ., Franco-Paredes C. Impact of climate variability in the occurrence of leishmaniasis in northeastern Colombia. The American Journal Tropical of Medicinal and Hygiene 2006; 75(2) 273–277.

[109] Field V., Gautret P., Schlagenhauf P., Burchard GD., Caumes E., Jensenius M., Castelli F., Gkrania-Klotsas E., Weld L., Lopez-Velez R., Vries P., Von Sonnenburg F., Loutan L., Parola P. Travel and migration associated infectious diseases morbidity in

Europe, 2008. BMC Infections Diseases 2010; 10(330). http://www.biomedcentral.com/1471-2334/10/330 (accessed 15 August 2013).

[110] Volpato H., Desoti VC., Cogo J., Panice MR., Sarragiotto MH., Silva SO., Ueda-Nakamura T., Nakamura CV. The Effects of N-Butyl-1-(4-dimethylamino)phenyl-1,2,3,4-tetrahydro- β -carboline-3-carboxamide against *Leishmania amazonensis* Are Mediated by Mitochondrial Dysfunction. Evidence-Based Complementary and Alternative Medicine 2013; 2013 (874367) 1-7. http://www.hindawi.com/journals/ecam/2013/874367/ (accessed 10 August 2013).

[111] Tolomeo M., Roberti M., Scapozza L., Tarantelli C., Giacomini E.; Titone L., Saporito L., Di Carlo P., Colomba C. TTAS a new stilbene derivative that induces apoptosis in *Leishmania infantum*. Experimental Parasitology 2013; 3(1) 37-43.

[112] Gohil VM., Brahmbhatt KG., Loiseau PM., Bhutani KK. Synthesis and anti-leishmanial activity of 1-aryl-b-carboline derivatives against *Leishmania donovani*. Bioorganic and Medicinal Chemistry Letters 2012; 22(12) 3905–3907.

[113] Bahar M., Deng Y., Zhu X., He S., Pandharkar T., Drew ME., Navarro-Vázquez A., Anklin C., Gil RR., Doskotch RW., Werbovetz KA., Kinghorn A.D. Potent antiprotozoal activity of a novel semi-synthetic berberine derivative. Bioorganic and Medicinal Chemistry Letters 2011; 21(9) 2606–2610.

[114] Miguel CD., Yokoyama-Yasunaka JKU., Uliana SRB. Tamoxifen Is Effective in the Treatment of *Leishmania amazonensis* Infections in Mice PLoS Neglected Tropical Diseases 2008; 2(6)249. http://www.ncbi.nlm.nih.gov/pmc/articles/PMC2398787/

[115] Hazra SJ., Ghosh S., Das SM., Sharma S., Mousumi Das, Saudagar P., Prajapati, VK., Dubey VK., Sundar S., Hazra B. Evaluation of a diospyrin derivative as antileishmanial agent and potential modulator of ornithine decarboxylase of *Leishmania donovani*. Experimental Parasitology 2013; 135(2) 407–413. http://www.sciencedirect.com/science/article/pii/S0014489413002075

[116] Balaña-Fouce R., Prada CF., Requena JM., Cushman M., Pommier Y., Álvarez-Velilla R., Escudero-Martínez JM., Calvo-Álvarez E., Pérez-Pertejo Y., Reguera RM. Indotecan (LMP400) and AM13-55: Two Novel Indenoisoquinolines Show Potential for Treating Visceral Leishmaniasis. Antimicrobial Agents and Chemotherapy 2012; 56(10) 5264-5270.

[117] Allahverdiyev AM., Abamor ES., Bagirova M., Baydar SY., Ates SC., Kaya F., Kaya C., Rafailovich M. Investigation of antileishmanial activities of Tio2@Ag nanoparticles on biological properties of *L. tropica* and *L. infantum* parasites, in vitro. Experimental Parasitology 2013; 135(1) 55–63.

[118] Abada Z, Cojean S, Pomel S, Ferrié L, Akagah B, Lormier AT, Loiseau PM, Figadère B. Synthesis and antiprotozoal activity of original porphyrin precursors and derivatives. European Journal of Medicinal Chemistry 2013; 67(12) 158-165.

[119] Shakya N., Sane SA., Vishwakarma P., Gupta S. Enhancement in therapeutic efficacy of miltefosine in combination with synthetic bacterial lipopeptide, Pam3Cys against experimental Visceral Leishmaniasis. Experimental Parasitology 2012; 131(3) 377-82.

Chapter 16

Nanoparticle Technology: An alternative approach for Leishmaniasis Treatment

Aldo Eloizo Job, Alexandre Fioravante de Siqueira,
Caroline Silva Danna, Felipe Silva Bellucci,
Flávio Camargo Cabrera,
Leandra Ernst Kerche Silva and
Pedro Henrique Benites Aoki

Additional information is available at the end of the chapter

http://dx.doi.org/10.5772/57283

1. Introduction

Leishmaniasis is an infection caused by a parasite from *Leishmania* genus, which can manifest itself through different forms: cutaneous (with skin ulcers) [1, 2], visceral (hepato and splenomegaly) [3], and diffuse integumentary form (injuries beyond the superficial skin barrier, hitting cartilages and deeper connective tissues) [4]. Leishmaniasis vectors are diptera from *Psychodida* family, which includes hematophagous from *Phlebotomus* genus (Old World) and *Lutzomuyia* genus (New World), with wide distribution in warm and temperate climates [5] (Figure 1).

In the New World, eight Leishmania species are responsible for men diseases: Leishmania braziliensis, Leishmania guyanensis, Leishmania panamensis, Leishmania lainsoni, Leishmania mexicana, Leishmania amazonensis, Leishmania venezuelensis and Leishmania chagasi [7]. Thus, leishmaniasis can be found in four continents, being considered endemic in 88 countries, of which 72 are in development [5].

Different protozoa species are able to live inside sand flies (insect vectors) from *Phlebotominae* subfamily and vertebrate hosts. This parasite lives between two different types of hosts due to its significant morphological changes. In vertebrate hosts, *Leishmania* is at amastigote form without flagella and inside the digestive tract of the sand flies, the parasite is flagellated and fusiform, and receives the name of promastigote, as shown in Figure 2.

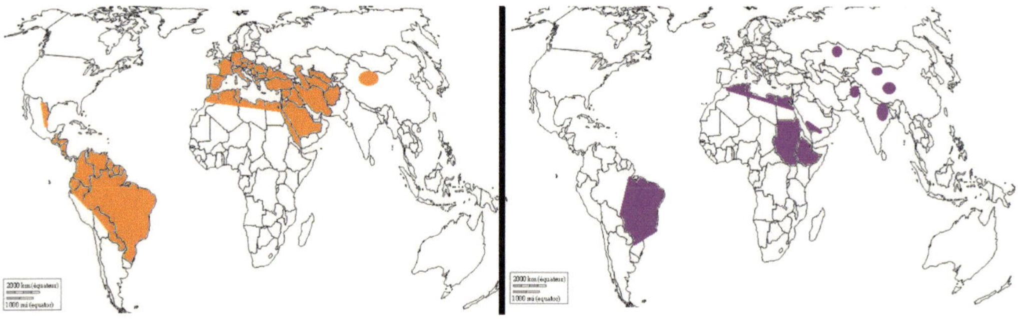

Figure 1. Distribution in Old World and New World of cutaneous (left, marked in orange) and visceral (right, marked in purple) leishmaniasis. Affected areas marked according to the World Health Organization [6].

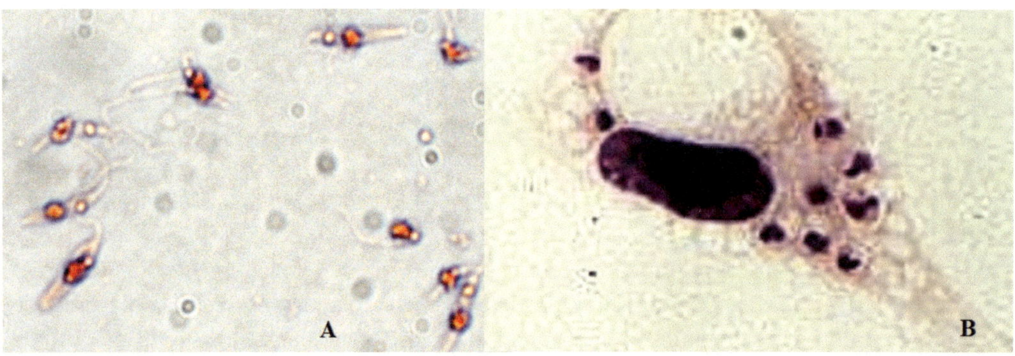

Figure 2. *Leishmania sp* (A) promastigote and (B) amastigote (right) forms.

In Figure 3, two important cellular structures used to identify the *Leishmania* parasites are highlited in the first image - the nucleus, indicated by the letter N and the kinetoplast, indicated by the letter K. These structures are kept in the distinct methacyclogenesis stages. After completing the cycle modifications, *Leishmania* becomes able to infect mammalian cells.

Different forms of leishmaniasis are transmitted through the bite of female sand flies. The transmission cycle begins when, during a bite, the mosquito ingests mammalian blood infected with amastigote forms. Once installed in the digestive tract of the host, *Leishmania* passes through the process of differentiation, methacyclogenesis, and the new form of the parasite, promastigote, can be inject in mammalian blood again during a bite, thus completing the disease transmission cycle (Figure 4).

http://dx.doi.org/10.5772/57283

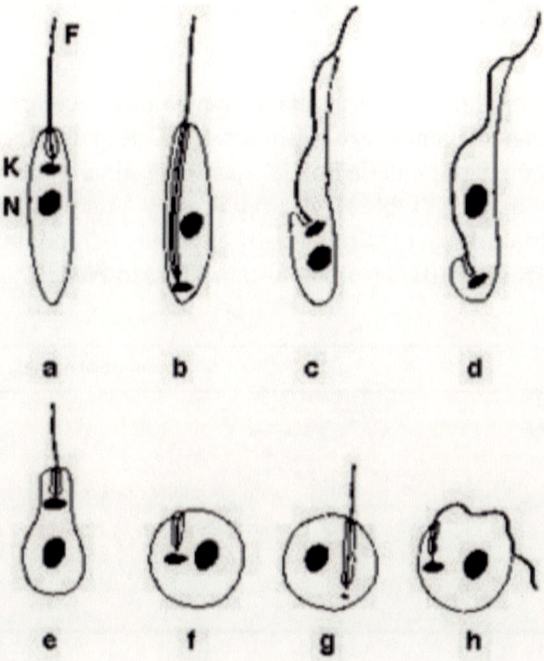

Figure 3. Different transition stages between (a) promastigote and (f) amastigote forms of *Leishmania braziliensis*.

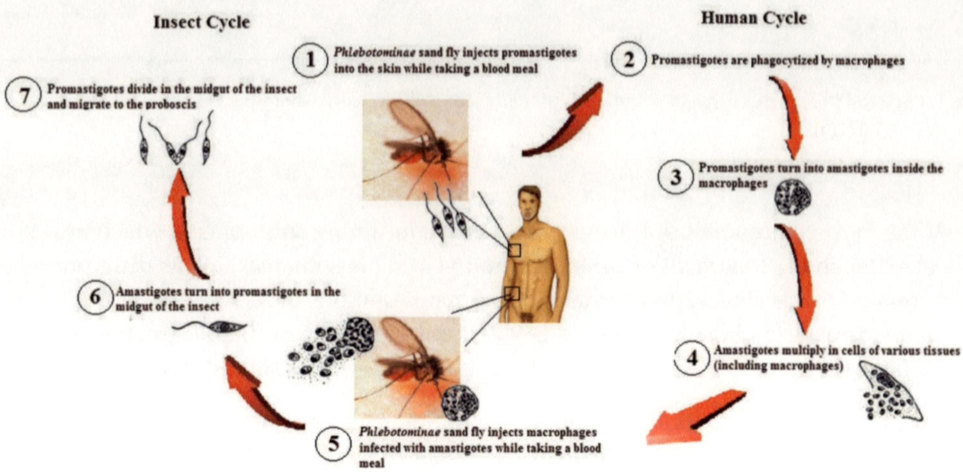

Figure 4. Life cycle of the parasite.

2. Current treatments

In 1912, Vianna [9] observed that the tartar emetic (an antimony compound) was effective in the treatment of American Integumentary Leishmaniasis. Due to toxicity and serious collateral damages associated to the tartar emetic use, i.e. gastrointestinal intolerance and cardiotoxic effects, the trivalent antimonials (Table 1) were replaced by quinquivalent compounds (Table 2). In 1936, Schmidt introduced in medical therapy antimony (V) sodium gluconate, commercially known as Solustibosan® (Bayer) or Pentostam® (Glaxo Wellcome) [10, 11].

Structural form	Chemical/commercial names
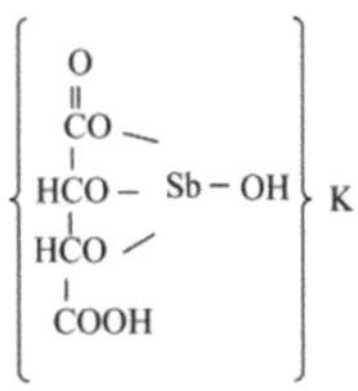	Antimony (III) potassium tartrate [11]/ Tartar emetic
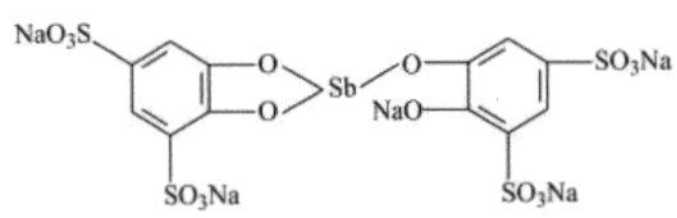	Sodium antimony (III) bis (catechol – 3,5 – disulfonate) [11]/ Stibophen, Repodral, Fuadina
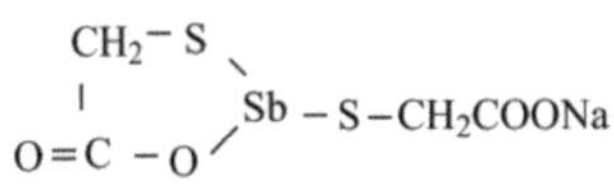	Antimony (III) sodium thioglicolate [11]

Table 1. Chemical structure of trivalent antimonials used in medical clinic, with their respective chemical and commercial names [5].

One of the most commonly used drugs is N-methylglucamine antimoniate, which are especially effective in the treatment of cutaneous and visceral leishmaniasis. This drug provokes fast regression of the clinical and hematological manifestations of the disease, as well as the dead of the parasite [5]. However, due to its low dosages and discontinuous treatments, some therapy failures, an increase of the resistant forms of the parasites started to show up [12-14].

The World Health Organization preconizes that antimonials dosages Should not trespass 20 mg/kg/day, and due to its elevated toxicity, the dosage of antimony ingested per day should not be higher than 850 mg [12]. However, the N-methylglucamine antimoniate is rapidly absorbed and about 90% of the antimony ingested is excreted through the kidneys in the firsts 48 hours [15]. Consequently, there is a necessity to administrate high doses of the drug, in continuous regimen, so an elevated dosage of antimony is assured in the tissues, and therefore the treatment efficacy is obtained.

http://dx.doi.org/10.5772/57283

Proposed structural form	Chemical/commercial name
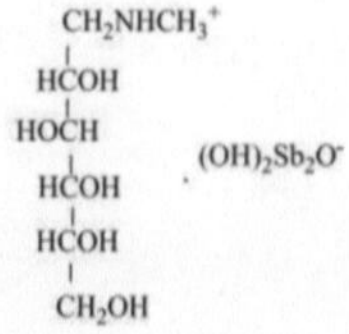	N-methylglucamine antimoniate [10]/ Glucantime®; Meglumine antimoniate
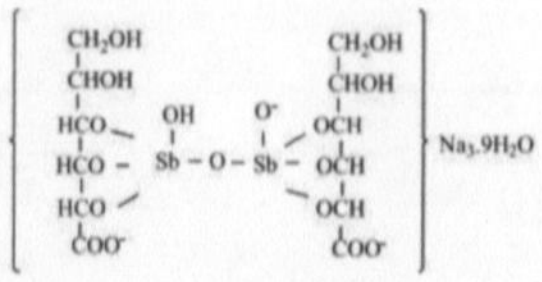	Antimony (V) Sodium Gluconate [10, 12] or Sodium Stibogluconate/ Pentostam®; Solustibosan®
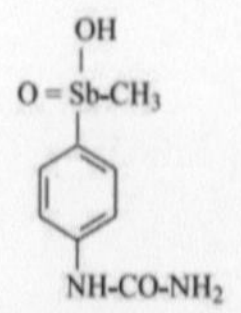	Urea estibamine [11]/ Estibamine®

Table 2. Chemical structure of quinquivalent antimonials used in medical clinic [5].

High doses of N-methylglucamine antimoniate generate a various diversity of collateral effects, such as nephritis, gastrointestinal, cardiovascular and respiratory disturbances. In some cases, besides destroying the parasites, some patients are led to death [11]. The antimony can still be detected in the hair of the patients a year after the treatment is finished [16]. The toxicity of antimony can be explained by the fact that there are some evidences describing that a metabolic conversion happens inside the macrophages transforming antimony V (Sb^{5+}) in antimony III (Sb^{3+}) [13] and the antimony III is proved to be more lethal to the *Leishmania* species [5]. So the hypothesis is that the antimony V works as prodrug, and the conversion to antimony III is what guarantee its efficacy after administration [17], and the antimony III interferes in the β-oxidation process of fat acids of the parasites, as so in the glycolysis, taking the ATP to a low level inside the cell [12]. This way, the antimony III would be responsible for the toxicity of the drug as well as its therapeutic activity [18].

Besides antimonials, other medicines have been used in the treatment of the various forms of leishmaniasis, among them can be found pentamidine, amphotericin B, paromomycin, and miltefosine (Table 3) [5]. Pentamidine is also effective in the trypanosomiasis treatment [19] and this drug is also highly toxic, showing as collateral effects hypoglycemia, hypotension, cardiologic changes, nephrotoxicity and even death [12]. Amphotericin B is an antibiotic produced by *Streptomyces* nodosus and can produce nephrotoxicity, depleting the potassium and magnesium levels of the organism [20]. Paromomycin is an aminoglycoside antibiotic active against *Leishmania* species in in vitro and in vivo forms. It is been highly tested in India, where antimonial standard treatments are not effective [5]. Miltefosine is an alkyl phospholipidic anticancer drug and it is in intensive tests also in India. It is showing excellent results and may be the first oral treatment against visceral leishmaniasis [21].

Structural form	Chemical/commercial name
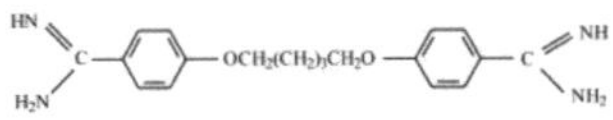	Pentamidine Isethionate [13]/ Lomidine
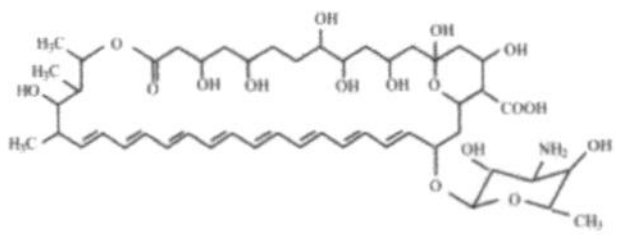	Amphotericin B [13]/ Fungizone
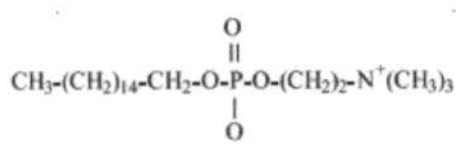	Miltefosine [21]
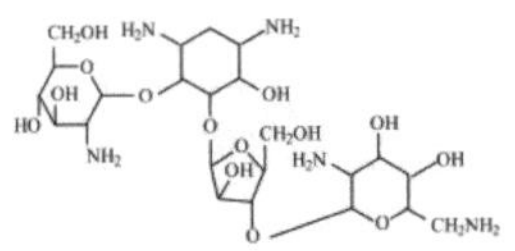	Paromomycin [13]/ Humatin

Table 3. Other chemicals used in leishmaniasis therapy, with their respective chemical and commercial names.

3. Alternative treatments

Association of some drugs used in leishmaniasis treatment within lipid vesicles called liposomes is one of the alternatives used to reduce the undesirable effects. This association increases the efficiency and the concentrations of these drugs in the tissues, reducing drastically their toxicity [22, 23]. The mechanism that could explain the effectiveness of liposomes is that they inhibit oxygen consumption by the parasite membrane [24].

One practical exemple of this association happens with Amphotericin B, a compound used for the treatment of calazar patients that are resistant to pentamidine. Amphotericin B can be toxic because they can associate with human cell cholesterol as they do to the ergosterol in the parasite plasmatic membrane [6]. To reduce this inappropriate recognition, there are some commercial formulations that associate the Amphotericin B to lipids (Ambisome, Abelcet, Amphotec). Besides their effectiveness in reducing this drug toxicity, they are very expensive and their use becomes basically impractical in poor countries [25].

However, there are some studies searching some low-cost methods of producing these drugs. One example is a formulation with a similar lipid composition to Abelcet, but with some different variables, such as conformation and molecular weight, that may influence the drug release and action in the organism [26]. This formulation was found to be much more effective and less toxic than Abelcet and, although it is less efficient than Ambisome, it is also less expensive for use in leishmaniasis treatment.

4. Vaccines against Leishmaniasis

Studies for the achievement of a vaccine for leishmaniasis immunization are accomplished since 1940 [27]. In the firsts vaccination process against this disease, scientists didn't know that they were dealing with a microbian ill. This vaccine method was based in the injection of the active wound secretion from one patient to another that was not ill.

From this vaccine, other techniques were developed aiming the raise of the prophylactic efficiency and to avoid some troubles caused by the emergence of a wound. Thus, specialized literature reports four types of vaccines against different types of leishmaniasis: the vaccine based on dead parasites, the vaccine based on living but attenuated parasites, the vaccine with antigenic fragments, and the genic vaccine based on DNA [28].

In a few countries, some clinical trials were already performed but none of the vaccines showed a level of efficiency higher than 80%, a fact that makes unfeasible human tests. This lack of security may be associated to the differentiation between *Leishmania* species [29], and this differentiation hampers the accomplishment of a wide immunization field.

New investments to the manufacture of a vaccine against leishmaniasis depend on an active biomass of these protozoa. This way, when in contact with the target it may generate an immunological response without generating the disease. But nowadays, the methods for obtaining this biomass [30, 31] are very expensive with low profitability, since it generates a very small sample with an inefficient outcome.

5. New treatment proposals

Due to intense collateral effects, lots of people who are infected with leishmaniases refuse treatment, and there is the need to new alternative treatments. One of the new possibilities in study nowadays uses natural rubber (NR) membranes with metallic nanoparticles (MNPs) such as silver and gold (SNPs and GNPs, respectively). NR membranes are used as an active support to the MNPs reduction process using precursor salts to obtain metallic particles, and that means that the NR membrane works as a reducing agent as well as a stabilizer for MNPs.

When a promastigote population of *Leishmania braziliensis* is in the presence of pure natural rubber membranes, there is a significant increase in the log phase of the cells, constituted by a large number of cells at the division process. In the 27th hour after inoculation, the parasite colony remains stable, without large variations in the population cells. In this phase, called stationary phase, the promastigote cells start morphophysiological transformations known as metacyclogenesis. With the end of the stationary phase, an environmental saturation happens with cell waste and lack of nutrients, resulting in the death of cells, phase known as fall.

This decrease could be explained by the natural dynamics of promastigotes in the culture medium. It is expected that after 150 hours, this decrease in the population number occurs because of nutritional deficit and saturation of the cellular environment with cellular excreta generated during the period of growth log and stationary phase, but the presence of nanoparticles anticipates the drop in the number of the parasites, probably because these metal components stop the absorption of nutrients of the environment through permeases and transplasmalema transport channels.

However, when promastigotes interact with natural rubber membranes impregnated with silver nanoparticles, a stretch of the first metabolic phase is seen, only with a non-significant growth. In figure 5 is possible to see that the decrease in *L. braziliensis* is proportional to the increase of silver concentrations in the NR membrane.

Silver nanoparticles toxicity is well known, and although death of the promastigotes may occur, it is believed that changes in the physiological maturation process, such as drastic changes in the surface glycoproteins, happen to the microorganism cell. In that way, the NR membranes with silver nanoparticles when put in the protozoa medium is capable of separating the cells without killing the whole population, eliminating only the ones which did not finalized their metacyclogenesis and are highly infective to the hosts (Figure 6). Immature cells that are not able to generate a disease are kept intact, and this process is what generates an important biomass to a future study focus a vaccine against this disease.

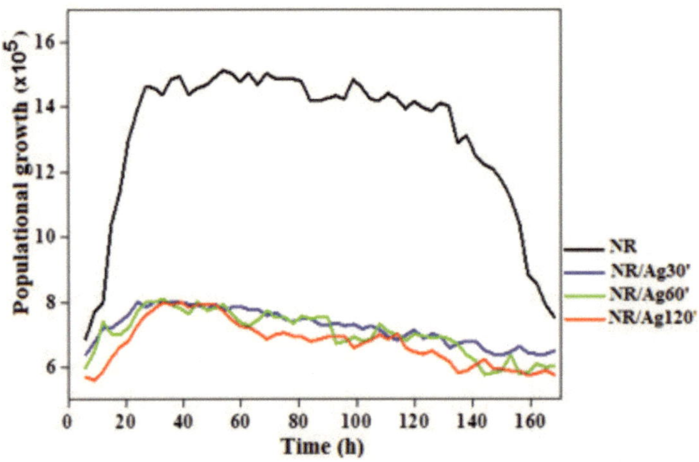

Figure 5. Populational growth of *Leishmania braziliensis* promastigotes in contact with natural rubber membranes and natural rubber membranes impregnated with silver nanoparticles using *in situ* reduction.

Natural rubber membranes containing GNPs (NR/Au) also decrease the population growth rate, showing a lower index of living promastigotes (attached to the membrane surface) depending on the amount of nanoparticles deposited in the membrane surface. Formation and growth of the GNPs within the NR membranes, by reduction of Au^{3+}, was monitored following the Plasmon absorption band. Reducing agents for GNPs formation are likely to be the carboxylic functional groups present in the NR. Nanoparticle, which produces an increase of the intensity of the distinctive plasmon absorption band of GNPs centered at approximately 560 nm, as shown in Figure 7 [33].

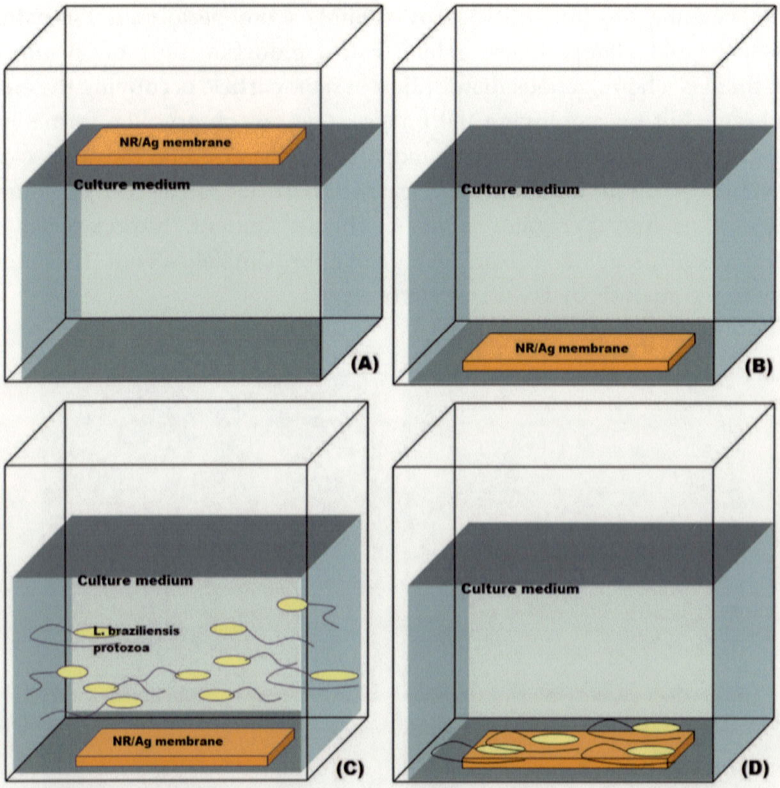

Figure 6. Separation Process of *Leishmania* in contact with NR membranes with silver (Ag) nanoparticles; (a) and (b) NR/Ag membranas in culture medium; (c) *Leishmania braziliensis* in contact to NR/Ag membranes; (d) Separated protozoa attached to NR/Ag membranes.

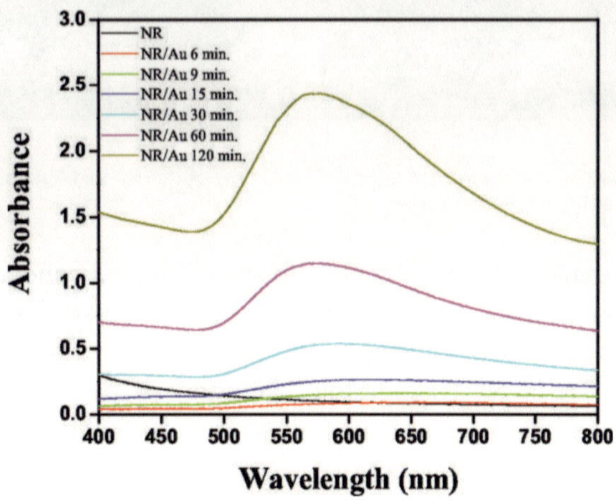

Figure 7. UV-Vis spectroscopy of natural rubber/gold nanoparticles prepared at different gold reduction times, compared to raw natural rubber membrane (preparation of the membrane annealed at 65 °C).

Analyses by scanning electron microscopy (ESEM) were performed for natural rubber membranes with gold nanoparticles, obtained at a reduction time of 30 min (Figure 8). Apparently, there is a homogenous distribution of nanoparticle occupying the entire surface of the membrane, but by amplifying the images, one can observe the formation of many nanoparticles in sites, and among them, nanoparticles dispersed on the surface of the polymeric matrix. In Figure 8 (d) the small spherical nanoparticles can be seen agglomerated over reduction sites, forming aggregates at an exorbitant amount. Nanoparticles sizes were measured and are very similar, with an average of approximately 48 nm. These results are in agreement with the analysis by UV-Vis spectroscopy.

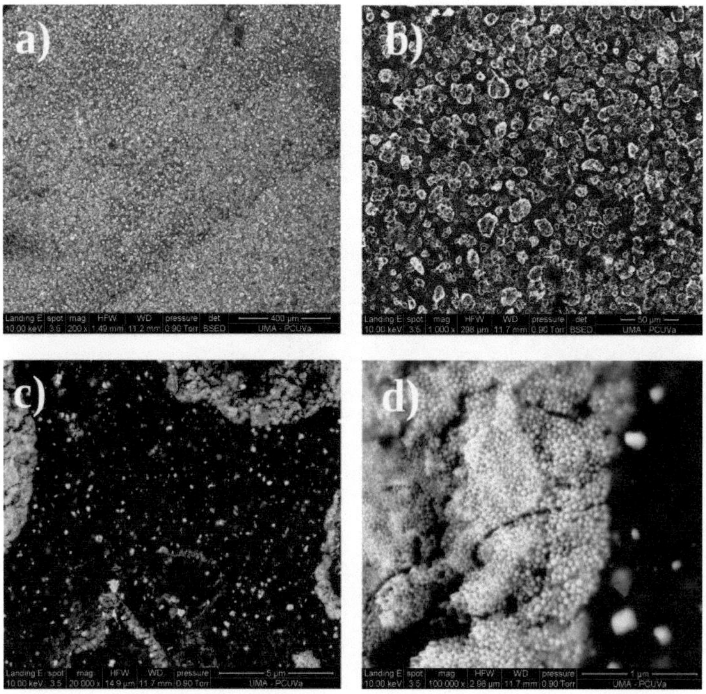

Figure 8. SEM analysis of NR/Au membrane obtained at 30 minutes of reduction. Magnification of (a) 200 times; (b) 1,000 times; (c) 20,000 times; (d) 100,000 times.

Natural rubber membranes, with colloidal incorporation of gold nanoparticles, were synthesized by *in situ* method (NR/Au) at different reduction times, in order to evaluate the physiological behavior of *L. braziliensis* promastigotes cultured in axenic medium, in a colony of seven weeks old, evaluating the increase kinetics in relation to the permanence time of the membranes in the culture medium as a function of reduction time and temperature of preparation of natural rubber membranes.

It was observed that the inclusion of NR/Au membrane in culture generates a delayed onset of growth in culture until about 24 hours, with a reduction in the development population proportional to the time reduction of the gold nanoparticles. It is also noted that the NR/Au

120 min. membrane presents the best results with regard to growth inhibition of promastigote population in culture medium. NR/Au 30 min membrane has a sharper decline in curve kinetics attributable to death of promastigotes from 120 hours. Upon analysis completion of growth medium, the membranes prepared for times of 30, 60 and 120 minutes showed similar results, with the number of promastigotes in solution smaller than inserted into the initial population.

According to the results the best allowed reduction time is 120 minutes, due to its greater population growth inhibition, and was then assessed the influence of the thermal treatment by the casting preparation method of membrane natural rubber annealed at 60, 80 and 120 °C, and then used as substrates for the reduction of nanoparticles. Results obtained for the kinetics of increase in solution are shown in Figure 9.

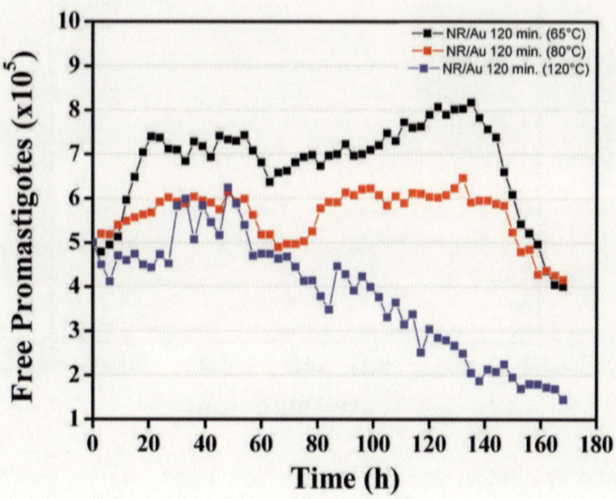

Figure 9. Analysis of the kinetics of increase of promastigotes in solution in the presence of natural rubber membranes prepared by the casting method, at temperatures of 65, 80 and 120 °C, and then incorporated gold nanoparticles to the time reduction of 120 minutes.

It is observed that with increasing of thermal treatment temperature in the preparation of NR membranes the population growth factor in culture decreases, reaching scores lower than $2x10^5$ promastigotes (less than half of the inoculum) to membranes prepared at 120 °C at a reduced nanoparticles to 120 minutes. It is known from promastigotes reactivity with carboxylic and nitrogenated groups, the same reactive groups and assigned to the reduction of nanoparticles. Higher the temperature of thermal treatment used in the preparation of NR membranes, smaller the amount of nanoparticles embedded in the membrane surface, attributed to the fact that there is further degradation of the active components of the membrane with increasing temperature. Thus, it is attributed the decrease in population growth in solution to generate more reactive nanoparticles or selective proteins contained in the culture medium, inhibiting the development of promastigotes, and may also be linked to decreasing of active cores on the membrane surface, or even liberation of radicals in the culture medium attributed to membrane preparation temperature, but the level of promastigotes in culture medium still remains considerable, so that in an attempt to develop a smart skin bandage incorporated into methylene blue molecules on Au particles to photodynamic treatment, due to the drug photosensitivity.

Membranes of pure natural rubber and with incorporation of gold nanoparticles and methylene blue were inserted in the culture medium and the behavior of *L. braziliensis* promastigotes were evaluated through the population growth kinetics and morphophysiological analysis. Results regarding to population growth obtained for protozoan eluted to membranes prepared at 120 °C of thermal treatment are presented in Figure 10.

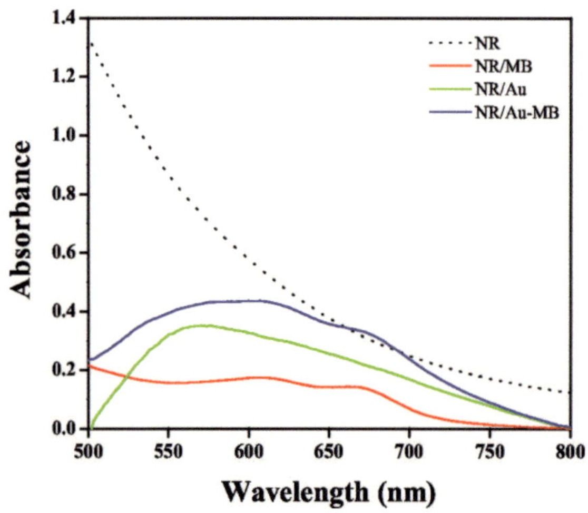

Figure 10. Molecular spectroscopy in UV-Vis region of natural rubber membranes with gold nanoparticles for reduction time of 120 min and functionalization with methylene blue molecules, compared to pure natural rubber membranes.

To improve the studies, blue methylene was incorporated to the NR membrane. This incorporation does not show toxic interaction with promastigotes, since the population growth usually develops when inserted NR/MB membranes. Moreover, when irradiated culture media containing BM molecules, a deficit in the population growth is observed. For NR/MB membranes irradiated with blue light total elimination of promastigotes is observed in about 120 hours, whereas when MB molecules deposited on gold nanoparticles this time decreases to about 60 hours. This fact is attributed to the amplification effect of surface commonly evaluated by micro-Raman spectroscopy, so that the metallic particles act as sites for amplification of energy absorbed by the anchored molecules.

The electrons assume an excited energy state, and during the release of the absorbed energy active radicals are generated, with interaction with the environment where are MB molecules. In the first instance, electrons from MB molecules, when returning to the ground state emit enough energy to excite the oxygen present in the medium converting to superoxides or peroxides radials. This transfer may occur also by interaction with hydrogen atoms present in other molecules to form radicals, e.g. hydroxyl, also with potential toxic to cells, or as in this case, the promastigotes. If the emission energy is derived from a transition to a triplet state of the photosensitizer, one can obtain the formation of a singlet oxygen molecule and an oxidizing agent more toxic to cells [34-38].

6. Conclusion

Membranes with metal nanoparticles significantly influences the development of the protozoan *L. braziliensis*, thus they can be used for different applications.

Membranes with SNPs can separate the cells at different stages of maturation. In this case, we obtain a biomass feasible to manufacture a vaccine for the purpose of immunization against leishmaniasis.

Membranes with GNPs can used for a possible treatment of cutaneous leishmaniasis, once the cell death is cause due to interaction between the gold and protozoan. NR/MB membranes can be direct to the photosensitive treatment of lesions and so accelerate the closing of the same. Thus, membranes with metallic nanoparticles are a viable and the low cost for both the immunization procedure and in the treatment process because the disease is already established. In addition, treatment with the application of membranes with MNPs dramatically reduces the side effects caused by conventional treatment.

Author details

Aldo Eloizo Job*, Alexandre Fioravante de Siqueira, Caroline Silva Danna, Felipe Silva Bellucci, Flávio Camargo Cabrera, Leandra Ernst Kerche Silva and Pedro Henrique Benites Aoki

*Address all correspondence to: job@fct.unesp.br

Department of Physics, Chemistry and Biology, Univ Estadual Paulista, Presidente Prudente, Sao Paulo, Brazil

References

[1] Tato Lmp Et Al. Colloids And Surfaces B: Biointerfaces. 2009;68: 55-60.

[2] Ministério Da Saúde, Secretaria De Vigilância Em Saúde. Manual De Vigilância Da Leishmaniose Tegumentar Americana. Brasília: Editora Do Ministério Da Saúde; 2007.

[3] Goto H, Lindoso Jal. Expert Review Of Anti-Infective Therapy. 2010; 8(4): 419-433.

[4] Späth Gf Et Al. Proceedings Of The National Academy Of Sciences (Usa). 2000; 97: 9258-9263.

[5] Rath S Et Al. Química Nova. 2003;26(4): 550-555.

[6] Santos Od. Parasitology Research. 2008;103: 1-10.

[7] Grimaldi, G.; Tesh, A. B.; Mcmahon, P. D. The American Journal Of Tropical Medicine And Hygiene, 41, 689, 1989.

[8] Http://Www.Dpd.Cdc.Gov/Dpdx/Html/Leishmaniasis.Htm

[9] Vianna, G. O. Anais Do 7º Congresso Brasileiro De Medicina E Cirurgia, 4, 426, 1912.

[10] Berman, J. D. Reviews Of Infectious Disease, 10, 560, 1988.

[11] Marsden, P. D. Revista Da Sociedade Brasileira De Medicina Tropical, 18, 187, 1985.

[12] Balaña-Fouce, R.; Reguera, R. M.; Cubría, C.; Ordóñez, D. General Pharmacology, 30, 435, 1998.

[13] Sereno, D.; Lemesre, J. L. Antimicrobial Agents And Chemotherapy, 41, 972, 1997.

[14] Berman, J. D.; Wyler, D. J. The Journal Of Infectious Diseases, 142, 83,1980.

[15] Limongi, J. P. In Farmacodinâmica; Corbett, C. E., Ed. Livraria Editora Artes Médicas, São Paulo, 1973, Cap. 61.

[16] D'Rea, J. G. Et Al. Clinical Chemistry, 33, 2081, 1987.

[17] Roberts, W. L.; Mcmurray, W. J.; Rainey, P. M. Antimicrobial Agents And Chemotherapy, 42, 1076, 1998.

[18] Miekeley, N.; Mortari, S. R.; Schubach, A. O. Analytical And Bioanalytical Chemistry, 372, 495, 2002.

[19] Doua, F. Et Al. American Journal Of Tropical Medicine And Hygiene, 55, 586, 1996.

[20] Rang, H. P.; Dale, M. M.; In Pharmacology, 2nd Edition, Churchill Livingstone: Uk, 1991.

[21] Fischer, C.; Voss, A.; Engel, J. Medical Microbiology And Immunology, 190, 85, 2001.

[22] Desjeux, P; Alvar, J. Annals Of Tropical Medicine And Parasitology, 97 (1), 3-15, 2003.

[23] Gontijo, B.; Carvalho, M. L. R. Revista De Sociedade Brasileira De Medicina Tropical, 36 (1), 71-80, 2003.

[24] Rosa, M. S. S. Et Al. Antimicrobial Agents And Chemotherapy, 47 (6), 1895-1901, 2003.

[25] Golenser, J. Et Al. Antimicrobial Agents And Chemotherapy, 43 (9), 2209-2214, 1999.

[26] Larabi, M. Et Al. Antimicrobial Agents And Chemotherapy, 47 (12), 3774-3779, 2003.

[27] Grimaldi Jr.,G. Memórias Do Instituto Oswaldo Cruz, 90, 553- 556, 1995.

[28] Handman, E. Parasitology Today, 13, 236-237, 1997.

[29] Antunes, C. M. F. Et Al. International Journal Of Epidemiology, 15, 572-579, 1986.

[30] Dórea, R. C. C., Et Al. Brazilian Journal Of Microbiology, 34, 1, 7-20, 2003.

[31] Kohri, M. Et Al, European Polymer Journal, 47, 2351-60, 2011.

[32] Barbosa-Filho, C.G. Et Al. Experimental Parasitology, 130, 152-158, 2012.

[33] Aroca, R. F.; Alvarez-Puebla, R. A.; Pieczonka, N.; Sanchez-Cortez, S.; Garcia-Ramos, J. V. Adv. Colloid Interface Sci., 116 (1-3), 45-61, 2005.

[34] Peloi, L. S. Et Al. Exp. Parasitol., 128 (4), 353, 2011.

[35] Prates, R. A. Et Al. Journal Of Photochemistry And Photobiology, 86 (1), 70-76, 2007.

[36] Wainwright, M. Journal Of Antimicrobial Chemotherapy, 42, 13-28, 1998.

[37] Miyabe, M. Braz. Oral Res., 25 (3), 230, 2011.

[38] Longo, J. P. F.; Azevedo, R. B. J. Dent. Clin. Res., 6 (3), 249-257, 2010.

Chapter 17

Treatment and Control of Leishmaniasis Using Photodynamic Therapy

Debora P. Aureliano, Martha S. Ribeiro,
José Angelo Lauletta Lindoso, Fabio C. Pogliani,
Fábio P. Sellera, Dennis Song and
Mauricio S. Baptista

Additional information is available at the end of the chapter

http://dx.doi.org/10.5772/57456

1. Introduction

Leishmaniasis is a chronic disease affecting the skin, mucosal and/or internal organs, caused by flagellate protozoa *Leishmania* of the *Trypanosomatidae* family. [1] It is among the six most important disease in terms of its impact in public health. The world incidence of leishmaniasis is very large with about half a million new cases per year. About 12 million people are infected with *Leishmania ssp* parasites worldwide. New treatment alternatives are highly needed. Our goal here is to critically revise the literature in order to show the potential of Photodynamic Therapy in the treatment and comprehensive control of this disease. We have separated this chapter in nine sections, besides this brief introduction, which are: Leishmaniasis: Background and treatment strategies; Mechanisms in Photodynamic Therapy; Treatment of animals infected with leishmaniasis using PDT; Vector control using PDT; PDT alternatives for Blood purification; PDT on the treatment of Old World Tegumentary Leishmaniasis; PDT - *In vitro* tests in species that cause Tegumentary Leishmaniasis; Conclusions; References.

2. Leishmaniasis — Background and treatment strategies

There are two main forms of leishmaniasis, visceral (VL) and tegumentary (TL) leishmaniasis, which are also respectively called Kala Azar and Bauru ulcer. The later, received its name because of the original high prevalence in Bauru, a city in the countryside of the State of São

Paulo, in Brazil. The tegumentary leishmaniasis is characterized by skin lesions (cutaneous-CL) and mucocutaneous lesions (such as, nasal and mouth regions) [2].

Leishmaniasis is a common zoonosis, with domestic (dogs and cats) and wild (rodents, marsupials, edentulous and wild canids) reservoirs. It is transmitted to humans by sand flies, which comprise the genus Lutzomyia and Phlebotomus. Details of the etiology and pathophysiology of the disease are out of the scope of this chapter and we suggest that the reader consult reviews that focus on these subjects [3].

The current scenario of leishmaniasis treatment is not promising. Therapeutic approaches include systemic administrations of anti-parasitic medications, which often present serious side effects. Few drugs are available in the clinic, mainly antimonials and amphotericin, and the frequency of resistance development is rising. Therefore, there is an urgent need to establish new and more effective treatments for both VL and TL. The treatment of TL (the focus of this chapter) urges new drugs and new therapeutic forms, that allows for more effective and conveniently administered treatments [4].

One of the promising approaches, and the one discussed in here, is photodynamic therapy (PDT). The main expectation of this approach is that it treats lesions in a localized manner, without damaging healthy tissues [5]. The few reports that are available in the literature have validated this hypothesis. In addition, no sign of systemic toxicity is reported in PDT, eliminating one of the major health issues related to existing TL treatments.[6] These points will be further discussed in this chapter.

The use of light as a therapeutic modality has gained strong impulse recently due to the development of efficient and affordable light sources. Consequently, photo-activated drugs (PhotoSensitizers-PS) play key roles in the present clinical portfolio, and more importantly, are the major lead in the development of new drugs to treat a variety of diseases such as cancer, microbial infections and tropical diseases. However, increasing the efficiency of PDT photosensitizers remains challenging [7-9].

The use of PDT in veterinary is much less common even considering the benefits that such strategies could bring in the treatment of high-value reproducing animals, as well as, in the treatment of animals that are reservoirs of human diseases [10].

In terms of developing effective treatments against leishmaniasis in endemic areas, it is important to think of comprehensive strategies that could cause a quick decrease in the pool of infected patients (Figure 1). It is also important to emphasize that leishmaniasis is a neglected tropical disease and, therefore, it is highly relevant to consider low-cost strategies that would serve as an alternative for public medicine in poor countries [9]. Developing efficient clinical protocols that would cure/control the disease would not only favor the patient itself, but also, would decrease the chance of this infection being transmitted to others by the vectors or by blood transfusion. In the next sections, we will explain how PDT can be helpful in the treatment of patients, as well as, of all the possible reservoirs and transmitting vectors that would favor the parasite infection cycle (Figure 1). Some of this potential has been attained and some are still in the step of hypothesis testing.

http://dx.doi.org/10.5772/57456

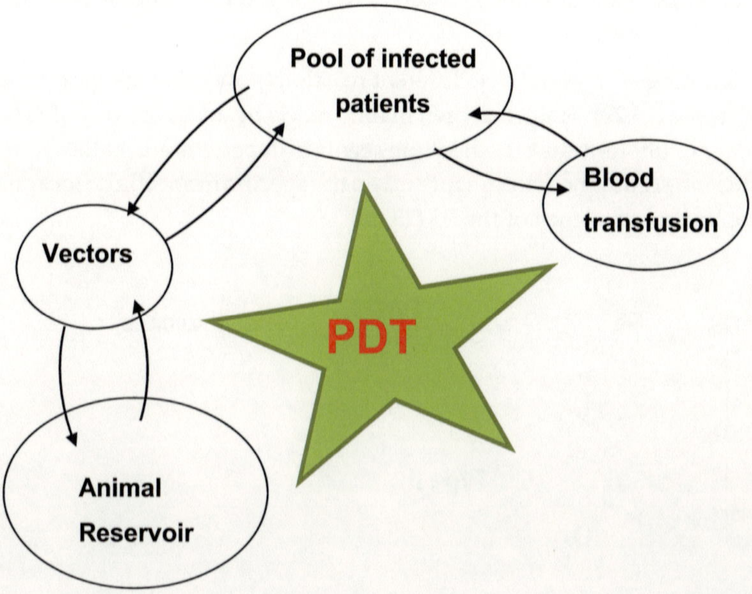

Figure 1. Schematic representation of a comprehensive strategy to control leishmania disease in endemic areas by using PDT. Besides treating patients and animals; killing vectors and disinfecting blood, should be considered in a PDT strategy to control leishmaniasis. The star represents the multi-target characteristic of the PDT strategy.

3. Mechanisms in photodynamic therapy

PDT is a clinical modality based on the damage caused in biological tissues or in infecting microorganisms by light-induced reactions, generically called photosensitization reactions. Photosensitization occurs when PS absorb light and transfer its energy to neighboring molecules, such that light converts into chemical reactivity [11-13]. After the end of a photocycle, PS returns to the ground state and may absorb another photon. The photophysical step that allows the formation of an efficient PS is the intersystem crossing (ICS), that converts singlet into triplet species, which are long lived and highly reactive (Figure 2) [13].

The photooxidation of biomolecules is responsible for changes in their structure and function. It can occur by two main mechanisms: electron transfer reaction (excited states are stronger oxidizing and reducing species than their respective ground states) catalyzing the formation of various radical species, including the highly reactive hydroxyl radical. These reactions are classified as type I. The photooxidation can also occur through energy transfer with molecular oxygen, catalyzing the formation of singlet oxygen, a mechanism called type II (Figure 2) [14].

It is considered that type II mechanism is the most relevant effector of photooxidation, because type I reactions usually lead to PS degradation [15]. However, in biological systems, there usually is shifts between these two mechanisms (type I versus type II), for several reasons, including local concentrations of oxygen and of reducing species, interaction of PS with other biomolecules and PS aggregation [17-21].

Free radicals and singlet oxygen have different reactivity towards biological targets, but both can react with them [14,22]. Singlet oxygen mainly reacts by addition to double bonds (Figure 2). The efficiency of photo-induced cell killing seems to depend more on the amount of PS that is located in the intracellular environment and on the specific intracellular location than on the *in-vitro* photophysical efficiency of the PS [23-28].

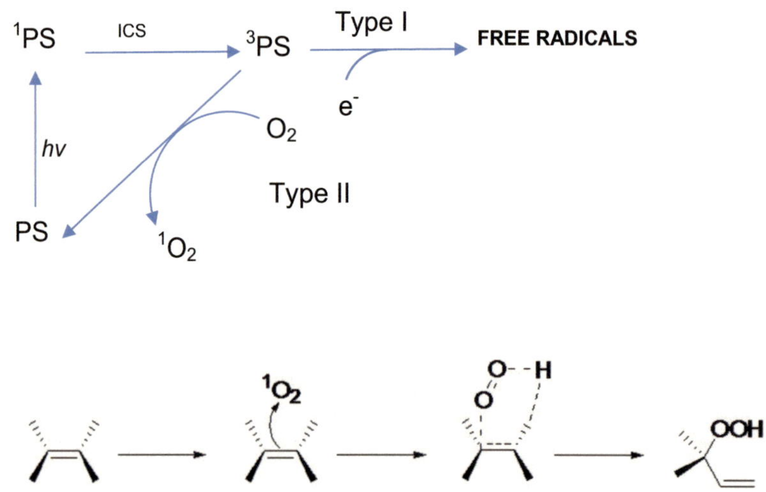

Figure 2. Top scheme. Main mechanisms of photooxidation. PS, ^{1}PS, ^{3}PS: photosensitizer ground state, singlet and triplet species, respectively. O_2 and $^1O_2$ correspond to oxygen in the ground state and the singlet excited state, respectively. *hv* represents light absorption at a specific wavelength and ICS is intersystem crossing between the singlet and the triplet states. Bottom scheme: Reaction of singlet oxygen with a double bond forming a hydroperoxide, which is the main reaction of singlet oxygen with lipid double bonds.

PDT combines three components to kill cells (eukaryotic and prokaryotic) and non-cellular organisms such as virus: PS, light and oxygen. PS is applied either topically or systemically and it must incorporate in the biological tissue to be treated, which is exposed to light in the presence of oxygen. The PS needs to absorb efficiently the incident light and form triplet species [14]. There are hundreds of PS molecules that have been synthesized and tested. In Figure 3 we present the chemical structures of few that are worth commenting in this chapter, because they either have been involved on treatments of leishmania or have the potential to be. Methylene Blue (MB) and Crystal Violet (CV) are positively charged and low-cost photosensitizers that enter cells and react mainly by type II and type I mechanisms, respectively. MB has been used to treat several diseases including leishmania [27], while CV should be tested since it has a great potential as a positively dye that mainly accumulates in mitochondria [28]. Riboflavin (RF, vitamin B2), is a natural PS that absorbs in the 400-500 nm region and has been used for blood disinfection as well as in test-tube leishmania killing assays [29]. Hypericin is another natural PS that is extract from St. John's wort and has been used in several PDT studies [30]. ALA is the first compound in the porphyrin synthesis pathway. Protoporphyrin IX is

http://dx.doi.org/10.5772/57456

formed intracellularly after the treatment with ALA and/or methyl ALA and is the most used PS in leishmaniasis treatment [31-35]. Chlorophyll is the main pigment of photosynthesis and their derivatives hold promising potential as low-cost PS [36].

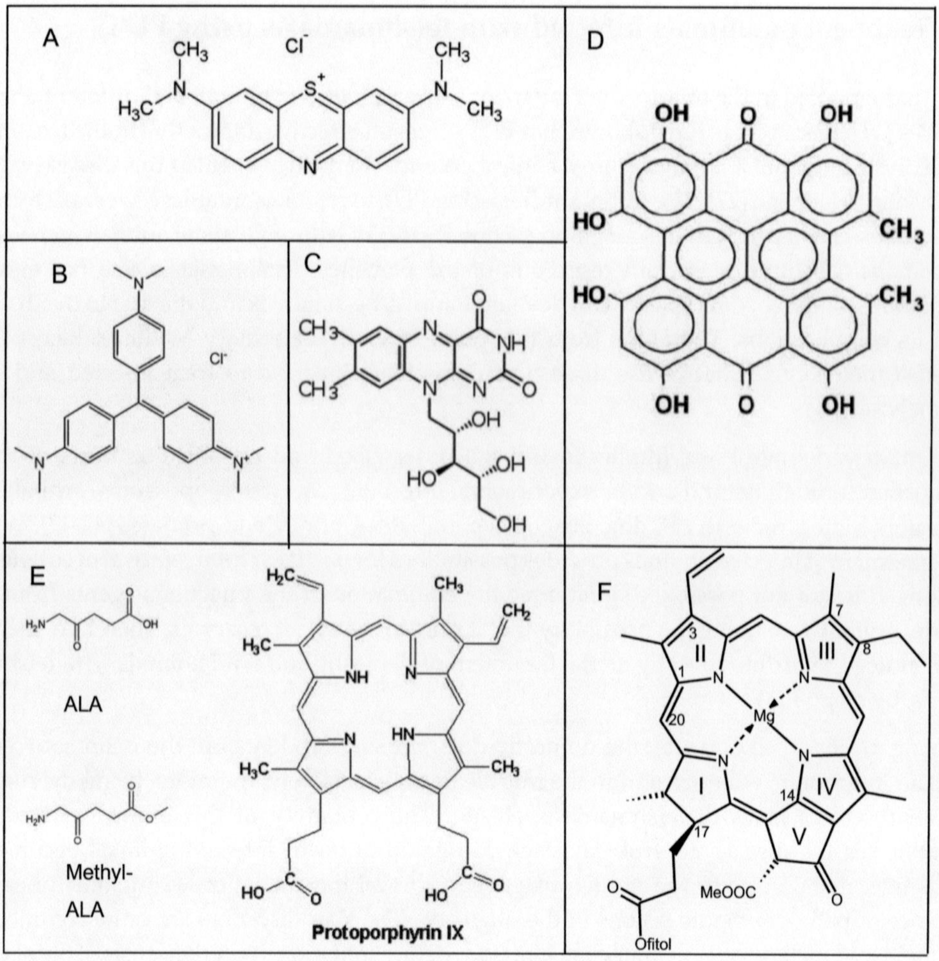

Figure 3. Molecular structure of relevant photosensitizers in PDT: (A) methylene blue; (B) crystal violet; (C) Riboflavin, (D) Hypericin; (E) ALA, Methl ALA and Protoporphyrin IX; (F) chlorophyll.

The ability of PDT to act as an anti-microbial treatment, i.e., to treat fungi, bacteria and virus infections, is well described in the scientific literature [37-39]. Many research groups have developed experiments that prove the effectiveness of this therapy for a large number of diseases, including certain parasitic diseases [40]. *In vitro* studies of photoinduced inactivation of parasites have been used to unravel important aspects of the therapy including, the action mechanisms, light dosimetry, structural-activity relationships, PS uptake and localization. PDT has been used in the treatment of human and experimental murine leishmaniasis of the Old and New Word. Despite the small number of cases related, literature highlights the ability of PDT to deliver better results compared to traditional treatments, emphasizing its better effectiveness in leading to amastigote-free lesions in a shorter time periods, in addition to its excellent esthetic results.

4. Treatment of animals infected with leishmaniasis using PDT

PDT has emerged in the treatment of cutaneous diseases among human and different animal species [41]. Researchers have shown that PDT offers an effective alternative in the treatment of CL indicating that it also has a great clinical potential in the treatment of this disease within Veterinary Medicine [27]. The initial studies using PDT to treat leishmaniasis were performed in humans and are further described on section 7 [31-35]. Although some animals, especially mammals, constitute important reservoirs of the parasites, leishmaniasis also has clinical importance because some species can develop injuries, become sick and die due to the disease and its complications. Therefore, from this point of view, Veterinary Medicine has special interest, not only to control the disease epidemiology, but also to treat infected and sick animals.

The main vertebrate hosts (domestic and wild) described and classified as hosts of these protozoan through natural and/or experimental infections, are: foxes, opossums, armadillos, anteaters, sloths, rodents, cat, dog, goat, sheep, buffaloes, horses and primates [42-47]. While the treatment of infected animals provides possibilities for partial or total removal of cutaneous lesions, it is still not possible to guarantee the elimination of the infectious agents from the carrier animal, remaining the possibility that it remains as a host reservoir. Therefore, there is a great need to further investigate the treatment of domestic and wild animals with leishmaniasis, by using PDT.

Among all involved animals, the domestic dog and some rodents are the main sources of human infection in America and in the Middle East, respectively; therefore, being the majors urban reservoir hosts of leishmaniasis [44,48]. The proximity of this animal to humans complicates the disease control. The lack of identification of infected animals becomes a challenge, mainly due to the numerous generic clinical manifestations, and sometimes the absence of pathognomonic lesions in the dogs [49]. The skin disorders are quite common in animals, and include opaque hair coat, alopecia, depigmentation, hyperkeratosis of nasal plan and digital cushions, mucocutaneous ulcers, intradermal nodules, onychogryphosis and excessive flaking [50,51] but the most common presentation of the cutaneous disease is a symmetrical alopecia accompanied by intense flaking with silvery appearance that often starts on the head and spreads to other parts of the body [52]. However, these symptoms are sometimes not correlated with leishmaniasis. Regarding the condition of the dogs as reservoir hosts in the epidemiology of the disease, clinical treatment is not recommended so far [51], making euthanasia of the infected animals mandatory in many countries [50] and keeping the controversial discussion among public health authorities, animal protectors and veterinarians [53,54]. Despite the importance of dogs in the epidemiology of the disease, the most used animal model and the one that has shown success in the treatment of the cutaneous disease are rodents, mainly mice and hamsters.

Several studies demonstrated the possibility of using PDT in animal models, especially on murines. In 2007 *Akilov et al.* reported an evaluation of the use of ALA (precursor of PpIX) in TL caused by Old World species in ears of Balb/c mice [55]. *Akilov et al.* also highlighted the action of ALA-PDT in murine with leishmaniasis compared to a control group treated with ALA [56]. The results showed a significant reduction of 24.5 folds in the parasite load compared with the control group. Nevertheless, they observed vascular damage in ears of the PDT-ALA group probably caused by PDT. According to the authors, a wide inflammatory and immunologic response was noted in Balb/c ears of ALA-PDT group, which correlated with the expressive decrease of parasite load and with the healing of the tissue.

Despite ALA, other classes of photosensitizers already widely used in PDT began to be tested. The phenothiazine 3,7-bis(di-n-butylamino)phenothiazin-5-ium bromide (PPA904) was tested by *Akilov et al.* in mice [57]. Ears of female Balb/c were infected with metacyclic parasites of *Leishmania* sp. Following infection, mice were treated with PPA904 cream and irradiated with a broad band light source. They tested the PS concentration, time of uptake and absorption site in the ear. The results showed that PPA904 applied during at least 90 min in consecutive sessions of PDT decreased parasite load around 5.2 log compared to the controls groups. However, PPA904 application also lead to skin irritation. Another study was carried out with female Balb/c infected with *L. major* parasites expressing green fluorescent protein (GFP) to monitor the parasitic load and the efficacy of PDT [58]. PPA904 was applied in the ears of the mice and the parasitic load was compared with control group (only infected). The fluorescence of GFP parasite in the ear of mice after the PPA-PDT decrease significantly, about 80%, compared to control group. The authors emphasized that this result was obtained after more than one PDT session.

*Peloi et al.*chosen a different murine, which is also considered an appropriate model to develop leishmaniasis caused by some New World *Leishmania* spp. Hamsters were used to investigate the effectiveness of PDT with methylene blue (MB) photosensitizer [59]. A light-emitting diode (LED) was chosen as light source. The footpads of hamsters were infected with *Leishmania* sp. The control presented an increase in thickness throughout the treatment. An opposite reaction occurred in the group A and B treated with oil/water lotion MB+LED and aqueous solution MB+LED, respectively. Statistically significant reductions on the thickness of the footpad and parasitic load were observed.

The scientific reports in PDT-treated animal models mentioned in this chapter show similar results to those reported in humans. In other words, PDT is capable to treat infected wounds reducing the parasitic load. In some cases, the complete disappearance of the parasite from tissue is achieved. Other aspect to highlight is its ability to inactivate both Old and New world *Leishmania* spp. Details of parameters from scientific studies using PDT on Old World and New World TL in murine models are described in table 1. However, treatment conditions of infected animals out of experimental controlled environment have not been described. Therefore, PDT has to become a more common procedure to be used in the clinical practice of Veterinary Medicine. It certainly has the unfulfilled potential to become a therapeutic alternative in veterinary medicine, and to help controlling the parasitic cycle in humans.

Author/year	Parasite	Animal	Photosensitizer	Uptake	Light source	Exposure time	wavelength	Irradiance	Fluence	Results
Akilov *et al*. 2007	*L. major*	BALB/c mice (age: 6–8 weeks) - ear	ALA (20%)	4 hours	Diode laser	#	635 nm	66 mW/cm2	50 J/cm2	1) Significant reduction in the parasitic load 2) Large tissue damage 3) Decrease of macrophages, increased levels of interleukin 6 in tissue
Akilov *et al*. 2009	*L. major*	BALB/c mice (age: 6–8 weeks) - ear	PPA 904 - 3,7-bis(N,N-dibutylamino) phenothiazinium bromide	30, 60 ,90 e 120 minutes	LC-122 non-coherent light source + broadband optical filte + fibra otica (665 ±15 nm)	#	665 ±15 nm at	50 mW/cm2	50 J/cm2 (50mW/cm2).	1) Best result of the treatment and cure in 90 min 2) Penetration of the PPA is dependent on time 3) Decreased parasite load and ulcer with 4 days of treatment
Latorre - Esteves *et al*. 2010	*L. major GFP*	BALB/c mice (age: 6–8 weeks) - ear	PPA 904 - 3,7-bis(N,N-dibutylamino) phenothiazinium bromide	60 minutes	LC-122A,non-coherent light source +fiber optic (665 ±15 nm)	11,6 minutes	665 ± 15 nm	30 mW/cm2	21 J/cm2	1) Significant reduction in parasite load in the ear of the animal compared to controls 2) After 4 days of PDT treatment appeared more effective 3) Decrease of parasites in limiting dilution
Peloi *et al*. 2011	*L. amazonensis*	Hamsters - footpad	CG - lotion MB and water+MB GA -oil/water (O/W) lotion 10 nM AM GB - aqueous solution 10nM AM	10 minutes	LED light system using 6 units (in series) that emit red light (663 nm)	1 hour	665 nm	5 mW/cm2	12 J/cm2	1) Significant reduction in parasite load in groups A and B 2) After 6 weeks of treatment absence of lesions in the GA and presence in 13.3% in the animals in GB 3) Decrease the size of the footpat in the group A and B compared to control

CG: control group / GA: group A / GB: group B

Table 1. Parameters used in PDT to the treatment of Old World tegumentary leishmaniasis and New World tegumentary leishmaniasis in murine models

5. Vector control using PDT

The field of insect photo-killing by administration of photosensitizer molecules and light exposition (usually sun light) is one of the areas of possible PDT application that has received small attention of the scientific community [60-63]. The few studies, which were mainly reported by Jori and co-authors, sustain that there is indeed great potential on this area. There are reports showing that the PS activity is a function of its log P_{OW} value and of its amphiphilic character [62,63]. PDT was also shown to be efficient for Larva control of dengue vector *Aedes aegypti* [60]. However, there is no scientific report on the use of PDT to control the vector (*Phlebotomus* sand flies) and its larva, which are responsible for the transmission the leishmania parasites. It is also important to emphasize that the amount of information available concerning larva development of phlebotomine sand flies is much less than what is known for the mosquitoes whose control have been studied by PDT. Nevertheless, for the matter of bringing new ideas to the field of *Leishmania* treatment, the concentration of photosensitizers that are needed to neutralize larva and to kill those mosquitoes is several orders of magnitude smaller than the concentrations of chemical insecticides, which are currently used for vectors control, causing great disturbance in the whole ecosystem. Therefore, it is up to our community to develop and test strategies to control vectors of *Leishmania* parasites using PDT.

6. Blood purification

The purification of blood products is critical to avoid disease transmittance through blood transfusion. Although this is not the main route of transmission of leishmaniasis, it is a possible one, and cases have been reported in the literature [64]. The focus of the disinfection strategy is to kill microorganisms without harming the cellular and plasma components. PDT offers great potential to be successful in blood disinfection, because it is a multi–target strategy, i.e, the reactive species that are formed (after light absorption and photosensitization reaction) are effective against viruses, bacteria, fungi, and parasites [37-40]. This strategy has even been proved effective to promote pathogen inactivation in the presence of fragile blood components, such as stem cells from blood of embryo's cord [65-68]. It is better than UV treatments, because it does not cause direct damage to blood components. Several PS have been used for blood disinfection including MB, CV and RF (Figure 2). Molecules that have intracellular targets such as MB and CV can be used to treat plasma derivatives but not whole cell blood, because they will cause extensive hemolysis. RF, however, is an aqueous based photosensitiser, which do not enter cells and can be used to disinfect whole blood derivatives. RF reacts either by type I or by type II mechanisms and is already in use. Several companies commercialize kits for blood and plasma decontamination, like Macopharma, whose technology for plasma decontamination is based on MB photosensitization (http://www.macopharmausa.com/). In the case of leishmaniasis, parasites remain mostly in the intracellular environment, except when they are in transit from a lysed cell to infect a macrophage or other phagocytic cell. We could think of using PDT to remove parasites in the plasma or to develop strategies to target PSs to destroy only infected cells of contaminated blood.

7. Photodynamic therapy on the treatment of old world tegumentary Leishmaniasis

There are several reports on the literature dealing with the treatment of leishmaniasis by PDT [5,6,33,34]. The first report was conducted by Enk's group in 2003 [5,6]. Both studies reported the use ALA and MAL, combined with red light. These authors performed the treatment of 32 TL lesions from 11 Israeli patients. The diagnostic was accomplished by verifying the amastigote presence in direct smear from the lesions [5]. This work showed that about 96% of the lesions healed, leaving some mild scars and pigment in place of the old lesions. Just one lesion presented amastigotes forms after PDT. Gardlo *et al.* published the case of a patient, aged 34, with CL confirmed by histology. According to the authors, the patient developed resistance to the treatment with sodium stibogluconate and presented 10 lesions, which were treated five times with PDT and five times with paromomycin sulfate ointment [6]. The result obtained is similar to the previous work and showed that the five ulcers treated with PDT healed without signs of amastigotes, while two ulcers treated with paromomycin partially responded to the drug, one of them did not respond and two lesions were shown to have no amastigotes. The ulcers that did not responded to paromomycin ointment were subsequently treated with PDT successfully.

Asilian and Davami developed a placebo-controlled, randomized clinical trial that provided definitive evidence of the efficacy of PDT in the treatment of CL [34]. 60 patients with confirmed CL by clinical and parasitological diagnosis were separated in 3 groups with different treatments. Group 1 was treated with PDT once a week, group 2 received twice daily paramomycin plus methylbenzethonium chloride ointment and in group 3 was used a paraffin-based ointment without active ingredients with same application time of the group 2. During four weeks, the groups received the treatments described above. At the end of the study healing was present in 93.5% of the patients of group 1, 41.2% of group 2 and 13.3% of group 3. At the same time, 100%, 64.7% and 20% of the lesions had parasitological cure in group 1, 2 and 3, respectively.

Other studies accomplished in Iran and German corroborated with the results described above. According to the authors, PDT showed to have the capacity to treat wounds caused by Old Word *Leishmania* species. We emphasize that most of the reports claim that this therapeutical modality can achieve results above 90% healing of wounds, however, a caveat must be held since some of these studies indicate that not all healed wounds become free of parasite [35,56]. The mechanism of ALA PDT in the case of leishmaniasis was shown to be due to the killing of infected host-cell killing (macrophages) instead of direct parasite killing (see further discussion about this issue on section 8).

One CL case of the New World leishmaniasis is described in the literature. Song *et al.* reported the case of a Brazilian patient presenting cutaneous leishmaniasis confirmed by smear stained by Giemsa. PDT was carried out using MB. In this specific case because of ethical concerns of possible development of evolution to mucocutaneou disease, the patient received at the same time a low dose of pentavalent antimony and PDT. The patient had two ulcers. One receive PDT and the other was only being treated with the low-dose pentavalent [27]. The treatment

http://dx.doi.org/10.5772/57456

showed 100% of cure in both lesions, but the lesion treated with PDT presented a faster wound recovery compared to the antimony alone (Table 2).

Author/year	Parasite	Photosensitizer	Uptake	Light source	wavelength	Irradiance	Fluence	Treatment sessions	Frequency	Patientes	Results
Enk *et al.* 2003	*L. major*	ALA*	4h	Curelight, Photocure	570-670 nm	150 mW/cm²	100 J/cm²	once weekly	until parasite was not detectable in the direct smear	11	96% cure 1 patiente with 1 lesion presented parasite
Gardlo *et al.* 2003	*Suspeita L. donovani*	MAL	5h	Curelight, Photocure	570-670 nm	150 mW/cm²	75 J/cm²	1° Twice weekly (12 weeks) + 2° once weekly (4 weeks)	1° 12 weeks / 2° 4 weeks	1	100% cure
Asilian et al. 2006	*L. major*	ALA	4h	Omnilux(visible red light)	633 nm	#	100 J/cm²	once weekly	4 weeks	20	93,5% cure
Ghaffarifar *et al.* 2006	*L. major*	ALA	4h	Red light	570-670 nm	150 mW/cm²	100 J/cm²	once weekly	4 weeks	5	100% cure
Sohl *et al.* 2007	*L. tropica*	MAL	3h	Waldman PDT 1200L	580-700 nm	#	100 J/cm²	once weekly	1 to 4 weeks	1	100% cure
Song *et al.* 2011	*L. amazonensis*	0.5 % Methilene Blue	#	RL 50 - LED	570-750 nm	35 mW/cm²	20 J/cm²	once weekly	4 weeks	1	100% cure

* First compound in the porphyrin synthesis pathway, precursor of Protoporphyrin IX (PpIX)

Table 2. Parameters used in PDT on the treatment of Old World and New World tegumentary leishmaniasis in humans

This brief account of the use of PDT for the treatment of CL demonstrates the ability of this therapeutic modality and encourages its use. It also stimulates research in the pursuit of new protocols with new PS, which could ensure not only healing but also clinical and parasitological cure of these patients.

Details of parameters from scientific studies using PDT on the treatment of Old World and New World tegumentary leishmaniasis in humans are described in Table 2.

8. Photodynamic therapy — *In vitro* tests in species which cause Tegumentary Leishmaniasis

The effectiveness of PDT on CL treatment was first conducted in humans and in animal models. *In vitro* tests began less than ten years ago to allow testing of PDT parameters like the efficiency of different types of photosensitizers, their respective uptakes and concentrations and accumulation sites.

Sujoy Dutta *et al.* began *in vitro* studies with the New World specie, *L. amazonensis* in 2005 [69]. The first part of that work evaluated *Leishmania* transfectants expressing GFPs. The PS tested was aluminum phthalocyanine chloride (AlPhCl) in different concentrations. The principal factor tested was the light-mediated cytolysis when cells were in the presence or pre-incubated with the AlPhCl. In the dark there was no phototoxicity for both promastigote and amastigote forms of the parasite. The opposite effect occurred when the photosensitizer received red light illumination, showing that promastigotes appear to be more sensible than amastigote forms. In addition, the loss of fluorescence of the GFP parasites indicated cell death. On the second part of the study, J774 cells (cell line immortalized murine Balb/c monocyte/macrophage) were tested at the same conditions reported above. The authors observed that they were 10-20 fold more resistant than promatigotes. According to the authors, the photosensitized *Leishmania* cells are susceptible to cytolysis, probably due to the generation of reactive oxidative species after illumination, an indicative of inefficiency of their antioxidant mechanisms. ALA did not induce protoporphyrin IX (PpIX) production in the *Leishmania* cells, because of a deficiency in the heme biosynthetic pathway in this parasite [57, 70].

Tests with other phthalocyanines were developed by Pinto *et al.* using species of Old and New world *Leishmanias*, *L. major* and *L. braziliensis*. The parasites were incubated with aluminum phthalocyanine tetrasulfonate (AlPcS4) at different concentrations and irradiated with a GaAlAs diode laser (λ= 659 nm, 40 mW). The experiments indicated a significant reduction of viable parasites in both species compared to controls, however *L. braziliensis* demonstrated higher mortality than *L. major* [71].

In Brazil, Song *et al.* performed tests to understand mechanism of action of PDT using MB in a case report. Promastigotes of *L. amazonensis* were incubated with different concentrations of MB, washed with PBS and illuminated using a home-built LED light source with a wavelength of maximum emission at λ= 650 nm. After the irradiation, cell survival was determined with MTT assay that detected cell toxicity after irradiation of light in the presence MB. There was an increase in the phototoxicity with the increase in the MB concentration indicating a concentration-dependent response [27]. Differently from PPIX induced by ALA and MAL, MB has parasite intracellular target. In fact, PS seems to be localized in mitochondria (Figure 4).

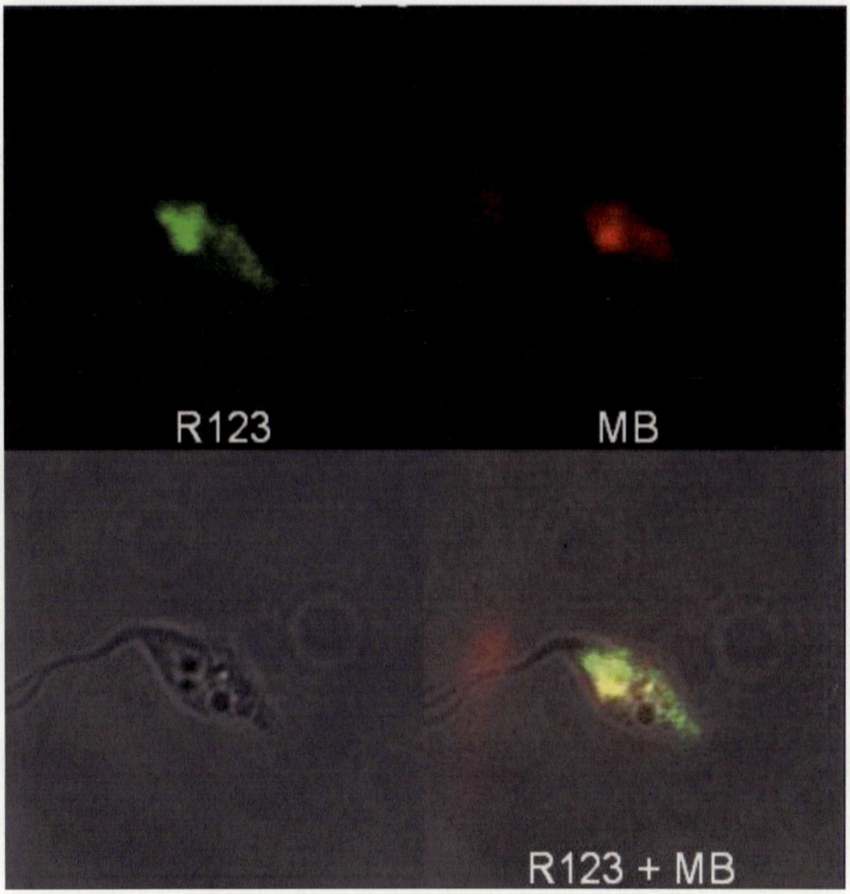

Figure 4. Top: Rhodamine 123 and Methylene blue fluorescences in promastigote parasites of *L. amazonensis.* Bottom: transmission image and colocalization of R123, MB and transmission images.

Other researchers have investigated the susceptibility of *L. amazonensis* regarding PDT. In order to verify the lethality of phenothiazine's derivatives on the promastigote forms, Barbosa *et al* [72] tested TBO (toluidine blue O), MB and a TBO/MB solutions. Irradiation was performed with a diode laser (λ= 660 nm, P= 40 mW). They tested different PS incubation time (5 and 60 min) and two energy densities (4.2 and 8.4 J/cm^2). The results showed a representative decrease on the viability of *L.amazonensis* promastigotes for all treated groups in comparison to their controls. The authors did not find statistical differences between the dyes, but reported that the best result was observed with TBO.

Dutta *et al.* published an article that described the use of a combination of photosensitizers. Uroporphyrin (URO1) and aluminum phthalocyanine chloride (AlPhCl) were used in uroporphyrinogenic mutants of *L. amazonensis* (RAT/ BA/ 74 /LV78) 12-1 clone, transfected with pX-alad and p6,5-PBGD [73]. This transfected *Leishmania* is able to absorb ALA and turns it into URO 1. The authors evaluated the combination of both drugs into promastigotes with and without irradiation of red light. Results showed photolysis of the irradiated parasites with both photosensitizers whereas non-irradiated parasites showed no damage.

Hernández *et al.* published another study that compared encapsulated chloroaluminum phthalocyanine (CLAlPc) in liposomes (UDL-CLAlPc) and free in solution. The experiments were conducted with two species of New World *Leishmania* in promastigote and amastigote forms and in THP1 cells. The experiments tried to verify the ability of the photosensitizer in reaching the *Leishmania* inside THP1 host cell. According to the authors, the UDL-ClAlPc photosensitizer was almost 10 times more photoactive than free ClAlPc on THP-1 cells as well as on promastigotes and with intracellular amastigotes of *L. chagasi* and *L. panamensis* [74].

9. Conclusions

- First reports of cutaneous leishmaniasis using PDT were performed in humans;
- Treatments using porphyrin precursors, ALA and MAL, showed positive results on the cure of patients with CL;
- The low-cost phenothiazine methylene blue and red light can be used to treat patients with CL;
- More than one PDT session is necessary to achieve wound healing.
- Both New and Old World *Leishmania* can be treated with PDT.
- Murine models of infection such as Balb/c and hamster show to be appropriate for PDT studies of CL treatment.
- *In vitro* tests demonstrate that Old and New world *Leishmania* species can be used to test new photosensitizers and to establish structure/activity relationships.
- PDT also has the potential to control leishmaniasis transmission by the treatment of vectors and infected animal reservoirs, although the development of these potentials will need further investigation.

http://dx.doi.org/10.5772/57456

Author details

Debora P. Aureliano[1,2], Martha S. Ribeiro[1], José Angelo Lauletta Lindoso[2,3], Fabio C. Pogliani[3], Fábio P. Sellera[4], Dennis Song[3,5] and Mauricio S. Baptista[5]

1 Centro de Lasers e Aplicações (CLA)/ IPEN- CNEN, Brazil

2 Laboratório de Soroepidemiologia (LIM38-HC-FMUSP) e Instituto de Medicina Tropical de São Paulo da Universidade de São Paulo, Brazil

3 Instituto de Infectologia Emilio Ribas-SES-SP, Brazil

4 Departamento de Clínica Médica, Faculdade de Medicina Veterinária e Zootecnia da Universidade de São Paulo, Brazil

5 Departamento de Bioquímica, Instituto de Química, Universidade de São Paulo, Brazil

References

[1] Farrell JD, World Class Parasites-Volume 4: Leishmania. Kluwer Academic Publisher, Boston, 2002.

[2] Peacock CS, Berriman M. Comparative genomic analysis of three Leishmania species that cause diverse human disease. *Nature Genetics* 2007, 39, 839.

[3] de Almeida MC, Vilhena V, Barral A, Barral-Netto M. Leishmanial infection: analysis of its first steps. A review. *Mem Inst Oswaldo Cruz* 2003, 98, 861.

[4] Santos DO, Coutinho CER, Madeira MF, Bottino CG, Vieira RT, Nascimento SB, Bernardino A, Bourguignon SC, Corte-Real S, Pinho RT, Rodrigues CR, Castro, HC. Leishmaniasis treatment—a challenge that remains: a review. *Parasitol Res* 2008, 103, 1.

[5] Enk CD, Fritsch C, Jonas F, Nasereddin A, Ingber A, Jaffe CL, Ruzicka T. Treatment of cutaneous leishmaniasis with photodynamic therapy. *Arch Dermatol American Medical Association*; 2003;139(4), 432.

[6] Gardlo K, Horska Z, Enk CD, Rauch L, Megahed M, Ruzicka T, Fritsch C. Treatment of cutaneous leishmaniasis by photodynamic therapy. *J Am Acad Dermatol*. 2003, 48(6), 893.

[7] Van der Snoek EM, Robinson DJ, van Hellemond JJ, Neumann HAM. A review of photodynamic therapy in cutaneous leishmaniasis. *J Eur Acad Dermatol Venereol* 2008, 22(8), 918.

[8] Demidova TN, Hamblin MR. Photodynamic therapy targeted to pathogens. *Int J Immunopathol Pharmacol.* 2011,17(3), 245.

[9] Tardivo JP, Del Giglio A, Oliveira CS, Gabrielli DS, Junqueira HC, Tada DB, Severino D, Turchiello R, Baptista MS. Methylene Blue in Photodynamic Therapy: From Basic Mechanisms to Clinical Applications. *Photodyag Photodyn Ther* 2005, 2/3, 175.

[10] Tesh RB. Control of zoonotic visceral leishmaniasis: is it time to change strategies? *Am J Trop Med Hyg.* 1995, 52(3), 287.

[11] Brown SB, Brown EA, Walker I. The present and future role of photodynamic therapy in cancer treatment. *The Lancet Oncology* 2004, 5, 497.

[12] Allison RR, Downie GH, Cuenca R, Hu X-H, Childs CJH, Sibata CH. *Photodiagn Photodyn Ther* 2004, 1, 27.

[13] Wilkinson F, Helman WP, Ross AB. Rate Constants for the Decay and Reactions of the Lowest Electronically Excited Singlet State of Molecular Oxygen in Solution. An Expanded and Revised Compilation *J Phys Chem* 1993, 22, 113.

[14] Foote CS. Mechanisms of photosensitized oxidations. *Science* 1968, 162, 963.

[15] Dougherty TJ. Photochemistry in the Treatment of Cancer. *Adv Photochem* 1992, 17, 275.

[16] Castano AP, Mroz P, Hamblin MR. Photodynamic therapy and anti-tumour immunity *Nature Rev* 2006, 6, 535.

[17] Junqueira HC, Severino D, Dias LG, Gugliotti M, Baptista MS. Modulation of the Methylene Blue Photochemical Properties Based on the Adsorption at Aqueous Micelle Interfaces. *Phys Chem Chem Phys* 2002, 4, 2320.

[18] Severino D, Junqueira HC, Gabrielli DS, Gugliotti M, Baptista MS. Influence of Negatively Charged Interfaces on the Ground and Excited State Properties of Methylene Blue *Photochem Photobiol* 2003, 77, 459.

[19] Gabrieli D, Belisle E, Severino D, Kowaltowski AJ, Baptista MS Binding, aggregation and photochemical properties of methylene blue in mitochondrial suspensions *Photochem Photobiol* 2004, 79, 227.

[20] Baptista MS, Indig GL. Effect of BSA Binding on Photophysical Photochemical Properties of Triarylmethane Dyes. *J Phys Chem B* 1998, 102, 4678.

[21] Baptista MS, Indig GL. Mechanism of Photobleaching of Ethyl Violet Non-Covalently Bound to Bovine serum Albumin *Chem Comm* 1997, 18, 1791.

[22] David R. Kearns. Physical and chemical properties of singlet molecular oxygen, *Chem Rev* 1971, 71 (4), 395.

[23] Pavani C, Uchoa AF, Oliveira CS, Iamamoto Y, Baptista MS. Effect of zinc insertion and hydrophobicity on the membrane interactions and PDT activity of porphyrin photosensitizers *Photochem Photobiol Sci* 2009, 8, 233.

[24] Pavani C, IamamotoY, Baptista MS. Mechanism and Efficiency of Cell Death of Type II Photosensitizers: Effect of Zinc Chelation, *Photochem Photobiol* 2012, 88, 774.

[25] Garcez AS, Núñez SC, Baptista MS, Daghastanli NA, Itri R, Hamblin MR, Ribeiro MS. Antimicrobial mechanisms behind photodynamic effect in the presence of hydrogen peroxide. *Photochem Photobiol Sci* 2011, 10, 483.

[26] Uchoa AF, Oliveira CS, Baptista MS. Relationship between structure and photoactivity of porphyrins derived from protoporphyrin IX. *J Porphyr Phthaloc* 2010, 14, 832.

[27] Song D, Lindoso JA, Oyafuso LK, Hatsumi E, Kanashiro Y, Cardoso JL, Uchoa AF, Tardivo JP, Baptista MS. Photodynamic therapy using methylene blue to treat cutaneous leishmaniasis. *Photomed Laser Surg* 2011, 29, 711.

[28] Oliveira C, Turchiello R, Kowaltowski AJ, Indig GL, Baptista MS. Major determinants of photoinduced cell kill: subcellular localization versus photosensitization efficiency *Free Radic Biol Med* 2011, 51, 824.

[29] Silva AV, López-Sánchez A, Rivas L, Baptista MS; Orellana G. Molecular Engineering of Riboflavin Derivatives for Enhanced Photodynamic Activity against Leishmania. *Tetrahedron*, submitted.

[30] Tardivo JP, Baptista MS. Treatment of Osteomyelitis in the Feet of Diabetic Patients by Photodynamic Antimicrobial Chemotherapy *Photomed Laser Surg* 2009, 27, 145.

[31] Gondim RMF, Vieira VCC, Veras MV, Ferreira MA, Caldini ETEG, Muñoz DR, Baptista MS. Protoporphyrin fluorescence induced by methyl–ALA in skin healing, *Photodiagn Photodyn Ther* in press.

[32] Kosaka S, Akilov OE, O'Riordan K, Hasan T. A Mechanistic Study of delta-Aminolevulinic Acid-Based Photodynamic Therapy for Cutaneous Leishmaniasis. *J Inv Dermatol* 2007, 127, 1546.

[33] Bristow C-A, Hudson R, Paget TA, Boyle RW. Potential of cationic porphyrins for photodynamic treatment of cutaneous Leishmaniasis. *Photodiagn Photodyn Ther* 2006, 3, 162.

[34] Asilian A, Davami M. Comparison between the efficacy of photodynamic therapy and topical paromomycin in the treatment of Old World cutaneous leishmaniasis: a placebo-controlled, randomized clinical trial. *Clin Exp Dermatol* 2006, 31(5), 634.

[35] Ghaffarifar F, Jorjani O, Mirshams M, Miranbaygi MH, Hosseini ZK.Photodynamic therapy as a new treatment of cutaneous leishmaniasis. *East Mediterr Health J* 2006, 12(6), 902.

[36] Bonnett R, Benzie R, Grahn MF, Salgado A, Valles MA. Photodynamic therapy photosensitizers derived from chlorophyll a. *Proc. SPIE* 1994, 2078, 171.

[37] Jori G, Fabris C, Soncin M, Ferro S, Coppellotti O, Dei D, Fantetti L, Chiti G, Roncucci G. Photodynamic therapy in the treatment of microbial infections: basic principles and perspective applications. *Lasers Surg Med* 2001, 34(1), 18.

[38] Wainwright M. Photodynamic antimicrobial chemotherapy (PACT) *J Antimicrob Chemother*, 1998, 42,13.

[39] Hamblin MR, Hasan T. Photodynamic therapy: a new antimicrobial approach to infectious disease? *Photochem Photobiol Sci* 2004, 3, 436.

[40] Baptista MS, Wainwright M. Photodynamic antimicrobial chemotherapy (PACT) for the treatment of malaria, leishmaniasis and trypanosomiasis. *Braz J Med Biol Res* 2011, 44, 1.

[41] Peplow PV, Chung T-Y, Baxter GD. Photodynamic Modulation of Wound Healing: A Review of Human and Animal Studies. *Photomed Laser Surg* 2012, 30, 118.

[42] Anjili CO, Ngichabe CK, Mbati PA, Lugalia RM, Wamwayi HM, Githure JI. Experimental infection of domestic sheep with culture-derived *Leishmania donovani* promastigotes. *Veter Parasitol*, 1998, 74, 315.

[43] Rey L. Principais grupos de protozoários e metazoários, parasitos do homem e seus vetores. In: Parasitologia. 3 ed. Rio de Janeiro: Guanabara Koogan, 2001. cap.9, p.123.

[44] Lainson R, Ishikawa EAY, Silveira FT. American visceral leishmaniasis: wild animal hosts. *Trans Royal Soc Trop Med Hyg* 2002, 96, 630.

[45] Garg RD, Ravendra A. Animal models for vaccine studies for visceral leishmaniasis. *Indian J Med Res* 2006, 123, 439.

[46] Vedovello FD, Jorge FA, Lonardoni MVC, Teodoro U, Silveira TGV. American cutaneous leishmaniasis in horses from endemic areas in the North-Central Mesoregion of Parana State, Brazil. Zoonoses and Public Health 2008, 55, 149.

[47] Bhattarai NR, Van Der Auwera G, Rijal S, Picado A, Speybroeck N, Khanal B, De Doncker S, DAS ML, Ostyn B, Davies C, Coosemans M., Berkvens D, Boelaert, M, Dujardin JC. Domestic animals and epidemiology of visceral leishmaniasis, *Nepal. Emerg Infect Dis* 2010, 16(2), 231.

[48] Faiman R, Abbasi I, Jaffe C, Motro Y, Nasereddin A, Schnur LF, Torem M, Pratlong F, Dedet JP, Warburg A. A newly emerged cutaneous leishmaniasis focus in northern Israel and two new reservoir hosts of Leishmania major. *PLoS Negl Trop Dis*. 2013, 7(2), 1.

[49] Singh S, Sivakumar R. Recent advances in the diagnosis of leishmaniasis. *J Postgrad Med* 2003, 49, 55.

[50] Ferrer L. Leishmaniasis. In: Kirk RW, Bonagura JD. Kirk's Current Veterinary Therapy XI. Philadelphia: W. B. Saunders, 1992, 266.

[51] Kontos VJ, Koutinas AF. Old world canine leishmaniasis. *Compendium on Continuing Education for the Practing Veterinarian* 1993, 15, 949.

[52] Noli C. Canine leishmaniasis. Waltham Focus, 1999, 9, 16.

[53] Oliveira CI, Teixeira MJ, Gomes R, Barral A, Brodskyn C. Animal models for infectious diseases caused by parasites: Leishmaniasis. *Drug Discovery Today: Disease Models* 2004, 1, 1.

[54] Esteves EL, Akilov OE, Rai1 P, Beverley SM, Hasan T. Monitoring the Efficacy of Antimicrobial Photodynamic Therapy in a Murine Model of Cutaneous Leishmaniasis using *L. major* expressing GFP. *J Biophotonics* 2010, 3, 328.

[55] kilov OE, Kosaka S, O'Riordan K, Hasan T. Parasiticidal effect of delta-aminolevulinic acid-based photodynamic therapy for cutaneous leishmaniasis is indirect and mediated through the killing of the host cells. *Exp Dermatol* 2007, 16, 651.

[56] Sohl S, Kauer F, Paasch U, Simon JC. Photodynamic treatment of cutaneous leishmaniasis. *J Dtsch Dermatol Ges* 2007, 5(2), 128.

[57] Akilov OE, Yousaf W, Lukjan SX, Verma S, Hasan T. Optimization of topical photodynamic therapy with 3,7-bis(di-n-butylamino)phenothiazin-5-ium bromide for cutaneous leishmaniasis. *Lasers Surg Med* 2009, 41(5), 358.

[58] Latorre-Esteves E, Akilov OE, Rai P, Beverley SM, Hasan T. Monitoring the efficacy of antimicrobial photodynamic therapy in a murine model of cutaneous leishmaniasis using L. major expressing GFP. *J Biophotonics* 2010, 3(5-6), 328.

[59] Peloi LS, Biondo CEG, Kimura E, Politi MJ, Lonardoni MVC, Aristides SMA, et al. Photodynamic therapy for American cutaneous leishmaniasis: the efficacy of methylene blue in hamsters experimentally infected with Leishmania (Leishmania) amazonensis. *Exp Parasitol* 2011, 128(4), 353.

[60] Lucantoni L, Magaraggia M, Lupidi G, Ouedraogo RK, Coppellotti O, Esposito F, Fabris C, Jori G, Habluetzel A. Novel, Meso -Substituted Cationic Porphyrin Molecule for Photo-Mediated Larval Control of the Dengue Vector *Aedes aegypti. Plos Neglect Trop Disease* 2011, 5, e1434.

[61] Coppellotti O, Fabris C, Soncin M, Magaraggia M, Camerin M, Jori G, Guidolin L, Porphyrin Photosensitised Processes in the Prevention and Treatment of Water- and Vector-Borne Diseases. *Curr Med Chem* 2012, 19, 808.

[62] Ben Amor T, Jori G. Sunlight-activated insecticides: historical background and mechanisms of phototoxic activity. *Insect Biochem Mol Biol* 2000, 30, 915.

[63] Ben Amor T, Bortolotto L, Jori G. Porphyrins and related compounds as photoactivatable insecticides. 3. Laboratory and field studies. *Photochem Photobiol* 2000, 71,124.

[64] Cardo LJ. Leishmania: risk to the blood supply. *Transfusion* 2006,46(9),1641.

[65] Wainwright M. Pathogen inactivation in blood products. *Curr Med Chem* 2002, 9, 127.

[66] Goodrich RP, Platz MS, Martin CB. Use of visible light to reduce of wavelengths of 500 to 550 nm to reduce the number of pathogen in the blood and blood components. Patent No. US patent 7,498,156 B2. 2009.

[67] Ruane PH, Edrich R, Gampp D, Keil SD, Leonard RL, Goodrich RP. Photochemical inactivation of selected viruses and bacteria in platelet concentrates using riboflavin and light. *Transfusion* 2004, 44, 877.

[68] Trannoy LL, van Hensbergen Y, Lagerberg JWM, Brand A. Photodynamic treatment with mono-phenyl-tri-(N-methyl-4-pyridyl)-porphyrin for pathogen inactivation in cord blood stem cell products. *Transfusion* 2008, 48, 2629.

[69] Dutta S, Ray D, Kolli BK, Chang K-P. Photodynamic sensitization of Leishmania amazonensis in both extracellular and intracellular stages with aluminum phthalocyanine chloride for photolysis in vitro. *Antimicrob Agents Chemother* 2005, 49(11), 4474.

[70] Chang CS, Chang KP. Heme requirement and acquisition by extracellular and intracellular stages of Leishmania mexicana amazonensis. *Mol Biochem Parasitol* 1985, 16(3), 267.

[71] Pinto JG, Soares CP, Mittmann J. Assessment of Leishmania major and Leishmania braziliensis promastigote viability after photodynamic treatment with aluminum phthalocyanine tetrasulfonate (AlPcS4). *J Venom Anim Toxins Incl Trop Dis* 2011, 17(3), 300.

[72] Barbosa AF, Sangiorgi BB, Galdino SL, Barral-Netto M, Pitta IR, Pinheiro AL. Photodynamic antimicrobial chemotherapy (PACT) using phenothiazine derivatives as photosensitizers against Leishmania braziliensis. *Lasers Surg Med* 2012, 44(10), 850.

[73] Dutta S, Waki K, Chang KP. Combinational sensitization of Leishmania with uroporphyrin and aluminum phthalocyanine synergistically enhances their photodynamic inactivation in vitro and in vivo. *Photochem Photobiol* 2012,88(3), 620.

[74] Hernández IP, Montanari J, Valdivieso W, Morilla MJ, Romero EL, Escobar P. In vitro phototoxicity of ultradeformable liposomes containing chloroaluminum phthalocyanine against New World Leishmania species. *J Photochem Photobiol B* 2012, 117, 157.

Chapter 18

Utilization of Composites and Nanocomposites Based on Natural Rubber and Ceramic Nanoparticles as Control Agents for *Leishmania braziliensis*

Aldo Eloizo Job, Alexandre Fioravante de Siqueira,
Caroline Silva Danna, Felipe Silva Bellucci,
Flávio Camargo Cabrera and
Leandra Ernst Kerche Silva

Additional information is available at the end of the chapter

http://dx.doi.org/10.5772/57211

1. Introduction

Nanoscience and Nanothecnology are revolutionizing the world of science and technology, bringing high expectations for technological innovation and the development of areas, such as: aerospace, agribusiness, defense, energy, environment, nanodevices, nanosensors, textiles, biotechnology and health. As part of its application to the health sciences, one of the priority targets are negligible diseases such as Leishmaniasis. In this context, the main objective of this chapter is to show the potential of some classes of ceramic nanoparticles and magnetic and ferroelectric nanocomposites based on natural rubber to modulate the growth of parasite colony of *Leishmania braziliensis* (LB) and to evaluate the toxicity of these materials against mammal cells.

1.1. Nanoscience and nanotechnology applied to neglected diseases

Materials with sizes ranging between $1x10^{-9}$ m and $100x10^{-9}$ m are called nanomaterials regardless of their nature, whether ceramic, polymer, metal or composite. When a material has dimensions on the nanometric scale, its surface properties and volume are differentiated in relation to material properties at a higher dimensional scale. These differences occur because the surface/volume ratio or high aspect ratios are not linear for different dimensional scales and this is in part responsible for the differentiated properties presented by nonascale materials. These differentiated properties can be transferred to other materials by the insertion of the nanomaterials in a matrix of a different nature and nanometric scale not generating a nanocomposite material[1, 2]. In general, the choice of polymer as a matrix or continuous phase is preferable since most have appreciable thermal and mechanical properties. Other properties must also be taken into account, such as hydrophobic/hydrophilic balance, chemical stability and biocompatibility. The nanometric component, generally inorganic, known as the dispersed phase, can provide a higher mechanical, thermal stability and also biological properties [3].

Multidisciplinary researches involving nanoscience, nanotechnology, materials science and engineering, biotechnology and health sciences have gained great strength in recent decades, aiming to increase the number of tools for addressing problems [4]. Each day new materials and methodologies are tested in fighting diseases such as cancer and diseases neglected by the pharmaceutical industry, for example, malaria, leishmaniasis and Chagas' disease. As a result of this innovation, nanocomposites and composites based in natural rubber filled with ceramic particle and nanoparticles can be used in biological applications, aiming at development of devices such as intelligent bandages or agents of control and reduction of parasitic colonies [5].

1.2. *Leishmania braziliensis*

Leishmaniasis is a endemic and parasitic infection caused by the Leishmania genus protozoa. Approximately 1.5 million people were affected by cutaneous leishmaniasis, which reaches 88 countries and has compulsory notification in only 30 of them. Presents itself throughout the Americas and Brazil is the country that has the highest prevalence of cases. Leishmaniasis is a typically tropical disease from Trypanosomatidae family, affecting the skin (cutaneous leishmaniasis, caused by *Leishmania braziliensis* protozoans) or viscera (visceral leishmaniasis, caused by *Leishmania donovani* protozoans), transmitted by the bite of the vector, a phlebotomine sand fly popularly known as "straw mosquito", which utilizes both animals and humans as host [6, 7].

Protozoans of Leishmania genus are unicellular, eukaryotic, heterotrophic, with asexual reproduction by binary fission, and feed via uptake of non-self-generated food. Within the human body, Leishmania protozoans feed of proteins present intracellularly or in blood plasma, and reproduce only within macrophages or similar cells of the immune system[6, 7].

1.3. Ceramic materials

Ceramic materials (in general, oxides, carbides or nitrides) are inorganic, non-metallic substances consisting of metallic and non-metallic elements connected together by covalent and/or ionic bonds. This class of materials displays a set of distinguished physical and chemical properties such as high mechanical strength, high hardness, low tenacity, low thermal and electrical conductivity, high melting point, among others. As a result of the variety of properties that ceramic materials exhibit, these materials has various industrial applications as, for example, bricks, crockery, refractory glass mortars, magnetic materials, electronic devices, fibers, abrasives and aerospace components.

Ceramic phases preparation processes can be classified primarily in chemical and physical routes, and the appropriate processing route selection depends on several aspects associated with the desired final product characteristics, such as desired dimensional scale, final product purity degree, ceramic phase complexity, amount of obtained material, desired physical and chemical properties and cost of the final product. Among several ceramic phases currently known, investigated and used, those with magnetic and ceramic properties with ferroelectric properties can be highlighted, e.g. ferrite with inverse spinel type structure and niobate potassium strontium with tetragonal tungsten bronze structure [8, 9].

1.3.1. Inverse spinel structure and the nickel-zinc ferrite

Among the materials with inverse spinel type structure, is highlighted the Ni-Zn ferrite paramagnetic or superparamagnetic ceramic phase, with cubic symmetry and space group Fd3m unit cell displaying an occupation represented by $(Zn_x^{2+}Fe_{1-x}^{3+})[Ni_x^{2+}Fe_{1+x}^{3+}]O_4^{2-}$ [10, 11]. In this formula the transition metal ions inside the parentheses occupy the tetrahedral site D, while the metal ions inside the brackets occupy the octahedral site E.

Considering the absence of Zn^{2+} cations in the ferrite, the amount of iron in both atomic sites would be equal and their contribution to the magnetic dipole moment would be canceled, and the formation of the material magnetic dipole moment would be responsibility for Ni^{2+} cations. Doping the ferrite with Zn^{2+} cations, there is a migration of Fe^{3+} cations from tetrahedral sites to octahedral sites, unbalancing initial equality of Fe^{3+} cations. Therefore there is an abrupt increase in magnitude of the magnetic dipole moment, because Fe^{3+} and Zn^{2+} cations are contributing to the dipole moment of the material. Thus, it is possible to produce a large number of intrinsically magnetic ferrite by appropriate substitution of metallic ions. Figure 1 presents a representation of a portion of nickel-zinc ferrite with $Ni_{0.5}Zn_{0.5}Fe_2O_4$ stoichiometry and structure type inverse spinel, with octahedral sites FeO_6 or NiO_6 in blue and tetrahedral sites FeO_4 or ZnO_4 in red.

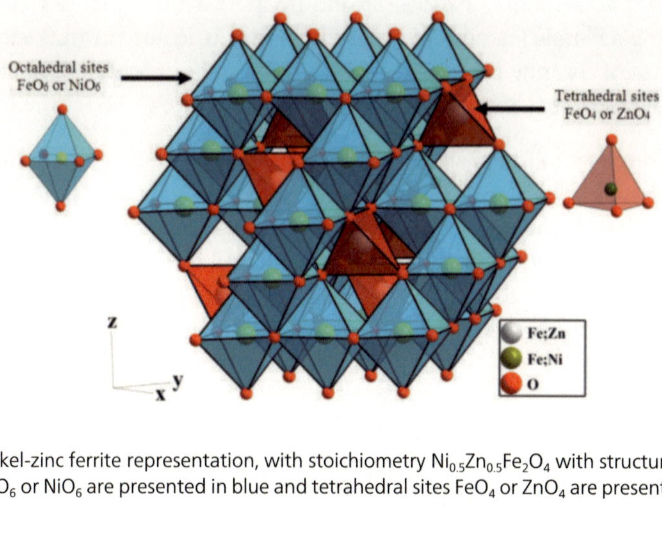

Figure 1. Oxide nickel-zinc ferrite representation, with stoichiometry $Ni_{0.5}Zn_{0.5}Fe_2O_4$ with structure type inverse spinel. Octahedral sites FeO_6 or NiO_6 are presented in blue and tetrahedral sites FeO_4 or ZnO_4 are presented in red.

Regarding magnetic ceramics, Ni-Zn ferrites stand out and attract scientific community interest, due to its high electrical resistivity, differentiated magnetic properties and several technological applications in electronics, telecommunications and biotechnology [8]. They are generally used in cores of transformers and inductors for high-frequency microwave devices, telecommunication systems and radars, high-speed read and recording magnetic heads, cellular telephony, hospital equipments, among others. In microwave-absorption devices (e.g. electromagnetic interference shielding), absorption capacity may be generated/potentiated by altering material magnetic or dielectric properties [12].

1.3.2. TTB structure and potassium-strontium niobate

Tetragonal tungsten bronze (TTB) crystalline structure is considered a structure derived from classic perovskite, where the central octahedral structure BO_6 is converted into three different types of cavities, tetrahedral and pentagonal tunnels similar to those found in perovskite structure which are favorable for substitution by cations, and trigonal tunnels are favorable for substitution by smaller cations and anions [9].

TTB structure can be described by chemical formula $A'_2B'_4C'_4Nb_{10}O_{30}$, where A', B' and C' represent different sites on the structure [13]. Depending on the number of sites available, TTB niobates are natural candidates to host structures, due to the possibility of a wide variety of cation substitutions, similar to what occurs with lead zirconate titanate ($PbZnTiO_3$). B' cavity has a cube-octahedral coordination of oxygen atoms; A' cavities have pentagonal prismatic coordinations, while C' cavities have trigonal prismatic coordinations. The size of these cavities decreases following the order A' > B' > C'. In TTB-type compounds, alkali and alkaline earth metals are located at A' and B' sites, while only cations with small atomic radius such as Li are located in C' site. TTB-type compounds with formula $A_6Nb_{10}O_{30}$, A'= Sr or Ba exhibit semiconductor characteristics which can be incremented when dopants are added.

Niobates with TTB-type structure such as $KSr_2Nb_5O_{15}$, $NaSr_2Nb_5O_{15}$, $KBa_2Nb_5O_{15}$, $NaBa_2Nb_5O_{15}$ and $K_3Li_2Nb_5O_{15}$ have created interest mainly by high anisotropy of the crystal structure. Among TTB-structure oxides, strontium potassium niobate oxide ($KSr_2Nb_5O_{15}$) stands out for being a classic ferroelectric material with Curie temperature close to 430 K[14], belonging to a class of ceramic composites which have great potential application as sensing devices, actuators, memories, transducers, filters and capacitors.

Figure 2 shows a representation of strontium potassium niobate oxide structure, with oxygen and niobium octahedra in blue and yellow dark, pentagonal sites with potassium atoms (K^{1+}), tetrahedral sites with strontium atoms (Sr^{2+}) and vacant trigonal sites. This type of structure has two niobium types, which differ from each other by crystallographic position, multiplicity and occupancy factor. Nb(I) leads to NbO_6 sites identified by their blue color, and Nb(II) leads to NbO_6 sites identified by dark yellow color. The ratio between Nb atoms is 4 Nb(I) to 1 Nb (II).

1.4. Natural rubber

Latex is extracted from rubber tree stem, more specifically, from lactiferous vessels located in the cortex, and is responsible for bringing food to the tree top. From a chemical point of view,

http://dx.doi.org/10.5772/57211

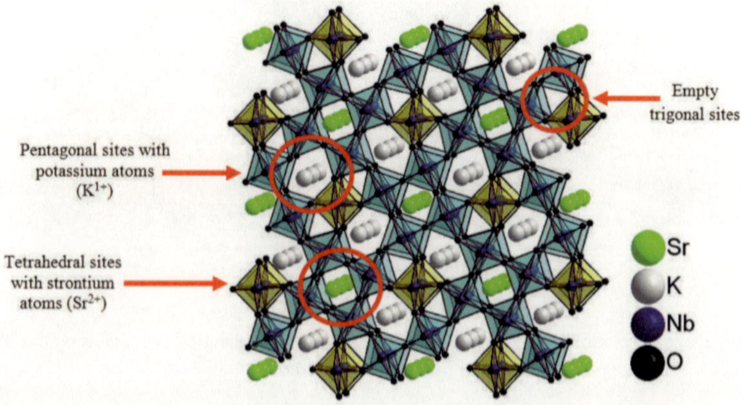

Figure 2. Representation of strontium potassium niobate oxide ($KSr_2Nb_5O_{15}$) with tetragonal tungsten bronze structure. Pentagonal sites occupied by atoms of potassium (K^{1+}), tetragonal sites occupied by atoms of strontium (Sr^{2+}) and trigonal vacant sites are highlighted.

latex is a stable colloidal dispersion of a polymer in an aqueous medium. The dispersed polymer is aggregated in the form of particles with approximately spherical geometry (natural rubber micelles), with typical diameters between 30 and 1, 000 nm [15].

The latex used in this work was collected from rubber trees of *Hevea brasiliensis* species, clone RRIM 600. This is a secondary clone developed by the Rubber Research Institute of Malaysia - RRIM, the most planted in the plateau region of São Paulo Brazilian state, due to its good performance and effect on production. This clone presents tall trees with vertical stem and fast growing when young. Its high production is highlighted, being one of the clones that has a higher dry rubber productivity.

Latex composition is, on average, 35% natural rubber (hydrocarbons), which compound is 2-methyl-1, 3-butadiene (C_5H_8), commercially known as isoprene. Recently-extracted latex is a neutral substance at room temperature with a pH between 6.0 and 7.2, depending on weather conditions, and density between 0.975 and 0.980 g/cm^3. When exposed to air for 12 - 24 hours, latex pH decreases to values close to 5.0 and spontaneous coagulation process begins, separating rubber and non-rubber fractions. Rubber fraction can be represented by $(C_5H_8)_n$, where n is the number of monomers in the chain (between 2, 000 and 10, 000), presenting an average molecular weight from 600, 000 to 950.000 g/mol.

Figure 3 presents the *Hevea brasiliensis* cultivation (a), the bleeding process, in order to collect latex (b), and dry natural rubber, "Brazilian pale crepe" type (*Crepe Claro Brasileiro - CCB*) (c).

1.5. Nanocomposite materials

As commented by P. M. Ajayan and co-workers [16], the field of nanocomposites involves the study of multiphase material where at least one of the constituent phases has one dimension less than 100 nm. The promise of nanocomposites lies in their multifunctionality, the possibility of realizing unique combinations of properties unachievable with traditional materials. The

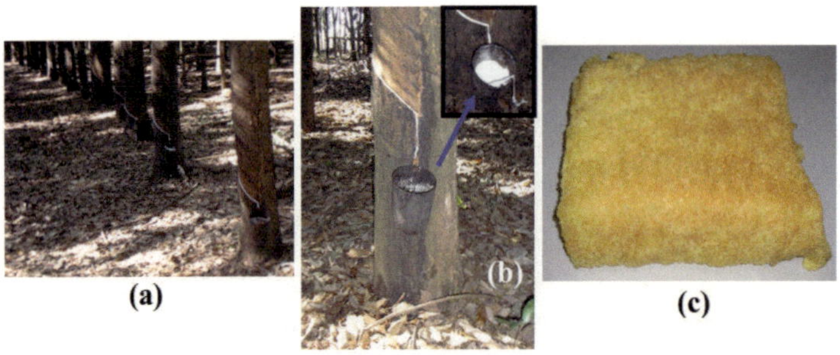

Figure 3. (a) Rubber tree plantation, *Hevea brasiliensis* species, (b) latex collection process using the bleeding method; detail: storage vessel, and (c) dry natural rubber, "Brazilian pale crepe" type.

challenges associate to this area are immense. They include control over the distribution in size and dispersion of the nanosize constituents, tailoring and understanding the role of interfaces between structurally or chemically dissimilar phases on bulk properties. Large scale and controlled processing of many nanomaterials has yet to be achieved.

An special class of composites and nanocomposites is the one formed by polymer and ceramic materials. In general, choosing a polymer as a matrix or continuous phase is interesting, since many of them have appreciable mechanical and thermal properties. Other properties are also regarded, e.g. hydrophobic/hydrophilic balance, chemical stability and bio-compatibility. The nanometric component is usually inorganic, and called dispersed phase. It can provide high mechanical and thermal stability and novel properties and functionalities that depend on component chemical nature, structure, size and crystallinity [17]. The dispersed phase provides or improves the redox properties, electronic, magnetic, density, refractive index, and others. In most cases, the main features of each of the components present in the nanocomposite is preserved or even improved and, in addition, one can obtain new properties resulting from the synergy of both components. Typical examples of polymer/ceramic nanocomposites of technological interest are formed by ceramic nanoparticles such as barium strontium titanate phase in a matrix with low dielectric loss [18] or nickel-zinc ferrite ($Ni_{0.5}Zn_{0.5}Fe_2O_4$ or NZF), dispersed in a polymeric matrix such as vulcanized natural rubber (NR) [19].

When mechanical properties of composites and nanocomposites are investigated, it is seen that the main contribution comes from the polymeric matrix. However, an appropriate nanoparticle engineering and dispersion process can act amplifying, reducing or creating new features in mechanical properties of nanocomposites. Interface and interaction between nanoparticles/matrix exert a significant influence on the mechanical properties, mainly due to the reorganization of chemical bonds and physical attractions of electrostatic nature. Therefore, properties of nanoparticles such as shape, size, surface activity, crystallinity and network microstrain become relevant. Depending on nanocomposites composition, external factors such as temperature, application of electric and magnetic fields can alter and modulate their properties, expanding application options for these materials. Thus, nanocomposites can be used in intelligent membranes, new catalysts and sensors, new generations of photovoltaic and fuel cells, intelligent micro-electronics systems, micro-optical and photonic components, and also therapeutic systems that combine marking, visualization, therapy and control of drug release [20, 21].

2. Employed methods

In the next topics, the preparation methods used in nanoparticles synthesis will be explored. The nanoparticles mentioned are magnetic (nickel-zinc ferrite, with stoichiometry $Ni_{0.5}Zn_{0.5}Fe_2O_4$ (NZF)), ferroelectric (strontium potassium niobate, stoichiometry $KSr_2Nb_5O_{15}$ (KSN)), besides magnetic and ferroelectric nanocomposites based on vulcanized natural rubber. Characterization techniques used are also covered, as well as biological testing of cell viability and against leishmaniasis.

2.1. Preparation of ceramic nanoparticles

Preparation of ceramic phases $KSr_2Nb_5O_{15}$ (KSN) and $Ni_{0.5}Zn_{0.5}Fe_2O_4$ (NZF) was performed using Modified Polyol Method [22, 23]. The main advantages of this method are high chemical homogeneity, the possibility of obtaining single phase powders and the large material portion produced in a single synthesis process (10 to 100g). Chemical formula and purity of starting reagents employed in oxides synthesis are listed in Table 1.

Component	Chemical formula	Purity
	Fuel for nanoparticles synthesis	
Ethylene glicol	$C_2H_4(OH)_2$	P.A.
Nitric acid	HNO_3	65%
	$KSr_2Nb_5O_{15}$ nanoparticles	
Strontium carbonate	$SrCO_3$	P.A.
Potassium carbonate	K_2CO_3	P.A.
Niobium complex salt	$NH_4H_2[NbO(C_2O_4)_3].3H_2O$	P.A.
	$Ni_{0.5}Zn_{0.5}Fe_2O_4$ nanoparticles	
Nickel oxide	Ni_2O_3	P.A.
Zinc oxide	ZnO	P.A.
Iron oxide	Fe_2O_3	P.A.

Table 1. Chemical formula and purity of the materials used in the preparation of ferroelectric and paramagnetic nanoparticles (respectively, $KSr_2Nb_5O_{15}$ and $Ni_{0.5}Zn_{0.5}Fe_2O_4$).

- **Description:** in a 2 L beaker, under stirring and heating, the dissolution in nitric acid of all precursor oxides was performed in proper proportion to the desired oxide stoichiometry. 50 g of niobate oxide and ferrite were prepared for each synthesis and stoichiometric calculations were based on this mass value. Upon dissolution of all starting materials, 100 ml of ethylene glycol were added. In a chapel, the temperature was raised to 180 °C using a magnetic stirrer. With the gradual increase of temperature occurred the emanation of a yellowish-brown coloured gas, due to decomposition of NO_3 groups, similar to the process developed in synthesis via Pechini method [24]. After this initial process, the material generated in the beaker was placed in a chamber-type oven.

- **Pre-calcining:** precursors pre-calcination was carried out in two stages, under an O_2 atmosphere with a flow of 500 ml/min for the niobate phase and under a N_2 atmosphere with a flow of 300 ml/min for the ferrite phase. In the first step, the temperature was increased from room temperature at a rate of 10 °C/min to 150 °C, which was held constant for 2 hours for elimination of low molecular mass molecules such as water vapor and some organic groups. In the following, keeping the same heating rate, temperature was raised to 300 °C and maintained for 1 h, in order to remove part of non-stoichiometric elements of the phase. During pre-calcination significant elimination of organic material fraction occurs, thus obtaining a black precursor powder for KSN and reddish-brown powder for NZF.

- **Calcination:** Both precursors were calcined with a final temperature of 450 °C. For niobate phase, a ten-hour threshold (600 m) was performed at 300 °C for disposal of organic wastes, and a two-hour threshold (120 m) in the final calcination temperature. A heating rate of 5 °C/min and nitrogen flow of 150 mL/min were used during heating, for avoiding sample oxidation in second phase formation. For ferrite, a three-hour threshold (180 minutes) was performed at final calcination temperature, in order to provide sufficient time for occurring of diffusional mass processes. A heating rate of 5 °C/min and air flow equal to 7 L/min were used during heating. For both phases, the cooling process was performed at a natural rate.

Figure 4 presents a flowchart of the steps for preparing and calcining the niobate and ferrite by modified Polyol method until to characterization stage.

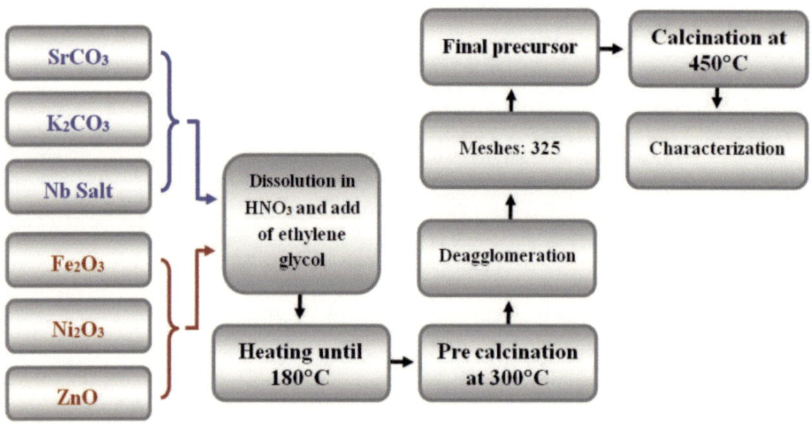

Figure 4. Flowchart of ferroelectric $KSr_2Nb_5O_{15}$ and paramagnetic $Ni_{0.5}Zn_{0.5}Fe_2O_4$ ceramic phases preparation by Modified Polyol Method. In blue, starting reactants from phase $KSr_2Nb_5O_{15}$ and in red, starting reactants from phase $Ni_{0.5}Zn_{0.5}Fe_2O_4$.

http://dx.doi.org/10.5772/57211

2.2. Nanocomposite magnetic and ferroelectric preparation

Magnetic and ferroelectric nanocomposites were obtained from mechanical blending of dry natural rubber, various concentrations of ceramic nanoparticles and vulcanization system. Chemical formula and purity of the starting reactants employed in preparation of vulcanized natural rubber nanocomposites are listed in Table 2.

Component	Chemical formula	Purity
	Nanocomposites	
Natural Rubber	$(C_5H_8)_n$	-
Zinc oxide	ZnO	P.A.
Stearic acid	$CH_3(CH_2)_{16}COOH$	P.A.
Mercaptobenzothiazole	$S_2NC_7H_5$	P.A.
Sulfur	S_8	P.A.

n: number of monomers in the polymer chain, between 2, 000 and 10, 000.

Table 2. Names, chemical formula, and purity of materials used in preparation of functional nanocomposites based on vulcanized natural rubber.

Nanocomposites preparation was initiated with dry mechanical mixing of the activation system in a open chamber mixer for 20 minutes. The activation system consists of 4 phr of zinc oxide and 3 phr of stearic acid with various concentrations of nanoparticles and 100 phr of dry natural rubber. At this stage the samples are called "activated samples". These samples were stored at a temperature of 25 °C and without light exposure for 24 hours.

After the storage step, vulcanization (2 phr of sulfur) and acceleration (1 phr of 2-mercapto-benzothiazole) agents were added to the activated samples by using the same mixing route. At this stage the samples are termed "accelerated samples". Accelerated samples were then thermo-conformated in thicknesses equal to 200 μm, 2 mm and 6 mm in a press with a heating system at 150 °C for 8 min and 30 s, and closing uniaxial pressure equal to 2.5 MPa. Vulcanization temperature and pressure used are indicated for natural rubber [25], and the vulcanization time parameter can be determined through rheometry test [26, 27].

Two sets of vulcanized natural rubber nanocomposites were prepared. The first set (NR/KSN) with $KSr_2Nb_5O_{15}$ ferroelectric nanoparticles, and the second set (NR/NZF) with $Ni_{0.5}Zn_{0.5}Fe_2O_4$ nanoparticles, both at various concentrations (1, 2, 3, 4, 5, 10, 20 and 50 phr). Figure 5 presents NR, NR/NZF and NR/KSN films and membranes with 5 phr of nanoparticles. Images of other samples with different concentrations and temperatures are visually similar and were not included in this section.

2.3. Main characterizations of nanoparticles and nanocomposites

- **XDR:** characterization by X-ray diffraction of KSN and NZF phases was performed on a X-ray diffractometer with Cu-Kα radiation ($\lambda = 1.54060$ Å), angular range of $5° \leq 2\theta \leq 80°$, and variation rate (or step) of 0.02°. Diffraction data were refined using the software FullProf

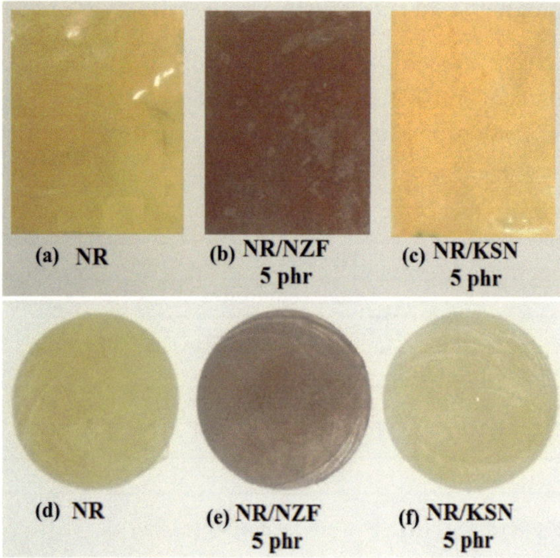

Figure 5. Thin films with a thickness of 200 μm (a, b and c) and membranes with a thickness of 2 mm (d, e and f) of NR, NR/NZF, NR/KSN and NR/KSN/NZF respectively, with 5 phr of nanoparticles.

[28]. KSN, with a bronze tungsten tetragonal structure was indexed to JCPDS-34-0108 and NZF, with a inverse spinel structure was indexed to JCPDS-08-0234 [29].

- **TEM:** images of transmission electron microscopy of KSN and NZF nanoparticles at a temperature of 25 °C were obtained from the supernatant fraction of the dispersion, nanoparticles and methanol, deposited on a polymer film. A field-emission (FEG) microscope with tungsten filament was used; accelerating voltage between 40 and 100 kV, CCD chamber.

- **SEM:** scanning electron microscopy images of vulcanized natural rubber and nanocomposites NR/KSN and NR/NZF were performed using a microscope with field emission (FEG) and energy dispersive analysis of x-ray analysis (EDX). Images were obtained on the sample and cryogenically fractured surfaces.

- **AFM:** atomic force microscopy AFM/STM was used in contact mode. AFM were performed to characterize nanoparticles morphology, vulcanized natural rubber and functional nanocomposites. The public domain software Gwyddion was used to generate the three-dimensional projection of the sample surface from the height mode AFM images (height).

2.4. Cell viability or toxicity assays

Assays of cell viability or the nanoparticles toxicity, vulcanized natural rubber and nanocomposites compared to mammalian cells were performed using "violet crystal method", as described by J. Moraes et al [30]. Mammalian cell lineage used in these experiments was of Vero cells ATCC CCL-81, originating from "American Type Culture Collection" (Manassas, VA, USA), a cell line from African green monkey *Cercopithecus aethiops (L.)* kidney. In the

http://dx.doi.org/10.5772/57211

experiments, Vero cells were grown in culture plates of 96 wells containing nanoparticles at concentrations between 15.6 and 1000 μg/mL or nanocomposites based on vulcanized natural rubber at concentrations between 250 and 4000 μg/mL in DMEM (Dulbecco's Modified Eagle Medium) environment, supplemented with 10% serum at 37 °C in an CO_2 atmosphere of 5%. Anova and Kruskal-Wallis tests were used to compare multiple normal or non-normal samples, respectively. Student's t-tests and Mann-Whitney test were used to compare two normal or non-normal samples, respectively. The BioEstat 5.0 software package [ACHO QUE ERA LEGAL COLOCAR UMA NOTA DE RODAPÉ FALANDO SOBRE ONDE OBTER O PROGRAMA] (Belém, Brazil, 2007) was used for performing the statistical tests and for graphical representations.

After 24 and 48 hours, supernatants were removed and adhered cells were fixed and stained with crystal violet 0.2% in methanol 20%v. It is noted that tests were carried out with concentrations of 150 mg/ml, concentrations significantly higher than those reported in the literature and no significant changes were observed as compared to essays up to 4000 μg/mL. Toxicity was evaluated from the absorbance of control wells containing cells in DMEM environment. Throughout the incubation period, cultures were monitored daily in inverted optical microscope. All assays were performed in triplicate and the obtained average standard deviation was less than 2%.

2.4. Leishmaniasis assays

In vitro population growth kinetics: In a BHI (brain heart infusion) environment supplemented with 10%v fetal bovine serum (FBS), 2% v human urine, 100 μg/ml potassium G penicillin and 100 μg/mL of streptomycin sulfate, a sample with rectangular dimensions 10x10x2mm of vulcanized natural rubber or nanocomposites with an inoculum of five hundred thousand parasites in the promastigote form of *Leishmania braziliensis* species, ARQ-1 strains isolated from clinical cases of Santa Cruz do Rio Pardo city, São Paulo state, in 1997.

From that instant, every three hours for a week, cell counts on the supernatant portion of the colony were performed using a Neubauer chamber. With data count a curve of parasite colony development was sketched. For comparison, control colonies, i.e. without the introduction of samples or natural rubber nanocomposites were also investigated. Throughout the tests, the temperature was maintained between 27 and 32 ºC, and hydrogen potential (pH) between 6.0 and 6.9. All assays were performed in triplicate and the average standard deviation obtained was less than 1%.

3. Main results and discussions

To support discussions related to the applications of nanoparticles and magnetic and ferroelectric nanocomposites in cultures of Leishmaniasis, morphological and structural characterization of nanometric materials were performed. Thus, information is obtained mainly about the interaction of the nanoparticles and nanocomposites with the biological material, cooperating in the understanding of the results.

3.1. Structural and morphological nanoparticle essays

Figure 6 presents the diffraction pattern at room temperature for KSN and NZF nanoparticles, calcined at 450 °C for 2 hours. Lines and vertical bars represent experimental data and diffraction patterns respectively, categorized in JCPDS database: 34-0108 (KSN) and 08-0234 (NZF).

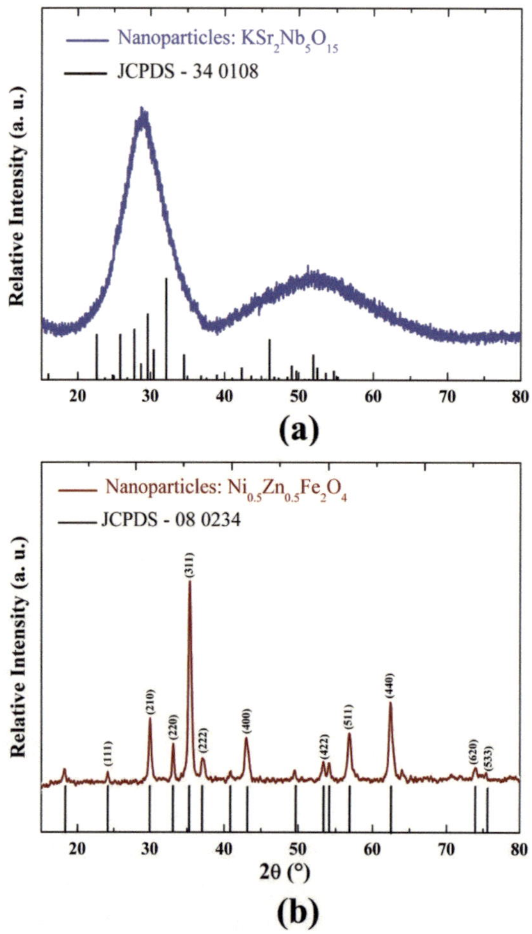

Figure 6. X-ray diffraction: (a) $KSr_2Nb_5O_{15}$ phase, calcined at 450 °C, together with experimental data, columns of the identity card JCPDS-34-0108 and (b) $Ni_{0,5}Zn_{0,5}Fe_2O_4$ phase, calcined at the temperature of 450 °C, together with experimental data, columns of the identity card JCPDS-08-0234.

As can be seen in Figure 6, and according to studies conducted previously by the authors [31], the diffraction pattern obtained for the KSN shows the typical profile of a material with short-distance ordering (amorphous), identifying only two large sets of overlapping diffraction lines indicating that the thermal energy supplied during the heat treatment was not sufficient for obtaining a crystalline material. Relative crystallinity obtained for KSN was equal to approximately 10%, compared with the same material calcined at 1150 °C.

A diffractogram obtained for NZF phase displays a set of well-resolved diffraction lines, indicating that heat treatment was suitable for the production of a material with a high crystallinity degree, relative crystallinity of 74% when compared with the same material calcined at 650 °C. For KSN phase, the formation of a tetragonal tungsten bronze structure (TTB) with P4bm spatial group (No. 100) was identified, while for phase NZF the formation of a inverse spinel structure with space group Fd3m (No. 227) was identified. Network parameters "a", "b" and "c" obtained from KSN phase and "a" for NZF phase are equal to "a" = 12.4585 Å, "b" = "c" = 3.9423 Å and "a" = 8.394 Å, respectively. The unit cell volume is equal to V = 611.90 $Å^3$ and V = 591.435 $Å^3$ to KSN and NZF.

Average crystallite size, obtained by Scherrer's equation, was equal to 2 nm for KSN and 14.7 nm for NZF. Network microstrain (γ), calculated by Williamson-Hall equation, was equal to 0.32 for KSN and 0.05 for NZF. Structural parameters obtained in this study are in agreement with values reported in previous publications [32, 33].

Figure 7 presents transmission electron microscopy (TEM) images at a temperature of 25 °C of KSN ferroelectric and NZF paramagnetic nanoparticles, both calcined at 450 °C, where (a) and (c) are 10, 000 times magnifications while (b) and (d) are 600, 000 times magnifications. The images (b) and (d) were generated from amplifications of specific regions of the images (a) and (c).

As can be seen in Figure 7 (b) and (d), for both types of primary particles, their geometry are approximately spherical due to nucleation-type particle growth mechanism, predominant in ceramic materials and also to the principle of surface energy minimizing. Average particle diameter of strontium potassium niobate is approximately 15 nm, while the average size for a primary particle of nickel-zinc ferrite is approximately 10 nm; both values are consistent with particle diameters in the scientific literature [32, 33] and agree with average-size crystallite values. As expected, KSN particle diameter for is larger than NZF particle diameter, due to the fact that tetragonal tungsten bronze structure (23 atoms/ minimal formula, pentagonal, tetragonal and trigonal sites) has greater complexity than cubic inverse spinel-type structure (7 atoms/minimal formula, octahedral and tetrahedral sites), thus the minimum cluster size to stabilize the particle tends to be higher for KSN than for NZF. Due to the difference of stage complexity, it is also expected that as both received the same heat treatment and then the same amount of thermal energy, NZF phase would be more crystalline than KSN phase, since NZF phase requires less energy to the atoms achieve their ideal atomic positions.

According to Figure 7 (a) and (c), one can identify that both ceramic phases present clusters even at nanometric scale, due to the action of secondary forces and coalescence phenomena. For KSN phase one can identify clusters with an average size of 80 nm or approximately 112 nanoparticles/cluster and for NZF phase, agglomerates with an average size of 100 nm or around 740 nanoparticles/cluster. For both estimates, clusters with spherical shape and a close-packing bundling type were considered [34]. In principle, magnetic properties displayed by NZF nanoparticles could contribute to formation of larger clusters when compared with non-magnetic phase clusters, as reported and discussed by E. M. A. Jamal et al., for nickel magnetic particles [35]. However, cluster formation is attributed essentially to preparation method used to synthesize ceramic nanoparticles; in this case, a chemical route.

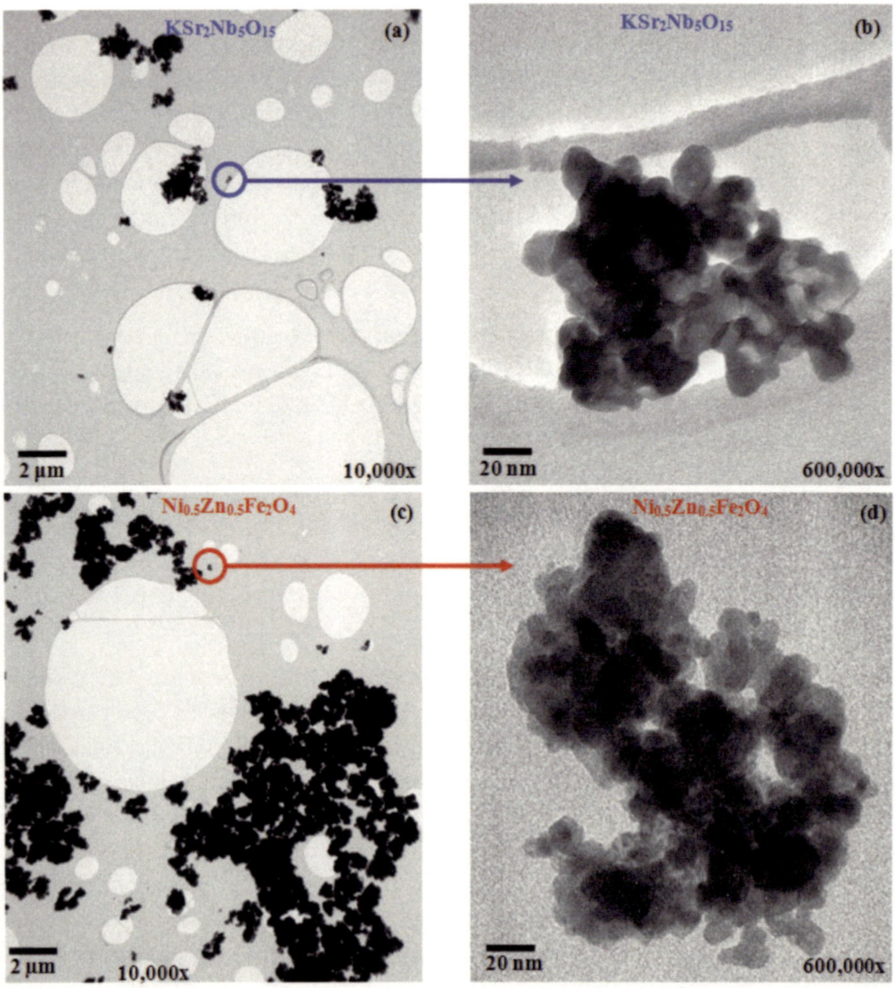

Figure 7. Transmission electron microscopy (TEM) at a temperature of 25 °C, of KSN ferroelectric [(a) and (b)] and NZF paramagnetic nanoparticles [(c) and (d)], calcined at 450 °C and at different magnifications.

Images acquired by Atomic Force Microscopy (AFM) at room temperature (25 °C) for KSN ferroelectric (a) and NZF paramagnetic nanoparticles (b) calcined at 450 °C are shown in Figure 8. Details on the grain boundary and the three-dimensional nanoparticle projection are given on the right.

According to Figure 8, structures on a nanometric scale were identified for both ceramic phases, in agreement with Figure 7. Images generated from amplitude data (main figure) provide qualitative information of nanostructure shape, while images generated from elevation data (three-dimensional projection) provide significant information about surface topography. Details on the grain boundary can be obtained from deflection data of the phase angle (image positioned in the third quadrant). For KSN ferroelectric nanoparticles, Figure 8 (a), a small

http://dx.doi.org/10.5772/57211

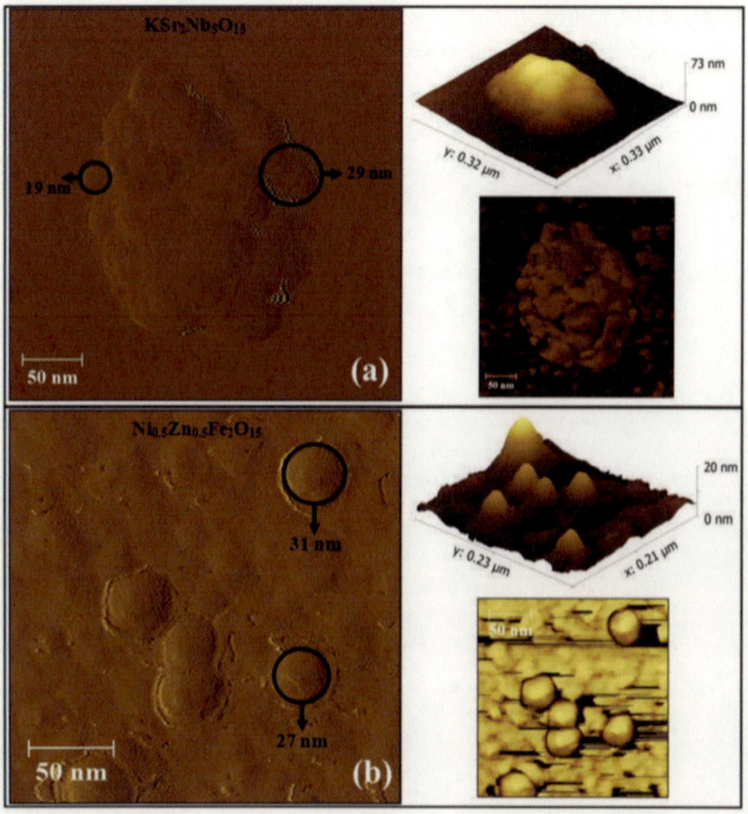

Figure 8. Atomic Force Microscopy (AFM) images generated from range, surface elevation and phase angle deflection data for KSN ferroelectric (a) and NZF paramagnetic nanoparticles (b). On the right, grain boundary details and three-dimensional nanoparticle projection.

cluster is observed in detail, with size approximately equal to 100 nm composed of nanoparticles with particle size distribution between 15 and 30 nm.

Small clusters formation is a typical feature of nanoscale materials processing using chemical routes. However, it is emphasized that the nanoparticles that compose the clusters are weakly linked together through secondary interactions of electrostatic origin. For NZF paramagnetic nanoparticles, Figure 8 (b), individual nanoparticles with approximately spherical geometry are identified, as well as the union of two or more nanoparticles by coalescence process. It is feasible to notice a particle size distribution between 25 and 40 nm for NZF phase. It should be noted that the particle size distribution for KSN and NZF is consistent with previously published work [36, 37].

3.2. Nanocomposite morphological study

Figure 9 presents scanning electron microscopy images obtained from the sample surface, a representation of the polymer chain and the EDX spectrum for the vulcanized natural rubber

NR/KSN-1phr ferroelectric and NR/NZF-1phr magnetic nanocomposites. Magnifications used were equal to 50, 000, 50, 000, and 150, 000 times.

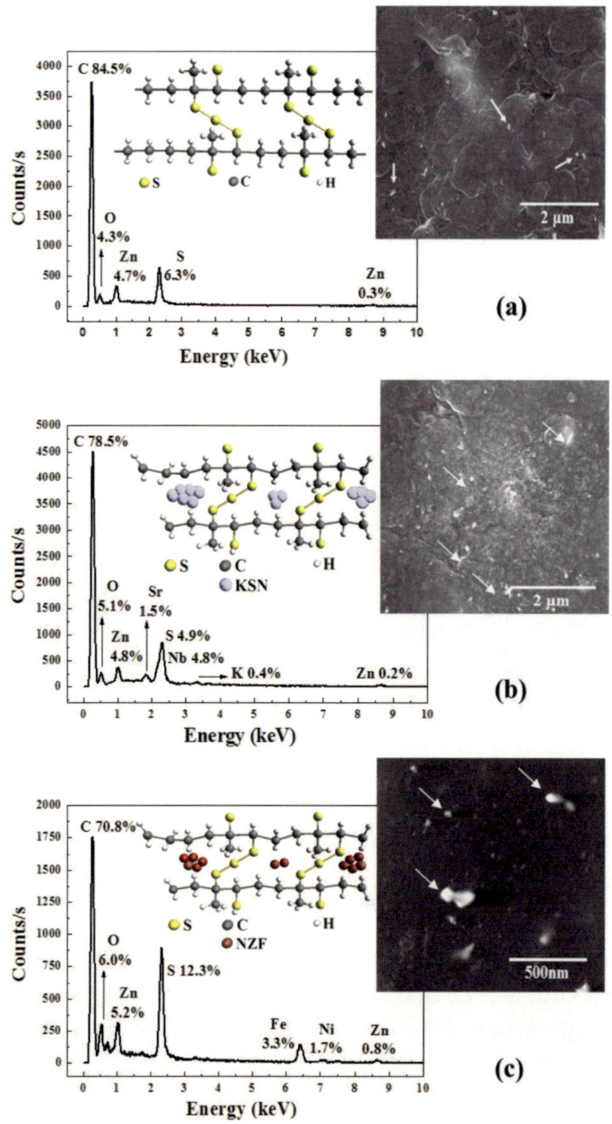

Figure 9. (a) Scanning electron microscopy images of the sample surface, polymer chain representation and EDX spectrum for vulcanized natural rubber, (b) ferroelectric nanocomposite NR/KSN-1phr and (c) magnetic nanocomposite NR/NZF-1phr.

In Figure 9 (a), a satisfactory surface homogeneity was observed, indicating that a vulcanization system in appropriate amounts and a efficient nanocomposite-preparing system was used. White spots were noticed and indicated with white arrows. Such points may be associated with the vulcanization system, in agreement with the results obtained by XRD, particularly zinc and sulfur with submicrometer dimensions (> 250 nm). According to Figure 9 (b) and (c), it is possible to identify a high dispersion of particles and small agglomerates with dimensions on the nanometer scale, between 20 nm and 80 nm, and a particle size in the submicron range.

It is suggested that the particles and small clusters are KSN and NZF nanoparticles, in accordance with the dimensional scale, dark grayish and reddish brown color in surface and inside of the nanocomposites, respectively. In EDX spectra, peaks of C, O, S and Zn were identified and are associated with the curing system and the polymer chains. EDX percentage differences observed for S and Zn among NR, NR/KSN-1phr and NR/NZF-1phr samples refer only to the position of the investigated sample and sample time exposure to X-ray.

Low percentages of K, Sr and Nb and Fe, Ni and Zn were found for samples of NR/KSN and NR/NZF and were assigned respectively to KSN and NZF nanoparticles. The values obtained are in agreement with the amount estimated by stoichiometric calculations. The difference in surface roughness observed in Figure 9 (a) and Figures 9 (b) and (c) may be associated to the mobility difference of the natural rubber polymer chain, due to the incorporation of nanoparticles, even in small mass quantities.

Images obtained by atomic force microscopy (AFM) for vulcanized natural rubber, NR/KSN-10phr ferroelectric nanocomposite and NR/NZF-10phr magnetic nanocomposite were performed directly on the surface of the samples, and their three-dimensional projections are presented in Figure 10, while Table 3 lists the values for NR surface roughness, NR/KSN ferroelectric and NR/NZF magnetic nanocomposites, depending on the nanoparticle concentration.

Sample	Superficial rugosity (nm)						
	NR	1 phr	3 phr	5 phr	10 phr	20 phr	50 phr
NR/KSN	0.45	0.68	0.83	0.70	0.55	0.50	0.58
NR/NZF	0.45	0.50	0.63	0.55	0.45	0.43	0.45

Table 3. Surface roughness values obtained from elevation mode AFM images, for vulcanized natural rubber (NR) and nanocomposites NR/KSN and NR/NZF.

According to Figure 10 and the data in Table 3, a satisfactory superficial homogeneity is noted for vulcanized natural rubber and both functional nanocomposites samples, suggesting that appropriate parameters and vulcanization system were used. Significant differences between the natural rubber nanocomposites were observed for surface roughness. At low nanoparticle concentrations, smaller than 3 phr, there is considerable roughness growth, followed by a reduction and stabilization of this parameter with increasing concentration of nanoparticles. This suggests that for low concentrations, local phenomena of elastomeric chain orientation as stress-induced crystallization [38, 39] can be significant.

Probably, differences in roughness identified between ferroelectric and magnetic nanocomposites are due to: (i) difference in interface between the nanoparticles that generate changes in polymer chains folding, (ii) different coefficients of thermal diffusion due to different ceramic phases and (iii) different anisotropies for polymer chains mobility [39].

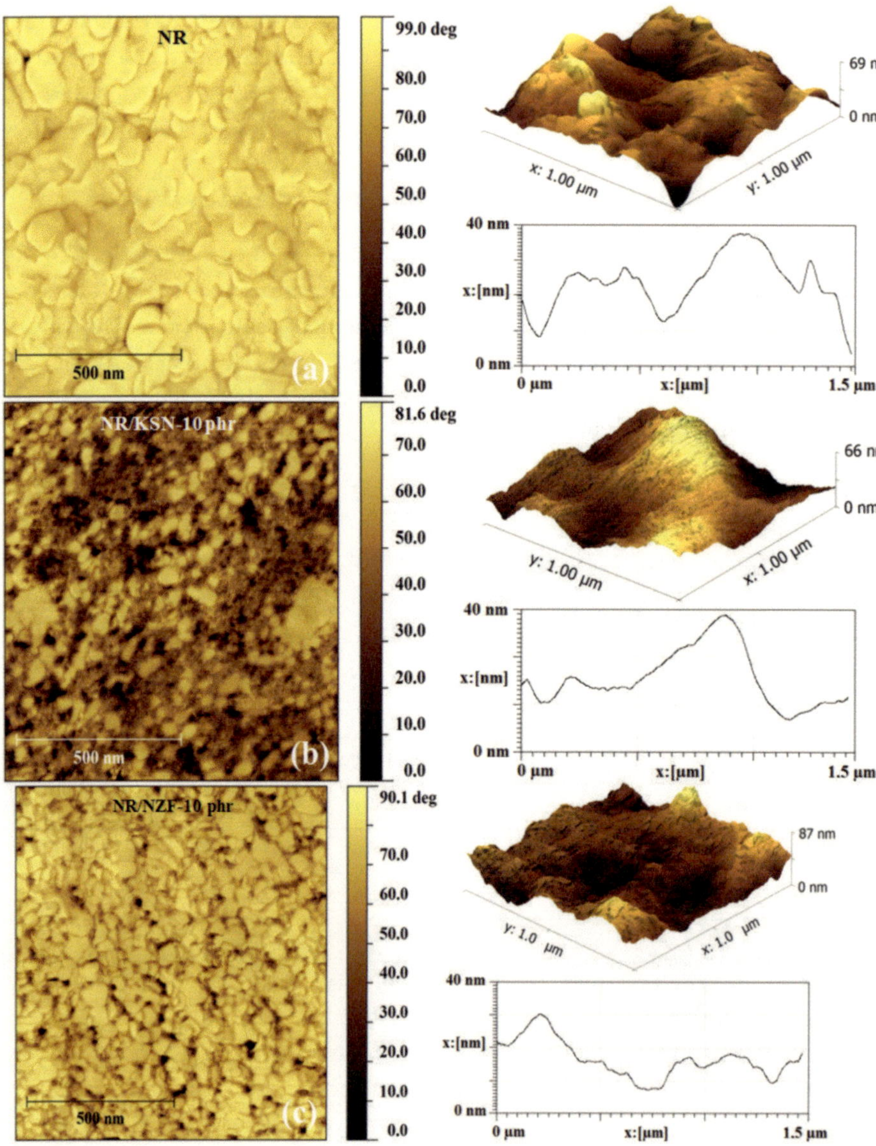

Figure 10. Images obtained using atomic force microscopy (AFM) to: (a) vulcanized natural rubber, (b) NR/KSN-10phr ferroelectric nanocomposite and (c) NR/NZF-10phr magnetic nanocomposite, performed directly on the surface of samples and their three-dimensional projections.

3.3. Polymer/ceramic composites and nanocomposites as an agent of control in Leishmaniasis colonies

Neglected diseases are illnesses that prevail not only in poverty conditions, but also contribute to the framework maintenance of economic and social inequality in the country (e.g. leishmaniasis, dengue, Chagas disease, schistosomiasis, leprosy and others [40]). As a result of this framework, multidisciplinary research involving materials science and biotechnology areas has gained significant strength, in order to develop new materials and methods to combat these diseases. For stimulating angiogenic processes [41] and due to its significant ability to disperse particulate fillers, natural rubber and its nanocomposites emerge as potential candidates for a new generation of bioactive agents with biocide character in biotechnology.

3.3.1. Biological study: toxicity evaluation

Due to great demand for innovation in biotechnology, nanoparticles and nanocomposites emerge as potential candidates for a new generation of biocides, and tests that assess the toxicity of these materials compared to mammalian cells comprises an important phase of the development process biotechnology.

Figure 11 presents the results of toxicity or viability evaluation of Vero cells after 48 h incubation in the presence of ceramic nanoparticles $KSr_2Nb_5O_{15}$ and $Ni_{0,5}Zn_{0,5}Fe_2O_4$ and their respective constituent elements, depending on particle concentration in the cellular environment [42].

According to Figure 11 for both ceramic phases and its constituent elements, except for potassium carbonate (K_2CO_3), there is no statistically significant decrease in cell viability at the end of the incubation period until the maximal concentration tested in this case (1000 μg/mL), compared to cells incubated only in the culture environment.

For cells culture in contact with potassium carbonate particles, there is clearly a statistically significant reduction ($P < 0.01$) in cell viability for concentration equal to or greater than 62.5 μg/mL. Potassium carbonate in aqueous environment tends to dissociate, originating potassium ions (K^+) that transform the extracellular environment, which should be hypotonic, in a highly hypertonic environment. Thus, cells pass for a excessive water-loss process through the cytoplasmic membrane and unbalances in key mechanisms for cell life maintenance, such as the sodium-potassium pump, mechanisms of nerve impulse conduction, protein synthesis and cell respiration. The combination of these processes is probably the responsible for the cell death observed for mammalian cells exposed to potassium carbonate particles. However, in $KSr_2Nb_5O_{15}$ ferroelectric phase, potassium ions (K^+) are isolated in the interstices of the crystallographic pentagonal structure (see Figure 4), which prevents the presence of these ions in the extracellular environment.

The results of toxicity or viability evaluation of Vero cells after 48 h incubation in the presence of vulcanized natural rubber NR/KSN ferroelectric and NR/NZF magnetic nanocomposites as a function of sample concentration in the cellular environment are shown in Figure 12. In detail, images generated by optical microscopy of cells exposed to NR/KSN-50 phr and NR/NZF-50 phr nanocomposites, and also the control sample.

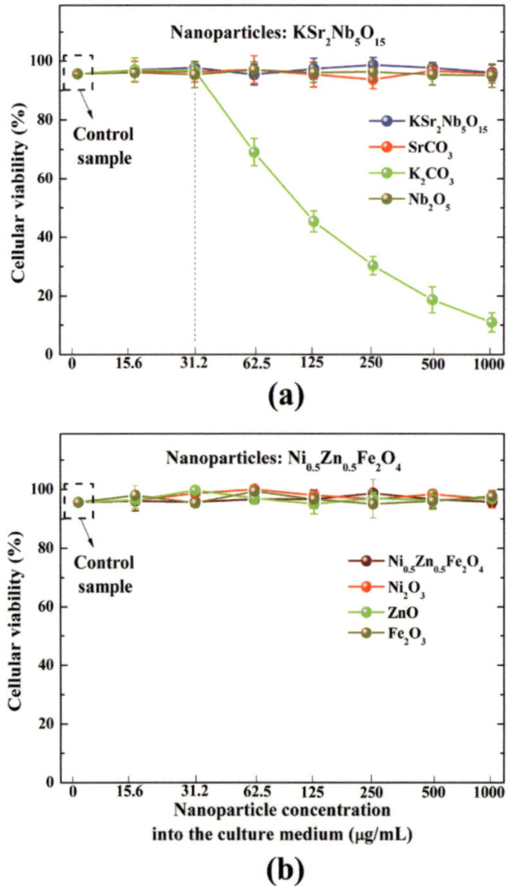

Figure 11. Cell viability in the presence of (a) ferroelectric nanoparticles, (b) magnetic nanoparticles and their respective constituents on the basis of the concentration of particles present in the culture environment. Vero-type mammalian cells cultured in particles presence were used.

As can be seen in Figure 12, for vulcanized natural rubber and both classes of nanocomposites, regardless of nanoparticles concentration, it is not possible to observe a statistically significant reduction in cell viability at the end of the incubation period until the maximal concentration tested (in this case 4000 μg/mL), compared to cells incubated only in the culture environment. In both images generated by optical microscopy, cells attached to the substrate are observed, indicating that cells remain biologically viable and comparing the cells exposed image to the two nanocomposites types with cells grown freely, it is not possible to identify significant morphological alterations, confirming that mammalian cells were not significantly affected due to nanocomposites presence. So as significant reductions were not identified in cell viability when mammalian cells were exposed to $KSr_2Nb_5O_{15}$ and $Ni_{0,5}Zn_{0,5}Fe_2O_4$ nanoparticles, vulcanized natural rubber and nanocomposites, one can consider that such systems have potential for using in biological systems composed by mammalian cells.

http://dx.doi.org/10.5772/57211

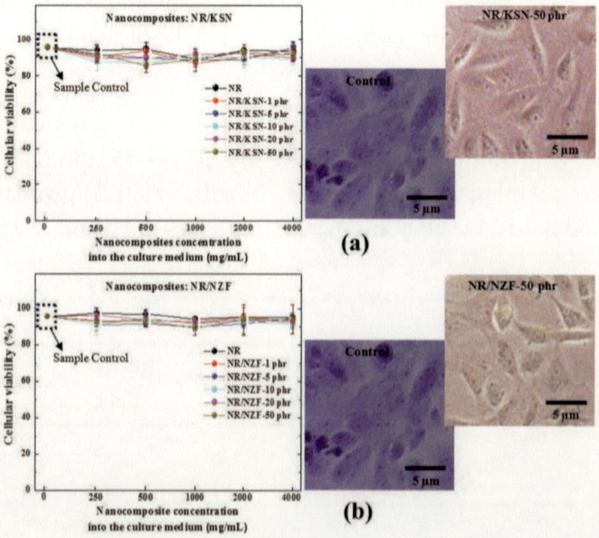

Figure 12. Cell viability in the presence of vulcanized natural rubber (a) NR/KSN ferroelectric and (b) NR/NZF magnetic nanocomposites as a function of sample concentration in the cell environment. In detail, images generated by optical microscopy of cells exposed and not exposed to nanocomposites. Vero-type mammalian cells were used, cultured in the presence of nanocomposites.

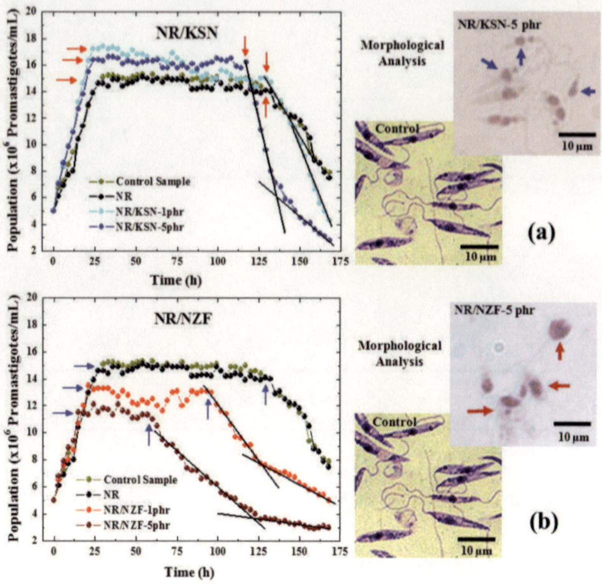

Figure 13. Population growth kinetics of Leishmania braziliensis (LB) parasite colony exposed to samples of vulcanized natural rubber, (a) NR/KSN and (b) NR/NZF nanocomposites. In detail, morphological comparison of parasites via optical microscopy.

Figure 13 presents the kinetics of colony population development of Leishmaniasis parasites exposed to vulcanized natural rubber samples, (a) NR/KSN ferroelectric and (b) NR/NZF magnetic nanocomposites in different nanoparticles concentrations. In detail, morphological comparison of the parasites after samples exposure.

Values for parameters maximum population density, phase duration, increase and decrease rates and also colony population of Leishmania braziliensis (LB) promastigotes exposed to samples of vulcanized natural rubber and nanocomposites are listed in Table 4.

Parameter	Sample								
	NR control	NR/KSN 1 phr	Δ%	NR/KSN 5 phr	Δ%	NR/NZF 1 phr	Δ%	NR/NZF 5 phr	Δ%
Generation time* (h)	14.4	9.3	-35%	9.7	-33%	13.1	-9%	12.0	-17%
Maximum population density (10^6 parasites/mL)	15.1	17.2	+14%	16.4	+9%	13.5	-11%	11.5	-24%
Length of logarithmic phase (h)	30	24	-20%	24	-20%	21	-30%	15	-50%
Average growth of logarithmic phase (10^6 cells/h mL)	0.3	0.51	+50%	0.48	+41%	0.4	+33%	0.4	+33%
Continuous phase duration (h)	102	108	+6%	93	-9%	75	-27%	42	-59%
Fall phase duration (h)	36	36	0%	51	+42%	72	+100%	111	+208%
Average rate of fall phase decrease (10^6 cells/h mL)	0.2	0.3	+50%	0.3	+50%	0.1	-50%	0.05	-75%

* Generation or double time: required time for doubling the cell population.

Table 4. Values for population development parameters of *Leishmania braziliensis* (LB) promastigotes colonies exposed to samples of natural rubber and vulcanized nanocomposites with different nanoparticle concentrations.

According to Figure 13 and data listed in Table 4, the increase curve evolution of LB promastigote population is similar for all samples studied, indicating that the presence of the samples did not change the colony global behavior. As expected, this evolution follows the standards of a colony of microorganisms grown in an artificial environment, being composed of three well-defined stages:

http://dx.doi.org/10.5772/57211

- **First stage:** denominated logarithmic phase, in which the pathogen has a large nutrient amount, conditions for their physiological maturation and mitotic cell division, a linear increase of promastigotes as a function of time is identified, and the average growth rate in this stage is higher for colonies exposed to samples. This suggests that the samples presence in the culture environment promotes the cell nutrition process;

- **Second stage:** denominated continuous phase, in which stabilize the processes of cell division, the parasites are mature and new members of the population do not arise; a constant number of promastigostas in function of time was identified. Oscillations in population density observed in this phase are due to cell death and reproduction, dependent on the environment nutritional availability or possible interaction between the parasite and the nanocomposite;

- **Third stage:** denominated fall phase, in which the nutritional resources of the culture environment are reduced and the process of cell death by depletion of internal micro-organism begins. A decreasing linear is identified, depending on time for control colony, and for the colonies exposed to vulcanized natural rubber samples and also linear decreasing for colonies exposed to samples of both nanocomposites and both nanoparticle concentrations, but with two different decrease rates, suggesting that there could be generations of parasites more resistant to the presence of samples in the colony, because they have already been evolved in nanocomposites presence.

Comparing the results for the control colony and the colony with a sample of vulcanized natural rubber samples, there is no statistically significant alterations in the of population growth kinetics, thus keeping unchanged the stages of cell development and maturation. However, for colonies exposed to nanocomposite samples having both nanoparticles, there are significant changes in microbial growth patterns. It should be mentioned that, regardless of the nanoparticle type associated with natural rubber, when the concentration of nanoparticles increases, the differences between the growth curves accentuate.

There is a progressive increase in the population of promastigotes in the logarithmic phase of the colonies exposed to NR/KSN nanocomposites (Figure 13 (a)), indicating that or KSN nanoparticles could come loose from nanocomposite surface, or something related to the interaction between the nanoparticles and the polymeric matrix is generating a change of or electronic nature significant structural proteins in the medium such that the parasites are able to ingest larger amounts of nutrients coming then to be reproduced more frequently. This hypothesis corroborates the reduction of over 30% in the generation time of the colonies.

The largest amount of immature parasites generated in logarithmic phase justifies the reduction in hours of the stationary phase, since the presence of large parasite quantities implies in a reduction of the amount of nutrients per parasite. It is worth mentioning that the population decrease noted in fall phase is intensified with increasing nanoparticles concentration in the nanocomposite, indicating that probably the same reason that is causing changes in culture proteins, facilitating their ingestion, is also hindering the absorption of these proteins by the parasites, accelerating nutritional starvation. Comparing the morphological characteristics of the parasites exposed to NR/KSN-5phr nanocomposites with colony control parasites [43, 44], one could clearly identify the kinetoplast and nucleus cell, but no significant morphological differences were observed, confirming the similarity of the curves in Figure 13 (a).

In the case of the colonies exposed to NR/NZF nanocomposite samples (Figure 13 (b)), one can identify a linear decrease in intensity of the logarithmic phase, depending of increasing concentration of nanoparticles, indicating that the presence of such nanoparticles difficult culture protein consumption and cell division by the parasite. However, a slight reduction (lower than 20%) can still be noticeable to the generation time of the colonies. With a smaller amount of parasites in culture and limited capacity of nutritional consumption in the environment, there is a smaller stationary phase and a fall phase greater than that of control colonies than the sample and exposed to natural rubber samples.

Comparing the morphological characteristics of the parasites exposed to NR/NZF-5phr nanocomposites with colony control parasites [43, 44], there is a clear morphological difference in cell design. Control parasites has elongated cell bodies, while for parasites in contact with NR/NZF-5phr, the cell body has approximately a circular shape.

Whereas both types of nanoparticles have nanometric sizes, the first factor to justify the identified differences is that the sum of factors such as differences in crystallinity, surface area, micro-deformations of the crystal lattice, cell volume and especially chemical composition that generate surface characteristics particular to each nanoparticle type is responsible for the differences noted in each colony. However, intrinsic interactions between cells and magnetic/ferroelectric nanoparticle properties, which would help to explain the high specificity exhibited by nanoparticles against leishmaniasis parasites and not against mammalian cells can not be discarded, although less likely.

4. Conclusions

Modified polyol method was used in the chemical synthesis of potassium strontium niobate ferroelectric oxide with stoichiometry $KSr_2Nb_5O_{15}$ and of nickel zinc ferrite paramagnetic oxide, stoichiometry $Ni_{0,5}Zn_{0,5}Fe_2O_4$. Single-phase ceramic phases with average crystallite size in nanometric scale were obtained. Using XRD and AFM essays, average crystallite size and particle surface parameters could be determined, mainly. We employed a method for the preparation of functional composites and nanocomposites based on vulcanized natural rubber, grounded in the dry mixing of the constituents using a open chamber mixing. A vulcanization system based on sulfur (S_8), suitable for natural rubber and ceramic nanoparticles was used. The development of a potential application for composites and nanocomposites based on vulcanized natural rubber was started and the preliminary results are encouraging, namely: use of paramagnetic and ferroelectric nanocomposites as modulating agents of the development of colonies of *Leishmania braziliensis* parasites.

http://dx.doi.org/10.5772/57211

Acknowledgements

The authors would want to acknowledge the Brazilian research agencies FAPESP, CAPES and CNPq for financial support, the graduate program of Materials Science and Technology, Carlos Gomes Barbosa-Filho and Dr. Josué de Moraes for the biological tests, Dr. José Antonio de Saja-Saéz, Prof. Dr. Miguel-Ángel Rodrigues-Pérez and Dr. Marcos Augusto de Lima Nobre for the scientific discussions and also Dr. Ricardo F. Aroca and Ariel Guerrero for the AFM measurements.

Author details

Aldo Eloizo Job*, Alexandre Fioravante de Siqueira, Caroline Silva Danna, Felipe Silva Bellucci, Flávio Camargo Cabrera and Leandra Ernst Kerche Silva

*Address all correspondence to: job@fct.unesp.br

Department of Physics, Chemistry and Biology, Univ Estadual Paulista, Presidente Prudente, Sao Paulo, Brazil

References

[1] Schneider P, Schmidt G. Nanocomposite polymer hydrogels. Colloid Polym Sci. 2009;287: 1-11.

[2] Bellucci FS et al. Preparation and structural characterization of vulcanized natural rubber nanocomposites containing nickel-zinc ferrite nanopowders. J. Nanosci. Nanotechnol. 2012; 12(3): 2691-2699.

[3] Oriakhi CO. Polymer nanocomposition approach to advanced materials. J. Chem. Educ. 2000; 77(9): 1138-1146.

[4] Moraes J et al. Schistosoma mansoni: In vitro schistosomicidal activity of piplartine. Exp. Parasitol. 2011; 127: 357-364.

[5] Joseph OH, Robert JN, Frank MC. Advantages of measuring changes in the number of viable parasites in murine models of experimental Cutaneous Leishmaniasis. Infect. Immun. 1983; 39(3): 1087-1094.

[6] Sepulveda C., editor. Leishmaniasis: Symptoms, Treatment and Potential Complications. Nova Publishers; 2013.

[7] Lindoso JAL et al. Review of the current treatments for leishmaniases. Research and Reports in Tropical Medicine. 2012;3: 69–77.

[8] Li XS et al. Synthesis and applications of functionalized magnetic materials in sample preparation. Trends Anal. Chem. 2013;45: 233-247.

[9] Lanfredi S et al. Síntese e Caracterização Estrutural do Niobato de Potássio e Estrôncio com Estrutura tipo Tetragonal Tungstênio Bronze (TTB). Cerâmica. 2005;51: 151-156.

[10] Zahi S. Synthesis, permeability and microstructure of the optimal nickel-zinc ferrites by sol-gel route. J. Electromagn. Anal. App. 2010;2: 56.

[11] Sharma S et al. Influence of Zn substitution on structural, microstructural and dielectric properties of nanocrystalline nickel ferrites. Mater. Sci. Eng., B. 2010;167: 189.

[12] Pessoa F. Síntese e caractarização de ferrita de níquel e zinco nanocristalina por combustão, para aplicação em compósito elastoméricoa absorvedores de micro-ondas. MSc dissertation. UFRJ; 2006.

[13] Lanfredi S. Structural characterization and Curie temperature determination of a sodium strontium niobate ferroelectric nanostructured powder. J. Solid State Chem. 2011;184(5): 990-1000.

[14] Das PS et al. Electrical properties of $Li_2BiV_5O_{15}$ ceramics. Physica B. 2007; 395: 98-103.

[15] Wititsuwannakul R et al. A rubber particle protein specific for Hevea latex lectin binding involved in latex coagulation. Phytochemistry. 2008;69(5): 1111-1118.

[16] Ajayan, P. M., Schadler, L. S. and Braun, P. V. Nanocomposite Science and Technology. Wiley-VCH GmbH & Co. KGaA. ISBN 3-527-30359-6, 2003.

[17] Calebrese C et. al. A review on the importance of nanocomposite processing to enhance electrical insulation. IEEE Trans. Dielectr. Electr. Insul. 2011; 18: 938.

[18] Zhou K et al. Dielectric response and tunability of a dielectric-paraelectric composite. Appl. Phys. Lett. 2008;93: 102908-102911.

[19] Ismail H et al. Properties of ferrite-filled natural rubber composites. Polym. Plast. Technol. Eng. 2007;46: 641-650.

[20] Spaldin NA. Magnetic materials: Fundamentals and device applications. Cambridge University Press; 2003.

[21] Malini KA et al. Magnetic and processability studies on rubber ferrite composite based on natural rubber and mixed ferrite. J. Mater. Sci. 2001;36: 5551.

[22] Daigle A et al. Structure, morphology and magnetic properties of $Mg_{(x)}Zn_{(1-x)}Fe_2O_4$ ferrites prepared by polyol and aqueous co-precipitation methods: a low-toxicity alternative to $Ni_{(x)}Zn_{(1-x)}Fe_2O_4$ ferrites. Nanotechnol. 2011;22(30): 305708.

[23] Feldman C. Polyol-mediated synthesis of nanoscale functional materials. Solid State Sci. 2005;7: 868-873.

[24] Nobre MAL. Varistores a Base de ZnO Obtidos a Partir das Fases $ZnSb_2O_6$ e $Zn_7Sb_2O_{12}$: Correlação entre as Fases, Microestrutura e Propriedades Elétricas. PhD thesis. Universidade Federal de São Carlos; 1999.

[25] Grison EC, Hoinacki E, Mello JB. Curso de tecnologia da borracha. Associação Brasileira de Química; 1984.

[26] Bellucci FS et al. Método de produção de nanocompósitos funcionais e produtos obtidos. Patent filing n° BR102012005278-4, 2012, international extension n° PCT/BR 2013/000063; 2013.

[27] Bellucci FS et al. Mechanical Properties of Vulcanized Natural Rubber Nanocomposites Containing Functional Ceramic Nanoparticles. Sci. Adv. Mater. 2013;5: 637.

[28] Rodriguez-Carvajal J. FullProf: A Program for Rietveld refinement and Pattern Matching Analysis. Collected Abstracts of Powder Diffraction Meeting, Toulouse, France, 1990;127.

[29] CPDS: Diffraction Data Base. Newton Square: International for Diffraction Data, CD-ROM, 1999.

[30] Moraes J et al. Schistosoma mansoni: In vitro schistosomicidal activity of piplartine. Exp. Parasitol. 2011;127: 357-364.

[31] Bellucci FS. Caracterização dielétrica de partículas nanométricas e nanoestruturadas de óxido de niobato da família tetragonal tungstênio bronze com estequiometria $KSr_2Nb_5O_{15}$. MSc dissertation. Univ Estadual Paulista; 2008.

[32] Lanfredi S, Cardoso CX, Nobre MAL. Crystallographic properties of $KSr_2Nb_5O_{15}$. Mater. Sci. Eng., B. 2004;112: 139-143.

[33] Ma R et al. Synthesis, characterization and electromagnetic studies on nanocrystalline nickel-zinc ferrite by polyacrylamide gel. J. Mater. Sci. Technol. 2008;24: 419-422.

[34] Desmond KW, Weeks ER. Random close packing of disks and spheres in confined geometries. Phys. Rev. E. 2009;80: 051305.

[35] Jamal EMA et al. On the magnetic, mechanical and rheological properties of rubber-nickel nanocomposites. Polym. Bull. 2010;64: 907.

[36] Lanfredi S. Thermistor behaviour and electricconduction analysis of Ni-doped niobate ferroelectric: the role of multiple β parameters. J. Phys. D: Appl. Phys. 2012;45: 435302.

[37] Ma R et al. Synthesis, characterization and electromagnetic studies on nanocrystalline nickel-zinc ferrite by polyacrylamide gel. J. Mater. Sci. Technol. 2008;24: 419.

[38] Trabelsi S, Albouy PA, Rault J. Stress-induced crystallization around a crack tip in natural rubber. Macromolecules. 2002;35: 10054-10061.

[39] Ozbas B et al. Strain-induced crystallization and mechanical properties of functionalized graphene sheet-filled natural rubber. J. Polym. Sci., Part B: Polym. Phys. 2012;50: 718-723.

[40] Departamento de Ciência e Tecnologia, Secretaria de Ciência, Tecnologia e Insumos Estratégicos, Ministério da Saúde. Doenças negligenciadas: Estratégias do Ministério da Saúde. Rev. Saúde Pública. 2010;44: 200.

[41] Ferreira M et al. Angiogenic properties of natural rubber latex biomembranes and the serum fraction of Hevea Brasiliensis. Braz. J. Phys. 2009;39(3): 564-569.

[42] Bellucci FS. Preparação e caracterização de nanocompósitos multifuncionais obtidos com nanopartículas ferroelétricas e paramagnéticas em filmes de borracha natural. PhD thesis. Univ Estadual Paulista and Universidad de Valladolid; 2013.

[43] Devorak G, Rovid-Spickler A, Roth JA. Handbook for zoonotic diseases of companion animals Interaction effects on the coercivity and fluctuation field in granular powder magnetic systems. Bayer Healthcare Animal Health; 2008.

[44] Barboza-Filho CG et al. The influence of natural rubber/Au nanoparticle membranes on the physiology of Leishmania brasiliensis. Exp. Parasitol. 2012;130: 152-158.

Chapter 19

Alkylphospholipids and Leishmaniasis

Faustino Mollinedo

Additional information is available at the end of the chapter

http://dx.doi.org/10.5772/58318

1. Introduction

Leishmaniasias is a complex of diseases caused by intracellular protozoan parasites that belong to the genus *Leishmania* (class: Kinetoplastida; order: Trypanosomatidae), for which there are more than 20 different species, and is transmitted by the bite of female phlebotomine sand flies (order: Diptera; family: Psychodidae; subfamily: Phlebotominae). Various species of phlebotomine sand flies of the genus *Phlebotomus* are responsible for transmission of leishmaniasis in the Old World, and of the genus *Lutzomyia* in the New World [1]. *Leishmania* parasite has a digenetic life-cycle alternating between a mammalian host and insect vectors, phlebotomine sand flies, which are small (1.5-2 mm body length) insects mainly found in tropical and subtropical regions. *Leishmania* lives extracellularly as flagellated promastigotes in the gut and salivary glands of the sand fly vector, and intracellularly as amastigotes in the vertebrate host macrophages. *Leishmania* promastigotes, transmitted to mammalian skin by the bite of a female phlebotomine sand fly, invade human macrophages as the main host for the parasites, where *Leishmania* transforms into amastigotes and replicate intracellularly. Leishmaniasis represents a major international health problem, has a high morbidity and mortality rate, and is classified as an emerging and uncontrolled disease by the World Health Organization (WHO). The disease burden of leishmaniasis is high, with about 350 million people in 98 countries considered at risk. Among parasitic diseases, leishmaniasis accounts for the second highest burden of disease after malaria, with a loss of about 2.4 million disability-adjusted life years (DALYs) [2, 3]. There are an estimated 1.5-2 million new cases per year, with 1.5 million cases of self-healing, but disfiguring, (muco-)cutaneous leishmaniasis, and 500,000 cases of life-threatening visceral leishmaniasis [2, 3]. However, more than 90% of the world's cases of visceral leishmaniasis are in India, Bangladesh, Nepal, Sudan, and Brazil. Some species tend to cause cutaneous leishmaniasis (e.g., *L. major* and *L.tropica*), whereas others lead to cause visceral leishmaniasis (e.g., *L. infantum* and *L. donovani*). Leishmaniases are usually classified based on the clinical manifestations, leading to three major clinical forms, namely:

- Cutaneous leishmaniasis. It is the most common form of the disease, leading to a skin sore at the bite site, which erupts weeks to months after the person affected is bitten by sand flies, and then heals in a few months to a year, leaving an unpleasant-looking scar.
- Mucocutaneous leishmaniasis. It occurs predominantly in the New World, starting with skin ulcers which spread, causing tissue damage and destruction, and certain *Leishmania* species migrate to the upper respiratory tract where destruction of the oropharynx and nose ensues, resulting in extensive midfacial destruction and, occasionally, in death.
- Visceral leishmaniasis. It is classically known as kala-azar, and also referred to as black fever, and Dumdum fever. It is the most serious and devastating form of the disease, where the parasites localize to the reticuloendothelial system, rather than to the skin, and migrate to and affect internal organs (usually spleen, liver, and bone marrow), producing a potentially lethal widespread systemic disease that is fatal if untreated. Visceral leishmaniasis is characterized by irregular bouts of fever, weight loss, substantial swelling of the spleen and liver, fatigue and anemia. The systemic infection of the liver, spleen and bone marrow leads to hepatomegaly, splenomegaly, lymph node enlargement, thrombocytopenia, and anemia.

Cutaneous leishmaniasis can be further divided into: a) localized (crusted papules or ulcers occur several weeks to months after sand fly bite inoculation on exposed skin, and lesions usually heal spontaneously); b) diffuse cutaneous (producing widespread skin lesions which resemble leprosy, being particularly difficult to treat; and patients cannot mount a cell-mediated immune response to the *Leishmania* parasite, developing multiple, widespread cutaneous papules and nodules); c) recidivans (appearing as a recurrence of lesions at the site of apparently healed disease years after the original infection; and occurring typically on the face as an enlarging papule, plaque, or coalescence of papules that heals with central scarring, leading to facial destruction in some cases); d) post-kala-azar dermal leishmaniasis (a complication of visceral leishmaniasis in areas where *L. donovani* is endemic, and characterized by a hypopigmented macular, maculopapular, and nodular rash that usually appears 6 months to 1 or more years after apparent cure of visceral leishmaniasis).

Another way to categorize leishmaniasis is based on geographic occurrence. Thus, Old World leishmaniasis, caused by *Leishmania* species found in Africa, Asia, the Middle East, and the Mediterranean, mainly leads to cutaneous or visceral forms of disease; and New World leishmaniasis, caused by *Leishmania* species found in endemic regions extending from southern USA to northern Argentina, mainly in Central and South America, generates cutaneous, mucocutaneous, and visceral forms of disease. It is interesting to note that distinct forms of leishmaniasis follow different clinical courses of the disease depending on the geographical location. Thus, post-kala-azar dermal leishmaniasis heals spontaneously in the majority of cases in Africa, but rarely in patients in India. This form of leishmaniasis, endemic to India and Sudan, is considered to have an important role in maintaining and contributing to transmission of the disease particularly in interepidemic periods of visceral leishmaniasis, acting as a reservoir for parasites. Post-kala-azar dermal leishmaniasis reflects the immune response of the individual to the *Leishmania* organism, and lesions may be numerous and persist for decades. Most forms of the disease are transmissible from non-human animals to people

http://dx.doi.org/10.5772/58318

(zoonotic transmission), but some can be spread between humans (anthroponotic transmission).

The chemotherapy currently available for the treatment of leishmaniasis is far from satisfactory and shows a series of problems, including toxicity, adverse side-effects, high costs and development of drug resistance [2, 4]. Thus, search for new antilesihmanial drugs is urgently needed.

2. Miltefosine as a new antileishmanial drug

The control of leishmaniasis in the absence of vaccine depends solely on the choice of chemotherapy. Additional complications in the treatment of leishmaniasis include intrinsic species-specific differences in drug susceptibility [5, 6] as well as differences in drug efficacy between geographical areas [7], which can reflect the genetic differences between *Leishmania* parasites at species and strain levels [8, 9]. The generation of drug resistance is a major concern in the treatment of leishmaniasis that can be worsened by the rather low number of drugs currently available in therapy, thus leading to the lack of a putative alternative for a drug to which resistance has arisen. In this regard, it is well known the increasing resistance against the widely used pentavalent antimonial compounds in India, where resistance rates have been shown to be higher than 60% in parts of the state of Bihar, in north-east India [10, 11]. Thus, search for novel anti-*Leishmania* drugs is desperately needed. In the last years a new drug has been included in the clinical arsenal of antileishmanial drugs named miltefosine (hexadecylphoshocholine) (Figure 1), which is orally administered and is effective against pentavalent antimonial compound-resistant *Leishmania* parasites. Following a number of successful clinical trials ranging from phase I/II to phase IV in the period 1996-2004, miltefosine was registered as a new antileishmanial drug in India in 2002 [12]. Miltefosine, registered under the trade name of Impavido®, is the first oral drug in leishmaniasis therapy, having being developed by Zentaris (Frankfurt, Germany) in close cooperation with WHO/Special Programme for Research & Training in Tropical Diseases (TDR), and currently being manufactured by Paladin (Quebec, Canada). The standard miltefosine treatment includes oral administration of 100-150 mg/day, depending on the body weight, for 28 days and is well tolerated, except for mild gastrointestinal side effects.

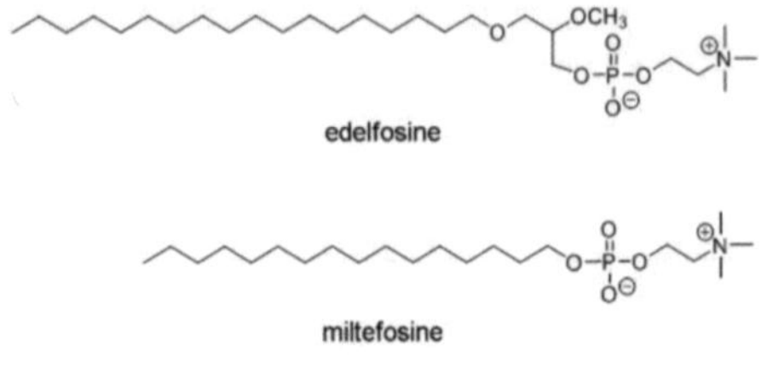

Figure 1. Chemical structures of edelfosine and miltefosine.

Miltefosine treatment leads to high cure rates in visceral leishmaniasis in India (*L. donovani*; 94% cure) [13]. However, different trials regarding the efficacy of miltefosine against cutaneous leishmaniasis in Colombia led to distinct outcomes ranging from a 90% cure [14] to an unsatisfactory cure rate of 69.8% [15]. Sensitivity to miltefosine is known to vary between *Leishmania* species [16]. In this regard, *L. braziliensis* seems to be somewhat refractory to miltefosine as shown in a number of clinical studies [14, 17-19]. Miltefosine efficacy against leishmaniasis lesions caused by *L. braziliensis*, which comprise more than 60% of cutaneous leishmaniasis in Colombia, fell to 49% [15], and was only 33% in Guatemala [14]. Additional clinical trials in Brazil showed a miltefosine cure rate of 75% and 71% for the treatment of cutaneous leishmaniasis caused by *L. braziliensis* [20] and *L. guyanensis* [21], respectively. Thus, these trials have challenged the therapeutical potential of miltefosine for the treatment of American cutaneous leishmaniasis. Miltefosine treatment has also led to approximately 70% cure rate for mucosal leishmaniasis due to *L. braziliensis* in Bolivia [18, 22], 53% for cutaneous leishmaniasis (33% for *L. braziliensis* infection, and 60% for *L. mexicana* infection) in Guatemala [14, 17, 23], and 63% for *L. tropica* infection in Afghanistan [23]. The above cure rates contrast with those reported for the treatment of visceral leishmaniasis (kala-azar) in India [12, 24] and Bangladesh [25] that were higher than 82%. These data highlight the great variability in the clinical outcome depending on the geographical area for reasons that are not well understood.

The main toxicity for miltefosine involves gastrointestinal organs in both animal and human studies. Thus, miltefosine frequently induces gastrointestinal side effects, such as anorexia, nausea, vomiting and diarrhea, that sometimes lead to drop out from treatment [2, 3, 24]. The testis and retina have been identified as target organs in rats, but the expected and corresponding effects and symptoms based on these observations have not been detected in clinical studies in humans [26]. Miltefosine distributes widely in body organs and is not metabolized by cytochrome P450 enzymes *in vitro*. Miltefosine has been found to be embryotoxic and fetotoxic in rats and rabbits, and teratogenic in rats, but not in rabbits [26]. Thus, miltefosine is potentially teratogenic, being contraindicated for use during pregnancy, and adequate contraception is required during treatment and for up to 3 months afterwards in women of child-bearing age [2, 3, 26]. An additional concern is the rapid *in vitro* generation of resistance to miltefosine [27-30] that could limit its clinical use.

Miltefosine is a member of a family of structurally-related compounds collectively known as synthetic alkylphospholipids (APLs), that target cell membranes and show pleiotropic actions with multiple biomedical applications in addition to their antitumor effect, which have been widely studied [31-35]. The advent of miltefosine as a new antileishmanial drug introduces APLs as putative novel drugs for the treatment of leishmaniasis. In addition, because of the numerous studies reported on the antitumor action of these compounds, it could be envisaged that the insight acquired for their antitumor action might be of use in the treatment of leishmaniasis.

http://dx.doi.org/10.5772/58318

3. Alkylphospholipids and leishmaniasis

As stated above miltefosine is a member of a series of synthetic lipids structurally related and known collectively as APLs, which in turn can be classified in two major categories [31]: a) the alkyl ether phospholipids (AEPs), widely referred to collectively as alkyl-lysophospholipid analogs (ALPs), containing ether bonds in the glycerol backbone of the phospholipid, as exemplified by 1-*O*-octadecyl-2-*O*-methyl-*rac*-glycero-3-phosphocholine (ET-18-OCH_3; edelfosine) (Figure 1); b) and the alkylphosphocholines (APCs), lacking the glycerol backbone and formed by a simple long-chain alcohol esterified to a phosphobase, as exemplified by hexadecylphosphocholine (HPC; miltefosine) (Figure 1). All of these APLs show low rates of metabolism both *in vitro* and *in vivo*. APLs were initially shown to elicit actions on the immune system and to kill cancer cells [31, 33, 35]. The first studies of the antiprotozoal activity of APLs in the 1980s against *Tetrahymena pyriformis* [36] and *L. donovani* [37, 38] were reported soon after their development as anticancer drugs [39-41]. APLs have been reported to be effective against different *Leishmania* species, including *L. donovani, L. infantum* (Old World)/*chagasi* (New World), *L. major, L. braziliensis, L. amazonensis, L. mexicana, L. panamensis, L. guyanensis, L. tropica, L. aethiopica* and *L. lainsoni* [16, 42-44].

In 1987, Croft *et al.* [38] reported the antiparasitic action of miltefosine against *L. donovani* amastigotes. Subsequently, *in vivo* studies showed the antileishmanial activity of miltefosine (10-20 mg/kg of body weight/day, orally administered) in mice infected with *L. donovani* and *L. infantum* [45]. Later on, following eight successful clinical trials [12], miltefosine (Impavido®) became the first oral treatment of visceral leishmaniasis and is the most recent drug to come to the market for the treatment of this disease.

Within APLs, edelfosine has been considered as the long-standing prototype of these compounds, and recent evidences have unveiled part of its mechanism of action as a promising antitumor drug. Another APL named perifosine, a miltefosine analog, is currently in clinical trials for different types of cancer. Thus, the insights gained in the last years on both the mechanism of action of APLs as antitumor agents, especially edelfosine, and the clinical experience acquired with some of these compounds, particularly miltefosine and perifosine, constitute an invaluable source of information for the putative use of APLs as antiparasitic drugs, as well as for the development of novel APL-related compounds as antileishmanial drugs. Very recently, edelfosine has been shown to be effective against different types of *Leishmania* parasites in *in vitro* and *in vivo* studies, displaying a better profile than miltefosine on the generation of drug resistance [30]. In addition, edelfosine exerts a potent anti-inflammatory effect [46], which is of importance as several of the clinical signs of leishmaniasis are due to an inflammatory response. In this regard, it is also worth mentioning that current evidence suggests that *Leishmania* parasites are initially engulfed by neutrophils, a major inflammatory cell type, and delivered to cytoplasmic neutrophil granules [47], where they survive and retain infectivity, thus using neutrophils as transport vehicles before they enter safely and silently their ultimate host cell, the macrophage [48, 49]. Increasing evidence suggests that APLs are new promising oral leishmanicidal drugs that could act either as single drugs or as combination therapy.

The antileishmanial efficacy of miltefosine in T cell-deficient athymic mice infected with *L. donovani* (25 mg/kg of body weight dissolved in a volume of 0.3 ml tap water, orally administered) was similar to that found in normal mice [50, 51]. These observations were extended in T and B-cell deficient severe combined immunodeficiency (SCID) mice, where miltefosine showed a similar effect to that detected in normal BALB/c mice [52]. These results raise the possibility that miltefosine may be of interest as an initial oral treatment approach to the growing problem of AIDS-associated visceral leishmaniasis in CD4 cell-depleted patients [53].

Currently, miltefosine is the only APL in the market for the treatment of leishmaniasis, but edelfosine and perifosine show promising and potent anti-*Leishmania* activity both *in vitro* and *in vivo* [30, 54, 55], warranting further studies for their putative clinical use in the future. The mechanism of action of miltefosine is not properly understood, but a clear correlation between the accumulation of the drug within the parasite and its toxic effects has already been described [27], this notion being identical to that previously advanced for edelfosine in its antitumor activity [32, 56-58], and therefore the ability of APLs to kill different *Leishmania* species and cancer cells is critically dependent on the drug uptake.

4. Mechanism of action of miltefosine as a leishmanicidal drug

The studies directed to unravel the underlying mechanism of miltefosine as an antiparasitic drug have followed to great extent the same trends previously reported and advanced in the analysis of the molecular and cellular pathways involved in the antitumor action of APLs. Thus, the insights generated from the antitumor action of APLs on cancer cells are being extrapolated to the APL killing action on *Leishmania* parasites. In this regard, a stark example lies in the direct induction of cell death by APLs in both tumor cells and *Leishmania* parasites. Following the studies reported simultaneously in 1993 by Diomede's group in Milan [59] and Mollinedo's group in Madrid [60], showing that the APL edelfosine induced apoptosis in a wide variety of tumor cells, subsequent studies extended this proapoptotic activity against cancer cells to other APLs, including miltefosine and perifosine [61, 62]. Later on in the new millennium, a number of studies have started to unveil the underlying mechanisms, signaling pathways and subcellular structures involved in the antitumor activity of APLs, including reorganization of lipid raft membrane domains, death receptors and mitochondria [32, 34, 63, 64]. These studies have provided a conceptual framework for a better understanding of the processes involved in the anti-*Leishmania* activity of APLs. Thus, two reports came out in 2004 showing that miltefosine induced a cell death process showing several features of metazoan apoptosis in *L. donovani* promastigotes and amastigotes [65, 66], including cell shrinkage, DNA fragmentation into oligonucleosome-sized fragments, and phosphatidylserine exposure. Then, subsequent studies have reported the miltefosine-mediated induction of an apoptosis-like cell death in promastigotes from different species of *Leishmania* promastigotes, including *L. amazonensis* [67], *L. infantum* [68], *L. tropica* [69], *L. major* [69], *L. panamensis* and many others [30]. The fact that an apoptosis-related process seems to be involved in the death of *Leishmania* parasites upon APL addition is further supported by the recent finding that tolerance to undergo apoptosis-like cell death in *Leishmania* is linked to multidrug resistance within the parasite *in vitro* [70]. This raises the concern that cross-tolerance to drug-induced apoptosis-like cell death, not only against a particular selective drug promoting resistance, but also against additional drugs sharing a similar mode of killing, might lead to a facilitated emergence of cross-resistance against other drugs that have different cellular targets but analogous ways of killing [70]. However the mechanism by which APLs induce an apoptosis-like cell death in *Leishmania* parasites remains to be fully elucidated.

One critical organelle that seems to be involved in the killing process in *Leishmania* is the mitochondrion. Miltefosine treatment has been found to lead to loss of mitochondrial membrane potential and the release of cytochrome *c* with consequent activation of cellular proteases in *L. donovani* promastigotes, even in arsenite-resistant L. *donovani* promastigotes displaying a multidrug resistance phenotype and overexpressing Pgp-like protein [71]. The finding that edelfosine-induced cell death in *L. infantum* promastigotes can be regulated by the ectopic expression of the antiapoptotic and proapoptotic members of the Bcl-2 family of proteins Bcl-X_L and Hrk, which affect mitochondria-related processes, suggests that this process shows certain similarities to apoptosis in eukaryotic cells and that mitochondria are involved in the killing process [72]. Furthermore, miltefosine inhibits mitochondrial cytochrome *c* oxidase in *L. donovani* promastigotes, and this enzyme was suggested to act as a target for this APL [73]. In this regard, cytochrome *c* oxidase has also been identified as a potential target of miltefosine from a genomic library screen of the model yeast *Saccharomyces cerevisiae* [74]. Miltefosine inhibited cytochrome *c* oxidase activity in a dose-dependent manner, and this inhibition most likely contributed to the miltefosine-induced apoptosis-like cell death in *S. cerevisiae* [74]. Figure 2 depicts a schematic view for the antileishmanial activity of miltefosine based on current data.

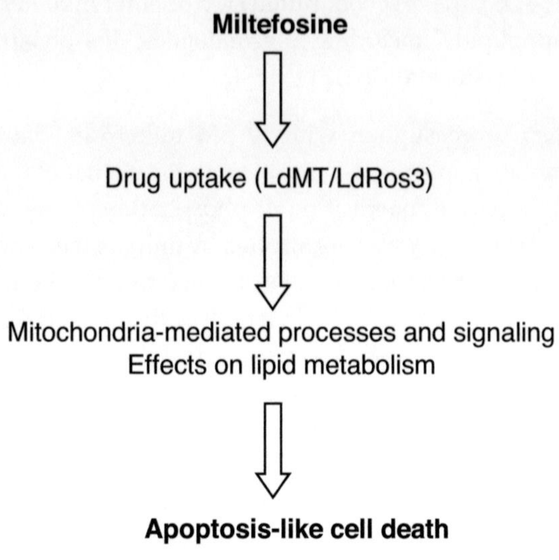

Figure 2. Schematic view of the antileishmanial mechanism of action of miltefosine. See text for further details.

5. Miltefosine effects on lipid metabolism

APLs, including miltefosine, have been found to interact with membrane lipids and affect lipid metabolism [75-77], these actions having been suggested being involved in their mechanism of action. In lipid monolayer studies, miltefosine molecules were inserted into the monolayer of lipids as monomers until the critical micellar concentration, and a high condensation was found between miltefosine and sterols showing a high affinity between miltefosine and sterols [78]. However, miltefosine did not act as detergent disturbing membrane integrity [78]. *Leishmania* parasites have high levels of ether-phospholipids [79-83], and these are mainly found in the glycosylphosphatidylinositol-anchored glycolipids and glycoproteins present on the surface of the parasites [84-86]. Because edelfosine and other APLs are ether lipids, it could be suggested that the biosynthesis of ether lipids occurring in the glycosomes of *Leishmania* might be affected. Miltefosine and edelfosine did not affect enzymes involved in early steps in ether lipid biosynthesis in *L. mexicana* promastigotes, including dihydroxyacetonephosphate acyltransferase, *sn*-l-acyl-2-*lyso*-glycero-3-phosphocholine and *sn*-l-alkyl-2-*lyso*-glycero-3-phosphocholine acyltransferases activities [87]. However, both miltefosine and edelfosine affected the later metabolism of alkyl-phosphatidylcholine intermediates by inhibiting the glycosomal located alkyl-specific-acyl-CoA acyltransferase in a dose-dependent manner with an inhibitory concentration of 50 μM, thus suggesting these drugs can perturb ether-lipid remodelling [87]. However, the fact that inhibition of alkyl-specific-acyl-CoA acyltransferase required drug concentrations higher than those showing cytotoxicity to *L. mexicana* (IC_{50}, 14 μM and 18 μM for miltefosine and edelfosine, respectively) [87] challenges the putative involvement of this pathway as the primary target of these drugs. In addition, the role of glycosylphosphatidylinositols and ether phospholipids in the survival of *Leishmania* amastigotes is questioned by the viability of *L. major* null mutants for alkyldihydroxyacetonephosphate synthase (ADS), the first committed step of ether lipid synthesis. These mutants lacked all ether phospholipids, including plasmalogens, lipophosphoglycan (LPG), and smaller glycosylphosphatidylinositols (GIPLs) [88].

Treatment of *L. donovani* promastigotes with 10 μM miltefosine significantly reduced the phosphatidylcholine content and enhanced the phosphatidylethanolamine content in parasite membranes, suggesting a partial inactivation of phosphatidylethanolamine-N-methyltransferase [89]. Phospholipase D activity was not affected by miltefosine, whereas the enhancement of the lysophosphatidylcholine content could be ascribed to phospholipase A2 activation. No effect was observed in the fatty acid alkyl chain length or the fatty acid unsaturation rate upon miltefosine treatment, whereas a two-fold increase was detected in the amount of cholesterol within the membranes [89]. Because cholesterol is not biosynthesized by the *Leishmania* parasite, but is taken from the external medium, it might be envisaged that miltefosine promotes cholesterol uptake in promastigotes perhaps by the condensation effect between miltefosine and cholesterol [78]. In contrast, a strong reduction of about two times in the C24 alkylated sterol content was detected in miltefosine-treated membranes, even though the level of the final C24 sterol alkylating product, ergosterol, the predominant plasma membrane sterol in fungi and *Leishmania*, was not changed [89].

Interestingly, the content of unsaturated phospholipid alkyl chains was lower in miltefosine-resistant parasite plasma membranes than in those of the wild type, suggesting a lower fluidity of miltefosine-resistant parasite membranes, and rendering the miltefosine interaction with the external monolayer of miltefosine-resistant parasites more difficult. Miltefosine-resistant parasite membranes displayed a higher content of short alkyl chain fatty acids, suggesting a partial inactivation of the fatty acid elongation enzyme system in miltefosine-resistant parasites, and the C24-alkylated sterol content was halved in miltefosine-resistant parasites, but this modification was not related to miltefosine sensitivity [90]. Thus, miltefosine resistance affects three lipid biochemical pathways: fatty acid elongation, the desaturase system responsible for fatty acid alkyl chain unsaturation, and the C-24-alkylation of sterols. [90]. Because of the differences detected in the lipid composition of miltefosine-treated *Leishmania* and miltefosine-resistant parasites, it could be hypothesized that continuous *in vitro* drug pressure affects the regulation of *Leishmania* lipid metabolism [89], but the real implication of these actions on parasite killing remains a topic of much debate.

6. Drug resistance

A major hurdle in successful leishmanial chemotherapy is emergence of drug resistance. Miltefosine, the first orally administrable anti-leishmanial drug, has shown the potential against drug-resistant strains of *Leishmania*. However, at the same time the readiness in generating miltefosine-resistant parasites *in vitro* in the laboratory [27-29] raises some concerns about the life span for an efficient use of miltefosine. The major underlying mechanisms involved in the generation of miltefosine-resistant parasites seem to reside in defective drug uptake into the parasite and increased drug efflux. In addition, its long half-life (approximately 150 hours) [91] might facilitate the emergence of resistance.

L. donovani promastigotes resistant to up to 40 μM miltefosine have been generated *in vitro* in the laboratory by continuous step-wise drug pressure, resulting in being 15-fold more resistant to miltefosine than wild-type promastigotes [28]. A drastic reduction (>95%) in the ability of resistant *L. donovani* promastigotes to internalize [^{14}C]miltefosine was detected, whereas binding of miltefosine to the plasma membrane and drug efflux from preloaded cells were similar in both drug-sensitive and -resistant cells, and no metabolism of [^{14}C]miltefosine was evident in either sensitive and resistant cells [92]. This miltefosine uptake was temperature and energy dependent and sensitive to the thiol-reactive agent N-ethylmaleimide [92]. Resistant parasites were also unable to take up other short-chain phospholipid analogs, independently of their polar head group, even though endocytosis remained unaltered [92]. The underlying basis for the generation of drug-resistant *L. donovani* promastigotes turned out to be a decrease in the uptake of miltefosine mediated by the plasma membrane P-type transporter *L. donovani* miltefosine transporter (LdMT) from the aminophospholipid translocase subfamily and by LdRos3 [93, 94]. LdMT is an inward-directed lipid translocase belonging to the P4 subfamily of P-type ATPases, which comprises lipid flippases that catalyze the translocation of phospholipids from the exoplasmic to the cytosolic leaflet of cell membranes; and LdRos3 is a non-catalytic subunit of LdMT that belongs to the CDC50/Lem3 family, which includes proteins proposed as likely beta subunits for P4-ATPases [93, 94]. LdMT and LdRos3 proteins are primarily localized to the *Leishmania* plasma membrane and required for the rapid intracellular uptake of miltefosine and additional related choline-bearing lipids. Likewise, in the budding yeast *S. cerevisiae*, members of the two protein families have been found to form stable transporter complexes that function in the translocation of phospholipids from the exoplasmic to the cytoplasmic leaflet of cellular membranes [95, 96]. Despite both LdMT and LdRos3 normally localize to the plasma membrane, they are retained at the endoplasmic reticulum in the absence of the other protein or in the presence of inactivating point mutations in LdMT [94]. Both LdMT and the Cdc50-like protein LdRos3 form a stable complex that plays an essential role in maintaining phospholipid asymmetry in the parasite plasma membrane [97], and constitute part of the same translocation machinery that determines flippase activity, responsible for miltefosine uptake, as well as miltefosine sensitivity in *Leishmania* [94]. Loss of either LdMT or LdRos3 blocks ATP-dependent transport of NBD-labeled phosphatidylethanolamine and phosphatidylcholine from the outer to the inner plasma membrane leaflet in *L. donovani* promastigotes and results in an increased cell surface exposure of endogenous phosphatidylethanolamine, whereas infectivity was not compromised [97]. A promastigote line, M-mutR, that shows mutations in LdMT, thus leading to defective miltefosine internalization, is infective to macrophages *in vitro* and in BALB/c mice *in vivo*, and displays a good correlation of *in vitro* resistance between promastigotes and intracellular amastigotes [29]. The fact that M-mutR parasites retain the resistant phenotype *in vivo* indicate that miltefosine-resistant *L. donovani* promastigotes transform to miltefosine-resistant amastigotes [29]. It was also observed no cross-resistance to other antileishmanial drugs in M-mutR amastigotes [29]. Some clinical studies have suggested, as indicated above, that miltefosine shows significantly less efficiency against the cutaneous and mucocutaneous leishmaniasis caused by *L. braziliensis* parasites, mainly due to their inability to internalize the drug because of the low expression levels of the beta subunit LbRos3 [98]. Overexpression of LbRos3 induced increased miltefosine sensitivity in both *L. braziliensis* promastigotes and intracellular amastigotes, further supporting the notion that miltefosine uptake is a major event in determining miltefosine antileishmanial potency [98]. Miltefosine-resistant promastigotes, displaying cross-resistance to the ether lipid edelfosine, but not to the standard anti-leishmanial drugs, shows no amplification of specific genes, including the multidrug resistance P-glycoprotein gene, and resistance has been found to be stable up to 12 weeks in drug-free culture medium [28].

The evidence gathered so far has shown that reduced miltefosine incorporation has always led to a resistant phenotype. This lower accumulation of miltefosine can be achieved by two processes: a) a decrease in drug uptake, rendered by inactivation of any one of the two proteins responsible for the miltefosine uptake, namely LdMT and its beta subunit LdRos3; b) an increase in drug efflux, mediated by the overexpression of the ABC transporter P-glycoprotein [27]. Thus, in addition to a flaw in the uptake of miltefosine as stated above, an increased efflux of miltefosine has also been implicated in miltefosine resistance. A multidrug resistance (MDR) *L. tropica* line overexpressing a P-glycoprotein-like transporter was found to display significant cross-resistance to the ALP miltefosine and edelfosine, with resistant indices of 9.2- and 7.1-fold, respectively [99]. This resistance was mediated through overexpression of an ABC transporter, namely the *Leishmania* P-glycoprotein-like transporter (*Leishmania* ABCB1 or

LtrMDR1) [99, 100]. ATP-binding cassette (ABC) transporters constitute one of the largest and most conserved protein families and have been considered major players in drug resistance during the treatment of cancer and infectious diseases. Interestingly, sesquiterpene C-3 completely sensitizes MDR parasites to APLs, acting as an inhibitor of LtrMDR1 [99]. In addition, overexpression of two *Leishmania*-specific ABC subfamily G (ABCG)-like transporters localized at the plasma membrane of *Leishmania* protozoan parasites, LiABCG6 and LiABCG4 half-transporters, conferred resistance to APLs in *Leishmania* parasites and *S. cerevisiae* [101, 102]. Overexpression of LiABCG6 not only leads to miltefosine resistance *in vitro*, but also to the antileishmanial oral drug 8-aminoquinoline analog sitamaquine [102].

Additional genes associated with miltefosine resistance have been identified by generating *L. major* promastigote mutants highly resistant to miltefosine (80-100 μM) in a step-by-step manner and subsequent analysis of the short-read whole genome sequencing [103]. In addition to the previously described P-type ATPase involved in phospholipid translocation, another new gene coding for pyridoxal kinase, involved in the formation of pyridoxal-5'-phophate (active vitamin B6), has been implicated in miltefosine susceptibility [103]. Following this genetic approach, it was clear the polyclonal nature of a resistant population with varying susceptibilities and genotypes, indicating that miltefosine resistance can be genetically and phenotypically highly heterogeneous [103].

7. Effects of APLs on the immune system

Even though miltefosine retains its antiparasitic activity against *Leishmania* infection in immunodeficient SCID mice, leading to similar levels of activity in both SCID and BALB/c mouse-*L. donovani* models [52], the immunomodulatory properties of miltefosine have been proposed as an additional factor to its antileishmanial action [104]. Thus, miltefosine's antileishmanial function has been reported to be significantly compromised in interferon-gamma (IFNγ)-deficient macrophages, suggesting the importance of endogenous IFNγ in the miltefosine-induced antileishmanial functions of macrophages. IFNγ responsiveness is reduced in *L. donovani*-infected macrophages but is significantly restored by miltefosine, as it induces IFNγ, enhances IFNγ receptors, and IFNγ induces STAT-1 phosphorylation but reduces activation of SHP-1, the phosphatase implicated in the downregulation of STAT-1 phosphorylation [104]. *L. donovani*-infected macrophages induced Th2 response, but miltefosine treatment reversed the response to Th1-type [104].

Miltefosine is able to form stable multilamellar vesicles (MLVs liposomes) to deliver the APL to monocytes/macrophages. Both micellar and liposomal miltefosine have been found to interact with human monocytes and upregulate specific adhesion molecules, including intracellular adhesion molecule-1 and class 1 major histocompatibility complex (MHC-1) antigen in a dose-dependent manner in U937 cells [105], used as a cell line model system to study human monocytes. These actions could be involved in the initial steps of miltefosine-mediated recruitment of macrophages [105]. Miltefosine, better in liposomal than in free (micellar) form, has also been reported to induce an increase in tumor necrosis factor (TNF) release and nitric oxide (NO) generation after *in vitro* co-culture of mouse peritoneal macrophages or U937 cells with lipopolysaccharide (LPS) [106-108]. Miltefosine has also been reported to enhance the immune response of IL-2-stimulated mononuclear cells resulting in granulocyte-macrophage colony-stimulating factor (GM-CSF) and IFNγ gene expression and IFNγ secretion [109].

However, recent studies on the effects of miltefosine on dendritic cells (DC) in *L. major* infection have challenged the putative role of the immunomodulatory action of miltefosine on its antiparasitic action, and suggest that miltefosine functions independently of the immune system, mostly through direct toxicity against the *Leishmania* parasite [110]. DC are critical for initiation of protective immunity against *Leishmania* through induction of Th1 immunity via interleukin 12 (IL-12), and when co-cultured with miltefosine for 4 days, most of the *in vitro*-infected DC were free of parasites. However, miltefosine treatment did not influence DC maturation (upregulation of major histocompatibility complex II [MHC II] or co-stimulatory molecules, e.g., CD40, CD54, and CD86), did not significantly alter cytokine release (IL-12, tumor necrosis factor alpha [TNF-α], or IL-10), antigen presentation, or NO production [110].

8. Canine leishmaniasis

Miltefosine is marketed as Milteforan® (Virbac, Carros, France) for the treatment of canine visceral leishmaniasis that is the result of infection with *L. infantum* in the Old World and *L. chagasi* in the New World. These two *Leishmania* species are considered sibling and indistinguishable species, and several genetic studies have shown evidence for the synonym of *L. infantum* and *L. chagasi*, and suggest the introduction of *L. infantum* from Southwest Europe into the New World in recent history [111-114]. Thus, *L. infantum* (Old World) and *L. chagasi* (New World) belong to the same species, and therefore *L. chagasi* has been synonymized with *L. infantum*. Dogs are considered the primary reservoir hosts *of L. infantum/chagasi*, and infection of dogs with *L. infantum/chagasi* involves cells of the lymphatic series resulting in visceralization of infection. The domestic dog seems to be a main reservoir for human visceral leishmaniasis, rendering canine disease control a critical issue. Unfortunately efforts to control leishmaniasis in dogs have been largely unsuccessful so far. Oral administration of miltefosine at a dose of 2 mg/kg body weight once a day for 28 days leads to significant reduction of parasite loads and clinical symptoms, whereas adverse reactions were not serious and observed in less that 12% of the dogs, the most frequent one being vomiting, which was transient, self-limiting, and reversible [115-117]. *Leishmania* DNA quantification by real-time PCR has shown that miltefosine treatment of dogs leads to a drastic and progressive reduction of parasite load in lymph node aspirates, but does not suppress the parasite in lymph nodes [118]. Miró et al. [119] has shown that the treatment of miltefosine-allopurinol combination therapy (2 mg/kg miltefosine orally once daily for 28 days and 10 mg/kg of allopurinol orally twice daily for 7 months) behaved similarly to the current reference combination therapy, namely meglumine antimoniate-allopurinol (50 mg/kg of meglumine antimoniate sub-cutaneously twice daily for 28 days and 10 mg/kg of allopurinol orally twice daily for 7 months), in promoting a significant reduction in total clinical score and parasite load over the 7-month study period. These

http://dx.doi.org/10.5772/58318

observations together with the lack of effect on renal and hepatic parameters and adverse reactions suggests that miltefosine, in combination with allopurinol, might offer a safe and effective alternative treatment option for canine leishmaniasis compared to the reference therapy [119]. A recent study [117], where dogs naturally infected with *L. infantum/chagasi* were treated with miltefosine using different therapeutic regimens, has shown that after treatment and during the following 24 months, there was progressive clinical improvement and complete recovery in 50% (7/14) of the treated animals. There was a decrease in the smear positivity of the bone marrow after treatment, and there was also a gradual and constant decrease in positive cultures at the end of the follow-up period. However, the PCR detection of parasite DNA remained positive, and the animals presented a significant increase in parasite load 6 months after treatment. Thus, the fact that the improvement in the clinical symptoms is not followed by total parasitological clearance, raises some doubts about the use of this drug in endemic areas where the dogs are involved in the maintenance of the parasite cycle.

9. Conclusions

At present the control of protozoan parasite *Leishmania* infections relies primarily on chemotherapy, but the armoury of drugs available for treating *Leishmania* infections is rather limited and includes a few drugs with unknown cellular targets and unclear mode of action. These drugs include pentavalent antimonials, pentamidine, amphotericin B, miltefosine, paromomycin, fluconazole, allopurinol, and few other drugs at various stages of their development process. The recent inclusion of miltefosine as a new antileishmanial drug has been a breakthrough in the treatment of leishmaniasis, as it constituted the first effective oral drug, thus facilitating medical access and making treatment more accessible to rural and remote areas. Interestingly, miltefosine belongs to a family of lipid compounds collectively known as APLs, some of them showing also interesting and promising antileishmanial activities in addition to their well known antitumor action. Thus, additional APLs or APL-related compounds might be of interest to identify novel drugs to combat *Leishmania* infections both in humans and animals, especially in dogs as major reservoirs for human visceral leishmaniasis (*L. infantum/chagasi*). Identification of the death signaling pathways activated in miltefosine-sensitive parasites will be essential for a better understanding of the molecular mechanisms of action and resistance in these parasites. In this regard, the knowledge acquired for the antitumor action of APLs is being and will be of further aid to unveil the mode of action of miltefosine and putative additional APLs with potent antileishmanial activities. Furthemore, elucidation of the molecular mechanisms underlying miltefosine- and APL-mediated cell death will facilitate the design of new therapeutic strategies against *Leishmania* parasites. The proneness to generate *in vitro* resistance to miltefosine raises some concerns about its putative life span in clinical use, thus favoring research on additional APLs that could improve the current antileishmanial features of miltefosine as well as on combination therapy regimens. APLs have shown themselves as potent antileishmanial drugs, and current evidence warrants further research on these promising lipid drugs that could make a difference in the clinical setting and medical care of leishmaniasis.

Author details

Faustino Mollinedo*

Address all correspondence to: fmollin@usal.es

Instituto de Biología Molecular y Celular del Cáncer, Centro de Investigación del Cáncer, CSIC-Universidad de Salamanca, Campus Miguel de Unamuno, Salamanca, Spain

References

[1] Bates PA. Transmission of *Leishmania* metacyclic promastigotes by phlebotomine sand flies. Int J Parasitol 2007;37:1097-106.

[2] Murray HW, Berman JD, Davies CR, Saravia NG. Advances in leishmaniasis. Lancet 2005;366:1561-77.

[3] WHO. Control of the leishmaniases. World Health Organization technical report series 2010;949:1-186.

[4] van Griensven J, Balasegaram M, Meheus F, Alvar J, Lynen L, Boelaert M. Combination therapy for visceral leishmaniasis. Lancet Infect Dis 2010;10:184-94.

[5] Croft SL. Monitoring drug resistance in leishmaniasis. Trop Med Int Health 2001;6:899-905.

[6] Croft SL, Sundar S, Fairlamb AH. Drug resistance in leishmaniasis. Clin Microbiol Rev 2006;19:111-26.

[7] Hailu A, Musa A, Wasunna M, Balasegaram M, Yifru S, Mengistu G, et al. Geographical variation in the response of visceral leishmaniasis to paromomycin in East Africa: a multicentre, open-label, randomized trial. PLoS Negl Trop Dis 2010;4:e709.

[8] Schonian G, Kuhls K, Mauricio IL. Molecular approaches for a better understanding of the epidemiology and population genetics of *Leishmania*. Parasitology 2011;138:405-25.

[9] Subba Raju BV, Gurumurthy S, Kuhls K, Bhandari V, Schnonian G, Salotra P. Genetic typing reveals monomorphism between antimony sensitive and resistant *Leishmania donovani* isolates from visceral leishmaniasis or post kala-azar dermal leishmaniasis cases in India. Parasitol Res 2012;111:1559-68.

[10] Sundar S. Drug resistance in Indian visceral leishmaniasis. Trop Med Int Health 2001;6:849-54.

[11] Sundar S, Chatterjee M. Visceral leishmaniasis - current therapeutic modalities. Indian J Med Res 2006;123:345-52.

[12] Sundar S, Jha TK, Thakur CP, Bhattacharya SK, Rai M. Oral miltefosine for the treatment of Indian visceral leishmaniasis. Trans R Soc Trop Med Hyg 2006;100 Suppl 1:S26-33.

[13] Sundar S, Jha TK, Thakur CP, Engel J, Sindermann H, Fischer C, et al. Oral miltefosine for Indian visceral leishmaniasis. N Engl J Med 2002;347:1739-46.

[14] Soto J, Arana BA, Toledo J, Rizzo N, Vega JC, Diaz A, et al. Miltefosine for new world cutaneous leishmaniasis. Clin Infect Dis 2004;38:1266-72.

[15] Velez I, Lopez L, Sanchez X, Mestra L, Rojas C, Rodriguez E. Efficacy of miltefosine for the treatment of American cutaneous leishmaniasis. Am J Trop Med Hyg 2010;83:351-6.

[16] Escobar P, Matu S, Marques C, Croft SL. Sensitivities of *Leishmania* species to hexadecylphosphocholine (miltefosine), ET-18-OCH_3 (edelfosine) and amphotericin B. Acta Trop 2002;81:151-7.

[17] Soto J, Berman J. Treatment of New World cutaneous leishmaniasis with miltefosine. Trans R Soc Trop Med Hyg 2006;100 Suppl 1:S34-40.

[18] Soto J, Toledo J, Valda L, Balderrama M, Rea I, Parra R, et al. Treatment of Bolivian mucosal leishmaniasis with miltefosine. Clin Infect Dis 2007;44:350-6.

[19] Minodier P, Parola P. Cutaneous leishmaniasis treatment. Travel medicine and infectious disease 2007;5:150-8.

[20] Machado PR, Ampuero J, Guimaraes LH, Villasboas L, Rocha AT, Schriefer A, et al. Miltefosine in the treatment of cutaneous leishmaniasis caused by *Leishmania braziliensis* in Brazil: a randomized and controlled trial. PLoS Negl Trop Dis 2010;4:e912.

[21] Chrusciak-Talhari A, Dietze R, Chrusciak Talhari C, da Silva RM, Gadelha Yamashita EP, de Oliveira Penna G, et al. Randomized controlled clinical trial to access efficacy and safety of miltefosine in the treatment of cutaneous leishmaniasis caused by *Leishmania* (*Viannia*) *guyanensis* in Manaus, Brazil. Am J Trop Med Hyg 2011;84:255-60.

[22] Soto J, Rea J, Valderrama M, Toledo J, Valda L, Ardiles J, et al. Efficacy of extended (six weeks) treatment with miltefosine for mucosal leishmaniasis in Bolivia. Am J Trop Med Hyg 2009;81:387-9.

[23] Soto J, Soto P. Oral miltefosine to treat leishmaniasis. Biomedica 2006;26 Suppl 1:207-17.

[24] Bhattacharya SK, Sinha PK, Sundar S, Thakur CP, Jha TK, Pandey K, et al. Phase 4 trial of miltefosine for the treatment of Indian visceral leishmaniasis. J Infect Dis 2007;196:591-8.

[25] Rahman M, Ahmed BN, Faiz MA, Chowdhury MZ, Islam QT, Sayeedur R, et al. Phase IV trial of miltefosine in adults and children for treatment of visceral leishmaniasis (kala-azar) in Bangladesh. Am J Trop Med Hyg 2011;85:66-9.

[26] Sindermann H, Engel J. Development of miltefosine as an oral treatment for leishmaniasis. Trans R Soc Trop Med Hyg 2006;100 Suppl 1:S17-20.

[27] Perez-Victoria FJ, Sanchez-Canete MP, Seifert K, Croft SL, Sundar S, Castanys S, et al. Mechanisms of experimental resistance of *Leishmania* to miltefosine: Implications for clinical use. Drug Resist Updat 2006;9:26-39.

[28] Seifert K, Matu S, Javier Perez-Victoria F, Castanys S, Gamarro F, Croft SL. Characterisation of *Leishmania donovani* promastigotes resistant to hexadecylphosphocholine (miltefosine). International journal of antimicrobial agents 2003;22:380-7.

[29] Seifert K, Perez-Victoria FJ, Stettler M, Sanchez-Canete MP, Castanys S, Gamarro F, et al. Inactivation of the miltefosine transporter, LdMT, causes miltefosine resistance that is conferred to the amastigote stage of *Leishmania donovani* and persists *in vivo*. International journal of antimicrobial agents 2007;30:229-35.

[30] Varela-M RE, Villa-Pulgarin JA, Yepes E, Muller I, Modolell M, Munoz DL, et al. *In vitro* and *in vivo* efficacy of ether lipid edelfosine against *Leishmania* spp. and SbV-resistant parasites. PLoS Negl Trop Dis 2012;6:e1612.

[31] Gajate C, Mollinedo F. Biological Activities, Mechanisms of Action and biomedical prospect of the antitumor ether phospholipid ET-18-OCH_3 (edelfosine), a proapoptotic agent in tumor cells. Curr Drug Metab 2002;3:491-525.

[32] Gajate C, Del Canto-Janez E, Acuna AU, Amat-Guerri F, Geijo E, Santos-Beneit AM, et al. Intracellular triggering of Fas aggregation and recruitment of apoptotic molecules into Fas-enriched rafts in selective tumor cell apoptosis. J Exp Med 2004;200:353-65.

[33] Mollinedo F, Gajate C, Martin-Santamaria S, Gago F. ET-18-OCH_3 (edelfosine): a selective antitumour lipid targeting apoptosis through intracellular activation of Fas/CD95 death receptor. Curr Med Chem 2004;11:3163-84.

[34] Gajate C, Mollinedo F. Edelfosine and perifosine induce selective apoptosis in multiple myeloma by recruitment of death receptors and downstream signaling molecules into lipid rafts. Blood 2007;109:711-9.

[35] Mollinedo F. Antitumor ether lipids: proapoptotic agents with multiple therapeutic indications. Expert Opin Ther Patents 2007;17:385-405.

[36] Tsushima S, Yoshioka Y, Tanida S, Nomura H, Nojima S, Hozumi M. Syntheses and antimicrobial activities of alkyl lysophospholipids. Chem Pharm Bull (Tokyo) 1982;30:3260-70.

[37] Achterberg V, Gercken G. Cytotoxicity of ester and ether lysophospholipids on *Leishmania donovani* promastigotes. Mol Biochem Parasitol 1987;23:117-22.

[38] Croft SL, Neal RA, Pendergast W, Chan JH. The activity of alkyl phosphorylcholines and related derivatives against *Leishmania donovani*. Biochem Pharmacol 1987;36:2633-6.

[39] Berdel WE. Membrane-interactive lipids as experimental anticancer drugs. Br J Cancer 1991;64:208-11.

[40] Berdel WE, Bausert WR, Fink U, Rastetter J, Munder PG. Anti-tumor action of alkyl-lysophospholipids. Anticancer Res 1981;1:345-52.

[41] Berdel WE, Fink U, Rastetter J. Clinical phase I pilot study of the alkyl lysophospholipid derivative ET-18-OCH_3. Lipids 1987;22:967-9.

[42] Croft SL, Neal RA, Thornton EA, Herrmann DB. Antileishmanial activity of the ether phospholipid ilmofosine. Trans R Soc Trop Med Hyg 1993;87:217-9.

[43] Croft SL, Seifert K, Duchene M. Antiprotozoal activities of phospholipid analogues. Mol Biochem Parasitol 2003;126:165-72.

[44] Yardley V, Croft SL, De Doncker S, Dujardin JC, Koirala S, Rijal S, et al. The sensitivity of clinical isolates of *Leishmania* from Peru and Nepal to miltefosine. Am J Trop Med Hyg 2005;73:272-5.

[45] Kuhlencord A, Maniera T, Eibl H, Unger C. Hexadecylphosphocholine: oral treatment of visceral leishmaniasis in mice. Antimicrob Agents Chemother 1992;36:1630-4.

[46] Mollinedo F, Gajate C, Morales AI, del Canto-Janez E, Justies N, Collia F, et al. Novel anti-inflammatory action of edelfosine lacking toxicity with protective effect in experimental colitis. J Pharmacol Exp Ther 2009;329:439-49.

[47] Mollinedo F, Janssen H, de la Iglesia-Vicente J, Villa-Pulgarin JA, Calafat J. Selective fusion of azurophilic granules with *Leishmania*-containing phagosomes in human neutrophils. J Biol Chem 2010;285:34528-36.

[48] Laskay T, van Zandbergen G, Solbach W. Neutrophil granulocytes--Trojan horses for Leishmania major and other intracellular microbes? Trends in microbiology 2003;11:210-4.

[49] van Zandbergen G, Klinger M, Mueller A, Dannenberg S, Gebert A, Solbach W, et al. Cutting edge: neutrophil granulocyte serves as a vector for *Leishmania* entry into macrophages. J Immunol 2004;173:6521-5.

[50] Murray HW. Suppression of posttreatment recurrence of experimental visceral leishmaniasis in T-cell-deficient mice by oral miltefosine. Antimicrob Agents Chemother 2000;44:3235-6.

[51] Murray HW, Delph-Etienne S. Visceral leishmanicidal activity of hexadecylphosphocholine (miltefosine) in mice deficient in T cells and activated macrophage microbicidal mechanisms. J Infect Dis 2000;181:795-9.

[52] Escobar P, Yardley V, Croft SL. Activities of hexadecylphosphocholine (miltefosine), AmBisome, and sodium stibogluconate (Pentostam) against *Leishmania donovani* in immunodeficient scid mice. Antimicrob Agents Chemother 2001;45:1872-5.

[53] Lawn SD, Wilkinson RJ. Immune reconstitution disease associated with parasitic infections following antiretroviral treatment. Parasite Immunol 2006;28:625-33.

[54] Cabrera-Serra MG, Lorenzo-Morales J, Romero M, Valladares B, Pinero JE. *In vitro* activity of perifosine: a novel alkylphospholipid against the promastigote stage of *Leishmania* species. Parasitol Res 2007;100:1155-7.

[55] Cabrera-Serra MG, Valladares B, Pinero JE. *In vivo* activity of perifosine against *Leishmania amazonensis*. Acta Trop 2008;108:20-5.

[56] Mollinedo F, Fernandez-Luna JL, Gajate C, Martin-Martin B, Benito A, Martinez-Dalmau R, et al. Selective induction of apoptosis in cancer cells by the ether lipid ET-18-OCH_3 (Edelfosine): molecular structure requirements, cellular uptake, and protection by Bcl-2 and Bcl-X_L. Cancer Res 1997;57:1320-8.

[57] Gajate C, Fonteriz RI, Cabaner C, Alvarez-Noves G, Alvarez-Rodriguez Y, Modolell M, et al. Intracellular triggering of Fas, independently of FasL, as a new mechanism of antitumor ether lipid-induced apoptosis. Int J Cancer 2000;85:674-82.

[58] Mollinedo F, Gajate C. Fas/CD95 death receptor and lipid rafts: New targets for apoptosis-directed cancer therapy. Drug Resist Updat 2006;9:51-73.

[59] Diomede L, Colotta F, Piovani B, Re F, Modest EJ, Salmona M. Induction of apoptosis in human leukemic cells by the ether lipid 1-octadecyl-2-methyl-*rac*-glycero-3-phosphocholine. A possible basis for its selective action. Int J Cancer 1993;53:124-30.

[60] Mollinedo F, Martinez-Dalmau R, Modolell M. Early and selective induction of apoptosis in human leukemic cells by the alkyl-lysophospholipid ET-18-OCH_3. Biochem Biophys Res Commun 1993;192:603-9.

[61] Konstantinov SM, Topashka-Ancheva M, Benner A, Berger MR. Alkylphosphocholines: Effects on human leukemic cell lines and normal bone marrow cells. Int J Cancer 1998;77:778-86.

[62] Konstantinov SM, Eibl H, Berger MR. BCR-ABL influences the antileukaemic efficacy of alkylphosphocholines. Br J Haematol 1999;107:365-80.

[63] Gajate C, Gonzalez-Camacho F, Mollinedo F. Lipid raft connection between extrinsic and intrinsic apoptotic pathways. Biochem Biophys Res Commun 2009;380:780-4.

[64] Gajate C, Mollinedo F. The antitumor ether lipid ET-18-OCH_3 induces apoptosis through translocation and capping of Fas/CD95 into membrane rafts in human leukemic cells. Blood 2001;98:3860-3.

[65] Paris C, Loiseau PM, Bories C, Breard J. Miltefosine induces apoptosis-like death in *Leishmania donovani* promastigotes. Antimicrob Agents Chemother 2004;48:852-9.

http://dx.doi.org/10.5772/58318

[66] Verma NK, Dey CS. Possible mechanism of miltefosine-mediated death of *Leishmania donovani*. Antimicrob Agents Chemother 2004;48:3010-5.

[67] Marinho Fde A, Goncalves KC, Oliveira SS, Oliveira AC, Bellio M, d'Avila-Levy CM, et al. Miltefosine induces programmed cell death in *Leishmania amazonensis* promastigotes. Memorias do Instituto Oswaldo Cruz 2011;106:507-9.

[68] Khademvatan S, Gharavi MJ, Saki J. Miltefosine induces metacaspase and PARP genes expression in *Leishmania infantum*. Braz J Infect Dis 2011;15:442-8.

[69] Khademvatan S, Gharavi MJ, Rahim F, Saki J. Miltefosine-induced apoptotic cell death on *Leishmania major* and *L. tropica* strains. The Korean journal of parasitology 2011;49:17-23.

[70] Moreira W, Leprohon P, Ouellette M. Tolerance to drug-induced cell death favours the acquisition of multidrug resistance in *Leishmania*. Cell death & disease 2011;2:e201.

[71] Verma NK, Singh G, Dey CS. Miltefosine induces apoptosis in arsenite-resistant *Leishmania donovani* promastigotes through mitochondrial dysfunction. Exp Parasitol 2007;116:1-13.

[72] Alzate JF, Arias A, Mollinedo F, Rico E, de la Iglesia-Vicente J, Jimenez-Ruiz A. Edelfosine induces an apoptotic process in *Leishmania infantum* that is regulated by the ectopic expression of Bcl-X_L and Hrk. Antimicrob Agents Chemother 2008;52:3779-82.

[73] Luque-Ortega JR, Rivas L. Miltefosine (hexadecylphosphocholine) inhibits cytochrome *c* oxidase in *Leishmania donovani* promastigotes. Antimicrob Agents Chemother 2007;51:1327-32.

[74] Zuo X, Djordjevic JT, Bijosono Oei J, Desmarini D, Schibeci SD, Jolliffe KA, et al. Miltefosine induces apoptosis-like cell death in yeast via Cox9p in cytochrome *c* oxidase. Mol Pharmacol 2011;80:476-85.

[75] Boggs K, Rock CO, Jackowski S. The antiproliferative effect of hexadecylphosphocholine toward HL60 cells is prevented by exogenous lysophosphatidylcholine. Biochim Biophys Acta 1998;1389:1-12.

[76] Boggs KP, Rock CO, Jackowski S. Lysophosphatidylcholine attenuates the cytotoxic effects of the antineoplastic phospholipid 1-*O*-octadecyl-2-*O*-methyl-*rac*-glycero-3-phosphocholine. J Biol Chem 1995;270:11612-8.

[77] Boggs KP, Rock CO, Jackowski S. Lysophosphatidylcholine and 1-*O*-octadecyl-2-*O*-methyl-*rac*-glycero-3-phosphocholine inhibit the CDP-choline pathway of phosphatidylcholine synthesis at the CTP:phosphocholine cytidylyltransferase step. J Biol Chem 1995;270:7757-64.

[78] Rakotomanga M, Loiseau PM, Saint-Pierre-Chazalet M. Hexadecylphosphocholine interaction with lipid monolayers. Biochim Biophys Acta 2004;1661:212-8.

[79] Beach DH, Holz GG, Jr., Anekwe GE. Lipids of *Leishmania* promastigotes. J Parasitol 1979;65:201-16.

[80] Herrmann H, Gercken G. Synthesis of phospholipids in *Leishmania donovani*. Hoppe-Seyler's Zeitschrift fur physiologische Chemie 1980;361:1735-42.

[81] Wassef MK, Fioretti TB, Dwyer DM. Lipid analyses of isolated surface membranes of *Leishmania donovani* promastigotes. Lipids 1985;20:108-15.

[82] Heise N, Opperdoes FR. The dihydroxyacetonephosphate pathway for biosynthesis of ether lipids in *Leishmania mexicana* promastigotes. Mol Biochem Parasitol 1997;89:61-72.

[83] Zufferey R, Ben Mamoun C. *Leishmania major* expresses a single dihydroxyacetone phosphate acyltransferase localized in the glycosome, important for rapid growth and survival at high cell density and essential for virulence. J Biol Chem 2006;281:7952-9.

[84] McConville MJ, Collidge TA, Ferguson MA, Schneider P. The glycoinositol phospholipids of *Leishmania mexicana* promastigotes. Evidence for the presence of three distinct pathways of glycolipid biosynthesis. J Biol Chem 1993;268:15595-604.

[85] McConville MJ, Ferguson MA. The structure, biosynthesis and function of glycosylated phosphatidylinositols in the parasitic protozoa and higher eukaryotes. Biochem J 1993;294 (Pt 2):305-24.

[86] Schneider P, Rosat JP, Ransijn A, Ferguson MA, McConville MJ. Characterization of glycoinositol phospholipids in the amastigote stage of the protozoan parasite *Leishmania major*. Biochem J 1993;295 (Pt 2):555-64.

[87] Lux H, Heise N, Klenner T, Hart D, Opperdoes FR. Ether-lipid (alkyl-phospholipid) metabolism and the mechanism of action of ether-lipid analogues in *Leishmania*. Mol Biochem Parasitol 2000;111:1-14.

[88] Zufferey R, Allen S, Barron T, Sullivan DR, Denny PW, Almeida IC, et al. Ether phospholipids and glycosylinositolphospholipids are not required for amastigote virulence or for inhibition of macrophage activation by *Leishmania major*. J Biol Chem 2003;278:44708-18.

[89] Rakotomanga M, Blanc S, Gaudin K, Chaminade P, Loiseau PM. Miltefosine affects lipid metabolism in *Leishmania donovani* promastigotes. Antimicrob Agents Chemother 2007;51:1425-30.

[90] Rakotomanga M, Saint-Pierre-Chazalet M, Loiseau PM. Alteration of fatty acid and sterol metabolism in miltefosine-resistant *Leishmania donovani* promastigotes and consequences for drug-membrane interactions. Antimicrob Agents Chemother 2005;49:2677-86.

[91] Maltezou HC. Drug resistance in visceral leishmaniasis. Journal of biomedicine & biotechnology 2010;2010:617521.

[92] Perez-Victoria FJ, Castanys S, Gamarro F. *Leishmania donovani* resistance to miltefosine involves a defective inward translocation of the drug. Antimicrob Agents Chemother 2003;47:2397-403.

[93] Perez-Victoria FJ, Gamarro F, Ouellette M, Castanys S. Functional cloning of the miltefosine transporter. A novel P-type phospholipid translocase from *Leishmania* involved in drug resistance. J Biol Chem 2003;278:49965-71.

[94] Perez-Victoria FJ, Sanchez-Canete MP, Castanys S, Gamarro F. Phospholipid translocation and miltefosine potency require both *L. donovani* miltefosine transporter and the new protein LdRos3 in *Leishmania* parasites. J Biol Chem 2006;281:23766-75.

[95] Saito K, Fujimura-Kamada K, Furuta N, Kato U, Umeda M, Tanaka K. Cdc50p, a protein required for polarized growth, associates with the Drs2p P-type ATPase implicated in phospholipid translocation in *Saccharomyces cerevisiae*. Mol Biol Cell 2004;15:3418-32.

[96] Furuta N, Fujimura-Kamada K, Saito K, Yamamoto T, Tanaka K. Endocytic recycling in yeast is regulated by putative phospholipid translocases and the Ypt31p/32p-Rcy1p pathway. Mol Biol Cell 2007;18:295-312.

[97] Weingartner A, Drobot B, Herrmann A, Sanchez-Canete MP, Gamarro F, Castanys S, et al. Disruption of the lipid-transporting LdMT-LdRos3 complex in *Leishmania donovani* affects membrane lipid asymmetry but not host cell invasion. PLoS One 2010;5:e12443.

[98] Sanchez-Canete MP, Carvalho L, Perez-Victoria FJ, Gamarro F, Castanys S. Low plasma membrane expression of the miltefosine transport complex renders *Leishmania braziliensis* refractory to the drug. Antimicrob Agents Chemother 2009;53:1305-13.

[99] Perez-Victoria JM, Perez-Victoria FJ, Parodi-Talice A, Jimenez IA, Ravelo AG, Castanys S, et al. Alkyl-lysophospholipid resistance in multidrug-resistant *Leishmania tropica* and chemosensitization by a novel P-glycoprotein-like transporter modulator. Antimicrob Agents Chemother 2001;45:2468-74.

[100] Perez-Victoria JM, Cortes-Selva F, Parodi-Talice A, Bavchvarov BI, Perez-Victoria FJ, Munoz-Martinez F, et al. Combination of suboptimal doses of inhibitors targeting different domains of LtrMDR1 efficiently overcomes resistance of *Leishmania* spp. to Miltefosine by inhibiting drug efflux. Antimicrob Agents Chemother 2006;50:3102-10.

[101] Castanys-Munoz E, Alder-Baerens N, Pomorski T, Gamarro F, Castanys S. A novel ATP-binding cassette transporter from *Leishmania* is involved in transport of phosphatidylcholine analogues and resistance to alkyl-phospholipids. Mol Microbiol 2007;64:1141-53.

[102] Castanys-Munoz E, Perez-Victoria JM, Gamarro F, Castanys S. Characterization of an ABCG-like transporter from the protozoan parasite *Leishmania* with a role in drug re-

sistance and transbilayer lipid movement. Antimicrob Agents Chemother 2008;52:3573-9.

[103] Coelho AC, Boisvert S, Mukherjee A, Leprohon P, Corbeil J, Ouellette M. Multiple mutations in heterogeneous miltefosine-resistant *Leishmania major* population as determined by whole genome sequencing. PLoS Negl Trop Dis 2012;6:e1512.

[104] Wadhone P, Maiti M, Agarwal R, Kamat V, Martin S, Saha B. Miltefosine promotes IFN-gamma-dominated anti-leishmanial immune response. J Immunol 2009;182:7146-54.

[105] Eue I. Hexadecylphosphocholine selectively upregulates expression of intracellular adhesion molecule-1 and class I major histocompatibility complex antigen in human monocytes. J Exp Ther Oncol 2002;2:333-6.

[106] Zeisig R, Rudolf M, Eue I, Arndt D. Influence of hexadecylphosphocholine on the release of tumor necrosis factor and nitroxide from peritoneal macrophages in vitro. J Cancer Res Clin Oncol 1995;121:69-75.

[107] Zeisig R, Eue I, Kosch M, Fichtner I, Arndt D. Preparation and properties of sterically stabilized hexadecylphosphocholine (miltefosine)-liposomes and influence of this modification on macrophage activation. Biochim Biophys Acta 1996;1283:177-84.

[108] Eue I, Zeisig R, Arndt D. Alkylphosphocholine-induced production of nitric oxide and tumor necrosis factor alpha by U937 cells. J Cancer Res Clin Oncol 1995;121:350-6.

[109] Hochhuth CH, Vehmeyer K, Eibl H, Unger C. Hexadecylphosphocholine induces interferon-gamma secretion and expression of GM-CSF mRNA in human mononuclear cells. Cell Immunol 1992;141:161-8.

[110] Griewank K, Gazeau C, Eichhorn A, von Stebut E. Miltefosine efficiently eliminates *Leishmania major* amastigotes from infected murine dendritic cells without altering their immune functions. Antimicrob Agents Chemother 2010;54:652-9.

[111] Mauricio IL, Howard MK, Stothard JR, Miles MA. Genomic diversity in the *Leishmania donovani* complex. Parasitology 1999;119 (Pt 3):237-46.

[112] Mauricio IL, Stothard JR, Miles MA. The strange case of *Leishmania chagasi*. Parasitology today (Personal ed 2000;16:188-9.

[113] Mauricio IL, Gaunt MW, Stothard JR, Miles MA. Genetic typing and phylogeny of the *Leishmania donovani* complex by restriction analysis of PCR amplified gp63 intergenic regions. Parasitology 2001;122:393-403.

[114] Kuhls K, Alam MZ, Cupolillo E, Ferreira GE, Mauricio IL, Oddone R, et al. Comparative microsatellite typing of new world *Leishmania infantum* reveals low heterogeneity among populations and its recent old world origin. PLoS Negl Trop Dis 2011;5:e1155.

[115] Woerly V, Maynard L, Sanquer A, Eun HM. Clinical efficacy and tolerance of miltefosine in the treatment of canine leishmaniosis. Parasitol Res 2009;105:463-9.

[116] Mateo M, Maynard L, Vischer C, Bianciardi P, Miro G. Comparative study on the short term efficacy and adverse effects of miltefosine and meglumine antimoniate in dogs with natural leishmaniosis. Parasitol Res 2009;105:155-62.

[117] Andrade HM, Toledo VP, Pinheiro MB, Guimaraes TM, Oliveira NC, Castro JA, et al. Evaluation of miltefosine for the treatment of dogs naturally infected with *L. infantum* (=*L. chagasi*) in Brazil. Veterinary parasitology 2011;181:83-90.

[118] Manna L, Gravino AE, Picillo E, Decaro N, Buonavoglia C. *Leishmania* DNA quantification by real-time PCR in naturally infected dogs treated with miltefosine. Ann N Y Acad Sci 2008;1149:358-60.

[119] Miro G, Oliva G, Cruz I, Canavate C, Mortarino M, Vischer C, et al. Multicentric, controlled clinical study to evaluate effectiveness and safety of miltefosine and allopurinol for canine leishmaniosis. Veterinary dermatology 2009;20:397-404.

Chapter 20

Metal-Based Therapeutics for Leishmaniasis

Ana B. Caballero, Juan M. Salas and
Manuel Sánchez-Moreno

Additional information is available at the end of the chapter

http://dx.doi.org/10.5772/57376

1. Introduction

1.1. Metal-based drugs and their growing application to the treatment of parasitic diseases

When we speak of metals in medicine, many of us still associate them almost unconsciously with toxic rather than curative effects. However, despite the known toxic effect of some metal ions in humans, many metal ions (in adequate dosages) are required for many critical functions in our organism. Scarcity of some of them even can lead to a disease. Well-known examples include anemia resulting from iron deficiency, growth retardation arising from insufficient zinc, and heart disease in children owing to copper deficiency.

Metals have been used for medicinal purposes since ancient times. The earliest evidence of their therapeutic application has been dated back to 1500BC in Ebers Papyrus, Egypt. Among 700 magical formulas and remedies, this ancient manuscript describes the use of copper to reduce inflammation and the use of iron to treat anemia. Later on, the alchemical practice in the Middle Age made a significant use of metals like gold or arsenic to prepare medicinal compounds and elixirs. In the 16th century, antimony was introduced by Paracelsus as a general panacea and was considered as one of the Seven Wonders of the World.

In the early 20th century, the physician Paul Elhrich (Nobel Prize 1908) discovered an impresive therapeutic effect of the compound arsenophenylglycine to treat sleeping sickness (Trypanosoma disease) and developed the first effective medicinal treatment for syphilis, also arsenium-containing drug Arshphenamine, which was commercialized under the name Salvarsan. The concept of chemotherapy was born. At this time, other metallodrugs appeared. Sodium vanadate and derivatives of bismaltolato oxovanadium(IV) complexes started to be applied to lower levels of blood sugar in diabetic patients, and gold(I) complexes such as Auranofin, sodium aurothiomalate and aurothioglucose were prescribed to treat rheumatoid arthritis

(Figure 1). In 1987, sodium aurothiomalate was also used to treat 10 patients with kala-azar and showed an excellent clinical response.[1]

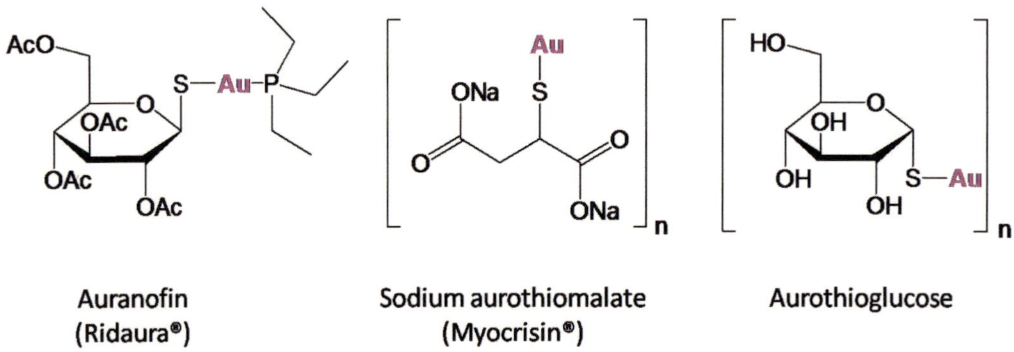

Figure 1. Gold-based drugs most commonly used for the treatment of rheumatoid arthritis. Sodium aurothiomalate has also shown chemotherapeutic effect against kala-azar.

Despite these early demonstrations of the potential of metals to treat diseases, organic drugs have traditionally dominated modern medicinal chemistry and pharmacology. It was the serendipitous discovery in 1969 of the anticancer properties of cisplatin, a Pt(II) complex, which propelled dramatically the research on metal ions in modern medicine until nowadays, not only in therapy but also in diagnosis. Examples of the latter are radiolabeling of compounds with ^{99m}Tc for X-ray imaging and use of Gd(III) complexes as MRI agents. Moreover, this event marked the change from an empirical discovery into a rational design of new metallodrugs and the consequent development of medicinal inorganic chemistry as a mature research discipline.

The increasing interest in the research of metal compounds with potential applications in medicine along the last decades has come along to a deeper understanding of the reactivity of metal ions and their interaction with a wide range of biomolecules such as DNA and proteins. [2] Scientific community has realized that either coordination or organometallic chemistry offer wide possibilities to develop novel metal-based drugs bearing quite different mechanisms of action aiming at different targets.

The dramatic incidence and economic impact of cancer diseases in modern world and especially in developed countries has led research on medicinal inorganic chemistry (and still is) to focus mainly on development of antitumoral compounds of different metals. This includes their design to specifically attack cancer cells and interact directly with DNA, with protein active sites or with smaller biomolecules of key importance in cancer development, as well as improving their biodistribution. As a result, a number of metal complexes with antitumoral potential have been developed in the last years, mostly of platinum and ruthenium, and some of them have provided excellent results. In fact, drugs like oxaliplatin are currently used to treat colorrectal cancer. Moreover, the antimetastatic drug NAMI-A is under the last phase of clinical evaluation.

http://dx.doi.org/10.5772/57376

On the other hand, a comparatively smaller progress has been made in the discovery of new metal compounds to treat tropical parasitic diseases, which has been mostly based on an empirical use. Various inorganic salts have been administered against the major tropical diseases, sometimes with very good results.

The best-known example is a series of antimony compounds such as sodium stibogluconate (Pentostam) and meglumine antimoniate (Glucantime). These compounds were developed more than 60 years ago and still constitute the treatment of choice for some forms of leishmaniasis. However, antimonial-based treatments usually present toxicity problems, limited efficacy and emerging resistance. This leads scientists to explore other metal ions in search of improved therapies. In addition no structure-function correlation studies have yet been performed on antiparasitic metal-based compounds. These arguments open the way to new mechanistic investigations in this research area for optimization of the identified metal leads and development of new ones.

But what can metals offer towards improved antiparasitic therapies? Metal ions offer a wide range of coordination numbers and geometries, redox states, and thermodynamic and kinetic characteristics. This, along with the possibility to rationally combine the intrinsic properties of a metal ion with a bioactive ligand/s bearing therapeutic interest, provides innumerable possibilities for drug design and an extremely wide spectrum of therapeutic activity not readily available to organic compounds.

One of the most used design approaches is grounded in the metal-drug synergism that results from the attachment of a metal moiety to the structure of an organic drug. [3] This synergy gives rise to two main effects:

a. An enhancement of biologic activity of the organic drug caused by the presence of the metal ion, possibly due to a longer time of residence of the drug in the organism allowing it to reach the biological targets more efficiently, or due to formation of reactive oxygen species (ROS), among other effects.

b. A decrease in the toxicity of the metal ion towards host cells due to the fact that complexation with organic drugs carries the metal ion to the specific site of action and makes it less readily available for undesired reactions such as inhibition of enzymes, or other damaging reactions leading to a malfunction in the organism.

The work of Williamson and Farrell in 1976 was the first in applying and demonstrate this concept for a tropical disease, trypanosomiasis. [4]

Among other illustrative examples of this approach, it should be mentioned the ferroquine (FQ), in which insertion of a Fe(II) ion in the form of ferrocene into the scaffold of the antimalarial drug chloroquine enhanced the pharmacology of the drug. [5] FQ is being developed by Sanofi-Aventis and entered phase II clinical trials in September 2007. Other example is a ruthenium(II) complex with the antitrypanocidal compound benznidazole, *trans*-[Ru(Bz)$(NH_3)_4SO_2](CF_3SO_3)_2$, which shows higher hydrosolubility and activity than the free antiparasitic drug. [6] (Figure 2)

Other advantages of using metal compounds are their pronounced selectivity for selected parasites biomolecules compared to the host biomolecules,[7] and the possibilities they offer to targeted therapies as targeting molecules may be reversibly appended and prodrugs can be developed to deliver highly reactive metal specia in the parasite target while minimising non-specific interactions.

In the last years, nanotechnology has revolutioned the medicine field by opening novel and promising approaches for drug design, in particular regarding use of nanoparticles (1-100 nm) as drug delivery vehicles. Despite being liposomes and polymeric particles the most investigated systems to deliver antiparasitic drugs, metal nanoparticles have also emerged as interesting alternative carriers. [8] Furthermore, use of nanoforms of antiparasitic metals like antimony and selenium as alternatives to molecular forms [9,10] has also been recently reported.

In summary, there is a clear need for research in this largely neglected area of medicinal chemistry that is tropical parasitic diseases, and use of metal complexes as possible chemotherapeutic agents arises as a very attractive alternative to tackle this immense problem. However, despite the obvious potential of metal complexes as diagnostic and chemotherapeutic agents, few pharmaceutical or chemical companies have serious in-house research programs that address these important bioinorganic aspects of medicine, which contrast tremendously with the case of purely organic drugs.

The following sections will focus on diverse examples of metal compounds with current or potential applications for leishmaniasis treatment.

2. Metal compounds as a new generation of leishmanicidal agents. Design strategies

2.1. Metal-based drugs for leishmaniasis

Currently, there is no vaccine against leishmaniasis yet, either purely organic or containing metals. Disease treatment relies solely on chemotherapy. After an intensive revision of the literature, we have found a wide range of metal-containing compounds that are currently used to treat different varieties of leishmaniasis or present a strong antileihsmanial activity and hence potential to be part of a new generation of chemotherapeutic agents with high efficacy and minimal toxicity for the patient. All of them are described in detail in this section.

2.1.1. Pentavalent antimonials: a (still) unbeatable classic in leishmanicidal therapy

Antimony-based compounds started to be used a century ago. Trivalent antimonials -Sb(III)- were first used, e.g. tartar emetic, which was first reported for treatment of cutaneous leishmaniasis in 1913. But the high toxicity of Sb(III) compounds and their unstability in tropical climate, led to discovery of pentavalent antimonials –Sb(V)- and in 1920 the Sb(V) compound urea stibamine emerged as an effective agent against visceral leishmaniasis (kala azar) while being less toxic than the trivalent antimonials.

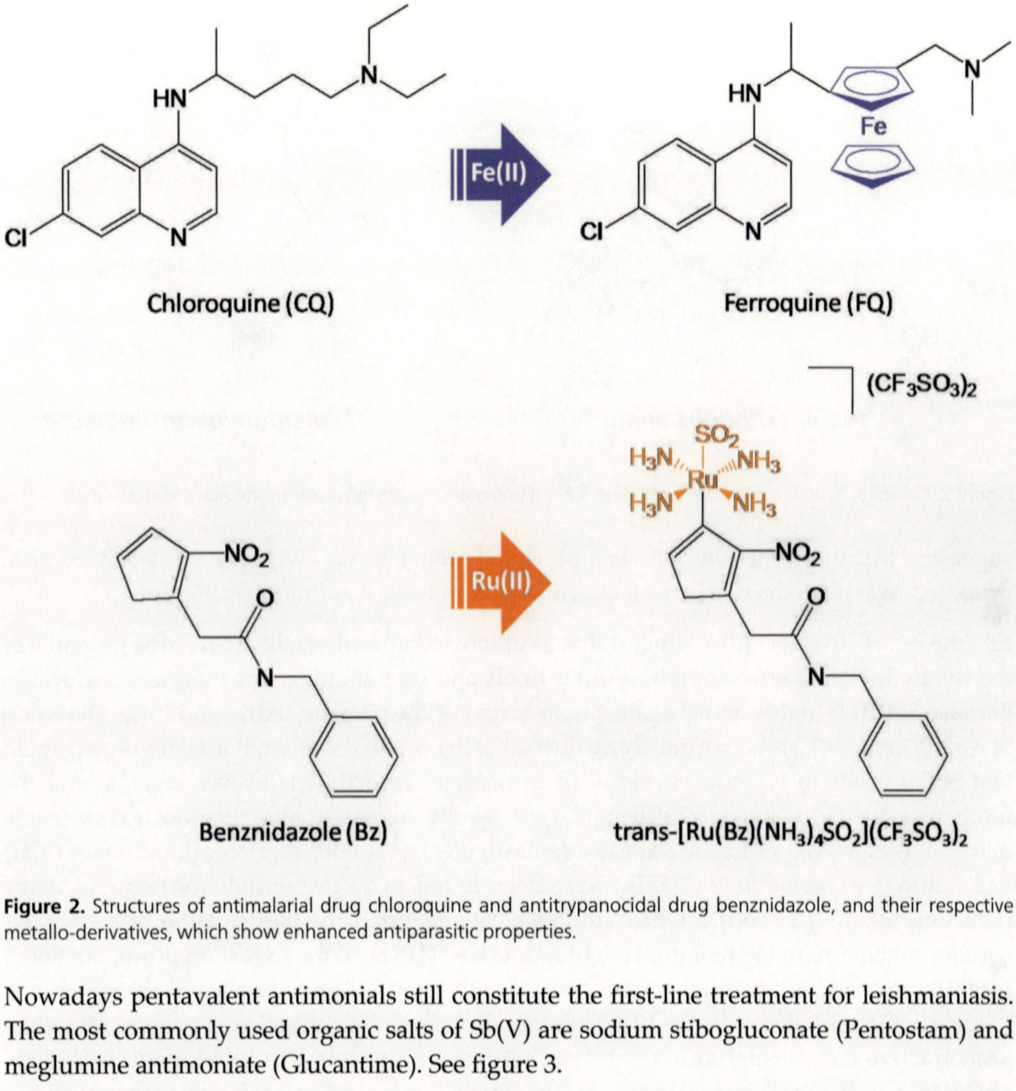

Figure 2. Structures of antimalarial drug chloroquine and antitrypanocidal drug benznidazole, and their respective metallo-derivatives, which show enhanced antiparasitic properties.

Nowadays pentavalent antimonials still constitute the first-line treatment for leishmaniasis. The most commonly used organic salts of Sb(V) are sodium stibogluconate (Pentostam) and meglumine antimoniate (Glucantime). See figure 3.

However, a significant increase in clinical resistance has been reported for this class of drugs in recent years. In some parts of the world like North East India, the percentage of cases of resistance development is so high (up to 65%) that these drugs are becoming obsolete.

Although acquired resistance is the most limiting factor for the application of pentavalent antimonials, these drugs present other important drawbacks such as low efficacy for some forms of leishmaniasis and toxic effects (e.g. cardiotoxicity, pancreatitis, anemia and leucopenia). Their toxicity is aggravated by usually required long periods of therapy (up to 4-6 weeks).

Even though antimonials have been in clinical use against leishmaniasis for more than 60 years, their molecular and cellular mechanisms of action are not well understood yet. [11] What is clear is that to be active, antimony has to enter the host cell, cross the phagolysomal membrane and act against the intracellular parasite. By analogy to pentavalent arsenate, it has been

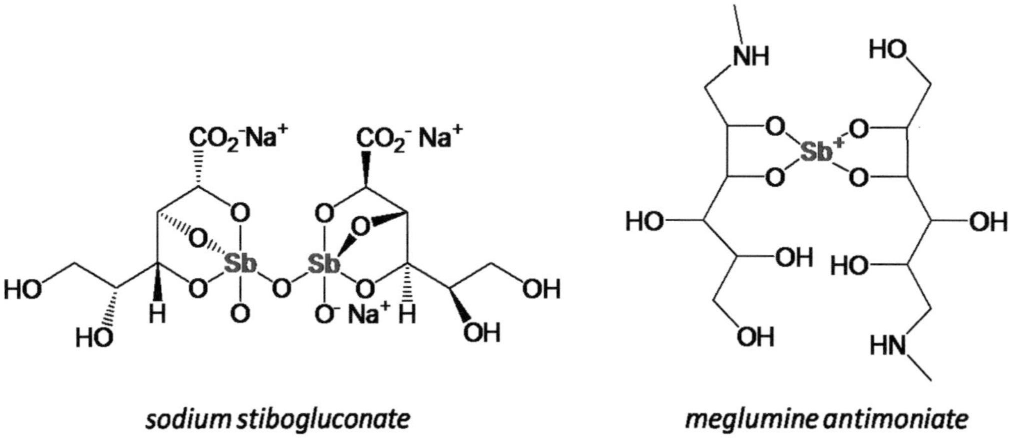

Figure 3. Chemical structure of sodium stibogluconate (Pentostam) and meglumine antimoniate (Glucantime).

suggested that they enter the cell via a phosphate transporter. Two main models have been proposed to explain the mechanism of action of pentavalent antimonials (Figure 4):

Prodrug model. Recent studies suggest that antimony compromises the thiol redox potential of the cell by inducing efflux of intracellular thiols and by inhibiting trypanothione reductase. Because Sb(III) is highly active against both stages of the parasite, extra- and intracellular on one hand, and Sb(V) is active mostly against amastigotes on the other, it is generally accepted that Sb(V) needs to be reduced to Sb(III) in order to be active. However, the site and the mechanism of reduction are unclear. Recent results suggest that activation occurs inside macrophages as well as inside parasites (amastigotes). [12] Both reduced glutathione (GSH) and reduced trypanothione ($T(SH)_2$) have been found to be responsible for non-enzymatic reduction of Sb(V) to Sb(III). Other studies have suggested the participation of a parasite-specific enzyme, namely thiol-dependent reductase (TDR1), in the reduction process of Sb(V) to Sb(III). Recent crystal structure studies display the mechanism of *Leishmania* trypanothione reductase (TR) inhibition by Sb(III). These studies show that trivalent antimony binds the protein active site with high affinity, and strongly inhibits enzyme activity. Metal binds directly to Cys52, Cys57, Thr335 and His461, thereby blocking hydride transfer and trypanothione reduction. Also evidence suggests that the active specia Sb(III) may interact with zinc-finger proteins by binding Cys residues. The interaction with TR would affect the metabolism of $T(SH)_2$ and induce rapid efflux of intracellular $T(SH)_2$ and GSH in *Leishmania* cells. [13] Moreover, the lowering of concentration of intracellular trypanothione in its reduced form $T(SH)_2$, increases the chances for oxidative damage and decreases the disposal of reducing equivalents for DNA synthesis. Sereno *et al.* found that Sb(III) induces DNA fragmentation after treating amastigotes of *L. infantum* at low concentrations of drug, which suggests appearance of late events of apoptosis.[14]

Active Sb(V) model. According to this model, Sb(V) would present intrinsic anti-leishmanial activity. It has been shown that sodium stibogluconate, but not Sb(III), specifically inhibits type I DNA topisomerase by binding the enzyme, thus inhibiting unwinding and cleavage.[15]

Formation of Sb(V) complexes with ribonucleosides has been reported, which would be kinetically favored in acidic biological compartments. Moreover, stability constants are consistent with the formation of such a complex in the vertebrate host following treatment with pentavalent antimonial drugs. It is hypothesized that formation of this complex might act as an inhibitor of the *Leishmania* purine transporters or that, once inside the parasite, this complex interferes with the purine salvage pathway. [16] The formation of these complexes with ribonucleosides might explain as well the depletion of ATP and GTP, as reported previously with sodium stibogluconate. [17]

When antimonials fail, amphotericin B and pentamidine are the recommended second-line treamtent for visceral, cutaneous and mucocutaneous leishmaniasis.However, they are not fully effective either and, additionally,produce toxic side effects. On the other hand, new formulations such as liposomal amphotericin B have been found to be very effective, but its high cost limits its availability to patients.

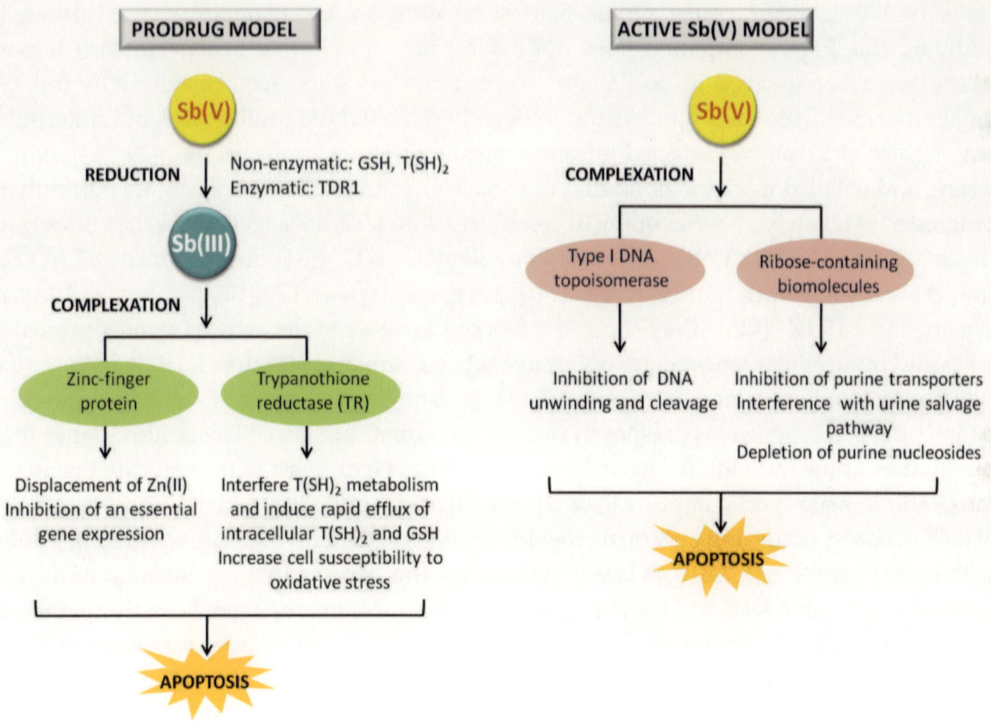

Figure 4. Main models proposed for the mechanism of action of pentavalent antimonials against leishmaniasis.

2.1.2. Metal complexes of organic drugs: Following the metal-drug synergism approach

Metal-drug synergism has led to several attempts to develop new potent antiparasitic agents. This approach involves combination of a compound of known antiparasitic activity and a metal in a single molecule. One example is complexation of antileishmanial drug pentamidine with

Rh(I) and Ir(I) to form binuclear complexes of general formula $[M_2(L_2)(\text{pentamidine})]^{2+}$, where L_2= 1,5-cyclooctadiene (COD), 1,3,1,5-cyclooctatetraene (COT) or $(CO)_2$. Some of these compounds were found to be more active than the uncomplexed drug pentamidine isethionate. The complex $[Ir(COD)(\text{pentamidine})][BPh_4]$ exhibits the same *in vitro* activity as free pentamidine, but its *in vivo* activity reaches 23% and 32% of parasite suppression for *L. donovani* and *L. major*, respectively, under conditions where pentamidine isethionate is inactive. The related compound $[Ir_2(COT)_2(\text{pentamidine})][\text{alizarin red}]_2$ showed to be at least twice as active as pentamidine isethionate against amastigotes of *L. donovani* and synergistic effect was observed when this complex was administered in combination with pentamidine, amphotericin B or paromomycin. [18]

Other metal-drug synergy-based strategies make use of diverse chemotherapeutic targets such as sterol 14-demethylases by attaching azole-type sterol biosynthesis inhibitors (SBIs) such as clotrimazole (CTZ) and ketoconazole (KTZ), to a metal-containing fragment. For example, compound $[Ru(\eta^6\text{-p-cymene})Cl_2(CTZ)]$ shows an enhancement of the activity of CTZ by a factor of 110 against *L. major* promastigotes, resulting in low nanomolar lethal doses. In addition, this Ru(II) compound does not exhibit any appreciable toxicity toward human osteoblasts when assayed up to 7.5 μM, which translates into excellent selectivity indexes higher than 500. This compound also significantly inhibited the proliferation of intracellular amastigotes of *L. major* in infected intraperitoneal mouse macrophages (IC_{70}=29 nM). *In vivo* testing and detailed mechanistic studies of these ruthenium–CTZ complexes are currently in progress.[19] Likewise, a series of Ru(II) complexes with KTZ have recently been synthesized: *cis,fac*-$[RuCl_2(DMSO)_3(KTZ)]$, *cis*-$[RuCl_2(bipy)(DMSO)(KTZ)]$, $[Ru(\eta^6\text{-p-cymene})Cl_2(KTZ)]$, $[Ru(\eta^6\text{-p-cymene})(en)(KTZ)][BF_4]_2$, $[Ru^{II}(\eta^6\text{-pcymene})(bipy)(KTZ)][BF_4]_2$, and $[Ru(\eta^6\text{-p-cymene})(acac)(KTZ)][BF_4]$. They showed a marked increase of the activity against promastigotes and intracellular amastigotes of *L. major* when compared with free KTZ or with similar ruthenium compounds not containing KTZ. Interestingly, selectivity of some of these compounds toward *Leishmania* parasites in relation to normal human cells was also higher than selectivities of the individual constituents of the drug. Hydrolysis of the chloride ligands to form cationic aqua species appears to be a prerequisite for biological activity, and dissociation of KTZ probably occurs but only on further interactions of the active species with biomolecules within the parasite cell. Authors relate the antiparasitic activity to a combination of the SBI action of dissociated KTZ and the ability of the nitrogen-containing ligands on the remaining ruthenium fragment to promote interactions with DNA through hydrogen bonding or by π–stacking interactions. [20]

Other metal ions like Pt(II), Rh(I) or Os(III) have been used to obtain organometallic compounds with ligands derived from benzothiazole, a compound of which some derivatives have shown promising antimicrobial, antifungus and antiparasite activity. The obtained compounds were active against promastigotes and amastigotes of *L. donovani* by targeting different biochemical pathways: [*cis*-$[Pt(da)(2,5\text{-dihydroxybenzenesulfonate})_2]$ (da = 1,2-diaminocyclohexane), $[Ru(CO)_2(2\text{-aminobenzothiazole})]$, $[Ru(CO)_2(2\text{-methylbenzothiazole})]$, [21] and a series of dithiocarbamate complexes with formula [Os(L)] where L= nitroimidazole, dinitroimidazole, benznidazole. Osmium complexes clearly inhibited DNA, RNA and protein synthesis, as well as enzymatic activities of succinate dehydrogenase, malate dehydrogenase and pyruvate kinase. [22]

Apart from vanadium compounds ability to exert different insulin-mimetic and antidiabetic effects, it has been recently proved that vanadium also offers interesting chemical and biochemical properties for the development of antiparasitic drugs. Noleto *et al.* combined the oxovanadium(IV) core with the antileishmanial compound galactomannan (GMPOLY), isolated from southern Brazil lichen *Ramalina celastri.* [23] Complexation highly increased leishmanicidal effect of galactomannan on amastigotes of *L. amazonensis* infecting peritoneal macrophages. This effect of GMPOLY on amastigotes could be attributed to the activation of the nitric oxide pathway. Nitric oxide is secreted by macrophages in response to IFN-γ (interferon γ) stimulation and it is regulated by tyrosine phosphatase events. Since the effect detected for GMPOLY oxovanadium(IV) complex occurred at concentrations where GMPOLY was non active, authors suggested the involvement of oxovanadium(IV) ion in the anti-parasite action.

2.1.3. Targeting cysteine proteases

Cysteine proteases have been found to play multiple roles in parasitic life cycles including nutrition, host invasion, protein processing, and evasion of the host immune response. In fact, there is an abundance of data to suggest that parasite cysteine proteases represent valid drug targets. For example, it was shown that an inhibitor of cathepsin B-like cysteine protease of *L. major*, cpB, inhibited parasite growth *in vitro* and ameliorated the pathology associated with a mouse model of leishmaniasis. [24] Since cysteine proteases found in *Leishmania* and *T. cruzi* have similarities to mammalian cathepsins B and L, the latter ones have been used as models to study the bioactivity of diverse metallic compounds. Cyclometallated gold, palladium, and rhenium derivatives have displayed cathepsin B inhibitory ability against cathepsin B and also similar order activity against the corresponding parasite enzyme cpB. These compounds have also shown growth inhibition of extracellular promastigotes of *L. major*, *L. mexicana* and *L. donovani* (see figure 5 and table 1). [25]

2.1.4. Vanadium compounds and their interaction with protein tyrosine phosphatases

Peroxovanadium compounds have shown potent inhibitors of protein tyrosine phosphatases and inducers of antileishmania effects like ROS and NO. Treatment of infected mice with bisperoxovanadium-1,10-phenanthroline or bis-peroxovanadiumpicolinate completely controlled progression of leishmaniasis in a NO-dependent manner. After injection, compounds rapidly triggered expression of inducible NO synthase in liver of mice infected with *L. major*. *In vivo* functional and immunological events associated with this peroxovanadium protective process have been identified. More recently, three dinuclear triperoxovanadate complexes, two mononuclear diperoxovanadate complexes with aminoacids or dipeptides as ancillary ligands and bis-peroxovanadate have been tested for their ability to kill *Leishmania* parasites *in vitro*, being $K[VO(O_2)_2(H_2O)]$ the most potent one. Combined administration of the latter with sub-optimal doses of sodium antimony gluconate on BALB/c mice experimentally

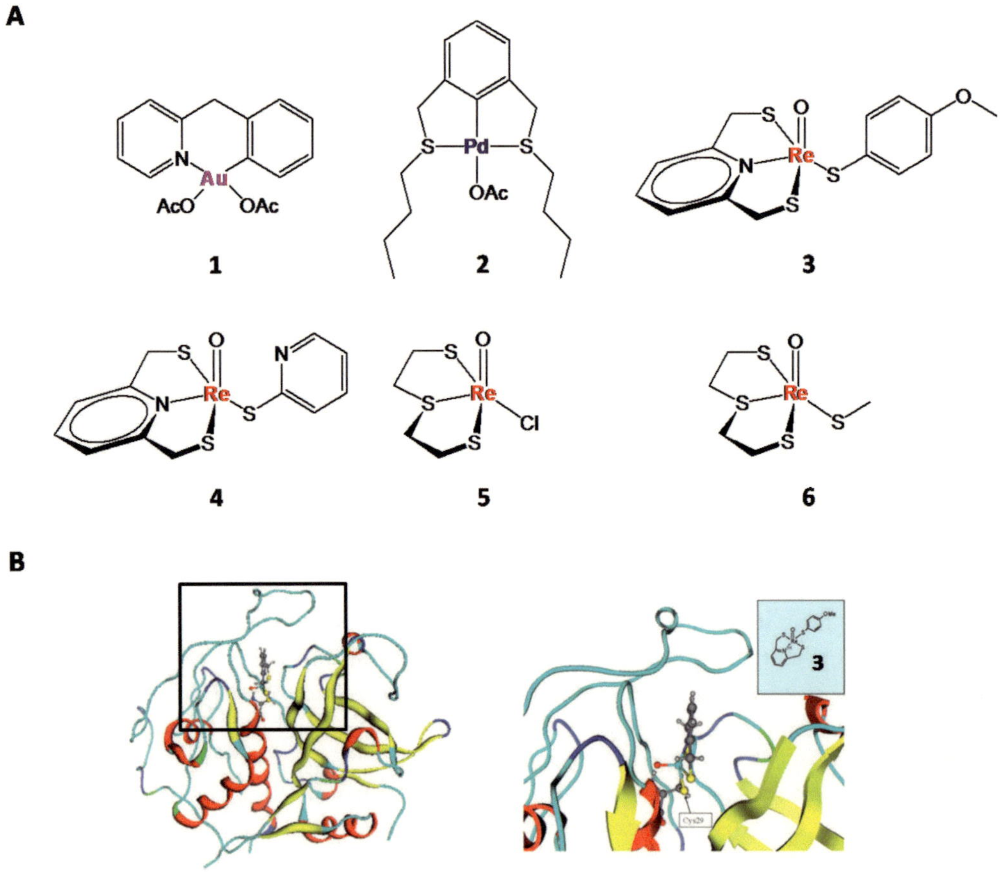

Figure 5. A) Structures of metal complexes with antileishmanial activity via inhibition of parasite cysteine proteases: (**1**) diaceto [2-[(2-pyridinyl-κ*N*)methyl] phenyl-κ*C*] gold(I), (**2**) aceto [2,6-bis [(butylthio-κ*S*)methyl]-phenyl-κ*C*] palladium(II), (**3**) (*p*-methoxyphenylthiolato-*S*) [2,6-bis[(mercapto-κ*S*)methyl] pyridine-κN^1] oxorhenium(V), (**4**) (2(1*H*)-pyridinethionato-κS^2)[2,6-bis [(mercapto-κ*S*)-methyl] pyridine-κN^1] oxorhenium(V), (**5**) chloro [2,2′-(thio-κ*S*)bis [ethanethiolato-κ*S*)]] oxorhenium(V), (**6**) (methanethiolato) [2,2′-(thio-κ*S*)bis [ethanethiolato-κ*S*)]] oxorhenium(V). B) Hypothetical model of oxorhenium(V) complex 3 binding to the active site cysteine of cathepsin B. Adapted from Ref. [25].

Compound	**1**	**2**	**3**	**4**	**5**	**6**
Cat B	1.29	0.40	6.51	0.12	0.0088	1.26
L. Major cpB	1.7	2.1	1.0	0.07	0.2	"/> 10

Table 1. Inhibitory effect of metal compounds 1-6 against mammalian cathepsin B and cathepsin B-like cystein protease of *L. major*. Results expressed as IC_{50} (μM). [25]

infected with antimony resistant *L. donovani* was highly effective in reducing the organ parasite burden. The effect was mainly associated with generation of ROS and nitrogen species that could kill intracellular parasites.

2.1.5. DNA-metallointercalators are not only to fight cancer

As the metabolic pathways of kinetoplastid parasites are similar to those of tumor cells, it has been proposed that compounds which efficiently interact with DNA in an intercalative mode could also show anti-trypanosomatid activity. [26] Based on this hypothesis, some work has been carried out on design of metallointercalators as anti-leishmania drugs, including metals of pharmacological interest. It has been found that certain DNA intercalating drugs which have potent trypanocidal action, such as ethidium, acriflavine, and ellipticines, inhibit the DNA topoisomerases. These enzymes thus may represent another potential target for DNA-intercalating trypanocidal metallodrugs.

DNA-intercalating metal complexes with potential leishmanicidal activity are generally made up of metals of known clinical application such as platinum, copper, silver and gold with planar polyaromatic ligands such as dppz (dipyrido[3,2-a:2′,3′-c]phenazine) and dpq (dipyrido[3,2-a:2′,3′-h]quinoxoline). Figure 6. Copper complexes with dppz and dpq ligands, $[Cu(L)_n(NO_3)_{2-n}](NO_3)_n$ where L = dppz or dpq (Fig. 6) have shown activity against *Leishmania braziliensis* (causative of the muco-cutaneous mode of the disease), and it has been demonstrated that their action is related to their ability to interact with DNA. $[Cu(dppz)_2](NO_3)_2$ was the most effective complex in this series, and the activity order was $[Cu(dppz)_2](NO_3)_2$>$[Cu(dppz)(NO_3)](NO_3)$ > $[Cu(dpq)_2](NO_3)_2$>$[Cu(dpq)(NO_3)](NO_3)$. [27]

Among the most effective complexes is $[Au(dppz)_2]Cl_3$. This complex induced a dose dependent antiproliferative effect with a minimal inhibitory concentration (MIC) of 3.4 nM and lethal doses LD_{26} of 17 nM at 48 h. This strong *in vitro* activity against *L. mexicana* could be related to their ability to interact with DNA through an intercalative mode. Also, preliminary ultrastructural studies using transmission electron microscopy carried out with treated parasites at a sublethal concentration (IC_7 = 0.34 nM for 24 h) showed polynucleated cells with DNA fragmentation and drastic disorganization of the mitochondria. [28]

Several years ago, a DNA metallointercalator (2,2′:6′2′′-terpyridine) platinum showed a remarkable antileishmanial activity, causing complete growth inhibition of *Leishmania donovani* amastigotes at 1 μM concentration.[29] This complex exploits simultaneous DNA intercalation of terpyridine and platinum(II) binding to the enzyme active site. The highest activity against *L. donovani* was found for the case of *p*-bromophenyl substituents in 4′-terpyridine position, and NH_3 as the ancillary hydrolysable ligand.[18]

Various DNA-intercalating organic ligands, have also been bound to vanadium ions. Although the potentiality of vanadium compounds in medicinal chemistry and medicinal applications has been extensively explored, work on vanadium compounds for treatment of some parasitic diseases of high incidence in human health has only arisen in a systematic way in recent years. [30] Benítez *et al.* obtained a series of oxovanadium complexes combining the aromatic planar polycyclic system 1,10-phenanthroline (phen) and tridentate salicylaldehyde semicarbazone derivatives as ligands, $[VO(L^1\text{-}2H)(phen)]$ and $[VO(L^2\text{-}2H)(phen)]$, where L^1 = 2-hydroxybenzaldehyde semicarbazone and L^2= 2-hydroxy-3-methoxybenzaldehyde semicarbazone. These compounds were active against *Leishmania* parasites showing low toxicity on mammalian cells. In addition, they showed cytotoxicicity on human promyelocytic leukemia HL-60 cells with

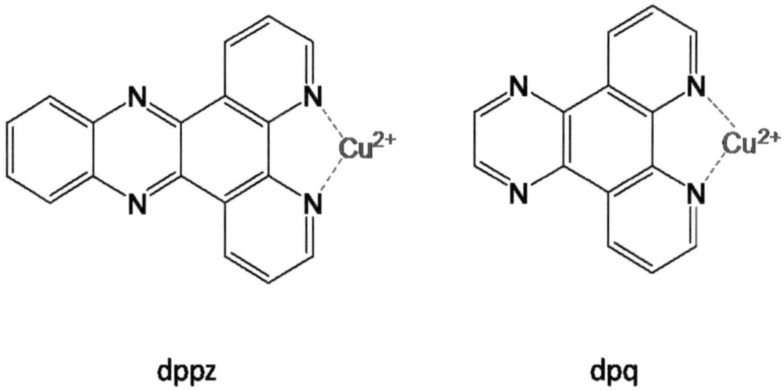

Figure 6. Structures of dppz (dipyrido[3,2-a:2′,3′-c]phenazine) and dpq (dipyrido[3,2-a:2′,3′-h]quinoxoline).

IC_{50} values of the same order of magnitude as cisplatin. Their interaction with DNA was demonstrated and studied by different techniques, suggesting that this biomolecule could be one of the potential targets for activity either in parasites or in tumor cells. [31]

2.1.6. *Zinc sulphate against cutaneous leishmaniasis: The privilege of simplicity*

Since zinc sulphate administered orally has been used in the last decades in medicine and dermatology, [32] then its use as an oral therapy for cutaneous leishmaniasis has appeared recently as an important addition to the armamentarium of antileishmanial drugs.

In vitro sensitivities of *L. major* and *L. tropica* strains to zinc were reported to be higher than those to pentavalent antimony, and these data were confirmed on mice. Zinc sulphate was also delivered intralesionally with success in cutaneous leishmaniasis. It is been suggested that oral zinc might not only affect directly to the parasite but also to macrophages function. Also it could have immunomodulatory effect (including T-lymphocytes), and help wound-healing. [33]

More recently, zinc sulphate was orally administered to Iraqi patients suffering from parasitologically confirmed cutaneous leishmaniasis. The species was not identified but it is known that only *L. major* and *L. tropica* are present in Iraq. This salt showed very promising cure rates (96.9%) against cutaneous leishmanaisis in a 45-days treatment with oral daily doses of 10 mg/kg. After a comparative study between oral zinc sulfate and meglumine antimoniate in the treatment of cutaneous leishmaniasis, it was suggested that systemic antimonial injections in cutaneous leishmaniasis treatment were better than zinc sulphate but oral administration of zinc sulphate makes it cheaper, more convenient its consumption, and nearly close cure percentage to systemic meglumine antimoniate injections without serious side effects. However at the moment zinc sulphate therapeutic effects should be confirmed by a greater sample volume. [34] Nevertheless, reported studies suggest that antileishmanial effect of zinc may result, partially or entirely, from inhibition of enzymes that are necessary for the parasites' carbohydrate metabolism and virulence. [35]

2.1.7. *Selenium and the key role of antioxidants in disease*

Selenium is an important and potent antioxidant in cells. Selenium compounds like selenites and selenates have strong inhibitory effects particularly on mammalian tumor cell growth. What is more, the nutritional deficiency of this essential trace metal may inhibit initiation and post-initiation phases of chemically induced mammary carcinogenesis and expression of some viruses, and it is important for optimal functioning of the immune system. [36]

Compounds of this metal have been reported to control human malaria if used in combination with vitamin E. [37] *In vitro* studies have shown that sodium selenite can inhibit *Leishmania donovani* growth although the mechanism of action is not clear yet. [38] Some authors have suggested that selenium has an important role in the pathophysiologic processes of cutaneous leishmaniasis, and that decreasing levels of this metal may be a host defense strategy of the organism against cutaneous leishmaniasis infection. Lack of selenium leads to a decrease of GSH-Px enzyme activity (it degrades H_2O_2), leading to increased amounts of hydroperoxides to kill protozoa as a host defense strategy.

2.1.8. *Triazolopyrimidines and their metal complexes: Mimicking the nature*

Triazolopyrimidines are purine analogues that have attracted much pharmaceutical interest during last decades. The most widely known derivative is the simple molecule Trapidil or Rocornal, a clinically used antiischemic and cardiatonic agent which acts as a platelet-derived growth factor (PDGF) antagonist and as a phosphodiesterase inhibitor. [39] This family of compounds have also found interesting applications as antipyretic, analgesic and anti-inflammatory, herbicidal, fungicidal agents with about 200 relevant patents. For example, 2-arenesulfonamido triazolopyrimidines were tested as leishmanicides showing some of them similar *in vitro* activity than pentamidine against *L. donovani* (Figure 7).

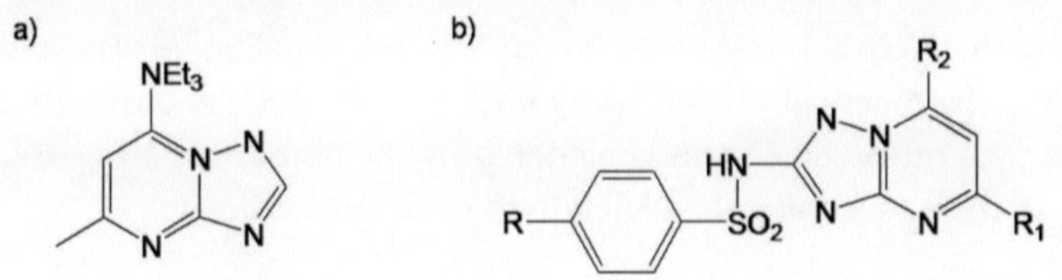

	R	R_1	R_2
a	CH_3	CH_3	CH_3
b	CH_3	C_6H_5	OH
c	Cl	C_6H_5	C_6H_5

Figure 7. Structures of triazolopyrimidine drugs: a) the anticoagulant drug Trapidil; b) a series of leishmanicidal derivatives.[39]

The biological activity of this family of organic compounds has led to investigating their coordination chemistry with the aim to develop new drugs with enhanced leishmanicidal activity and selectivity towards the parasites. Recently our group developed a series of transition metal complexes containing 1,2,4-triazolo[1,5-a]pyrimidines with high antiproliferative activity and extremely high selectivity indexes (see section 3). Studies revealed that apart from being all of them active *in vitro* against both extracellular and intracelular forms of *L. infantum* and *L. braziliensis*, these compounds are not toxic towards the host cells and are effective at lower concentrations than the drug used as a reference, Glucantime.[40] In the following section, we will present a case study in which our latest findings of our research with triazolopyrimidine metal complexes are described.

2.1.9. Nanoparticles: a promise for the future

A vast array of intriguing nanoscale particulate systems capable of targeting different cells and extracellular elements in the body to deliver drugs, genetic materials and diagnostic agents have been developed in the last years. Currently, antiparasitic delivery via nanosized particles is at the forefront of the research in this area. Liposomes and polymeric nanoparticles are the best studied nanosystems for evaluating antileishmania activity of compounds like amphotericin B or pentamidine. [41]

But nanosized metal particles are also emerging as promising antiparasitic agents. In recent studies it was determined that metal nanoparticles possess effective antimicrobial activities due to their unique properties and large surface areas. Moreover, metal nanoparticles are capable of producing reactive oxygen species (ROS), which would be able to kill parasites and other infectious agents.

Use metal of metal nanoparticles against *Leishmania* has followed two main approaches:

a. As antiparasitic drug carriers. Nano-bioconjugate gold has recently been conceived as a stratagem against macrophage-infested leishmanial infections. One example is the functionalization of gold nanoparticles with the flavonoid quercetin, reported as one of the most powerful leishmanicidal among all plan flavonids tested so far. [8] This flavonoid inhibits synthesis of parasite DNA by inhibition of topoisomerase II mediated linearization of kDNA. Quercetin in addition can chelate iron and then limit availability of this metal for ribonucleotide reductase during DNA synthesis. On the other hand, gold nanoparticles as such can cause impairments in parasite oxygen metabolism.

Quercetin functionalized gold nanoparticles showed to be effective against *L. donovani* promastigotes and amastigotes. They were also effective against drug resistant strains with a very high selectivity index. A synergistic effect was considered by the authors as a possible reason for the higher activity of the nanoconjugate related to the free quercetin.

b. As antiparasitic administration nanoforms. Because of the larger surface area of nanoparticles, they are more reactive and thus chemotherapeutic properties of a metal with antiparasitic activiy would be enhanced for its nanoform.

Selenium, for example, is a bioactive metal as it has antioxidant, cancer preventing, and antiviral activities. [37] Beheshti *et al.* prepared biogenic selenium nanoparticles, in this case, biosynthesized by *Bacillus sp.* MSh-1 and tested their *in vitro* and *in vivo* activity against *Leishmania major*. The particles showed antiproliferative activity against promastigote and amastigote forms of *L. major* and limited localized cutaneous leishmaniasis in animal model. These results present this kind of particles as novel therapeutic agents for treatment of the localized lesions typical of cutaneous leishmaniasis. However further studies are needed to investigate the mechanism of action of these Se NPs.[9]

http://dx.doi.org/10.5772/57376

Antimony sulfide NPs (Sb_2S_5), obtained also by green synthetic methods, proved to be effective on proliferation of promastigote forms of *L. infantum* and can induce apoptosis in promastigotes. [10]

The capability of metal nanoparticles to generate ROS and their potential use as leishmanicidal agents have also been explored. This is the case of silver nanoparticles, which have shown to be able to produce high amounts of ROS independently of the host cells. *In vitro* effects of AgNPs against promastigotes and amastigotes of *Leishmania tropica* were investigated. In order to increase the amount of ROS that are generated, AgNPs were irradiated with UV light which enhanced their antileishmanial effects without affecting host cells. [42]

2.2. Strategies for the design of new metal-based leishmanicidal drugs

To address the need for new, cost-effective metal-based leads for chemotherapy of leishmaniasis, different strategies of structure-based drug design have been applied so far. Four main strategies may be identified along revision in section 2.1:

2.2.1. Antitumoral activity implies antiparasitic activity

This strategy is based on the knowledge that highly-proliferative cells such as kinetoplastid parasites and tumor cells show metabolic similarities that lead in many cases to a correlation between antitrypanosomal and antitumor activities.[4] In this sense, use of metal complexes which have previously shown antitumoral activity, or synthesis of new metal complexes with ligands bearing activity could be a promising approach towards development of new agents against protozoa like *Leishmania*. A good correlation between antitumor and trypanostatic properties of several metal-based drugs has already been observed.

2.2.2. Metal-drug synergism approach

Perhaps one of the most popular strategies to develop new antiparasitic drugs consists on using an established antiparasitic drug as scaffold for the inclusion of a metal centre, either via direct coordination to the drug or by binding a metal complex. This way an enhancement of the drug pharmacological properties is pursued and resistance mechanism might be circumvented. See section 2.1.2.

2.2.3. Delivery nanovehicles

In finding innovative parasite-specific formulations, established but deficient drugs might be optimised by using drug delivery systems, in order to enhance their efficiency and reduce negative side effects at relatively low cost. Antiparasitic efficacy of drugs already in clinical use might be significantly improved by the adaptation of a new drug formulation. Use of nanocarriers to deliver established metal-based drugs such as antimonials would be both cost-effective and the quickest way to produce effective results. New drug formulations like liposomes for other drugs like amphotericin B (Ambisome) have been successfully developed for treating visceral leishmaniasis.

On the other hand, use of metal-based nanosystems as drug carriers, e.g. noble metal nanoparticles, might provide additional advantages such as the possibility for diagnosis by imaging techniques and the combined effect of producing ROS as it is the case for silver. ROS can induce oxidative stress, DNA damage, alkylation of target proteins and eventually apoptosis of the parasite.

In order to inhibit *Leishmania* parasites with a ROS-based treatment, these oxygen derivatives must be produced in a physical way rather than in an enzymatic way that can be blocked by parasites. Metal nanoparticles are able to produce high amounts of ROS, as they are more reactive than the corresponding bulk metal (see example of AgNPs in section 2.1.9).

Nanocarriers also offer the possibility to specifically target the parasites by attaching appropiate targeting molecules onto their surface. This way side effects to the host would be minimised. In addition, drug delivery vehicles such as nanoparticles allow prompt interactions with biomolecules present within as well as on the surface of the cell and may be tuned into different sizes to get the optimal uptake rate and blood circulation times of the drug.

2.2.4. Specifically targeted drugs: Metal inhibitors of parasite enzymes and DNA-binders

Recent advancements in molecular biology have identified a few parasite targets that are likely to be very sensitive to metal-based compounds. These targets usually are enzymes, some of them bearing free thiols at their active sites that manifest a high propensity to react with soft Lewis acids, i.e. metal ions such as Ag(I), Au(III) or Zn(II). Therefore these parasite targets will be susceptible to strong and selective inhibition by this kind of metals. This is the case of dithiol reductases like trypanothione reductase ($T(SH)_2$), which have been shown to play a key role in the *Leishmania* metabolism (see Section 2.1.1) and therefore constitute primary targets for metal compounds. Cysteine proteases, such as cathpesin L-like or cathepsin B-like, are another example of proteins with thiol-containing active sites and thus responsive to inhibition by metal compounds. Inhibitors that would effectively target both types of cysteine proteases in *Leishmania,* while maintaining some selectivity versus homologous host enzymes, would be ideal drug leads.

Regarding DNA interaction, previous studies have shown that DNA-binding metal compounds such as cisplatin display antiparasitic activity. These findings along with the observation that many antiparasitic drugs bind to DNA, have led to propose that in general every DNA interacting compound is potentially active against parasites.

Therefore DNA-intercalating molecules have been used as ligands to form metal complexes showing antiparasitic activity. Intercalating ligands are usually polyaromatic systems with two or more donor atoms in close disposition to "chelate" metal ions. These ligands would not only be responsible for interaction of the metal compound with DNA but also they could act as carriers of the metal, increasing interaction of complexes with DNA by minimizing exposure of metal to inactivating cellular nucleophiles such as thiols.

3. Case study: Evaluation of the chemotherapeutic potential of metal complexes containing nucleobase-analogues against *Leishmania infantum* and *Leishmania braziliensis*

In this section we will describe some of our latest findings, which have been published recently. [40] Through this case study, we seek to provide the reader with an useful insight on our research, which is aimed at the rational design of new biomimetic metal-based systems as potential antiparasitic agents. Our research activity can be summarized in the following tasks:

a. Study of the interaction of a series of purine analogs, namely 1,2,4-triazolopyrimidines, with a wide range of metal ions, mainly from the first and second transition series.

b. Based on the coordination properties of triazolopyrimidine derivatives, design and synthesize new metal complexes showing structural and physical properties such as photoluminescent or magnetic properties that might be of interest for further applications.

c. Evaluate their *in vitro* activity against *Trypanosoma cruzi* and different species of *Leishmania* spp. Studies with *T. cruzi* are complemented with *in vivo* assays (murine model) for the most active compounds.

d. Analyze possible structure-activity correlations and investigate mechanism of action.

3.1. Transition metal complexes with 1,2,4-triazolo[1,5-a]pyrimidines

1,2,4-triazolopyrimidines are bicyclic heterocycles that are formed from the condensation of a ring of 1,2,4-triazole and another one of pyrimidine. Depending on the relative orientation of both rings, four different isomeric families can arise: 1,2,4-triazolo[1,5-a]pyrimidines, 1,2,4-triazolo[1,5-c]pyrimidines, 1,2,4-triazolo[4,3-a]pyrimidines, and 1,2,4-triazolo[4,3-c]pyrimidines. Among them, 1,2,4-triazolo[1,5-a]pyrimidine derivatives are the most stable thermodynamically and, because of this, the object of our present studies.

In previous works, 1,2,4-triazolo[1,5-a]pyrimidines have proved to be excellent ligands for a wide range of transition metal ions. [43] This fact is due to their, at least, three coordination positions, N1, N3 and N4, which can lead to several coordination modes. The coordination capability of these derivatives can be increased by the presence of heteroatoms as ring-substituents. However, a systematic revision on the existing results indicates a clear trend of these ligands to coordinate monodentately by N3, followed by N3,N4-bidentate and N1,N3-bidentate bridging modes (Figure 8).

The rich coordination chemistry of these derivatives has led in the last years to a great variety of multidimensional coordination compounds showing interesting properties, especially from the magnetic and biological viewpoints.

In addition, the biomimetic character of 1,2,4-triazolo[1,5-a]pyrimidines with purine nucleobases confers a potential biological activity to these derivatives and to their metal complexes, which can be used for therapeutic aims. Our studies have revealed the high potential of this kind of compounds for acting as leishmanicidal agents.

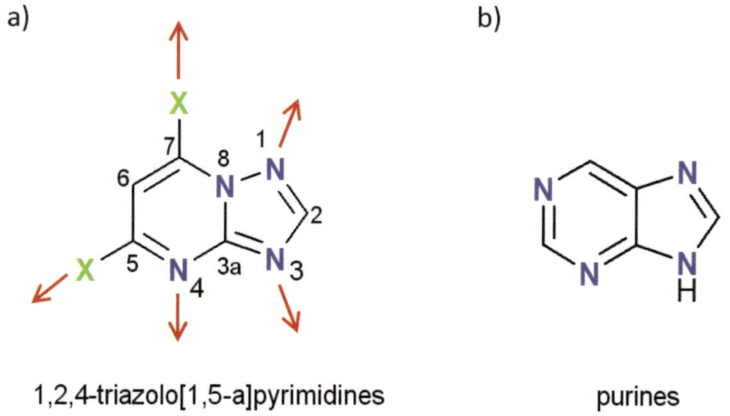

Figure 8. Basic structure of 5,7-substituted 1,2,4-triazolo[1,5-a]pyrimidines (a) and purines (b). Numbering scheme and possible binding sites to metal ions are also depicted for triazolopyrimidines. X=donor atom (N, O, S, etc.)

Herein we report the results obtained with three of the most promising metal compounds we have obtained so far: $[Cu(HmtpO)_2(H_2O)_3](ClO_4)_2$ H_2O (1), $\{[Cu(HmtpO)_2(H_2O)_2](ClO_4)_2$ $2HmtpO\}_n$ (2) and $\{Co(HmtpO)(H_2O)_3](ClO_4)_2$ $2H_2O\}_n$ (3), Figure 9. All of them contain the neutral form of 5-methyl-1,2,4-triazolo[1,5-a]pyrimidin-7(4*H*)-one (HmtpO) and perchlorate as counteranion. The three compounds show different topology and dimensionality. Compound 1 is a monomeric complex in which HmtpO shows both N3 monodentate and N1,O71 bidentate modes; compound 2 is a two-dimensional framework in which HmtpO ligand shows an N3,O71 bidentate bridging mode; and the structure of compound 3 consists of one-dimensional chains in which HmtpO displays an N1,N3,O71 tridentate bridging mode. The structural diversity of these compounds is mainly due to the mode of the triazolopyrimidine ligand.

As depicted in Figure 9, the compounds 1-3 were synthesized by mixing their corresponding metal perchlorate salts with HmtpO derivative in aqueous media and bringing to reflux for 30 min before acidification with HCl. In all cases, compounds were isolated as crystals from their respective solution after several days standing at room temperature. Obtention of single crystals allowed to determine their crystal structure by X-ray analysis and their characterization was completed by elemental and thermal analysis (thermogravimetry and differential scanning calorimetry), and spectroscopic techniques such as FTIR and UV-Vis. Magnetic studies indicate that compound 1 exhibits simple paramagnetism in 2-300 K while the overall behaviour of 2 and 3 corresponds to weak ferromagnetically and antiferromagnetically coupled systems, respectively. [44]

3.2. *In vitro* antiproliferative activity against promastigote forms (extracellular forms) and toxicity against a mammalian host cell model

Firstly we evaluated the toxic activity of the free triazolopyrimidine compound HmtpO and its Cu(II) and Co(II) complexes 1-3 against promastigotes of two species of *Leishmania* (*L.*

http://dx.doi.org/10.5772/57376

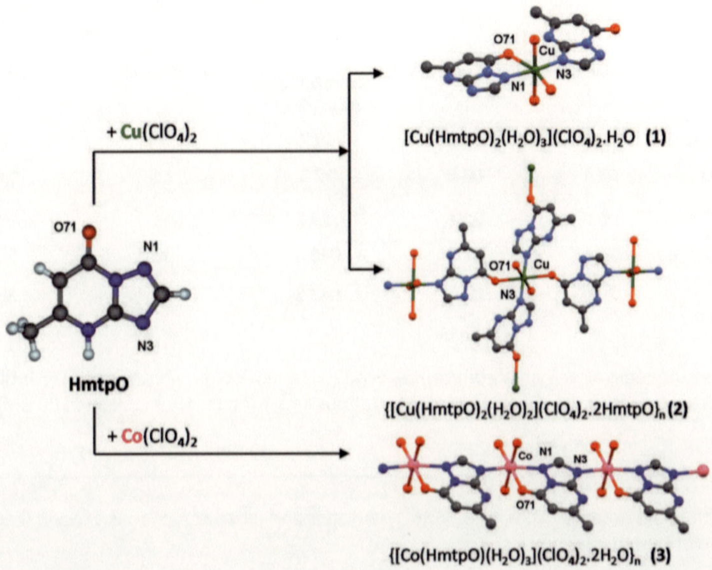

Figure 9. Synthetic scheme and structures of triazolopyrimidine derivative HmtpO and its metal complexes 1-3. Please note that the graphs of 1-3 correspond only to the cationic part of the metal compounds.

infantum and *L. braziliensis*). IC_{50} values registered after 72 h of exposure are shown in Table 2, including Glucantime as reference drug. Antileishmanial activity of metal complexes 1-3, expressed as IC_{50}, was similar to that found for Glucantime for both *L. infantum* and *L. braziliensis*. In contrast, the free derivative HmtpO is significantly less active than its metal compounds.

To evaluate toxicity on the host, J774.2 macrophages (mammalian cells) were used as cell model. Cytotoxic studies showed that metal complexes 1-3 are much less toxic than Glucantime and the free HmtpO derivative (Table 2).

On the other hand, selectivity and thus efficacy of assayed compounds towards parasite cells was evaluated and quantified by using the selectivity index (SI). This parameter is defined as the cocient between IC_{50} for cells and IC_{50} for parasites. A value greater than 1 is considered more selective for activity against parasites, and a value less than 1 is considered more selective for activity against cells.[45] SI of these derivatives was 30-fold or more higher than SI of Glucantime and HmtpO. These results are indicative of the higher potential of metal compounds 1-3 as antiparasitic agents compared with the current treatments, in this case Glucantime. Moreover it is evident that the presence of the metal ion in the scaffold enhances significantly triazolopyrimidine derivative activity and selectivity. This example constitutes another proof of the validity of the metal-drug synergism approach.

3.3. Effects on the infection rate and the intracellular replication of the amastigote forms

Most studies on *in vitro* biological activity of new compounds against *Leishmania* spp. are performed on promastigote forms because it is much easier to work with these forms *in vitro*.

Compound	IC50 (μM) L. infantum	IC50 (μM) L. braziliensis	Toxicity J774.2 macrophages IC_{50} (μM) [a]	SI [b] L. infantum	SI [b] L. braziliensis
Glucantime	18.0	25.6	15.2	1	1
HmtpO	63.4	60.6	99.8	1.6	1.6
1	20.0	22.1	723.8	36	33
2	24.4	31.5	945.5	39	30
3	29.0	23.5	843.3	29	36

[a] Towards J774.2 macrophages after 72 h of culture. IC_{50} is the concentration required to give 50% inhibition, calculated by linear regression analysis from the K_c values at concentrations employed (1, 10, 25, 50 and 100 μM).

[b] Selectivity index (SI) =IC_{50} macrophages/IC_{50} parasite

Table 2. *In vitro* activity of reference drugs, free HmtpO derivative and metal compounds 1, 2 and 3 against promastigote forms of *Leishmania* spp.

However, in our studies we also include the effects of these compounds on the forms that develop in the host (amastigotes). This study is of great importance to determine effects in the definitive host and thus it gives a better idea of the potential application as antiparasitic drugs.

To predict the effect of metal complexes 1-3 on the capacity for infection and growth inhibition of intracellular forms of *L. infantum* and *L. braziliensis*, adherent J774.2 macrophages (1×10^5 macrophages) were incubated for two days and then infected with 1×10^6 promastigote forms of *L. infantum* and *L. braziliensis* for 12 h. Non-phagocytosed parasites were afterwards removed and culture was kept in fresh medium for 10 days. Parasites invaded cells and then converted into amastigotes within one day after infection. On the 10th day, the rate of host-cell infection reached the maximum. When drugs 1-3 were added at their respective IC_{25} concentration to macrophages infected with *Leishmania* spp. promastigote forms in exponential growth phase, infection rate decreased significantly after 12 h with respect to control measurements, following the trend 1>3>2 for *L. infantum* and 3>1>2 for *L. braziliensis*, with percentages of infestation-inhibition capacity of 84%, 79% and 67%, respectively, in the case of *L. infantum* and 86%, 79% and 75%, respectively, in the case of *L. braziliensis*. These values are remarkably higher than those for inhibition by Glucantime (56% and 36% for *L. infantum* and *L. braziliensis*, respectively). The three complexes inhibited *Leishmania* spp. amastigote replication in macrophage cells *in vitro*, following a similar pattern to that for infection rate inhibition and again being more effective than reference drug. Although not always it is possible to establish a direct relationship between drug action on extracelular promastigote and intracellular amastigote forms, in case of compound 3, it was effective against both forms.

3.4. Studies on the mechanism of action

In order to investigate the possible mechanism of action of metal compounds 1-3 on the parasite, their effect on metabolite excretion is analyzed, and microscopy studies on the treated parasites are carried out to visualize any ultrastructural alteration that may be provocked by the compounds.

3.4.1. *Metabolite excretion effect*

To the best of our knowledge, none of the trypanosomatids studied is capable of completely degrading glucose to CO_2 under aerobic conditions, so they excret a great part of the carbon skeleton into medium as fermented metabolites, which can differ according to the employed species.[46] *Leishmania* spp. have a high rate of glucose consumption, thereby acidifying culture medium due to incomplete oxidation to acids. ^{1}H-NMR spectra enable us to determine fermented metabolites that are excreted by the parasites during their *in vitro* culture. One of the major metabolites excreted by *Leishmania* spp. is succinate, the main role of which is probably to maintain the glycosomal redox balance by providing two glycosomal oxidoreductase enzymes. These enzymes allow reoxidation of NADH that is produced by glyceraldehyde-3-phosphate dehydrogenase in the glycolytic pathway. Succinic fermentation offers one significant advantage, since it requires only half of the produced phosphoenolpyruvate (PEP) to maintain the NAD^+/NADH balance. The remaining PEP is converted into acetate, depending on the species being considered. Figure 10 (on the left) shows ^{1}H-NMR spectrum of cell-free medium four days after inoculation with *L. infantum*. Additional peaks, corresponding to the major metabolites that were produced and excreted during growth, could be detected when this spectrum was compared with the one made in fresh medium. Taking into account that *L. infantum* excretes mainly succinate and acetate, ^{1}H-NMR spectra show that only compound 2 significantly altered excreted metabolites by *L. infantum*. When promastigote forms of *L. infantum* were treated with compound 2 at IC_{25} doses, the excretion of catabolites (succinate and acetate) was clearly disturbed and a new peak, identified as pyruvate, appeared (Figure 10). These results mean that compound 2 inhibits glycosomal enzymes, causing pyruvate to be excreted as a final metabolite. On the other hand, compounds 1 and 3 inhibite excreted metabolites only slightly. In the case of *L. braziliensis*, compounds 1-3 showed a similar behavior as for *L. infantum*, being again compound 2 the most inhibitory.

3.4.2. *Ultrastructural alterations*

Transmission electron microscopy images showed that compounds 1-3 induced morphological alterations in *L. infantum* and *L. braziliensis* promastigotes when parasites were treated with the respective IC_{25}. Compound 2 was the most effective against both parasite species.

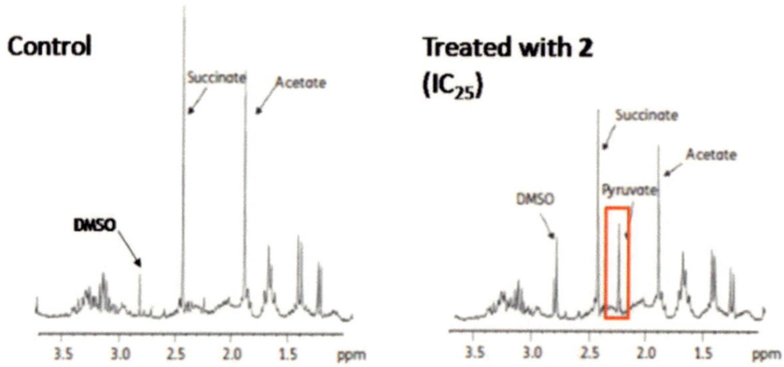

Figure 10. NMR spectra of promastigote forms of *L. infantum*, which show the characteristic peaks of the major excreted metabolites of non-treated parasites (left) and parasites that have been treated with IC_{25} of compound 2 (right) for four days.

http://dx.doi.org/10.5772/57376

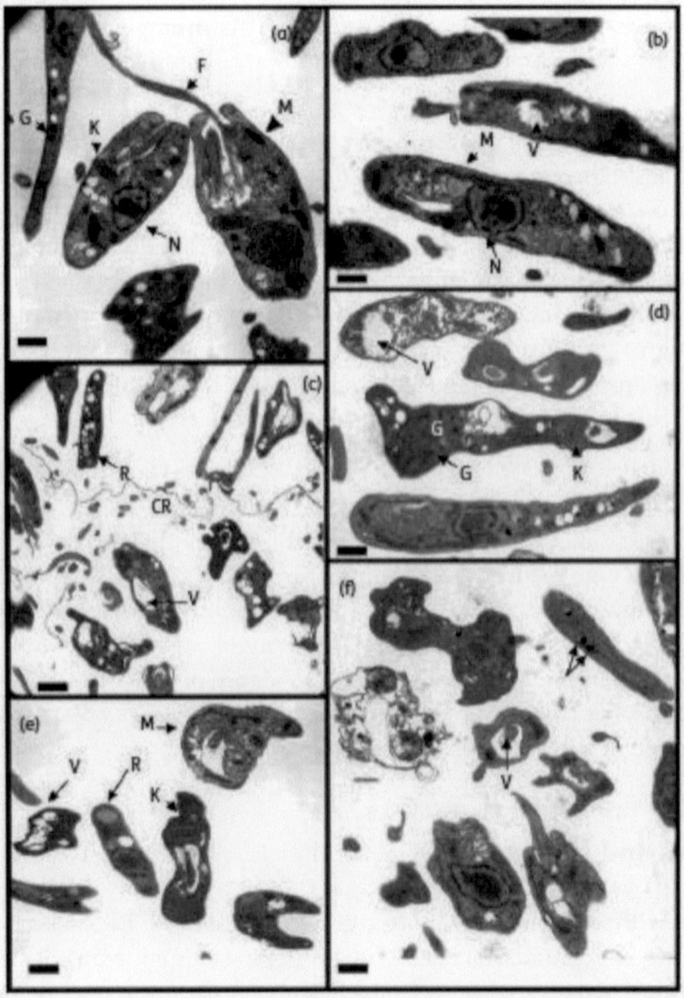

Figure 11. TEM images showing ultrastructural alterations in *L. infantum* and *L. braziliensis* after being treated with compounds 1, 2 and 3 (at IC_{25} concentrations) for 72h. (a) Control parasite of *L. infantum* showing organelles with their characteristic aspect, such as nucleus (N), kinetoplast (K), flagellum (F), glycosomes (G) and mitochondrion (M). Bar=1.00 µm. (b) Control parasite of *L. braziliensis* with structures such as nucleus (N), vacuoles (V) and mitochondrion (M). Bar=1.00 µm. (c) *L. infantum* treated with compound 2, showing cellular rest (CR), intense vacuolization (V) and reservosomes (R). Bar=1.59 µm. (d) *L. infantum* treated with compound 3, showing electrodense cytoplasm, vacuoles (V), glycosomes (G) and kinetoplast (K). Bar=1.00 µm. (e) *L. braziliensis* treated with compound 1, showing intense vacuolization (V), giant reservosomes (R) and kinetoplast (K) and swelling mitochondrion (M). Bar=1.00 µm. (f) Promastigotes of *L. braziliensis* treated with compound 2, with vacuoles (V) and electrodense organelles (arrows). Bar=1.00 µm.

After treating *L. braziliensis* promastigotes with compound 2, many of the parasites appeared dead and others adopted distorted shapes, while in others a uniformly electrodense cytoplasm was formed, in which no cytoplasmic organelles were visible. Parasites vacuolization was pronounced and many of these vacuoles contained strongly electrodense inclusions. In case of *L. infantum*, compound 2 led mostly to cell destruction (Figure 11c), which was evident from the presence of a great quantity of cell remains in supernatant. Likewise parasites had strongly electrodense cytoplasm with intense vacuolization, with both empty vacuoles and membranes, and reservosomes, which appeared in greater numbers than in non-treated promastigotes (Figure 11a).

On the other hand, compound 1 was again very effective against *L. braziliensis* as some parasites appeared dead and others completely altered (Figure 11e), replete with reservosomes and enormous vacuoles. Some promastigotes appeared to be distorted and strongly electrodense, and showed condensed kinetoplast and very swollen mitochondria. In contrast, compound 3 was effective against *L. infantum* (Figure 11d), whose alterations were similar to those already described, with unrecognizable parasites, filled with vacuoles, which distorted their morphology, as well as a great quantity of reservosomes that occupied practically the entire cytoplasm. In these parasites kinetoplast and mitochondria also appeared swollen, resulting in a strongly electrodense cytoplasm. Dead parasites were also visible.

3.5. Final remarks

In addition to these studies, it should be noted that compounds 1-3 have displayed a high *in vitro* activity against both extra and intracellular forms of *T. cruzi* and are effective at concentrations similar to those of benznidazole. At the same time, they are much less toxic for host cells than the latter. Moreover antileishmanial activity of metal compounds is much higher than that of isolated HmtpO ligand, which is an evidence of the critical role of metal ions in antiparasitic activity. Furthermore, promising *in vivo* activity was observed for all of them, with results consistent with those observed *in vitro*.

4. Conclusion and future trends

In comparison with economically more attractive diseases like cancer, cardio-vascular problems and allergies, commercial interest in developing new antiparasitics is still rather low. Low income of most of the people affected by leishmaniasis, as it is the case for other tropical diseases, discourages big pharmaceutical companies from investing in developing new therapies. Therefore there is an urgent need to investigate into new drugs with low cost of production but also with high efficacy and selectivity.

Research on metal-based compounds to treat leishmaniasis has resurged in the last years and significant progress has been made. The possibility to finely tune their reactivity through a change of the metal ion and appropiate choice of the ligand/s makes of metal compounds promising alternatives to fight this disease in a cost-effective way.

Optimization of currently available metal-based drugs such as antimonials through use of nanovehicles and attachment of targeting moieties may be an interesting option to overcome antimonials resistance problems and maybe the quickest way to produce effective results. Therapeutic effects might be enhanced by using e.g. metal nanoparticles as delivery carriers, which depending on the metal, might be able to produce high amounts of reactive oxygen species and induce oxidative stress to the parasites.

http://dx.doi.org/10.5772/57376

On the other hand, significant advances in parasite genoma sequences and identification of targets in the last years along with an increasing understanding of metals interactions with a wide range of biomolecules, will contribute to development of highly efficient target-specific metal-based drugs in the future while avoiding recurring to time-consuming drug screening methodologies.

Meanwhile some authors have pointed at the metal-drug synergism approach as a very useful alternative for drug design at the moment.

Author details

Ana B. Caballero[1], Juan M. Salas[2] and Manuel Sánchez-Moreno[3]

1 School of Chemistry, University of Birmingham, Birmingham, United Kingdom

2 Department of Inorganic Chemistry, School of Sciences, University of Granada, Granada, Spain

3 Department of Parasitology, School of Sciences, University of Granada, Granada, Spain

References

[1] Singh MP, Mishra M, Khan AB, Ramdas SL, Panjiyar S. Gold treatment for kala-azar. Br. Med. J. 1989; 299 1318.

[2] Bruijnincx PC, Sadler PJ. New Trends for Metal Complexes with Anticancer Activity. Curr Opin Chem Biol. 2008; 12(2) 197–206.

[3] Sánchez-Delgado RA, Anzellotti A. Metal complexes as chemotherapeutic agents against tropical diseases: trypanosomiasis, malaria and leishmaniasis. Mini-Reviews in Medicinal Chemistry 2004; 423-30.

[4] Farrell NP. Transition Metal Complexes as Drugs and Chemotherapeutic Agents. In: R. Ugo, B. R. James (eds.) Catalysis by Metal Complexes. Vol 11. Dordrecht: Kluwer Academic Publishers; 1989. p. 222-242.

[5] Dubar F, Khalife J, Brocard J, Dive D, Biot C. Ferroquine, an Ingenious Antimalarial Drug –Thoughts on the Mechanism of Action. Molecules 2008; 13 2900-2907.

[6] Nogueira-Silva JJ, Pavanelli WR, Salazar Gutierrez FR, Chagas Alves Lima F, Borges Ferreira da Silva A, Santana Silva J, Wagner Franco D. Complexation of the anti-*Trypanosoma cruzi* Drug Benznidazole Improves Solubility and Efficacy. J. Med. Chem. 2008; 51 4104–4114.

[7] Navarro M, Gabbiani C, Messori L, Gambino D. Metal-based drugs for malaria, trypanosomiasis and leishmaniasis: recent achievements and perspectives. Drug Discovery Today 2010; 15 1070-1078.

[8] Das S, Roy P, Mondal S, Bera T, Mukherjee A. One pot synthesis of gold nanoparticles and application in chemotherapy of wild and resistant type visceral leishmaniasis. Colloids and Surfaces B: Biointerfaces 2013; 107 27-34.

[9] Beheshti N, Soflaei S, Shakibaie M, Yazdi MH, Ghaffairfar F, Dalimi A, Shahverdi AR. Efficacy of biogenic selenium nanoparticles against *Leishmania major*: *In vitro* and *in vivo* studies. Journal of Trace Elements in Medicine and Biology 2013; 27 203-207.

[10] Soflaei S, Dalimi A, Ghaffarifar F, Shakibaie M, Shahverdi AR, Shafiepour M. In Vitro Antiparasitic and Apoptotic Effects of Antimony Sulfide. Nanoparticles on Leishmania infantum. Journal of Parasitology Research 2012; doi 10.1155/2012/756568.

[11] Ouellette M, Drummelsmith J, Papadopoulou B. Leishmaniasis: drugs in the clinic, resistance and new developments. Drug Resistance Updates 2004; 7 257-266.

[12] Ashutosh, Sundar S, Goyal N. Molecular mechanisms of antimony resistance in *Leishmania*. Journal of Medical Microbiology 2007; 56 143-153.

[13] Baiocco P, Colotti G, Franceschini S, Ilari A. Molecular Basis of Antimony Treatment in Leishmaniasis. J. Med. Chem. 2009; 52 2603–2612.

[14] Sereno D, Holzmuller P, Mangot I, Cuny G, Ouaissi A, Lemesre J. Antimonial-mediated DNA fragmentation in *Leishmania infantum* amastigotes Antimicrob. Agents Chemother. 2001;45 2064-2069.

[15] Chakraborty AK, Majumder K. Mode of action of pentavalent antimonials: Specific inhibition of type I DNA topoisomerase of Leishmania donovani. Biochemical and Biophysical Research Communications 1988; 152(2) 605-611.

[16] Haldar AK, Sen P, Roy S. Use of Antimony in the Treatment of Leishmaniasis: Current Status and Future Directions. Molecular Biology International 2011, Article ID 571242. DOI: 10.4061/2011/571242

[17] Berman, J.D.; Waddell, D.; Hanson, B.D. Biochemical mechanisms of the antileishmanial activity of sodium stibogluconate. Antimicrob. Agents Chemother. 1985, 27, 916-920.

[18] Sánchez-Delgado RA, Anzellotti A, Suárez L. Metal complexes as chemotherapeutic agents against tropical diseases: malaria, trypanosomiasis and leishmaniasis. In: Sigel A and Sigel H (eds). Metal Ions in Biological Systems Volume 41: Metal Ions and Their Complexes in Medication. FontisMedia and Marcel Dekker; 2004, p. 379-420.

[19] Martinez A, Carreon T, Iniguez E, Anzellotti A, Sanchez A, Tyan M, Sattler A, Herrera L, Maldonado RA, Sanchez-Delgado RA. Searching for New Chemotherapies for Tropical Diseases: Ruthenium–Clotrimazole Complexes Display High in Vitro Activ-

ity against *Leishmania major* and *Trypanosoma cruzi* and Low Toxicity toward Normal Mammalian Cells. J Med Chem 2012; 55 3867–3877.

[20] Iniguez E, Sanchez A, Vasquez MA, Martınez A, Olivas J, Sattler A, Sanchez-Delgado RA, Maldonado RA. Metal–drug synergy: new ruthenium(II) complexes of ketoconazole are highly active against *Leishmania major* and *Trypanosoma cruzi* and nontoxic to human or murine normal cells. J Biol Inorg Chem 2013. DOI 10.1007/s00775-013-1024-2

[21] Mesa-Valle CM, Moraleda-Lindez V, Craciunescu D, Osuna A. Antileishmanial Action of Organometallic Complexes of Pt(II) and Rh(I). Mem. Inst. Oswaldo Cruz, Rio de Janeiro 1996, 91, 625-633.

[22] Castilla JJ, Mesa-Valle MC, Sánchez-Moreno M, Arnedo T, Rosales MJ, Mascaro C, Craciunescu D, Osuna A. In vitro activity and biochemical effectiveness of new organometallic complexes of osmium(III) against *Leishmania donovani* and *Trypanosoma cruzi*. Arzneim.-Forsch.-Drug Res. 1996, 46, 990-996.

[23] Noleto GR, Mercê ALR, Iacomini M, Gorin PAJ, Soccol VT, Oliveira MBM. Effects of a lichen galactomannan and its vanadyl (IV) complex on peritoneal macrophages and leishmanicidal activity. Mol. Cell. Biochem. 2002; 233 73-83.

[24] Selzer PM, Pingel S, Hsieh I, Ugele B, Chan VJ, Engel JC, Bogyo M, Russell DG, Sakanari JA, McKerrow JH. Cysteine protease inhibitors as chemotherapy: Lessons from a parasite target. Proc. Natl. Acad. Sci. U. S. A. 1999; 96 11015–11022.

[25] Fricker SP. Cysteine proteases as targets for metal-based drugs. Metallomics 2010; 2 366–377.

[26] a) Kinnamon K, Steck EA, Rane ES. Activity of antitumor drugs against African trypanosomes. Antimicrob. Agents Chemother. 1979; 15 (2) 157-160. (b) Farrell NP, Williamson J, McLaren DJM. Trypanocidal and antitumour activity of platinum-metal and platinum-metal-drug dual-function complexes. Biochem. Pharmacol. 1984; 961-971.

[27] Navarro M, Cisneros-Fajardo EJ, Sierralta A, Fernández- Mestre M, Silva P, Arrieche D, Marchán E. Design of copper DNA intercalators with leishmanicidal activity. J. Biol. Inorg. Chem. 2003;8 401-408.

[28] Navarro M, Hernandez C, Colmenares I, Hernandez P, Fernandez M, Sierraalta A, Marchan E. Synthesis and characterization of $[Au(dppz)_2]Cl_3$. DNA interaction studies and biological activity against *Leishmania (L) Mexicana*. Journal of Inorganic Biochemistry. 2007; 101 111–116.

[29] Lowe G, Droz AS, Vilaivan T, Weaver GW, Tweedale L, Pratt JM, Rock P, Yardley V, Croft SL. Cytotoxicity of (2, 2′:6′, 2′′-terpyridine) platinum (II) complexes to *Leishmania donovani, Trypanosoma cruzi* and *Trypanosoma brucei*. J. Med. Chem. 1999; 42, 999–1006.

[30] Gambino D. Potentiality of vanadium compounds as anti-parasitic agents.Coordination Chemistry Reviews 2011; 255 (19–20) 2193–2203.

[31] Benítez J, Becco L, Correia I, Milena Leal S, Guiset H, Costa Pessoa J, Lorenzo J, Aviles F, Escobar P, Moreno V, Garat B, Gambino D. Vanadium polypyridyl compounds as potential antiparasitic and antitumoral agents: new achievements. J. Inorg. Biochem. 2011; 105 303-312.

[32] Neldner KH, Hambidge KM, Walravens PA. Acrodermatitis enteropathica. Int J Dermatol. 1978;17(5) 380-387.

[33] Minodier P, Parola P. Cutaneous leishmaniasis treatment. Travel Medicine and Infectious Disease 2007; 5, 150–158.

[34] Yazdanpanah MJ, Banihashemi M, Pezeshkpoor F, Khajedaluee M, Famili S, Rodi IT, Yousefzadeh H. Comparison of Oral Zinc Sulfate with Systemic Meglumine Antimoniate in the Treatment of Cutaneous Leishmaniasis. Dermatology Research and Practice 2011, doi 10.1155/2011/269515.

[35] Al-Mulla Hummadi YM, Al-Bashir NM, Najim RA. The mechanism behind the antileishmanial effect of zinc sulphate. II. Effects on the enzymes of the parasites. Annals of Tropical Medicine and Parasitology 2005; 99(2) 131-139.

[36] Combs Jr GF. Selenium and cancer. In: Garewal HS, editor. Antioxidants and disease prevention. New York, NY: CRC Press; 1997. p. 97–113.

[37] Levander OA. Selenium and sulfur antioxidant protective systems, relationships with vitamin E and malaria. Proc Sot Exp Biol Med 1992; 200 255-259.

[38] Mukhopadhyay R, Madhubala R. Effect of antioxidants on the growth and polyamine levels of *Leishmania donovani*. BiochemicalPharmacology 1994; 47(4) 611-615.

[39] Fischer G. Recent Progress in 1, 2, 4-Triazolo[1, 5-a]pyrimidine Chemistry. Adv. Heterocycl. Chem. 2008; 95 143-219.

[40] Ramirez-Macias I, Marin C, Salas JM, Caballero A, Rosales MJ, Villegas N, Rodriguez-Dieguez A, Barea E, Sanchez-Moreno M. Biological activity of three novel complexes with the ligand 5-methyl-1, 2, 4-triazolo[1, 5-a]pyrimidin-7(4H)-one against *Leishmania* spp. J Antimicrob Chemother 2011; 66 813–819.

[41] Venier-Julienne MC, Vouldoukis I, Monjour L, Benoit JP. In vitro study of the antileishmanial activity of biodegradable nanoparticles.*Journal of Drug Targeting* 1995; 3(1) 23–29. (b) Durand R, Paul M, Rivollet D, Fessi H, Houin R, Astier A, Deniau M. Activity of pentamidine-loaded poly (D, L-lactide) nanoparticles against *Leishmania infantum* in a murine model, " *Parasite 1997;* 4(4) 331–336.

[42] Allahverdiyev AM, Abamor ES, Bagirova M, Ustundag CB, Kaya C, Kaya F, Rafailovich M. Antileishmanial effect of silver nanoparticles and their enhanced antiparasit-

ic activity under ultraviolet light. International Journal of Nanomedicine 2011; 6 2705–2714.

[43] a) Salas JM, Romero MA, Sánchez MP, Quirós M. Metal complexes of [1, 2, 4]triazolo-[1, 5-a]pyrimidine derivatives. Coord. Chem. Rev. 1999; 193-195 1119-1142. (b) Caballero AB, Maclaren JK, Rodríguez-Diéguez A, Vidal I, Dobado JA, Salas JM, Janiak C. Dinuclear silver(I) complexes for the design of metal-ligand networks based on triazolopyrimidines. Dalton Trans. 2011; 40(44) 11845-55; (c) Caballero AB, Rodríguez-Diéguez A, Barea E, Quirós M, Salas JM. Influence of pseudohalide ligands on the structural versatility and properties of novel ternary metal complexes with 1, 2, 4-triazolo[1, 5-a]pyrimidine. CrystEngComm 2010; 12 3038; (d) Abul Haj M, Quirós M, Salas JM, Dobado JA, Molina J, Basallote MG, Máñez MA. Structurally different dinuclear copper(II) complexes with the same triazolopyrimidine bridging ligand. Eur. J. Inorg. Chem. 2002; 811-818.

[44] Caballero AB, Rodriguez-Dieguez A, Lezama L, Barea E, Salas JM. Structural and magnetic properties of three novel complexes with the versatile ligand 5-methyl-1, 2, 4-triazolo[1, 5-a]pyrimidin-7(4H)-one. Dalton Transactions 2011; 40(19), 5180-5187.

[45] Tiuman TS, Ueda-Nakamura T, Garcia Cortez DA, Dias Filho BP, Morgado-Díaz JA, de Souza W, Nakamura CV. Antileishmanial activity of parthenolide, a sesquiterpene lactone isolated from *Tanacetum parthenium*. Antimicrob. Agents Chemother. 2005; 49 176-182.

[46] Bringaud F, Riviere L, Coustou V. Energy metabolism of trypanosomatids: adaptation to available carbon sources. Mol BiochemParasitol 2006; 149 1–9.

Chapter 21

Novel Therapeutic Approaches to Leishmania Infection

Levi H.C. Makala and Babak Baban

Additional information is available at the end of the chapter

http://dx.doi.org/10.5772/58167

1. Introduction

1.1. Leishmaniasis

Leishmaniasis is a parasitic disease transmitted by phlebotomine sandflies. Approximately 1.2 million cases of cutaneous leishmaniasis (CL) and 500,000 cases of visceral leishmaniasis (VL), which is lethal if untreated, occur annually across the globe as per world health organization (WHO) estimates [1-3]. Current statistics and information relevant to leishmaniasis are summarized in Table 1. Leishmaniasis currently affects about 12 million people and it is estimated that approximately 350 million people live in risk of infection [1-3].The number of cases of leishmaniasis is probably underestimated because only 40 of the 88 countries where diseases frequently occur report them on a regular basis [4]. Leishmaniasis, is caused by several *leishmania* spp., that are obligate intracellular and unicellular kinetoplastid protozoan flagellate that establish themselves within the phagolysosome of host immune competent cells, especially macrophages and dendritic cells (DCs). In 1903, W.B. Leishman and C. Donovan reported this new parasite at the turn of the century [5,6]. Ronald Ross christened the new genus leishmania and the new species donovani in year 1903 [7]. *L. major* infection (leishmaniasis) in mice is a widely used model of human infection that has yielded critical insights into the immunobiology of leishmaniasis [8-10]. Leishmaniasis as a parasitic disease manifests itself mainly in 3 clinical forms; visceral leishmaniasis (VL), cutaneous leishmaniasis (CL) and mucocutaneous leishmaniasis (MCL), of which VL is the most severe form of the disease. VL is lethal if untreated and spontaneous cure is extremely rare. Cutaneous leishmaniasis usually has milder course and often results into a self-healing of ulcers. Resolution of leishmanial infection is dependent on the coordinated interactions between components of cell mediated immune response, specifically the activation of targeted T-cell populations for appropriate cytokine production and activation of macrophages. *L. major* infection of B6 and BALB/c mouse strains drives predominantly T_H1 and T_H2 responses, respectively [11-14]. In murine model, the development of Th1 response is associated with control of infection, and Th2 response is associated with disease progression. However, Th1 and Th2 dichotomy in the human system is not as distinct as in mice and the murine model does not strictly apply to human leishmaniasis.

Parameter	Statistic or Information
Geographical location	Worldwide tropical and subtropical regions
Population at risk in 2013	~350 million
Number of people affected	~12 million
Number of deaths in 2013	~20,000 – 30,000
Number of new cases in 2013	~1.3 million
Global disease burden in 2013 (DALYs)	~1.7 million
Multidrug-resistance in 2013	Resistance to antimonials only
Visceral Leishmaniasis (VL)	~200 000 to 400 000 new cases of VL occur worldwide each year. Over 90% of new cases occur in six countries: Bangladesh, Brazil, Ethiopia, India, South Sudan, and Sudan.
Cutaneous Leishmaniasis (CL)	~One-third of CL cases occur in the Americas, the Mediterranean basin, and the Middle East and Central Asia. An estimated 0.7 million to 1.3 million new cases occur worldwide annually
Mucocutaneous Leishmaniasis	Reported in Bolivia, Brazil and Peru.
Major risk factors	Socioeconomic conditions, Malnutrition, Population mobility, Environmental changes, Climate change
Prevention and control	Early diagnosis and effective case management, Vector control, Effective disease surveillance, Control of reservoir hosts, Social mobilization and strengthening partnerships

Abbreviations: CL, cutaneous leishmaniasis; DALYs, disability-adjusted life years; NK, not known; VL, visceral leishmaniasis, WHO, World Health Organization.

Table 1. Factfile: WHO leishmaniasis statistics for 2013 (Adapted from http://www.who.int/mediacentre/factsheets/fs375/en/)

2. Conventional treatment strategies and limitations

Chemotherapy is the primary method used to control leishmaniasis. Despite the existence of several drugs for chemotherapy of human leishmaniasis, many of them are new formulations of ancient drugs repurposed in the last decade [15,16]. The treatment options for leishmaniasis are limited and include penta-valent antimonials, pentamidine, amphotericin B (AmB) and its lipoidal formulations and miltefosine, which have been introduced recently in the group of antileishmanial drugs (Table 2). Among all of these drugs, pentavalent antimonials are the first choice drugs in most of the developing countries as in these countries treatment strategy is governed by economic factors. But a large number of incidences of resistance have been observed for antimonials, particularly in India where the failure rate has been reported up to 65% [17,18]. AmB is very effective against leishmania parasite but frequent and severe adverse effects associated with it limit its application.

Drugs	Admin Route	Dosage	Known Toxicities	Mechanism of Action	Resistance	Comment	References
Antimonial drugs (sodium stibogluconate and meglumine antimoniate (Pentostam)	IM, IV	28 mg/kg/day (28-30 days)	Cardioto-xicity, nephroto-xicity, hepatotoxicity, pancreati-tis (frequent and severe)	Activated within the amastigote, but not in the promastigote, by conversion to a lethal trivalent form. Activation. Mechanism not known. Antileishmanial activity might be due to action on host macrophage.	Failure rates up to 65% (in India)	First line drugs but high incidences of resistance has been emerged	[16,19-22]
Amphotericin B (AmB) or Polyene antibiotic	IV	0.75-1 mg/kg/day (15-20 days, daily or alternately)	Severe nephrotoxicity, infusion-related reactions (frequent and severe)	Complexes with 24-substituted sterols, such as ergosterol in cell membrane, thus causing pores which alter ion balance and result in cell death	-	Severe toxicity	[16,22,23]
Lipoidal formulations of AmB (Amphotec or Amphocil; AmBisome; Abelcet and dimyristoyl phosphatidyl glycerol with AMB)	IV	10-30 mg/kg total dose (single dose 3-5 mg/kg/ dose)	Mild nephrotoxicity (infrequent and mild)	Am**B** formulation, act by binding to the sterol component cell membranes, leading to alterations in cell permeability and cell death. They bind to the	-	High market price	[16,22,24,25]

Drugs	Admin Route	Dosage	Known Toxicities	Mechanism of Action	Resistance	Comment	References
				cholesterol component of the mammalian cell.			
Miltefosine (Hexadecylphosphocholine)	Oral	100 mg/day (28 days)	GIT problems, nephrotoxicity, hepatotoxicity, chances of teratogenicity (frequent, mild and transient)	Primary effect uncertain, possible inhibition of ether remodelling, phosphatidylcholine biosynthesis, signal transduction and calcium Homeostasis.	Common in laboratory isolates	Effective orally but its long half-life may encourage emergence of resistance on prolonged use	[16,22,26,27]
Paromomycin (Monomycin or Aminosidine	IM	15 mg/day (21 days)	Nephrotoxicit-ototoxicity and hepatotoxicity (infrequent)	In bacteria, paromomycin inhibits protein synthesis by binding to 30S subunit ribosomes, causing misreading and premature termination of mRNA translation. In Leishmania, paromomycin also affects mitochondrion.	Common in laboratory isolates	Low cost; being investigated by non-profit groups	[16,22,26]

Adapted with modifications from Jain and Jain, 2013 and van Griensven, J. and Diro, E. 2012)

Abbreviations: AmB, Amphotericin B; IM, Intramascular; IV, Intravenous;

Table 2. Standard treatment protocols for leishmaniasis, characteristics and mechanisms of action

The development of lipoidal formulations of AmB reduced the severity and frequency of adverse effects but resulted in high cost of formulation [22-25]. The conventional treatment schedule for visceral leishmaniasis suffers from a lot of problems like invasive route of administration (parenteral), long treatment course, severe toxicity (nephrotoxicity, cardiotoxicity, among others), high cost of treatment, few treatment regimens, emergence of resistance and variable patient response [17,28,29]. Thus there is continuous need for alternative new treatment strategies, vaccine candidates and new chemotherapeutic agents to provide complete cure from leishmaniasis taking into account the fatality of disease, high toxicity, high cost and inefficiency of current treatment protocols.

2.1. Nano-based antileishmanial agents

Currently, the pharmaceutical industry has undergone a profound transformation with the advent of nano-science. With a rapid growth of nanotechnology, different nanoparticles have been presented for medical science applications. Nanomaterials have unique chemical and physical properties, and may be used in the treatment of different severe or chronic diseases in the future [30]. Hitherto, it has been shown that some metal and metal oxide nanoparticles have antimicrobial activities [31]. It has long been demonstrated that silver ions, silver nanoparticles (Ag NPs), and nanosilver-containing complexes have antimicrobial behavior with high ability to inactivate bacteria and viruses [32]. Other reports indicate that gold nanoparticles (Au NPs), titanium dioxide nanoparticles (TiO2 NPs), zinc oxide nanoparticles (ZnO NPs), magnesium oxide nanoparticles (MgO NPs), etc. have antibacterial properties [33-37]. Nanotechnology has enabled the creation of nano-particle formulations such as liposomes, microemulsions and microcapsules [34]. Liposomes are microscopic vesicles composed of one or more concentric lipid bilayers separated by aqueous media. They can encapsulate hydrophilic and lipophilic substances in the aqueous compartment of the membrane respectively. Since liposomes are biodegradable, biocompatible and non-immunogenic, they are highly versatile for research, therapeutic and analytical applications [38]. In spite of the reported antileishmanial properties of nanoparticles under UV, IR, and dark conditions, these nanoparticles have the some cytotoxicity on immune competent cells such as macrophages and other antigen presenting cells and this must be considered in future applications and studies.

2.2. Leishmaniasis vaccines

Despite the knowledge about various life stages of the parasite and the ongoing work, designing an effective vaccine against leishmaniasis is still a matter of research, there are hundreds of potent vaccine candidates but issues regarding the cost, antigenic complexity along with the variability of organisms and the mixed type of responses produced in the host are limiting the progress in the relevant direction. Thus the technical challenges and the complexity in the immunity against the parasites clearly contribute to the absence of vaccines. There are three vaccines known: two in Brazil and one in Europe out of which one is highly efficient in treating VL and CL, thus still enlightening the ray of hope for progress in this field [39]. A glimpse of various antigens that has been used as vaccine candidates in last two decades are summarized in (Figure 1).

These candidates include major surface, intracellular, stress responsive molecules, as well as other biomolecules of various metabolic pathways that can be the targets for vaccine development. Vaccine design and development has focused on all the forms of leishmania because of the conserved nature of molecules in all the species of leishmania that have been selected as the targets. Many of these targets have been studied in mice models while others in humans during diseased state producing promising results (Table 3). The availability of complete

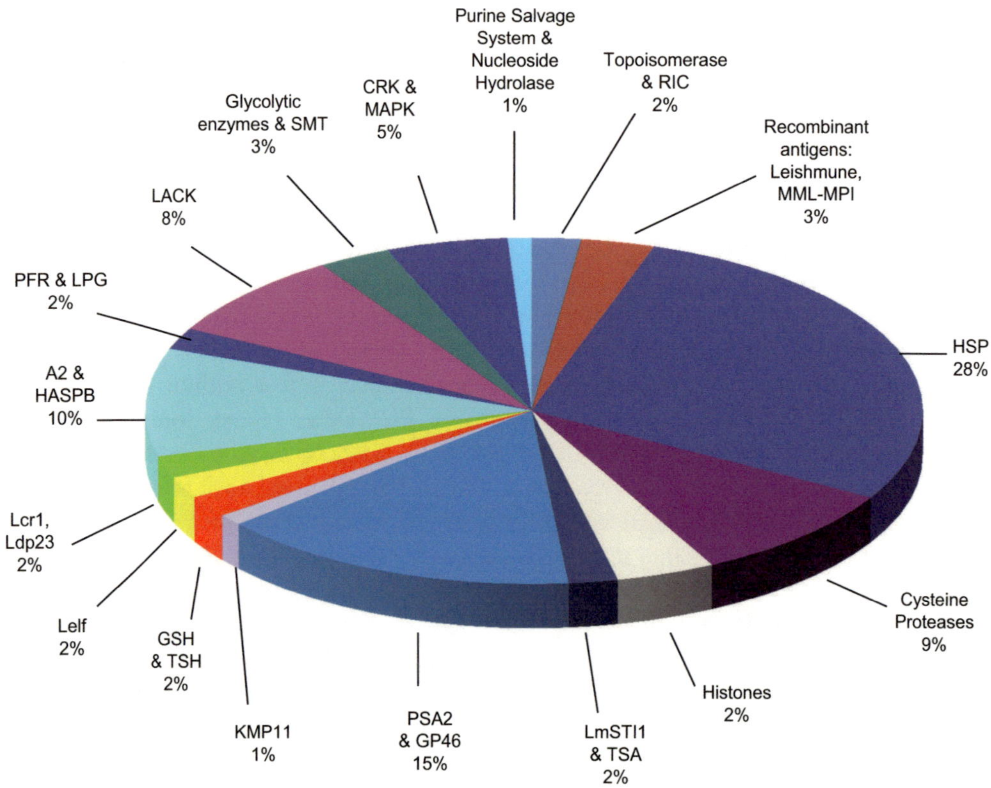

Figure 1. A glimpse of various antigens that have been used as vaccine candidates in past ten years (Adapted and modified with permission from Singh, and Sundar, 2012).

genome sequence of leishmania has provided hope for researchers to work with novel molecules as vaccine candidates [40]. The history of vaccination with the virulent forms of leishmania termed as "leishmanization" dates back to early 20th century but has since been banned for trials due safety concerns in human models [41]. First generation vaccines were limited in terms of the conferred immunity [42]. Second generation vaccines are currently in trial and are useful in providing protection of varying levels in different species along with the DNA and other subunit vaccines. The main hurdle in developing a potent vaccine stems from lack of multiple experimental study models necessary to provide all facets of immune responses in humans as well as safety issues [43].

2.3. Potential drug targets

Notwithstanding the significant progress of leishmanial research in the last few decades, identification and characterization of novel drugs and drug targets are far from satisfactory. The digenetic life cycle of leishmania consists of motile flagellated, extracellular promastigote forms which survive and multiply within the phagolysosomal compartments of macrophages and other antigen presenting cells. Therefore, the search for new

Antigenic Molecule	Vaccine type	Experimental model	References
LPG, gp 63, A2	Native antigen	Mouse	[44-47]
gp 63	Protein expressed in BCG	Mouse	[48]
gp63, gp 46, PSA-2, A2, KMP11	DNA Vaccine	Mouse	[49-53]
p36, LACK	DNA vaccine + protein expressed in vaccinia virus	Mouse	[54]
p36, LACK	Recombinant protein + IL12	Mouse	[55,56]
LmSTI1, TSA, HASPB1, CPB	Recombinant protein	Mouse	[57-59]
gp 63, KMP11	DC pulsed with native antigen	Mouse and Monkey	[60]
gp 63, LCR 1	Protein expressed in BCG	Mouse	[61,62]
Leish 111f	Recombinant polyprotein of TSA, LmSTI1 and LeIF + MPL-SE	Mouse	[63,64]
IDO 1	IDO Inhibitors / IDO specific vaccines	Mouse and Human	[65-68]

DC – dendritic cells CP – cysteine proteinase; BCG Mycobacterium bovis bacillus Calmette–Guerin; IDO, Indoleamine pyrrole 2,3-dioxygenase, IL, interleukin; MPL-SE, monophosphoryl lipid A soluble emulsion; TSA, thiol-specific-antioxidant antigen.

Table 3. Current Potent/effective vaccines against leishmaniasis

potential drug targets mainly focuses on biochemical and metabolic pathways essential for parasite survival [69-71]. The strategy to target more than one enzyme of a metabolic pathway simultaneously may prove more useful and effective. Important biochemical and enzymatic machineries that are utilized as putative drug targets for generations of true antileishmanial drugs are as follows: enzymes of polyamine synthesis [72,73], enzymes of the glycosomal machinery [74,75], enzymes of thiol-metabolic cyclin dependent kinases, enzymes of sterol biosynthesis [76,77], Pepsidases, Mitogen activated protein kinases (MAPK), dihydrofolate reductases (DHFR) [78], topoisomerases metacaspases [79,80]; and leishmanial antigens that modulate host immune functions [81].

Polyamines are not only involved in parasite growth and differentiation, but also down regulate lipid peroxidation generated by oxidant compounds to make the environment compatible for survival [82-84]. The leishmania genome has 154 peptidases namely serine, cysteine, aspartic, threonine and metallopeptidases. These enzymes play a role in reducing viability and induction of morphological changes [85,86]. Roles of other enzyme systems include but limited to roles in metabolic activities like glycolysis, oxidation of fatty acids, lipid biosynthesis and purine salvage pathways [87-103]. Other Functions of the above mentioned biochemical and metabolic pathways include: Cell division cycle, transcription, apoptosis, cell proliferation, cell differentiation and innate immunity to activation of adaptive immunity [104-113]. All these functions are essential for parasite survival, hence can be targeted to disrupt the unique targeting signal sequences.

3. Phytotherapy

Phytotherapy is the study of the use of extracts from natural origin as medicines or health-promoting agents. The main difference of phytotherapy medicines from the medicines containing the herbal elements is in the methods of plant processing. Methods of plant processing to receive medicines containing herbal elements are aimed on extraction of the chemical clean active substances, but methods of plants processing to obtain phytotherapy medicines are aimed to preserve all complex of active substances of plant in the most simple and close to the natural form. The biological activity of plant extracts has been attributed to compounds belonging to diverse chemical groups including alkaloids, flavonoids, phenylpropanoids, steroids, and terpenoids. [114-116]. Phytotherapy can be an important tool in the search for novel antileishmanial agents with fewer side effects and low cost. Firstly, the chemical diversity of plants makes them a valuable source of metabolites with pharmacological relevance [117]. Secondly, metabolites isolated from plants extracts or essential oils can be used in several different ways in the development of drugs. To obtain a herbal medicine or an isolated active compound, different research strategies can be employed, among them, investigation of the traditional use, the chemical composition, the toxicity of the plants, or the combination of several criteria [118]. In the extraction processes, different plant parts and different solvents have generally been used. In screening for biological activity, there is clearly substantial room for improvement in the extraction methodologies, since a variety of techniques can be used to prepare extracts [119-121]. Usually, solvents of different polarity are employed for the extractions. For purification and isolation, the active extracts of the plant are sequentially fractionated, and each fraction and/or pure compound can be evaluated for biological activity and toxicity. This strategy is called bioactivity-guided fractionation, which allows tests that are simple, reproducible, rapid, and low-cost [120,121]. In the last two decade, much attention has been given to the search of novel drug delivery systems for herbal drugs. The development of nanoparticles loaded with herbal drugs presents several advantages including: increase of drug solubility and bioavailability, protection against the toxicity, enhancement of pharmacological activity, increase of stability, and protection against degradation [122]. The tendency of nanoparticules, especially liposomes, to be captured by the mononuclear phagocyte system may be an additional advantage in the treatment of a variety of intracellular infectious diseases. Intraperitoneal and intravenous administration of liposomes proved to be a good bio-distribution system for drugs in the treatment of visceral leishmaniasis, since it allows increasing of drug accumulation in macrophage-rich tissues such as liver and spleen thus reducing the level of toxicity to other tissues and organs [123].

In vitro screenings are only the first steps to prove the efficacy and safety of medicinal plants for application in the treatment of leishmaniasis. In addition, variation in the efficacy of drugs in treating leishmaniasis may often result from differences in the drug sensitivity of leishmania species, the immune status of the patient, or the pharmacokinetic properties of the drug [4]. A review of the literature on the use of natural products, including plant crude extracts, fractions, isolated compounds, and essential oils, shows that there is a massive effort by scientists around the world to identify and characterize natural plant compounds with antileishmanial activity [124-126]. These efforts are now bearing fruit,

http://dx.doi.org/10.5772/58167

obtaining good results and validating natural products as genuine sources for drug discovery. A fitting example would be essential oils that are known to possess a wide variety of hydrophobic compounds with antimicrobial potential. The ability to diffuse across cell membranes certainly gives to those molecules some advantage in targeting cellular components, being a valuable research option for the search of bioactive compounds [124-126]. The *Ocimum gratissimum* essential oil and eugenol, its major component, was tested on the growth, viability, and ultrastructural alterations of the amastigote and promastigote forms of *L. amazonensis*, as well as on the interaction of these flagellates with mouse peritoneal macrophages, concomitant with nitric oxide production stimulation by the infected macrophages. Significant mitochondrial alterations occurred at the ultrastructural level of the parasite, such as remarkable swelling, disorganization of the inner membrane, and an increase in the number of cristae after treatment of parasites with *O. gratissimum* essential oil [125, 126]. Additionally, the linalool-rich essential oil extracted from the leaves of *Crotoncajucara*, also has effects on *L. amazonensis* parasites, on the interaction of these flagellates with mouse peritoneal macrophages and on nitric oxide production by the infected macrophages [125].

3.1. Alternative synthetic compounds

Screenings of synthetic compounds and their derivatives for antileishmanial activity has been carried out. In the last 10 years several compounds have been tested to identify potential new drugs, with the desirable characteristics. Most of the compounds exhibited antileishmanial activity against the promastigote form of L. major at non-cytotoxic concentrations and these compounds are also effective against intracellular L. major, and significantly decrease the infectivity index [127,128].

The stilbene trans-3,4 0,5-trimethoxy-3 0 -amino-stilbene (TTAS) has potent effect with low toxicity on *Leishmania infantum* (LD 50 value of 2.6 g/mL). The mechanism of action involves the disruption of the mitochondrial membrane potential and the ability to block leishmania parasites in the G2–M phase of the cell cycle [129,130]. N -Butyl-1-(4-dimethylamino) phenyl-1,2,3,4- tetrahydro- β -carboline-3-carboxamide is effective against *Leishmania amazonensis*.

BTB 06237 (2-[(2,4-dichloro-5-methylphenyl)sulfanyl]-1,3-dinitro-5-(trifluoromethyl) benzene) and its analogues, a compound previously identified through quantitative structure-activity relationship (QSAR) has also been shown, to possesses potent and selective activity against leishmania parasites. This compound and its analogues has the ability to reduce parasitemia levels in immune competent cells especially peritoneal macrophages, and additionally possess the ability to generate reactive oxygen species (ROS) in L. donovani promastigotes [131]. The in vitro antileishmanial activity of 44 derivatives of 1,3,4-thiadiazole and related compounds against promastigote forms of L. donovani have also been tested. Micromolar concentrations of these agents were used to study the inhibition of multiplication of promastigotes. Seven compounds were identified as potential anti-growth agents against the parasite [132]. Additionally, a series of 2,4,6-trisubstituted pyrimidines and 1,3,5-triazines following synthesis and screening display antileishmanial activity against L. donovani. Nitroimidazolyl-1,3,4-thiadiazole-based antileishmanial agents against L. major also exhibits antileishmanial activity against the promastigote form of L. major at non-cytotoxic concentrations [128]. Other compounds with antileishmanial activity, both in vitro and in vivo include a series of 1- phenylsubstituted b-carbolines containing an N-butylcarboxamide group at C-3 of the b-carboline nucleus, tetrahydrobenzothieno-pyrimidines, R(+)-limonene derivatives, quinoline tripartite hybrids from chloroquine, ethambutol, and isoxyl drugs, and (4-butoxyphenyl)-N0-{2-[(7-chloroquinolin-4-yl)amino]ethyl}urea [133,136]. The urgent need to develop cost-effective new drugs and to discover novel molecules with potent antiparasitic activity and improved pharmacological characteristics cannot be overemphasized. Although many advances have been made in the treatment of leishmaniasis, much still remains to be understood.

3.2. A potential role of indoleamine 2,3-dioxygenase-specific T cells in leishmania vaccination

IDO is an immunoregulatory enzyme implicated in immunity under normal and pathological settings [137,138], and provides a potential mechanism for the development of dendritic cell (DC)–mediated T-cell tolerance [139]. IDO1 DCs inhibit T-cell proliferation due to tryptophan depletion and accumulation of toxic tryptophan metabolites [138]. 1-Methyl-D-tryptophan is an inhibitor of the enzymes IDO and INDOL1 (indolamine 2,3-dioxygenase 1 and 2) with selectivity for INDOL1 [140-142]. The enzymes perform similar transformations and are responsible for catalyzing the rate-limiting step of oxidative tryptophan catabolism in the kynurenine pathway. IDO activity is correlated with an induction of tolerance and immune-suppression through activation of regulatory T cells by metabolites generated from tryptophan catabolism. Inhibition of IDO by 1-Methyl-D-tryptophan blocks this induced immune suppression, which has shown utility in suppressing acquired immunities of tumors and indicates potential for chemical intervention of chronic inflammatory diseases [143-145]. In a recent report, Makala and colleagues [65, 66] elegantly showed that IDO is implicated in suppressing T-cell immunity to parasite antigens, and IDO inhibition reduced local inflammation and parasite burdens. The findings by Makala and colleagues support a counter-regulatory role for IDO that benefits the pathogen, not the host. In this regard, an interesting aspect of IDO is that systemic inactivation at the organism level, either pharmacologically or genetically, does not appear to cause autoimmunity [65-68,138]. A conceptual model of IDO-mediated activation and effector T cell suppression following *L. major* infection is summarized in Figure 2 [Makala, 2012].

The model depicts interactions between IDO+ DCs, Tregs and naïve T cells that drive suppressive and non-suppressive outcomes under IDO-sufficient (+) and IDO-deficient (-) conditions in response to *L. major* infection. Induced IDO activity in DCs triggers cell stress responses blocks IL6 production by pDCs themselves, and by other cells (e.g. macrophages) capable of producing IL6. Under conditions of IDO ablation the same stimuli do not create suppression, and instead DCs stimulate naïve T cells, and express IL6, which converts Tregs to TH17 T cells or promotes TH17 differentiation from naïve CD4+ T cells. The chemical structures of IDO and its inhibitors are shown in Figure 3.

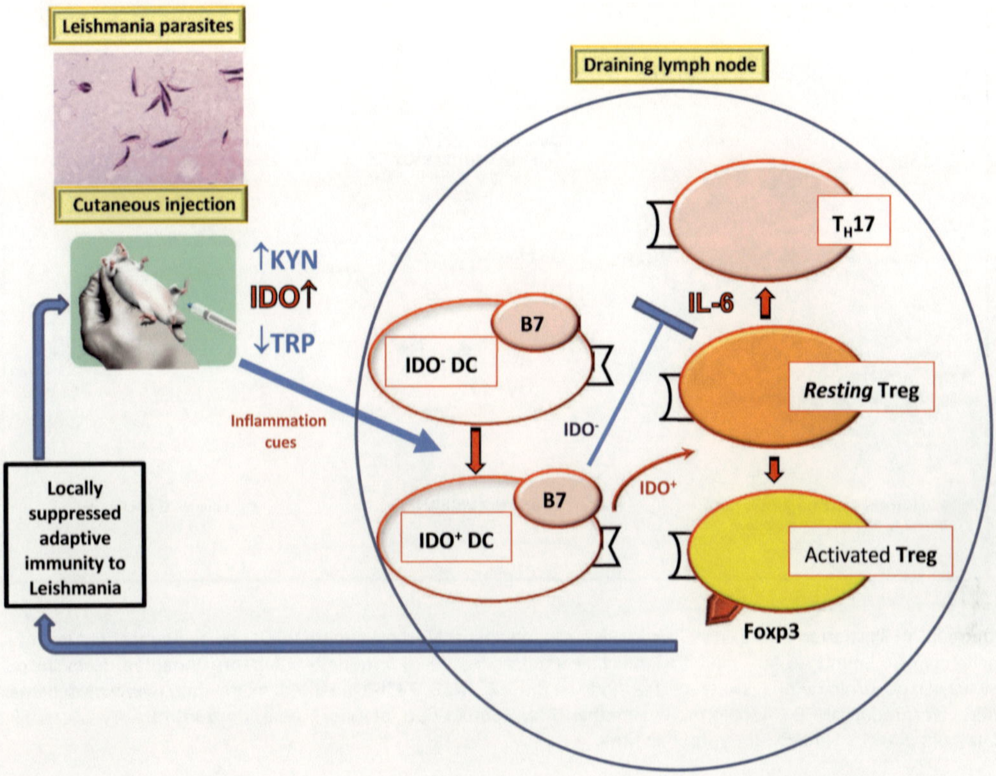

Figure 2. A conceptual model of IDO-mediated activation and effector T cell suppression following *L. major* infection. The model depicts interactions between IDO+ DCs, Tregs and naïve T cells that drive suppressive and non-suppressive outcomes under IDO-sufficient (+) and IDO-deficient (-) conditions in response to *L. major* infection. Induced IDO activity in DCs triggers cell stress responses blocks IL6 production by pDCs themselves, and by other cells (e.g. macrophages) capable of producing IL6. Under conditions of IDO ablation the same stimuli do not create suppression, and instead DCs stimulate naïve T cells, and express IL6, which converts Tregs to TH17 T cells or promotes TH17 differentiation from naïve CD4+ T cells (Adapted and modified from Makala, 2012).

To examine the possible effects (and/or side effects) of the induction of IDO-specific T cells, a phase I vaccination study is ongoing at the Center for Cancer Immune Therapy, Copenhagen University Hospital, in which patients with non-small-cell lung cancer are vaccinated with an IDO-derived peptide with Montanide adjuvant (www.clinicaltrials.gov; NCT01219348). Different species of leishmania are responsible for cutaneous, mucocutaneous, or visceral leishmaniasis infections in millions of people and animals. Adverse reactions caused by antileishmanial drugs, emergence of resistance, and lack of a vaccine have motivated the search for new therapeutic options to control this disease. There have been notable advances in molecular diagnostics, in the understanding of host immune responses to infection, and in vaccine development. The fact that IDO may be involved in tolerance to non-self-antigens, may have key attractive implications for IDO-based immune therapy as boosting immunity to neo-antigens, but not normal self-antigens, by the activation of IDO-specific T cells. Makala and colleagues [65-68, 138] demonstrated that IDO suppresses adaptive immunity, supporting

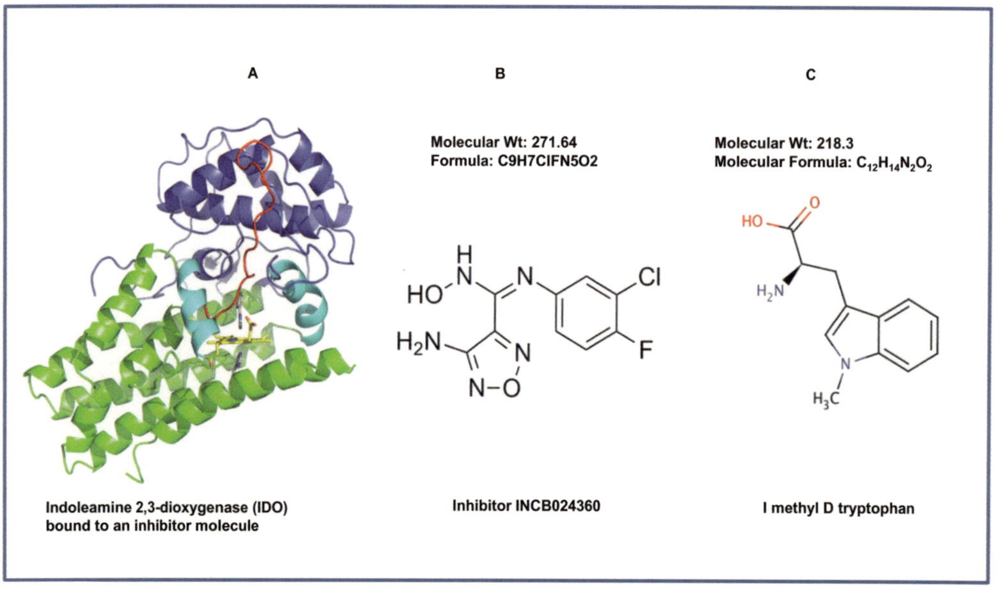

Figure 3. An illustration of the crystal structure for Indoleamine 2,3-dioxygenase (IDO) and chemical structures of its Inhibitors. A. bound to an inhibitor molecule.Indoleamine-2,3-dioxygenase inhibitors. Adapted from http://www.riken.go.jp/biometal/7_structures.files/index-e.htm. B. INCB024360 adapted from http://www.medchemexpress.com/product/INCB024360.html. C. I methyl D tryptophan (Ido inhibitor). Adapted from http://www.scbt.kr/datasheet-200313-1-methyl-d-tryptophan.html.

the notion that in clinical setting, the targeting of IDO could have synergistic effects in leishmania vaccine development. Thus, the induction of IDO-specific immune responses by therapeutic measures could function synergistically with additional immune therapy. Almost any successful immune therapy strategy aims at inducing immunological activation and inflammation. Since IDO-expressing cells might antagonize the desired effects of other immunotherapeutic approaches, targeting IDO-expressing cells by vaccination would be easily implementable and compatible with such therapeutic measures.

3.3. Multidrug treatment strategy

Combination therapy has increasingly been explored, particularly in highly endemic regions, aiming to identify a short, cheap, well-tolerated combination regimen that can preferably be given in an ambulatory way and requiring minimal clinical monitoring. To date combination therapy has shown promising results including improved treatment efficacy with reduced side effects, shorter duration of therapy, reduced cost as well as reduced incidence of resistance in phase 2 clinical trial, as has been used for diseases like malaria, tuberculosis, and HIV. [1,3,146]. A 17-day combination of antimonials with paromomycin was found effective in east Africa (93% efficacy). Owing to such fascinating results numerous phase 3 clinical trials are progressively being conducted in Asian and African continents to further investigate the clinical efficacy of combination therapy in treatment of leishmaniasis. Researchers have continued to study the effect of immunotherapy using combinations of two or more antileishmanial drugs

[146-149]. A list of completed or currently in progress clinical trials for treatment of leishmaniasis are shown in (Table 4). Sundar et al. [150] investigated the efficacy and safety of three combinations of three effective antileishmanial drugs (lipo-somal AmB, miltefosine, paromomycin) and compared their efficacy as duration of treatment with the standard monotherapy in India, that is, AmB infusion in an open-label, parallel-group, non-inferiority, randomized control trial conducted in two hospitals at Bihar, India. Combination regimens including liposomal amphotericin B (5 mg/kg single dose), paromomycin and/or miltefosine were also found highly effective (98%–99%) and safe, and are now included in WHO recommendations for the Indian subcontinent [3,146,147]. The multidrug treatment has been found equally effective as standard monotherapy even with fewer side effects and shorter course of administration [150]. Combination treatment approaches for leishmaniasis have been advocated by many scientists but they are also enforcing the simultaneous development of other measures in the control of this parasitic disease in the endemic regions of Asia and Africa including control of sandflies, clinical monitoring of treatment, advances in case detection and rapid methods of diagnosis as well as proper evaluation of various leishmania control programs [146,151,152]. The clinical efficacy of multidrug therapy has been confirmed and so far the results are convincing and give hope for the future in terms of treatment.

Condition	Intervention	Study Phase	Study Objective
ML MCL	• Meglumine antimoniate (MA)	2 3	To compare efficacy of the standard recommended schedule with an alternative regimen of MA in the treatment of ML /MCL
CL	• Paramomycin • WR279, 396 (Paramomycin / Gentamycin)	3	To determine if WR279, 396 results in statistically superior final clinical cure rates compared to Paramomycin alone
VL	• Antimoniate of N-Methylglucamine (Fungizone) • Amphotericin B Deoxycholade (Anforicin) • Liposomal Amphotericin B (Ambisome)	4	To compare efficacy and safety of medications in Brazil
L	• Sodium Stibogluconate (SSG) (Pentosam)	2	To collect safety and efficacy data on the use of Pentosam
VL	• AmBisome + Miltefosine • AmBisome + Paromomycin sulfate • Miltefosine + Paromomycin sulfate • Amphotericin B Deoxycholate	3	To identify a safe and effective combination for short course treatment of visceral leishmaniasis with reduced risk of parasite resistance

Condition	Intervention	Study Phase	Study Objective
VL	• Sodium stibogluconate • Paromomycin sulfate • Sodium stibogluconate + Paromomycin sulfate	3	To assess the efficacy and safety of sodium stibogluconate 30 days alone, paromomycin sulfate 21 days alone and sodium stibogluconate and paromomycin sulfate as a combination course of 17 days in the treatment of patients with visceral leishmaniasis
VL	• Ambisome • AmBisome + Miltefosine • AmBisome + Paromomycin • Miltefosine + Paromomycin	3	To evaluate efficacy and safety of various combinations of the three drugs; AmBisome, paromomycin and miltefosine at reduced total dosage against the standard treatment with a total dose of 15 mg/kg of AmBisome
VL	• AmBisome + Sodium stibogluconate • AmBisome + Miltefosine • Miltefosine	2	To assess combinations of sodium stibogluconate plus single dose AmBisomeW, miltefosine plus single dose AmBisomeW and miltefosine alone in treatment of visceral leishmaniasis in Eastern Africa
VL	• Miltefosine + AmBisome	2	To sequential design to combine miltefosine and AmBisome in different doses
VL	• AmBisome + Miltefosine	2	To evaluate the final cure after six months on sequential administration of both drugs. AmBisome will be given on day 1, followed by miltefosine for 14 days
VL	• Sitamaquine	2	To evaluate the final cure after six months on sequential administration of both drugs. AmBisome will be given on day 1, followed by miltefosine for 14 days

Mucosal Leishmaniasis (LM), Mucocutaneous Leishmaniasis (MCL), Cutaneous Leishmaniasis (CL), Visceral Leishmaniasis (VL), Meglumine antimoniate (MA), Leishmaniasis (L).

Table 4. Clinical trial completed or currently recruiting for treatment of leishmaniasis (at: http://clinicaltrials.gov/ (accessed 10-10-2013))

4. Concluding remarks

Leishmaniasis is one of the major neglected infectious diseases. Progress has been achieved in terms of treatment, including the development of combination therapy as well as our understanding of the molecular nature of potential vaccine candidates following the completion of the genome sequence. The occurrence of drug resistance in disease-endemic countries is concerning and should be closely monitored. In spite of all these drawbacks, there is presently rapid progress in our understanding of the molecular nature of potential vaccine candidates. There is a need to develop more potent, cost effective drugs and vaccine candidates. Total eradication of leishmaniasis will depend on the combined efforts of governments, the scientific research community, the pharmaceutical industry and people with a view to reduce the

http://dx.doi.org/10.5772/58167

transmission of disease, rapid diagnosis and appropriately targeted treatment of the various forms of leishmanisis. Understanding of the molecular nature of potential vaccine candidates could potentially lead to novel gene-based, plant-based and synthetic-based therapeutic approaches or a dependable cure for leishmaniasis.

Abbreviations

LM: Mucosal leishmaniasis

MCL: Mucocutaneous leishmaniasis

CL: Cutaneous leishmaniasis,

VL: Visceral leishmaniasis

MA: Meglumine antimoniate

AmB: Amphotericin B

IM: Intramascular

IV: Intravenous

DC: dendritic cells

CP: cysteine proteinase

BCG: Mycobacterium bovis bacillus Calmette–Guerin

IDO: Indoleamine-pyrrole 2,3-dioxygenase

IL: Interleukin

MPL-SE: monophosphoryl lipid A soluble emulsion

TSA: thiol-specific-antioxidant antigen

pDC: Plasmacytoid Dendritic Cell

HSP: Heat Shock Proteins

LmSTI1: L. major stress-inducible 1

LeIF: Leishmania elongation initiation factor

KMP-11: Kinetoplastid membrane protein-11

GSH: Glutathione complex

TSH: thyroid - stimulating hormone

LACK: Leishmania analogue of the receptor kinase C

Lcr1: T-cell antigens from an amastigote of L. chagasi containing homologous 67-amino-acid repeats

Ldp23: 23 kDa highly hydrophilic protein rich in lysine residues present on the surface of L. donovani and L. major

LPG: Leishmania major lipophosphoglycan

T(SH)2: trypanothione;

CRK: cdc-2 related kinase

RIC: RNA import complex

A2: amastigote stage-specific protein family in L. donovani

HASPB: hydrophilic acylated surface protein B

PFR-2paraflagellar rod protein

MAPK: Mitogen-activated Protein (MAP) kinases

SMT: sterol 24-cmethyltransferase

GPI/GP46: glycosylphosphatidylinositol

PSA: Promastigote surface antigen

MML: multi-subunit recombinant leishmanial vaccine

Author details

Levi H.C. Makala[1*] and Babak Baban[2]

*Address all correspondence to: lmakala@gru.edu

1 Georgia Regents University, Medical College of Georgia, Department of Pediatrics, Hematology/Oncology Section, Georgia, USA

2 Georgia Regents University, Medical College of Georgia, Department of Oral Biology, College of Dental Medicine, Georgia, USA

References

[1] World Health Organization. First WHO report on neglected tropical diseases. 2012. WHO. 1-172. Available at: http://whqlibdoc.who.int/publications/2010/9789241564090_eng.pdf.

[2] Aguilar-Be I Zardo RS, Souza EP, Borja-Cabrera GP, Rosado-Vallado M, Mut-Martin M, García-Miss MR, Sousa CBP, Dumonteil E. Cross-Protective Efficacy of a Prophylactic *Leishmania donovani* DNA Vaccine against Visceral and Cutaneous Murine Leishmaniasis. Infection and Immunity. 2005;73(2) 812–819.

[3] World Health Organization. Control of the leishmaniasis. Report of a meeting of the WHO Expert Committee on the Control of Leishmaniases. Geneva (Switzerland): World Health Organization; 2010. Available at: http://whqlibdoc.who.int/trs/WHO_TRS_949_eng.pdf. (Accessed October 10, 2013).

[4] Croft SL, Sundar S, Fairlamb AH. Drug resistance in leishmaniasis. Clinical Microbiology Review 2006;19(1) 111–126.

[5] Leishman W.B: "On the possibility of the occurrence of trypanomiasis in India". *The British Medical Journal* 1903

[6] Donovan C: "Memoranda: On the possibility of the occurence of trypanomiasis in India.".The British Medical Journal 1903.

[7] Ross R: "Further notes on Leishman's bodies". Ibid 1903;(ii) 1401.

[8] Peters N, Sacks D. Immune privilege in sites of chronic infection: Leishmania and regulatory T cells. Immunological Reviews 2006;213 159–179.

[9] Liese J, Schleicher U, Bogdan C: The innate immune response against Leishmania parasites. Immunobiology 2008;213 377–387.

[10] Sharma U, Singh S: Immunobiology of leishmaniasis. Indian Journal of Experimental Biology 2009;47 412– 423. 161.

[11] Moll H, Röllinghoff M. Resistance to murine cutaneous leishmaniasis is mediated by TH1 cells, but disease-promoting CD4+ cells are different from TH2 cells. *European Journal of Immunol*ogy 1990;20(9) 2067-2074.

[12] Lohoff M, Sommer F, Solbach W, Röllinghoff M. Coexistence of antigen-specific TH1 and TH2 cells in genetically susceptible BALB/c mice infected with Leishmania major. *Immunobiology*. 1989;179(4-5) 412-421.

[13] Locksley RM, Heinzel FP, Holaday BJ, Mutha SS, Reiner SL, Sadick MD. Induction of Th1 and Th2 CD4+ subsets during murine Leishmania major infection. *Research in Immunol*ogy 1991;142(1) 28-32.

[14] Scott P. IFN-gamma modulates the early development of Th1 and Th2 responses in a murine model of cutaneous leishmaniasis. *Journal of Immunol*ogy 1991;147(9) 3149-3155.

[15] Croft SL, Yardley V. Chemotherapy of leishmaniasis. Current Pharmaceutical Design 2002;8 319-342.

[16] Jain K, Jain NK. Novel therapeutic strategies for treatment of visceral leishmaniasis. Drug Discovery Today 2013 [Epub ahead of print].

[17] Sane, S.A. Shakya N, Gupta S. Immunomodulatory effect of picroliv on the efficacy of paromomycin and miltefosine in combination in experimental visceral leishmaniasis. Experimental Parasitology 2011;127(2) 376–381.

[18] Ait-Oudhia K. Gazanion E, Oury B, Vergnes B, Sereno D. The fitness of antimony-resistant Leishmania parasites: lessons from the field. Trends in Parasitology 2011;27 141–142.

[19] Roberts WL, McMurray WJ, Rainey PM. Characterization of the antimonial antileishmanial agent meglumine antimonate (glucantime). Antimicrobiol Agents of Chemotherapy 1998;42(5) 1076-1082.

[20] Zilberstein,D. and Ephros, M. (2002) Clinical and laboratory aspects of Leishmania chemotherapy in the area of drug resistance. In World Class Parasites (Vol. 4) (Black, S.J. and Seed, J.R., eds), pp. 115–136, Kluwer Academic Press, London.

[21] Pathak, M.K. and Yi, T. (2001) Sodium stibogluconate is a potent inhibitor of protein tyrosine phosphatases and augments cytokine responses in hemopoietic cell lines. J. Immunol. 167, 3391–3397.

[22] Croft SL, Coombs GH. Leishmaniasis--current chemotherapy and recent advances in the search for novel drugs. Trends in Parasitology 2003;19(11) 502-508.

[23] Roberts CW, McLeod R, Rice DW, Ginger M, Chance ML, Goad LJ. Fatty acid and sterol metabolism: potential antimicrobial targets in apicomplexan and trypanosomatid parasitic protozoa. Molecular Biochemical Parasitology 2003;126(2) 129-142.

[24] Clemons KV, and Stevens DA Comparative efficacies of four amphotericin B formulations--Fungizone, amphotec (Amphocil), AmBisome, and Abelcet--against systemic murine aspergillosis. Clemons KV, Stevens DA. Antimicrobiol Agents of Chemotherapy 2004;48(3) 1047-50.

[25] Daftarian PM, Stone GW, Kovalski L, Kumar M, Vosoughi A, Urbieta M, Blackwelder P, Dikici E, Serafini P, Duffort S, Boodoo R, Rodríguez-Cortés A, Lemmon V, Deo S, Alberola J, Perez VL, Daunert S, Ager AL. A Targeted and Adjuvanted Nanocarrier Lowers the Effective Dose of Liposomal Amphotericin B and Enhances Adaptive Immunity in Murine Cutaneous Leishmaniasis. Journal of Infectious Diseases 2013 [Epub ahead of print].

[26] el-On J, Halevy S, Grunwald MH, Weinrauch L. Topical treatment of Old World cutaneous leishmaniasis caused by Leishmania major: a double-blind control study. Journal of the American Academy of Dermatology 1992;27(2 Pt 1) 227-231.

[27] Croft SL, Seifert K, Duchêne M. Antiprotozoal activities of phospholipid analogues. Molecular Biochemical Parasitology 2003;126(2) 165-172.

[28] Akendengue B, Ngou-Milama E, Laurens A, Hocquemiller R. Recent Advances in the fight against leishmaniasis with natural products. Parasite 1999;6 3-8.

[29] Singh S.K. Bimal S, Narayan S, Jee C, Bimal D, Das P, Bimal R.. Leishmania donovani: assessment of leishmanicidal effects of herbal extracts obtained from plants in the visceral leishmaniasis endemic area of Bihar, India. Experimental Parasitology 2011;127(2) 552–558.

[30] Angeli E, Buzio R, Firpo G. Nanotechnology applications in medicine. Tumori 2008;94 206–215.

[31] Elechiguerra J.L, Burt JL, Morone, JR. Interaction of silver nanoparticles with HIV-1. Journal of Nanobiotechnology 2005;3 6.

[32] Shrivastava S, Bera T, Roy A, Singh G, Ramachandrarao P, Dash D. Characterization of enhanced antibacterial effects of novel silver nanoparticles. Nanotechnology 2007;18 1–9.

[33] AshaRani PV, Low Kah Mun G, Hande MP. Cytotoxicity and genotoxicity of silver nanoparticles in human cells. ACS Nano 2009;3 279–290.

[34] Chen M, Yang Z, Wu H, Pan X, Xie X, Wu C. Antimicrobial activity and the mechanism of silver nanoparticle thermosensitive gel. International Journal of Nanomedicine 2011;6 2873–2877.

[35] Li WR, Xie X., Sh, QS, Zeng H., OU-Yan, YS, Chen YB. Antibacterial activity and mechanism of silver nanoparticles on Escherichia coli. Appl. Microbiolology and Biotechnology 2010;85 1115–1122.

[36] Xia T, Kovochich M, Brant J. Comparison of the abilities of ambient and manufactured nanoparticles to induce cellular toxicity according to an oxidative stress paradigm. Nano Letters 2006;6 1794–1807.

[37] Zheng J, Wu X, Wang M, Ran D, Xu W, Yang J. Study on the interaction between silver nanoparticles and nucleic acids in the presence of cetyltrimethylammonium bromide and its analytical application. Talanta 2008;74 526–532.

[38] Edwards KA, Baeumner AJ. Liposomes in analyses. Talanta. London, 2006;68(5) 1432-1441.

[39] Singh B, Sundar S. Leishmaniasis: vaccine candidates and perspectives. Vaccine, 2012 30(26) 3834-3842.

[40] Kumari S, Kumar A, Samant M, Singh N, Dube A. Discovery of novel vaccine candidates and drug targets against visceral leishmaniasis using proteomics and transcriptomics. Current Drug Targets 2008;9(11):938–947.

[41] Noazin S, Modabber F, Khamesipour A, Smith PG, Moulton LH, Nasseri K, et al. First generation leishmaniasis vaccines: a review of field efficacy trials. Vaccine 2008;26 (52) 6759–6767.

[42] Rafati S, Nakhaee A, Taheri T, Taslimi Y, Darabi H, Eravani D, et al. Protective vaccination against experimental canine visceral leishmaniasis using a combination of DNA and protein immunization with cysteine proteinases type I and II of L. infantum. Vaccine 2005;23(28) 3716–25.

[43] Okwor I, Liu D, Uzonna J. Qualitative differences in the early immune response to live and killed Leishmania major: implications for vaccination strategies against Leishmaniasis. Vaccine 2009;27(19) 2554–62.

[44] Mitchell GF, Handman E, Spithill TW. Examination of variables in the vaccination of mice against cutaneous leishmaniasis using living avirulent cloned lines and killed promastigotes of Leishmania major. International Journal of Parasitology 1985;15(6) 677–684.

[45] McConville MJ, Bacic A, Mitchell GF, Handman E. Lipophosphoglycan of Leishmania major that vaccinates against cutaneous leishmaniasis contains an alkylglycerophosphoinositol lipid anchor. Proceedings of the National Academy of Science U S A 1987;84(24) 8941–8945.

[46] Rivier D, Bovay P, Shah R, Didisheim S, Mauel J. Vaccination against Leishmania major in a CBA mouse model of infection: role of adjuvants and mechanism of protection. Parasite Immunology 1999;21(9) 461–473.

[47] Soong L, Duboise SM, Kima P, McMahon-Pratt D. Leishmania pifanoi amastigote antigens protect mice against cutaneous leishmaniasis. Infection and Immunity 1995;63(9) 3559–3566.

[48] Abdelhak S, Louzir H, Timm J, Blel L, Benlasfar Z, Lagranderie M, et al. Recombinant BCG expressing the leishmania surface antigen Gp63 induces protective immunity against Leishmania major infection in BALB/c mice. Microbiology 1995;141(Pt 7) 1585–1592.

[49] Xu D, McSorley SJ, Chatfield SN, Dougan G, Liew FY. Protection against Leishmania major infection in genetically susceptible BALB/c mice by gp63 delivered orally in attenuated Salmonella typhimurium (AroA- AroD). Immunology 1995;85(1) 1–7.

[50] Walker PS, Scharton-Kersten T, Rowton ED, Hengge U, Bouloc A, Udey MC, et al. Genetic immunization with glycoprotein 63 cDNA results in a helper T cell type 1 immune response and protection in a murine model of leishmaniasis. Human Gene Therapy 1998;9(13) 1899–1907.

[51] Ahmed SB, Bahloul C, Robbana C, Askri S, Dellagi K. A comparative evaluation of different DNA vaccine candidates against experimental murine leishmaniasis due to L. major. Vaccine 2004;22(13–14) 1631–1639.

[52] Ghosh A, Zhang WW, Matlashewski G. Immunization with A2 protein results in a mixed Th1/Th2 and a humoral response which protects mice against Leishmania donovani infections. Vaccine 2001;20(1–2) 59–66.

http://dx.doi.org/10.5772/58167

[53] Basu R, Bhaumik S, Basu JM, Naskar K, De T, Roy S. Kinetoplastid membrane protein-11 DNA vaccination induces complete protection against both pentavalent antimonial – sensitive and – resistant strains of Leishmania donovani that correlates with inducible nitric oxide synthase activity and IL – 4 generation: evidence for mixed Th1 – and Th2 – like responses in visceral leishmaniasis. Journal of Immunology 2005;174(11) 7160–7171.

[54] Dondji B, Perez-Jimenez E, Goldsmith-Pestana K, Esteban M, McMahon-Pratt D. Heterologous prime – boost vaccination with the LACK antigen protects against murine visceral leishmaniasis. Infection and Immunity 2005;73(8) 5286–5289.

[55] Mougneau E, Altare F, Wakil AE, Zheng S, Coppola T, Wang ZE, et al. Expression cloning of a protective Leishmania antigen. Science 1995;268(5210) 563–566.

[56] Gurunathan S, Prussin C, Sacks DL, Seder RA. Vaccine requirements for sustained cellular immunity to an intracellular parasitic infection. Nature Medicine 1998;4(12) 1409–1415.

[57] Campos-Neto A, Porrozzi R, Greeson K, Coler RN, Webb JR, Seiky YA, et al. Protection against cutaneous leishmaniasis induced by recombinant antigens in murine and nonhuman primate models of the human disease. Infection and Immunity 2001;69(6) 4103–4108.

[58] Stager S, Smith DF, Kaye PM. Immunization with a recombinant stage – regulated surface protein from Leishmania donovani induces protection against visceral leishmaniasis. Journal of Immunology 2000;165(12) 7064–7071.

[59] Rafati S, Kariminia A, Seyde-Eslami S, Narimani M, Taheri T, Lebbatard M. Recombinant cysteine proteinases – based vaccines against Leishmania major in BALB/c mice: the partial protection relies on interferon gamma producing CD8(+) T lymphocyte activation. Vaccine 2002;20(19–20) 2439–2447.

[60] Berberich C, Ramirez-Pineda JR, Hambrecht C, Alber G, Skeiky YA, Moll H. Dendritic cell (DC) – based protection against an intracellular pathogen is dependent upon DC – derived IL – 12 and can be induced by molecularly defined antigens. Journal of Immunology 2003;170(6) 3171–3179.

[61] Connell ND, Medina-Acosta E, McMaster WR, Bloom BR, Russell DG. Effective immunization against cutaneous leishmaniasis with recombinant bacille Calmette–Guerin expressing the Leishmania surface proteinase gp63. Proceedings of the National Academy of Science U S A 1993;90(24) 11473–11477.

[62] Streit JA, Recker TJ, Donelson JE, Wilson ME. BCG expressing LCR1 of Leishmania chagasi induces protective immunity in susceptible mice. Experimental Parasitology 2000;94(1) 33–41.

[63] Coler RN, Goto Y, Bogatzki L, Raman V, Reed SG. Leish-111f, a recombinant polyprotein vaccine that protects against visceral Leishmaniasis by elicitation of CD4+ T cells. Infection and Immunity2007;75 (9) 4648–4654.

[64] Chakravarty J, Kumar S, Trivedi S, Rai VK, Singh A, Ashman JA, et al. A clinical trial to evaluate the safety and immunogenicity of the LEISH-F1 + MPL-SE vaccine for use in the prevention of visceral leishmaniasis. Vaccine 2011;29(19) 3531–3537.

[65] Makala LH, Baban B, Lemos H, El-Awady AR, Chandler PR, Hou DY, Munn DH, Mellor AL. Leishmania major attenuates host immunity by stimulating local indoleamine 2,3-dioxygenase expression. Journal of Infectious Diseases 2011; 203:715–725.

[66] Makala LH. The role of indoleamine 2, 3 dioxygenase in regulating host immunity to leishmania infection. Journal of Biomedical Science 2012;(9)19:5.

[67] Thor-Straten P, Andersen MH. A potential role of indoleamine 2,3-dioxygenase-specific T cells in leishmania vaccination. (Comment on Leishmania major attenuates host immunity by stimulating local indoleamine 2,3-dioxygenase expression. Journal of Infectious Diseases 2011;204(3) 488-489. doi: 10.1093/infdis/jir274.

[68] Mellor AL, Munn DH. Creating immune privilege: active local suppression that benefits friends, but protects foes. Nature Reviews Immunology 2008; 8:74–80.

[69] Gil ES, Cunha LC, Paula JR, Bezerra JCB, Aguiar, FA. Leishmaniasis: Therapeutic Options and Molecular Targets. Vita et Sanitas, Trindade/Go 2007;1(01).

[70] Melos JLR, Echevarria A. Sistemas Enzimáticos de Tripanossomatídeos como Potenciais Alvos. Quimioterápicos. Revista Virtual de Quimíca 2012;4(4) 374-392.

[71] Van-Griensven J, Diro E, Lopez-Velez R, Boelaert M, Lynen L, Zijlstra E, Dujardin JC, Hailu A. HIV-1 protease inhibitors for treatment of visceral leishmaniasis in HIV-co-infected individuals. Lancet Infectious Diseases 2013;13(3) 251-259. doi: 10.1016/S1473-3099(12) 70348-1.

[72] Reguera MR, Tekwani BL, Balaña-Fouce R. Poliamine transport in parasites: A potential target for new antiparasistic drug development. Comparative Biochemistry and Physiology 2005 Part C(140) 151-164.

[73] Roberts, S. C. (2013). Genetic manipulation of Leishmania parasites facilitates the exploration of the polyamine biosynthetic pathway as a potential therapeutic target. In K.V. Urbano (Ed.), Advances in Genetics Research, v.10, p. 29-54.

[74] Genestra M, Guedes SD, Souza WJS, Cysne-Finkelstein L, Soares-Bezerra RJ, Monteiro, FP, Leon LL. Nitric Oxide Synthase (NOS) Characterization in Leishmania amazonensis Axenic Amastigotes. Archives of Medical Research 2006;37(3) 328-333.

[75] Dias SS, Hogan C, Ochocka AM, Meek DW. Polo-like kinase-1 phosphorylates MDM2 at Ser260 and stimulates MDM2-mediated p53 turnover. *FEBS Lett.* 2009;583(22) 3543-3548. doi: 10.1016/j.febslet.2009.09.057.

[76] Lepesheva GI, Hargrove TY, Anderson S, Kleshchenko Y, Furtak V, Wawrzak Z, Villalta F, Waterman M. Sterol 14 α-demethylase as a potential target for antitrypanosomal therapy: enzyme inhibition and parasite cell growth. Chemistry and Biology 2007;14 1283–1293.

[77] Zhang K, Beverle SM. Molecular & Biochemical Parasitology Phospholipid and sphingolipid metabolism in Leishmania - Review Article. Molecular and Biochemical Parasitology 2010;170(2) 55-64.

[78] Gangjee A, Jain HD, Kurup S. Recent advances in classical and non-classical antifolates as antitumor and antiopportunistic infection agents: part I. Anticancer Agents in Medicinal Chemistry. 2007;7(5):524-42.

[79] Libusová L, Sulimenko T, Sulimenko V, Hozák P, Dráber P. Gamma- Tubulin in *Leishmania*: cell cycle-dependent changes in subcellular localization and heterogeneity of its isoforms, Experimental Cell Research 2004;295 (2) 375-386.

[80] Najwa, M. J, Abu-Mejdad A.; Athraa A, Al-Hilfy A. Evaluation of therapeutic effects of vicine against leishmania donovani. in vitro. Journal American Science 2013;9(5) 115-120.

[81] Singh N, Kumar M, Singh RK. Leishmaniasis: current status of available drugs and new potential drug targets. Asian Pacific Journal Tropical Medicine 2012;5(6) 485-497. doi: 10.1016/S1995-7645(12)60084-4.

[82] Takele Y, Abebe T, Weldegebreal T, Hailu A, Hailu W, Hurissa Z, Ali, J, Diro E, Sisay Y, Cloke T, Modolell M, Munder M, Tacchini-Cottier F, Müller I, Kropf P. Arginase activity in the blood of patients with visceral leishmaniasis and HIV infection. PLoS Neglected Tropical Diseases 2013;7(1):e1977. doi: 10.1371/journal.pntd.0001977.

[83] Vannier-Santos MA, Menezes D, Oliveira MF, de Mello FG The putrescine analogue 1,4-diamino-2-butanone affects polyamine synthesis, transport, ultrastructure and intracellular survival in Leishmania amazonensis. Microbiology 2008;154(Pt 10) 3104-3111.

[84] Roberts SC, Jiang Y, Gasteier J, Frydman B, Marton LJ, Heby O, Ullman B. Leishmania donovani polyamine biosynthetic enzyme overproducers as tools to investigate the mode of action of cytotoxic polyamine analogs. apy 2007;51(2) 438-445.

[85] Withers-Martinez C, Jean L, Blackman MJ. Subtilisin-like proteases of the malaria parasite. Molecular Biology 2004;53(1) 55-63.

[86] Silva-Lopez RE, Morgado-Díaz JA, Chávez MA, Giovanni-De-Simone S.Effects of serine protease inhibitors on viability and morphology of Leishmania (Leishmania) amazonensis promastigotes. Parasitolgy Research 2007;101(6) 1627-1635.

[87] Plewes KA, Barr SD, Gedamu L. Iron superoxide dismutases targeted to the glycosomes of Leishmania chagasi are important for survival. Infect Immun. 2003 Oct; 71(10):5910-20.

[88] Luz, N. F.; Andrade, B. B.; Feijó, D. F.; Araújo-Santos, T.; Carvalho, G. Q.; Andrade, D.; Abánades, D. R.; Melo, E. V.; Silva, A. M.; Brodskyn, C. I.; Barral-Netto, M.; Barral, A.; Soares, R. P.; Almeida, R. P.; Bozza, M. T.; Borges, V. M. Heme oxygenase-1 promotes the persistence of Leishmania chagasi infection. The Journal of Immunology 2012;188(9):4460-7. doi: 10.4049/jimmunol.1103072.

[89] Kaur PK, Dinesh N, Soumya N, Babu NK, Singh S. Identification and characterization of a novel Ribose 5-phosphate isomerase B from Leishmania donovani. Biochemical and Biophysical Research Communications 2012;421(1) 51-56. doi: 10.1016/j.bbrc.2012.03.107.

[90] Cordeiro AT, Feliciano PR, Pinheiro MP, Nonato MC. Crystal structure of dihydroorotate dehydrogenase from Leishmania major. Biochimie 2012;94(8) 1739-48. doi: 10.1016/j.biochi.2012.04.003.

[91] Silva AM, Tavares J, Silvestre R, Ouaissi A, Coombs GH, Cordeiro-da-Silva A. Characterization of Leishmania infantum thiol-dependent reductase 1 and evaluation of its potential to induce immune protection. Parasite Immunology 2012;34(6) 345-350. doi: 10.1111/j.1365-3024.2012.01361.

[92] Rotella, D. P. (2012) Recent results in protein kinase inhibition for tropical diseases. Bioorg Med Chem Lett. Nov 15;22(22):6788-93. doi: 10.1016/j.bmcl.2012.09.044.

[93] Wetzel DM, McMahon-Pratt D, Koleske AJ. The Abl and Arg kinases mediate distinct modes of phagocytosis and are required for maximal Leishmania infection. 2012; 32(15) 3176-86. doi: 10.1128/MCB.00086-12.

[94] Cummings HE, Barbi J, Reville P, Oghumu S, Zorko N, Sarkar A, Keiser TL, Lu B, Rückle T, Varikuti S, Lezama-Davila C, Wewers MD, Whitacre C, Radzioch D, Rommel C, Seveau S, Satoskar AR. Critical role for phosphoinositide 3-kinase gamma in parasite invasion and disease progression of cutaneous leishmaniasis. Proceedings of the National Academy Sciences. U S A. 2012;109(4) 1251-6. doi: 10.1073/pnas.1110339109.

[95] Gilroy C, Olenyik T, Roberts SC, Ullman B. Spermidine synthase is required for virulence of Leishmania donovani. Infection and Immunity 2011;79(7) 2764-9, doi: 10.1128/IAI.00073-11

[96] Grover A, Katiyar SP, Singh SK, Dubey VK, Sundar D. A leishmaniasis study: structure-based screening and molecular dynamics mechanistic analysis for discovering potent inhibitors of spermidine synthase. Biochimica et Biophysica Acta 2012;1824(12):1476-83.2012doi: 10.1016/j.bbapap.2012.05.016.

[97] Mahmoudzadeh-Niknam H, McKerrow JH. Leishmania tropica: cysteine proteases are essential for growth and pathogenicity. Experimental Parasitology 2004;106 158-163.

[98] Silva-Lopez RE. Proteases de Leishmania: novos alvos para o desenvolvimento racional de fármacos. Química Nova [online] 2010;33(7) 1541-1548.

[99] Swenerton RK, Zhang S, Sajid M, Medzihradszky KF, Craik CS, Kelly BL, McKerrow JH. The oligopeptidase B of Leishmania regulates parasite enolase and immune evasion. The Journal Biology Chemistry 2011;286(1) 429-440. doi: 10.1074/jbc.M110.138313.

[100] Jäger W, Santag S, Weidner-Glunde M, Gellermann E, Kati S, Pietrek M, Viejo-Borbolla A, Schulz TF. The ubiquitin-specific protease USP7 modulates the replication of Kaposi's sarcoma-associated herpesvirus latent episomal DNA. Journal of Virology 2012;86(12) 6745-6757, doi:10.1128/JVI.06840-11.

[101] Schetelma RA, Decuypere S, T"Kindt R, Dujardin JC, Coombs GR, Breitling G. The potential of metabolomics for Leishmania research in the post-genomics era. Parasitology 2010;137: 1291–1302.

[102] Ogungbe VI, Setzer, WN. In-silico Leishmania Target Selectivity of Antiparasitic Terpenoids. Molecules 201318(7); 7761-7847; doi:10.3390/molecules18077761.

[103] Urbina JA. Specific chemotherapy of Chagas disease: relevance, current limitations and new approaches. Acta Tropica 2010;115(1-2) 55-68.

[104] Schneider E, Hsiang YH, Liu LF. DNA topoisomerases as anticancer drug targets. Advances in Pharmacology 1990;21 149-183.

[105] Heisig P. Inhibitors of bacterial topoisomerases: mechanisms of action and resistance and clinical aspects. Planta Medica 2001;67(1) 3-12.

[106] Singh G, Jayanarayan KG, Dey CS. Novobiocin induces apoptosis-like cell death in topoisomerase II over-expressing arsenite resistant Leishmania donovani. Molecular Biochemical Parasitology 2005;141(1) 57-69.

[107] Rosypal AC, Tripp S, Lewis S, Francis J, Stoskopf MK, Larsen RS, Lindsay DS. Survey of antibodies to Trypanosoma cruzi and Leishmania spp. in gray and red fox populations from North Carolina and Virginia. Journal of Parasitology 2010;96(6) 1230-1241. doi: 10.1645/GE-2600.1.

[108] Kosec G, Alvarez VE, Agüero F, Sánchez D, Dolinar M, Turk B, Turk V, Cazzulo JJ. Metacaspases of Trypanosoma cruzi: possible candidates for programmed cell death mediators. Molecular Biochemical Parasitology 2006 Jan;145(1) 18-28.

[109] Lee N, Gannavaram S, Selvapandiyan A, Debrabant A. Characterization of metacaspases with trypsin-like activity and their putative role in programmed cell death in the protozoan parasite Leishmania. Eukaryot Cell 2007;6(10) 1745-57.

[110] Denise H, Poot J, Jiménez M, Ambit A, Herrmann DC, Vermeulen AN, Coombs GH, Mottram JC. Studies on the CPA cysteine peptidase in the Leishmania infantum genome strain JPCM5. BMC Molecular Biology 2006;13;7 42.

[111] González IJ, Desponds C, Schaff C, Mottram JC, Fasel N. Leishmania major metacaspase can replace yeast metacaspase in programmed cell death and has arginine-specific cysteine peptidase activity. International Journal of Parasitology 2007;37(2) 161-72.

[112] Meslin B, Zalila H, Fasel N, Picot S, Bienvenu AL. Are protozoan metacaspases potential parasite killers? Parasitology Vectors 2011;4:26. doi: 10.1186/1756-3305-4-26.

[113] Fritsche C, Sitz M, Wolf M, Pohl HD. Development of a defined medium for heterologous expression in Leishmania tarentolaeogy 2008;48(6) 488-95. doi: 10.1002/jobm. 200700389.

[114] Iwu MM, Jackson JE, Schuster BG. Medicinal plants in the fight against leishmaniasis. Parasitology Today 1994;10 65–68.

[115] Rocha LG, Almeida JR, Mace^do RO, Barbosa-Filho JM. A review of natural products with antileishmanial activity. Phytomedicine 2005;12 514–535.

[116] Wang J, Peng Q, Li G. New compounds of natural resources in 2008. African Journal of Biotechnology 2009;8 4299–4307.

[117] Basso LA, Silva LHP, Fett-Neto AG, Junior WFA, Moreira IS. Palma MS, Calixto JB, Astolfi Filho S, Santos RR, Soares MBP, Santos DS. The use of biodiversity as source of new chemical entities against defined molecular targets for treatment of malaria, tuberculosis, and T-cell mediated diseases – A Review. Memórias do Instituto Oswaldo Cruz 2005;100(6) 575-606.

[118] Rates SM. Plants as source of drugs. Toxicon 2001;39 603–613.

[119] Eloff JN. Which extractant should be used for the screening and isolation of antimicrobial components from plants? Journal of Ethnopharmacology 1998;60 1–8.

[120] Beutler JA. Natural products as a foundation for drug discovery. Current Protocols in Pharmacology 2009;46(9.11) 1-9. 11.21.

[121] Sereno D, Cordeiro da Silva A, Mathieu-Daude F, Ouaissi A. Advances and perspectives in Leishmania cell based drug-screening procedures. Parasitology International 2007;56 3–7.

[122] Ajazuddin SS. Applications of novel drug delivery system for herbal formulations. Fitoterapia 2010;81(7) 680-689.

[123] Harvier P, Désormeaux A, Gagne N, Tremblay M, Poulin L, Beauchamp D, Bergeron MG. Lymphoid tissues targeting of liposome-encapsulated 2',3'-dideoxyinosine. AIDS 1995;9 701-707.

[124] Wink M. Medicinal plants: a source of anti-parasitic secondary metabolites. Molecules 2012;17(11):12771-12791.

[125] Alviano DS, Alviano CS. Plant extracts: search for new alternatives to treat microbial diseases. Current Pharmaceutical Biotechnology 2009;10(1) 106-121.

[126] Alviano DS, Barreto ALS, Dias FA, Rodrigues IA, Rosa MSS, Alviano CS, Soares RMA. Conventional therapy and promising plant-derived compounds against trypanosomatid parasites. Frontiers in Microbiology 2012;3 283. doi: 10.3389/fmicb.2012.00283. eCollection 2012.

[127] Brenzan MA, Nakamura CV, Dias Filho BP, Ueda-Nakamura T, Young MC, Coˆrrea AG, et al. Structure–activity relationship of (_) mammea A/BB derivatives against Leishmania amazonensis. Biomedical Pharmacotherapy 2008;62 651–658.

[128] Poorrajab F, Ardestani SK, Emami S, Behrouzi-Fardmoghadam M, Shafiee A, Foroumadi A. Nitroimidazolyl-1,3,4 thiadiazole-based anti-leishmanial agents: synthesis and in vitro biological evaluation. European Journal of Medicinal Chemistry 2009;44 1758–1762.

[129] Tolomeo M, Roberti M, Scapozza L, Tarantelli, C, Giacomini E, Titone L, Saporito L, Di Carlo P, Colomba C. TTAS a new stilbene derivative that induces apoptosis in *Leishmania infantum*. Experimental Parasitology 2013;133(1) 37-43. doi: 10.1016/j.exppara.(2012) 10.006.

[130] Volpato H, Desoti VC, Cogo J, Panice MR, Sarragiotto MH, Silva SO, Ueda-Nakamura T, Nakamura CV. The Effects of N-Butyl-1-(4-dimethylamino)phenyl-1,2,3,4-tetrahydro- β -carboline-3-carboxamide against *Leishmania amazonensis* Are Mediated by Mitochondrial Dysfunction. Evidence Based Complement Alternatives in Medicine 2013; 2013 874367. doi: 10.1155/2013/874367.

[131] Delfı´n DA, Morgan RE, Zhu X, Werbovetz KA. Redox-active dinitrodiphenylthioethers against Leishmania: synthesis, structure–activity relationships and mechanism of action studies. Bioorganics and Medicinal Chemistry 2009;17 820–829.

[132] Al-Qahtani A, Siddiqui YM, Bekhit AA, El-Sayed OA, Aboul-Enein HY, Al-Ahdal MN. Inhibition of growth of Leishmania donovani promastigotes by newly synthesized 1,3,4-thiadiazole analogs. Saudi Pharmacology Journal 2009;16 227–232.

[133] Srinivas N, Palne S, Nishi, Gupta S, Bhandari K. Aryloxy cyclohexyl imidazoles: a novel class of antileishmanial agents. Bioorganic Medicinal Chemical Letters 2009;15 324–327.

[134] Tonin LT, Panice MR, Nakamura CV, Rocha KJ, Santos AO, Ueda-Nakamura T, et al. Antitrypanosomal and antileishmanial activities of novel N-alkyl-(1- phenylsubstituted-beta-carboline)-3-carboxamides. Biomedical Pharmacotherapy 2010;64: 386–389.

[135] Aponte JC, Vaisberg AJ, Castillo D, Gonzalez G, Estevez Y, Arevalo J, et al. Trypanoside, anti-tuberculosis, leishmanicidal, and cytotoxic activities of tetrahydrobenzothienopyrimidines. Bioorganic Medicinal Chemistry 2010;18 2880–2886.

[136] Graebin CS, Madeira MF, Yokoyama-Yasunaka JK, Miguel DC, Uliana SR, Benitez D, et al. Synthesis and in vitro activity of limonene derivatives against Leishmania and Trypanosoma. European Journal of Medicinal Chemistry 2010;45 1524–1528.

[137] Baban B, Hansen AM, Chandler PR, Manlapat A, Bingaman A, Kahler DJ, Munn DH, Mellor AL. A minor population of splenic dendritic cells expressing CD19 mediates IDO-dependent T cell suppression via type I IFN signaling following B7 ligation. International Immunology 2005;17 909–919.

[138] Munn DH, Mellor AL. Indoleamine 2,3- dioxygenase and tumor-induced tolerance. Journal of Clinical Investigations 2007;117 1147–54.

[139] Sharma MD, Baban B, Chandler P, Hou DY, Singh N, Yagita H, Azuma M, Blazar BR, Mellor AL, Munn DH. Plasmacytoid dendritic cells from mouse tumor-draining lymph nodes directly activate mature Tregs via indoleamine 2,3-dioxygenase. Journal of Clinical Investigations 2007;117 2570–2582.

[140] Ball HJ, Yuasa HJ, Austin CJ, Weiser S, Hunt NH. Indoleamine 2,3-dioxygenase-2; a new enzyme in the kynurenine pathway. International Journal of Biochemistry & Cell Biology 2009;41(3) 467-471. doi: 10.1016/j.biocel.2008.01.005. Epub 2008 Jan 11.

[141] Metz R, Duhadaway JB, Kamasani U, Laury-Kleintop L, Muller AJ, Prendergast GC. Novel tryptophan catabolic enzyme IDO2 is the preferred biochemical target of the antitumor indoleamine 2,3-dioxygenase inhibitory compound D-1-methyl-tryptophan. Cancer Research 2007;67(15) 7082-7087.

[142] Chen W, Liang X, Peterson AJ, Munn DH, Blazar BR. The indoleamine 2,3-dioxygenase pathway is essential for human plasmacytoid dendritic cell-induced adaptive T regulatory cell generation. Journal of Immunology 2008;181(8) 5396-5404.

[143] Hou DY, Muller AJ, Sharma MD, DuHadaway J, Banerjee T, Johnson M, Mellor AL, Prendergast GC, Munn DH. Inhibition of indoleamine 2,3-dioxygenase in dendritic cells by stereoisomers of 1-methyl-tryptophan correlates with antitumor responses. Cancer Research 2007;67(2) 792-801.

[144] Johnson BA 3rd, Baban B, Mellor AL. Targeting the immunoregulatory indoleamine 2,3 dioxygenase pathway in immunotherapy. Immunotherapy. 2009;1(4) 645-661. doi: 10.2217/IMT.09.21.

[145] Cady SG, Sono M.1-Methyl-DL-tryptophan, beta-(3-benzofuranyl)-DL-alanine (the oxygen analog of tryptophan), and beta-[3-benzo(b)thienyl]-DL-alanine (the sulfur analog of tryptophan) are competitive inhibitors for indoleamine 2,3-dioxygenase. Archives of Biochemistry and Biophysics 1991;291(2) 326-333.

[146] van Griensven, J. Balasegaram M, Meheus F, Alvar J, Lynen L, Boelaert M. Combination therapy for visceral leishmaniasis. Lancet Infectious Diseases 2010;10(3) 184–194.

[147] van Griensven, J. and Diro E. Visceral leishmaniasis. Infectious Disease Clinics of North America 2012;26, 309–322.

[148] Bimal S. Sinha S, Singh SK, Narayan S, Kumar V, Verma N, Ranjan A, Sinha PK, Das VN, Pandey K, Kar SK, Das P. Leishmania donovani: CD2 biased immune response skews the SAG mediated therapy for a predominant Th1 response in experimental infection. Experimental Parasitology 2012;131 274–282.

[149] Shakya N. Sane SA, Vishwakarma P, Gupta S. Enhancement in therapeutic efficacy of miltefosine in combination with synthetic bacterial lipopeptide, Pam2Cys against experimental Visceral Leishmaniasis. Experimental Parasitology 2012;131 377–382.

[150] Sundar S. Sinha PK, Rai M, Verma DK, Nawin K, Alam S, Chakravarty J, Vaillant M, Verma N, Pandey K, Kumari P, Lal CS, Arora R, Sharma B, Ellis S, Strub-Wourgaft N, Balasegaram M, Olliaro P, Das P, Modabber F. Comparison of short-course multi-drug treatment with standard therapy for visceral leishmaniasis in India: an open-label, non-inferiority, randomized controlled trial. Lancet 2011;377 477–486.

[151] Matlashewski G, Arana B, Kroeger A, Battacharya S, Sundar S, Das P, Sinha PK, Rijal S, Mondal D, Zilberstein D, Alvar J. Visceral leishmaniasis: elimination with existing interventions. Lancet Infectious Diseases 2011;11(4) 322–325.

[152] van Griensven J. and Boelaert M. Combination therapy for visceral leishmaniasis. Lancet 2011;377(9764) 443–444.